Surgical
Pathology
of the
Thyroid

Virginia A. LiVolsi, M.D.

Professor of Pathology, University of Pennsylvania
Director of Surgical Pathology
Department of Pathology and Laboratory Medicine
Hospital of the University of Pennsylvania
Philadelphia, Pennsylvania

Surgical Pathology of the Thyroid

Volume 22 in the Series
MAJOR PROBLEMS IN PATHOLOGY

JAMES L. BENNINGTON, M.D., *Consulting Editor*

Chairman, Department of Pathology
Children's Hospital of San Francisco
San Francisco, California

1990

W.B. SAUNDERS COMPANY

Harcourt Brace Jovanovich

Philadelphia   London   Toronto   Montreal   Sydney   Tokyo

W. B. SAUNDERS COMPANY
Harcourt Brace Jovanovich, Inc.

The Curtis Center
Independence Square West
Philadelphia, PA 19106

Library of Congress Cataloging-in-Publication Data

Livolsi, Virginia A.

Pathology of the thyroid / Virginia A. Livolsi.

p. cm.—(Major problems in pathology; v. 22)

1. Thyroid gland—Tumors—Histopathology.   2. Thyroid
   gland—Histopathology.   I. Title.   II. Series.
   [DNLM: 1. Thyroid Diseases—pathology. 2. Thyroid
   Neoplasms—pathology. W1 MA492X v. 22 / WK 200
   L788p]

RC280.T6L54 1990   616.4'407—dc20   89–70101

ISBN 0–7216–5782–6

Editor: Richard Zorab
Designer: Joanne Carroll
Production Manager: Ken Neimeister
Manuscript Editor: George Vilk
Illustration Coordinator: Cecelia E. Kunkle
Indexer: Susan Thomas

SURGICAL PATHOLOGY OF THE THYROID   ISBN 0-7216-5782-6

Printed in the United States of America.

Last digit is the print number: 9   8   7   6   5   4   3

This book is dedicated to my mother,
Mary LiVolsi,
who epitomized the definition of the word "teacher."

Foreword

The thyroid gland generates a challenge for pathologists out of all proportion to the numbers of thyroid specimens examined. The types of distinctions that the surgical pathologist is called upon to make, e.g., neoplastic or hyperplastic, benign or malignant, follicular variant of papillary carcinoma or follicular carcinoma, and so on, are generally determined on the basis of subtle morphologic differences, and as such frequently represent very difficult diagnostic decisions.

Dr. LiVolsi, in PATHOLOGY OF THE THYROID, has produced an authoritative reference work covering all aspects of the surgical pathology of the thyroid gland. This book is a must for anyone interested in thyroid disease, but will be appreciated particularly by the surgical pathologist as a guide to dealing with the difficult-to-diagnose thyroid lesion.

The last chapter should be perused by the prospective buyer, and read first by the owner. It is representative of the direct and practical approach by the author, and of the wealth of useful information to be found in the other chapters. In my opinion, the last chapter alone makes PATHOLOGY OF THE THYROID invaluable to the pathologist.

JAMES L. BENNINGTON, M.D.
Consulting Editor

Preface

This monograph discusses thyroid disease from a predominantly morphologic viewpoint, although for completeness a brief review of clinicopathologic data and laboratory evaluation of thyroid function and thyroid disease is included.

The book is divided into three areas: (1) nonneoplastic (chiefly inflammatory) conditions; (2) proliferative (neoplastic and hyperplastic) lesions, and (3) descriptions of morphologic techniques in the diagnosis of thyroid disorders.

Chapter headings in the first two sections are divided chiefly into pattern recognition groups. This division is presented solely as a way to enable the reader faced with thyroid lesions of varying morphology to seek out such lesions as characterized by their histologic features. Within the subgroups an attempt is made to describe the gross and microscopic pathology, including use of ancillary morphologic techniques. Histogenetic, pathophysiologic, and prognostic data are included.

The division of the various chapters along these lines is solely the author's responsibility. The author has found that in studying thyroid diseases of various types it has been convenient to divide them into these pattern recognition groups, and this has been of great help in teaching thyroid pathology.

VIRGINIA A. LiVOLSI

Acknowledgments

Many people assist an author in any work of this size. I wish to express my thanks to some of them.

To Drs. Raffaele Lattes, Karl Perzin, and Carl Feind, who taught me early on in my pathology career to appreciate the fascinating lesions of the thyroid;

To Drs. Maria Merino and David Lowell, for inspiring ideas and asking disconcerting questions that made me search for answers;

To Dr. Chester Andrzejeweski, for help in understanding the immunologic aspects of autoimmune thyroid disease;

To Dr. David Hicks, who taught me about the molecular biologic techniques to discern clonality of neoplasms;

To Dr. Jacki Abrams for helping me understand thyroid cytology;

To Dr. Renato Iozzo, for electron photomicrographs;

To Claudia Catan, who helped with gross photography; and to Robert Specht for some of the photomicrography;

To Nancy Brago, for untiring patience in typing multiple revisions; and

To the editorial staff of W. B. Saunders, for their patience, professionalism, and assistance.

Contents

HISTORICAL REVIEW AND INTRODUCTION

The thyroid gland, the largest endocrine organ, has been recognized as a neck structure since ancient times. Goiter was known in ancient China where seaweed was used to treat it;[1] the Egyptians illustrated goitrous females in some of their art; and the Hindus apparently recognized that large goiters can produce difficulties in respiration and loss of voice.[1] Greek and Roman physicians also described thyroid enlargement, although they probably did not separate the gland from cervical lymph nodes.

Until the late 17th century, medical theorists considered the thyroid as a gland which secreted material needed to lubricate the larynx and its cartilages. Goiter was known to affect chiefly women and became a symbol of beauty as reflected in the art of the Middle Ages. During the late Middle Ages, the relationship between endemic goiter and idiocy was recognized, especially by anatomists and physicians in Alpine regions of Europe.

Naming the gland "thyroid," derived from the Greek word *thyreos* meaning "oblong shield," is attributed to Thomas Wharton in the 17th century.[1–4]

In the modern era, following the carefully documented anatomic dissections of Vesalius, Morgagni, and others, and the observations of the extensive vascularity in the gland, some scholars attributed to the thyroid the function of protecting the brain from sudden onrush of blood.[1–4]

In the 18th and 19th centuries, hyperthyroidism with exophthalmos was described first by Parry, later by Graves and von Basedow.[1–6] Other authors documented the thyroid's relationship to cretinism and adult myxedema. The classical descriptions of thyroiditis by Hashimoto, DeQuervain, and Riedel appeared during the late 19th and early 20th centuries.[7–9]

Finally, in the early part of this century, the role of iodine in thyroid physiology was established.[1–3]

In recent times, interrelationships among the thyroid, pituitary, and hypothalamus have been defined. Thyroid function testing has rapidly progressed from measurement of basal metabolic rate to precise radioimmunoassays to define small quantities of hormones involved in thyroid secretion and regulation. Chronic lymphocytic thyroiditis serves as a model for immunobiologists in the study of autoimmune diseases.

The definitions and descriptions of clinical aspects of a variety of thyroid neoplasms have evolved over the past 30 years; recent advances in immunohistology have been helpful in understanding the histogenesis of these tumors. The advent of fine needle aspiration cytology has changed the approach to thyroid nodule diagnosis dramatically in only a decade.

This monograph discusses thyroid disease from a predominantly morphologic viewpoint, although for completeness a brief review of clinicopathologic data and laboratory evaluation of thyroid function and thyroid disease is included.

REFERENCES

1. Medvei, V. C.: The History of Endocrinology. Lancaster, Kluwer Academic Publishers, 1982.

2. Werner, S. C.: Historical Resumé. Chapter 1. *In*: Ingbar, S. H., and Braverman, L. E. (eds.): Werner's The Thyroid, 5th edition. Philadelphia, J. B. Lippincott, 1986, pp. 3–6.
3. Thompson, J.: Historical Notes. *In*: Smithers, D. (ed.): Tumours of the Thyroid. Vol. 6, Neoplastic Diseases at Various Sites. Edinburgh, Livingstone, Ltd., 1970.
4. Rolleston, H. D.: The Endocrine Organs in Health and Disease. Oxford University Press, 1936.
5. Graves, R. J.: Clinical lectures. Lond. Med. Surg. J. (Part II), 7:516, 1935.
6. Von Basedow, C. A.: Exophthalmos durch Hypertrophe des Zellgewebes in der Augenhohle. Wochenschr. Heilk. *6*:197, 1840.
7. Hashimoto, H.: Zur Kenntniss der lymphomatoser Veranderung der Schildruse (Struma lymphomatosa). Arch. Klin. Chir. *97*:219, 1912.
8. DeQuervain, F., and Giordanengo, G.: Die akute und subakute nichteitige Thyroiditis. Mitt. Grenzgeb. Med. Chir. *44*:538, 1936.
9. Riedel, B.: Vorstellung eines Kranken mit chronischen Strumitis. Verh. Dtsch. Ges. Chir. *26*:127, 1897.

Nonneoplastic Conditions

INTRODUCTION

Both neoplastic and nonneoplastic diseases affect the thyroid. Inflammatory conditions, collectively termed thyroiditides, can be appropriately classified as acute, subacute (granulomatous), or chronic.

The first part of this monograph reviews nonneoplastic conditions in the thyroid. In seven chapters, the following topics are discussed: normal development and morphology, disorders associated with thyroid hyper- or hypofunction, including thyroid function tests, the true thyroiditides (acute infectious, granulomatous, and chronic autoimmune types), fibrosing lesions affecting the gland, crystal deposition and pigmentary disorders, and a brief review of systemic diseases and drug reactions that can influence thyroid morphology.

1

DEVELOPMENTAL BIOLOGY AND ANATOMY OF THE THYROID, INCLUDING THE ABERRANT THYROID

This chapter reviews the embryology, development, and normal anatomy of the thyroid. During this discussion, anomalous development, including the problem of interpretation of the medial and lateral aberrant thyroid tissue, is described.

EMBRYOLOGY

The embryologic development of the human thyroid gland can be understood by distinguishing between the origins of the medial portions of the gland and the lateral lobes.

The Medial Anlage[2, 76, 98, 105]

The median anlage of the thyroid arises as a bilobated vesicular structure at the foramen cecum of the tongue; it is attached to the tongue by the thyroglossal duct. Identifiable at approximately 17 days of fetal life, the thyroid precursor is seen as a circumscribed area of proliferating entoderm in the floor of the fetal pharynx in close association with the heart. In the 24 day embryo, the median thyroid anlage resembles a deep cup; this soon forms a flask-like vesicle with a narrow neck connecting it to the pharynx.

Synchronously, the narrow strand of tissue elongates as the thyroglossal duct. In normal circumstances, the duct atrophies, and remnants of thyroid tissue may persist anywhere along this pathway of descent. If the duct persists, it may become cystic, dilated, and, in some instances, infected. With the normal involution of the thyroglossal duct, the median thyroid anlage, now a bilobed solid structure, begins to expand laterally. During weeks five to seven of fetal life, the thyroid descends as the heart and great vessels move caudally. At this stage, approximately seven weeks of embryologic life, the median portion has reached the level of the lateral thyroid (Fig. 1–1).

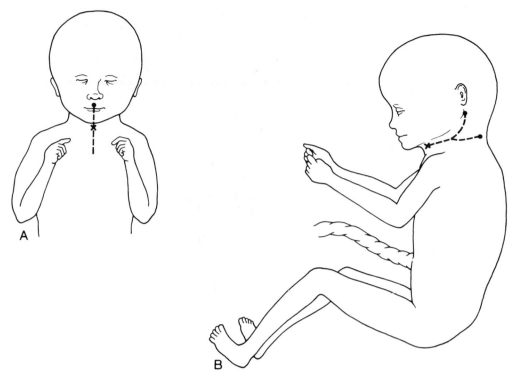

Figure 1–1. *A,* Normal development of the thyroid. *B,* Migration of thyroid anlagen during embryogenesis.

In the ninth week of fetal life, the solid thyroid differentiates into cords and plates a few cells thick. Bead-like enlargements develop along the cords throughout the gland and a tiny lumen appears in most of these enlargements by the 10th week. Thus the follicles develop. At 12 weeks, colloid formation begins, especially at the periphery of the gland. At this time active formation of iodocompounds begins. By week 14, the gland consists of colloid-containing follicles and interfollicular cells. As fetal growth continues, the follicles increase in size and number.

The histologic differentiation of the human fetal thyroid can be divided into three stages: from weeks 7 to 13, the precolloid stage; weeks 13 to 14, beginning colloid formation; and, finally, after 14 weeks, the follicular phase (Fig. 1–2). By the seventh week of gestation, the thyroid cells contain intracellular canaliculi which, with maturation, become dilated, migrate toward the apex of the cell, discharge their contents extracellularly, and then fuse. Desmosomes, which hold the apical edges of juxtaposed cells together, limit the spread of the extruded material to a central lumen, the colloid space. During the third or follicular phase there is a progressive increase in the diameter of the follicles and increasing storage of colloid with histologic resemblance to the adult thyroid (Fig. 1–2). The onset of follicle formation in the fetal thyroid has generally been considered evidence of initiation of thyroid function; however, function may begin as early as the 29th day of gestation when the thyroid is still a simple cell mass attached to the buccal floor. Radioactive carbon–labeled amino acid studies suggest that thyroglobulin synthesis can be established this early, about five to seven weeks before the onset of colloid formation. The stimulus to thyroglobulin secretion is unknown since thyrotropin (TSH) cannot be detected until the 13th week of fetal life. When the thyroid follicles begin to accumulate colloid, the gland simultaneously starts to trap iodide, binding it to tyrosine, and forming the thyroid hormones, thyroxine (T_4) and triiodothyronine (T_3).[27, 33, 92, 93, 101]

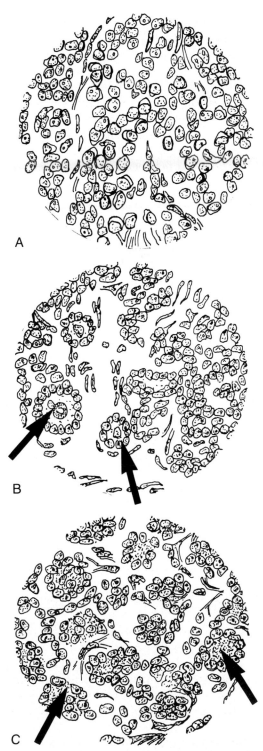

Figure 1–2. Stages of development—histologic changes: *A,* precolloid, 9 weeks; *B,* beginning colloid formation, 13 weeks (arrows); *C,* follicular phase, more than 14 weeks (arrows).

The Lateral Thyroid Anlage

Dispute has arisen among embryologists as to the number of branchial pouches present during human fetal development; some purists believe that comparison of human embryology with that of other mammals may be misleading.[60, 77] Thus, authors such as Norris[77] indicate that in human fetal development, only four pouches can be recognized and the structure called the "lateral thyroid" is derived from the caudal end of the fourth branchial pouch.

Other authors extrapolate from the more detailed embryologic studies of other animals and use the term "ultimobranchial body" for the fifth branchial pouch, which gives rise to the lateral thyroid;[105] doubt is expressed as to whether the caudal end of the fourth pouch need be designated as the fifth branchial pouch or not. Sugiyama[98] settles this issue diplomatically and refers to "the fourth-fifth branchial pouch complex."

While these issues continue to be debated, it is clear that in human fetal life, the lateral anlage of the thyroid is derived from the fifth (or tail of the fourth) branchial pouch or ultimobranchial body. The latter, still connected to the pharynx, gradually loses this connection in the seventh week of life. Its lumen is obliterated by proliferating cells and it appears as a solid mass surrounding the median thyroid tissue. The ultimobranchial bodies give rise to the parafollicular or C cells. Since the ultimobranchial bodies fuse with the medial anlage in its upper lateral aspects, the C cells are found in this area in the adult human thyroid.

Does the ultimobranchial body give rise to more than the C cells? Does the rest of the structure disappear in postfetal life? The literature contains various answers to these questions. Some authors "illustrate" that the lateral anlage gives rise to structures indistinguishable from follicles.[77] Hence, cords of cells from the medial thyroid migrate and enwrap themselves around the solid ultimobranchial body. Fusion occurs between the two anlagen and follicles develop. Whether some of these follicles are actually of lateral anlage derivation is unclear.

In humans with thyroid nondescent (or unilateral aplasia),[40] there are no recognizable thyroid follicles in these usual locations. Hence, it appears unlikely that the ultimobranchial body alone contributes to thyroid follicle development. It still may be possible, however, that specific interactions between medial and lateral anlagen could lead to an ultimobranchial component to thyroid follicles.

Sugiyama's studies indicate that the ultimobranchial body, after it fuses with the medial thyroid, divides into a central thick-walled stratified epithelial cyst and a peripheral part composed of cell groups dispersed among follicles—the C cells.[98] In postnatal life, the central epithelial cyst may disappear. Sugiyama found it in 14 percent of thyroid lobes he examined. It corresponds to so-called solid cell nests (see below).[48, 55, 97]

Estimates of the relative contributions to thyroid weight from the lateral anlagen range from less than 1 to 30 percent.[60, 77, 101, 105]

The fusion of medial and lateral thyroid anlagen in humans differs from that which occurs in some species. Birds, for example, maintain complete separation of thyroid gland from ultimobranchial bodies.[48] The physical forces and/or chemical attraction leading to fusion in some mammals, including man, remain unknown.[2, 60]

Expansion of the medial thyroid caudally and laterally appears to inhibit further growth of the ultimobranchial body; similarly, the ultimobranchial body's migration may control development of the medial anlage.[98]

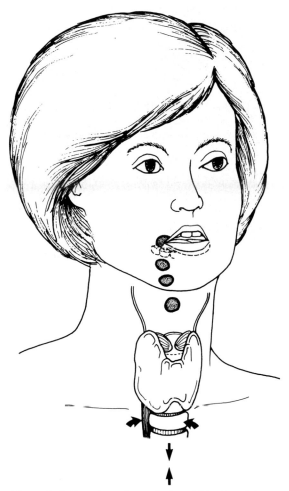

Figure 1–3. Location of ectopic thyroid in the adult.

ABNORMAL DEVELOPMENT (Fig. 1–3)

Abnormalities of development can be understood by considering the medial and lateral thyroid anlagen separately. Very rare instances of total or partial thyroidal agenesis have been recorded;[10, 29, 40, 69, 82] more often disordered migration during fetal life leads to maldevelopment.

The median anlage can give rise to aberrant thyroid rests in two ways. These include (1) failure of descent and (2) differentiation in abnormal positions. Lingual thyroid results from a failure of the median anlage to descend from the pharynx.[4, 74, 85, 95, 96] The thyroid retains its primitive topography and differentiates into thyroid at the base of the tongue. Such a thyroid can function; indeed, it may represent the only functional thyroid in an affected individual. The removal, therefore, of a "mass" present in the base of the tongue without appropriate evaluation for normally located thyroid may lead to severe acute hypothyroidism postoperatively.

Maldescent may result in the finding of thyroid tissue along the pathway of the thyroglossal duct.[1, 14, 35, 36, 63, 66, 71, 78] The thyroglossal duct or tract is found in the midline attached to the isthmus and extending upward for varying distances up

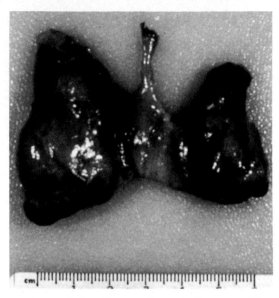

Figure 1–4. Gross appearance of normal thyroid; centrally projecting upward from isthmus is pyramidal lobe.

to the base of the tongue at the foramen cecum (Fig. 1–3). In one study, 63 percent of thyroglossal duct cysts contained thyroid tissue in their walls.[66] Ectopic thyroid may also be found in the larynx or trachea, where it may produce respiratory difficulties in young children or even in adults.[7, 21, 41, 73, 87]

Median aberrant thyroid also includes the development of a pyramidal lobe or tract (Fig. 1–4) which extends from the thyroid isthmus forward and upward through the thyroid cartilage and into the lower border of the hyoid bone.

Accentuated descent of the median anlage may lead to location of thyroid tissue substernally in the preaortic area, in the pericardium, or even in the heart itself.[3, 17, 19, 58, 83, 91] Rare instances of thyroid tissue, apparently normal, have been reported in the porta hepatis, gallbladder,[16, 56] and groin.[88] The embryological twists necessary to explain this finding are unclear,[16] although teratomatous origin must be considered.

In rare instances where the ultimobranchial body remnants fail to fuse with the medial thyroid, nests of solid and cystic squamous-appearing cells associated with lymphocytes may be found in the neck.[55, 98, 101] In avian species, this is the normal pattern of development.[48] When the development of the third and fourth branchial pouches is arrested, parathyroids, thymus, and C cells are absent (DiGeorge syndrome).[9] Associated cardiac abnormalities are frequently found.[61] (See also Chapter 10.) For further discussion of thyroid in unusual sites, see Chapter 16.

FINDINGS OF IMPORTANCE FROM THYROID EMBRYOLOGY: THE ABERRANT THYROID, IMPORTANCE FOR THE SURGICAL PATHOLOGIST

From the embryologic developmental sequences described above, it can be appreciated that the thyroid itself may contain inclusions of various types and that thyroid inclusions may be found outside the gland itself.

Since the thyroid develops in conjunction with the branchial or pharyngeal pouches, derivatives of these structures can sometimes be found in the gland.

Thus, intrathyroidal parathyroid tissue, salivary gland remnants, and thymic tissue can be seen.[13, 97, 105] So-called solid cell nests, probably representing rests of the ultimobranchial bodies, can also be found; these have been reported in 7 to 28 percent of serially sectioned glands[97, 98, 105] (Figs. 1–5 to 1–7).

In addition, the intimate development of the thyroid with the mesodermal structures of the neck may lead to the finding of normal thyroid tissue in the muscle or fat of the cervical soft tissue (Figs. 1–8 to 1–10).[6, 13, 72] This should not be mistaken for neoplastic growth, but merely a variant in thyroid anatomy. Since aberrantly placed thyroid tissue may undergo all the changes that occur in the normally located gland, especially nodule formation, these considerations must be remembered so as not to overdiagnose malignancy.

Similarly, fat, cartilage, and/or muscle may occasionally be found within the thyroid gland capsule. This is also not surprising because of the intimate associations of these various tissues during fetal life.[26, 30]

The problem of lateral aberrant thyroid has plagued pathologists and surgeons for many years.[6, 28, 72, 104] In modern times, our understanding of thyroid pathology should allow us to put this problem to rest. Lateral aberrant thyroid is defined as thyroid tissue located lateral to the jugular vein. *If unassociated with lymph node, lateral aberrant thyroid may be seen as part of anomalous development, especially in a gland involved by a diffuse process such as thyroiditis or nodular goiter, or following surgery or trauma to the neck wherein dislodged portions and bits of thyroid tissue may implant in the neck.*[6, 62, 72, 90] The apparently unique case reported by Rubenfeld et al.[90] described a patient in whom the only thyroid present was ectopically located in the carotid area.

Normal-appearing thyroid tissue anywhere within lymph nodes lateral to the jugular vein represents metastatic papillary thyroid carcinoma and is not a developmental anomaly. The

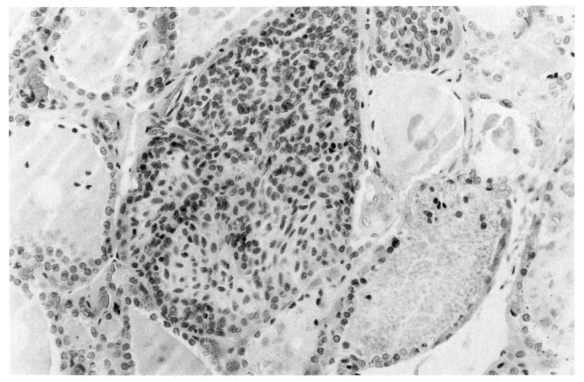

Figure 1–5. Solid cell nest (SCN). Note transitional cell appearance of these masses interspersed among follicles. Occasionally associated lymphoid tissue is seen. × 200, H & E.

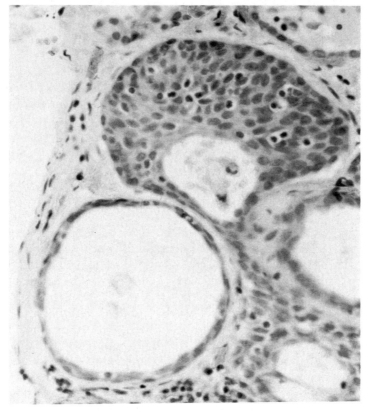

Figure 1–6. Occasionally cystic changes in or near SCN can be found. × 200, H & E.

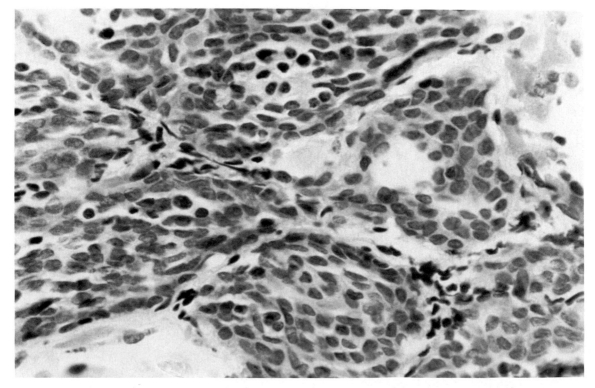

Figure 1–7. Higher power of SCN shows spindly appearance of the cells. × 350, H & E.

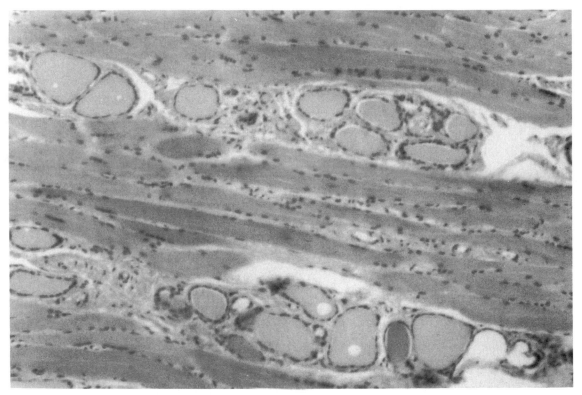

Figure 1–8. Normal thyroid "interdigitates" into cervical muscle. × 100, H & E.

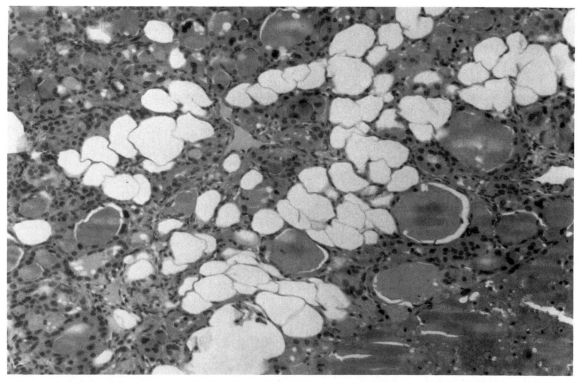

Figure 1–9. Fat and thyroid are admixed at edges of gland. Note lack of a "fibrotic response" helping to distinguish this finding from an invasive cancer. × 100, H & E.

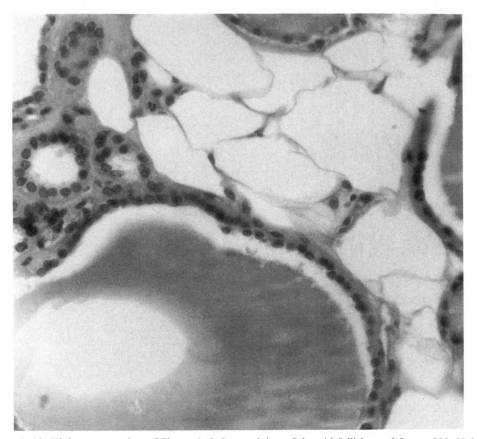

Figure 1–10. Higher power view of Figure 1–9. Intertwining of thyroid follicles and fat. × 300, H & E.

possibility that normal thyroid follicles may be present as an embryologic rest within *capsules* of medially located nodes (analogous to benign nevus cells in lymph nodes) remains disputed, although many pathologists accept this possibility.[32, 49, 66, 70, 89] Meyer and Steinberg[70] noted normal thyroid follicles in cervical nodes in five of 106 autopsies; serial sectioning of the thyroids in these cases showed thyroid carcinoma in only one case. These authors concluded such nodal thyroid inclusions are benign.[70] The authors who accept the medial aberrant thyroid in nodes as benign insist that the thyroid tissue look like normal follicles, that no papillae or psammoma bodies be found, and that the location of the tissue be in the nodal capsule and not within the node itself.[66, 70] Other authors consider any thyroid follicles present in a lymph node, regardless of the location, to represent metastatic thyroid cancer to that node.[12, 56] Butler et al.[12] noted thyroid tissue in 22 of 120 patients who had head, neck, or lung cancer. In 15 of the 22, a cancer was found in the thyroid (the gland was incompletely evaluated in the remaining seven). These authors concluded that thyroid tissue in nodes represents metastatic cancer.[12] The problem of carcinoma's arising in ectopic thyroid will be discussed in Chapter 16.

ANATOMY OF THE THYROID

Macroscopic Appearance

The normal adult thyroid consists of two lobes connected by an isthmus. The individual lobes have a pointed superior pole and a blunt inferior pole. Each lobe measures 2 to 2.5 cm. wide by 4 cm. long.[53] The gland is loosely attached to the anterior trachea by loose connective tissue. The lobes lie along the lower halves of the lateral margins of the thyroid cartilage. Laterally lie the carotid sheaths and the sternocleidomastoid muscles; the recurrent laryngeal nerves lie between the lateral lobes and the trachea.[31] Two parathyroids are normally situated on the posterior aspect of each lobe.[53] Among normal variants are included discrepancy in the sizes of the lobes, or the presence of a pyramidal lobe.[42]

Normal weights of the adult gland have been estimated to range from 16 to 25 grams and depend upon functional state, sex, hormonal status, and size of the individual, as well as appropriate iodine intake.[22, 45, 81] Recent studies published in 1985 give lower weights for normal thyroid (women 14.5 g.; men 18 g.).[81] In women, thyroid volume changes correlate with the menstrual cycle; increased volumes (up to 50 per cent) can be seen during the early secretory phase of the cycle.[44]

The thyroid is encapsulated by thin fibrous tissue, which invaginates into the gland, forming pseudolobules. Thyroid tissue is light brown in color, firm in consistency, and often glistening on its cut surface. The normal gland is loosely attached to neighboring structures, but fascial planes are distinct. Nodules are not uncommon in the adult gland and can be found grossly in about 10 percent of the endocrinologically normal population.[8]

The vascular supply of the thyroid is derived from the superior and inferior thyroidal arteries. Venous blood drains through the two sets of thyroidal veins: superior and medial veins drain into the external jugular vein, whereas the inferior thyroid vein joins the brachiocephalic vein (Fig. 1–11). The rich intraglandular capillary network courses to the capsule of the gland and gives rise to collecting trunks within the thyroid capsule.[15, 51, 52] The collecting trunks are closely associated with the blood supply of the gland and follow the veins.[42] The thyroid contains a rich lymphatic network;[79] intraglandular and subcapsular lymphatics drain into the internal jugular lymph nodes. Feind[25] has divided the lymphatics into groups. The superior group drains the upper gland and medial isthmus; these empty into the internal jugular nodes. On the other hand, the inferior group drains the lower gland and empties into pre- and paratracheal nodes.[25]

The nerves are nonmedullated postganglionic fibers originating from superior and middle cervical sympathetic ganglia. These nerve fibers are vasomotor and influence thyroid secretion indirectly by their action on blood vessels. In addition, a network of adrenergic fibers exists which ends near the follicular basement membrane. Adrenergic receptors are present in follicular cells as well.[102] Hence, it is believed that direct neural influences as well as indirect vasomotor nerve signals can influence thyroid hormone secretion.[53, 67, 100] Mast cells, normally found in the thyroid interstitium, may influence thyroid blood flow and secretion by release of vasoactive compounds.[68]

Light Microscopic Appearance

Microscopically (Figs. 1–12 to 1–14), the thyroid is divided into lobules composed of about 20 to 40 follicles. It is estimated that approximately three million follicles are present in the thyroid of an adult man. Each lobe or lobule is supplied by an intralobular artery and vein. The follicles are lined by epithelial cells, which surround central deposits of colloid. In general, the follicles range from uniform to variable size (varying from 50 to 500 micra); however, the plane of section may give the appearance of small follicles interspersed with large ones.[86, 97] Follicular

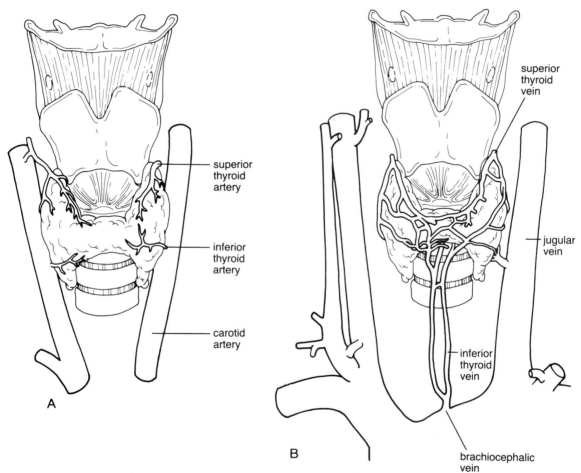

Figure 1–11. Normal thyroid—arterial (A) and venous (B) anatomy.

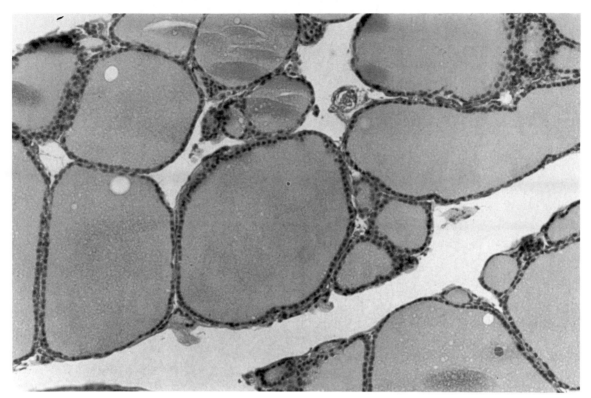

Figure 1–12. Normal thyroid; follicles of more or less uniform size replete with colloid. × 100, H & E.

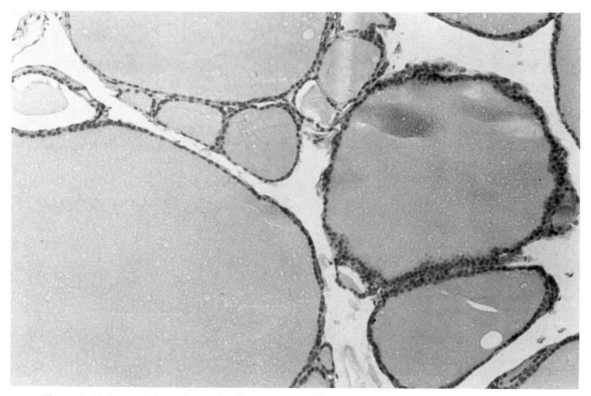

Figure 1–13. Normal thyroid; occasionally one or more follicles are larger (lower left). × 100, H & E.

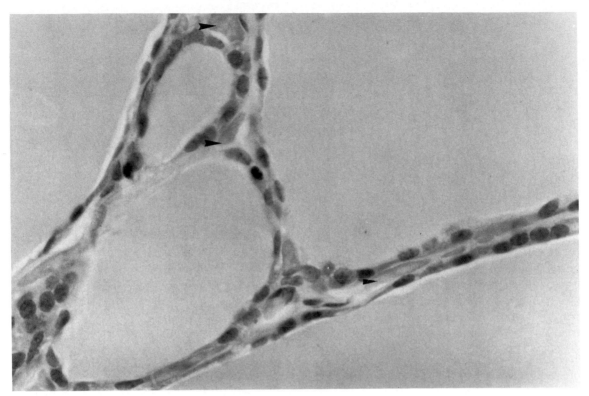

Figure 1–14. Normal thyroid follicular epithelium is low cuboidal in the resting state; colloid fills central lumina. Interfollicular stroma contains many capillaries (arrowheads). × 250, H & E.

cells have a definite polarity, with their apices directed toward the lumen of the follicle and their bases toward the basement membrane.[75] The total number of acini in the gland does not change with age; hence, volume changes must reflect changes in the sizes of the individual acini. The presence of microscopically visible nodules increases with age in endocrinologically normal individuals.[8] As noted above, the normal thyroid may occasionally contain thymic rests, parathyroid tissue, muscle, and adipose tissue.

In the interfollicular stroma, and occasionally abutting between the follicular epithelial cells, are individual or small groups of parafollicular (C) cells. On ordinary hematoxylin and eosin stain, it is difficult to identify C cells and distinguish them from tangentially cut follicular epithelium; they may appear as polygonal elements larger than follicular cells and contain pale-staining granular cytoplasm and central oval nuclei.[97] Immunostaining for calcitonin may be necessary to disclose these cells.[18, 43, 64, 65] It is estimated that they constitute 0.1 percent of the mass of the adult normal human thyroid. Some studies have indicated that C cells are more abundant in children's than in adults' thyroids.[106, 107] In the latter, they are scattered individually or in groups of three to five cells in the interfollicular stroma.[65, 107] However, in older patients (over age 50), nodules of C cells may be a normal finding, perhaps related to hormonal and calcium metabolic alterations.[47, 80] (See also Chapter 10.)

Solid cell nests (SCN) are a not uncommon finding in the posterolateral or posteromedial portion of the lateral lobes of the thyroid.[97] They can be found in up to 28 percent of glands.[55, 108] Most authors believe these SCN represent rests of ultimobranchial body;[55, 97] indeed, finding immunoreactive calcitonin-containing cells near or within solid cell nests seems to be evidence of such a relationship.[38, 39, 55] (However, Sugiyama could not confirm this association.[97])

Histologically, epithelial cells in nests and cords are seen. Occasionally, central cystic structures are noted; within the cysts clumps of eosinophilic material may be seen.[38, 39] The cyst lining is low cuboidal; the nests themselves exhibit an epidermoid or transitional cell appearance[55, 97, 108] The present author has noted the resemblance of these cell groups to endometrial morules or Walthard rests. (See Figs. 1–5 to 1–7.)

Antigen-presenting dendritic cells can be identified (by immunostaining for S100 and/or class II major histocompatibility determinants) outside thyroid follicles in normal glands.[37, 57] These cells are increased in autoimmune thyroid disorders, wherein they are in intimate contact with intrathyroidal lymphocytes.

Ultrastructural Appearance (Figs. 1–15 and 1–16)

Ultrastructural studies[34, 46, 59] of normal thyroid disclose that the follicular cells are arranged in a single layer around the central colloid. Microvilli are easily found projecting from the apical portions of the cell. One to four cilia project from the central portion of each follicular cell. By scanning electron microscopy, the microvilli are prominent, especially in smaller follicles.[94] Within the cytoplasm, liposomes are prominent; endoplasmic reticulum and small mitochondria are also seen. The nuclei are round with homogeneous chromatin; nucleoli are rarely seen.[34] The basal surface is separated from the interfollicular space by a basement membrane, which is approximately 350 to 400 Å thick. Well-developed desmo somes and terminal bars are found between cells near the lumina. In the interstitium, fenestrated capillaries and collagen fibers are noted. Elastic fibers are not seen surrounding the normal follicles.[34, 99]

In normal physiologic states, iodide trapped from the circulation is transported through follicular epithelial cells, chemically joined to peroxidase, and is incorporated into tyrosyl groups of thyroglobulin at the luminal surface. In thyroglobulin, these iodotyrosines couple to form thyroid hormones thyroxine and triiodothyronine, T_4 and T_3. These compounds are stored as colloid.[23, 103]

When stimulated by thyrotropin from the pituitary, this process is reversed. Portions of colloid (thyroglobulin) are actively enwrapped by pseudopodia[5, 24, 50, 54] of follicular cells, transported into the cytoplasm wherein thyroxine and triiodothyronine are released. At the basal end of the cell the hormones are released in the rich capillary network and hence into the circulation.[54] The ultrastructural morphology conforms to this sequence.

The C cells are always separated from the follicular epithelium by a basement membrane, although at the light microscopic level the C cells may appear in intimate contact with the follicle. The cytoplasm of the parafollicular cells is occupied by numerous double membrane-bound neurosecretory granules, which, by immunoelectron microscopic studies, have been shown to contain calcitonin.[34, 43] (See Chapter 10.)

Immunohistochemistry

Immunostaining studies[11, 20] have shown that normal follicular epithelium contains thyroglobulin and low molecular weight keratin and may coexpress vimentin. Sex hormone receptors have been demonstrated in human thyroid tissue;[84] these probably play a role in physiologic responses of thyroid epithelial cells. C cells

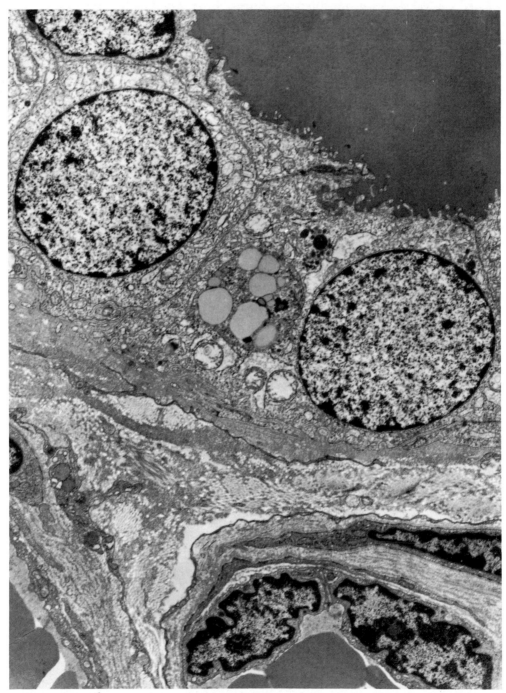

Figure 1–15. Electron micrograph of normal thyroid follicle. Colloid at upper right. Note uniform low cuboidal follicular epithelium and round nuclei. At outer edge of follicle is basement membrane and collagen; capillary is seen close by in interfollicular stroma. × 6800, Uranyl acetate–lead.

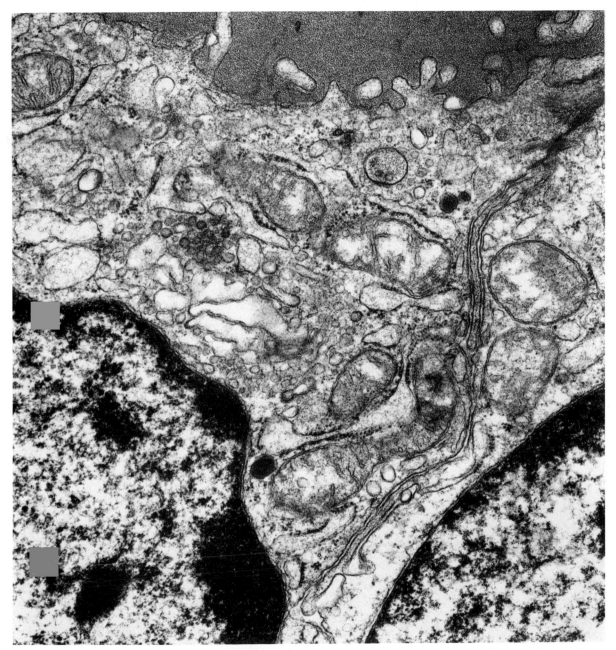

Figure 1–16. Luminal cilia are seen jutting into colloid (top). Note intracytoplasmic organelles including endoplasmic reticulum, ribosomes, and scattered mitochondria. Note cell-to-cell junction near lumen (upper right corner). × 38,000, Uranyl acetate-lead.

stain for calcitonin and carcinoembryonic antigen. The utility of immuno-staining for hormones and keratins in the distinction and diagnosis of thyroid tumors is discussed in Chapter 18.

SUMMARY

This chapter has reviewed embryologic aspects of the human thyroid in order to focus on abnormalities that may result from aberrant development. The anatomy, histology, and ultrastructure of the normal thyroid are also summarized.

REFERENCES

1. Allard, R.H.B.: The thyroglossal cyst. Head Neck Surg. 5:134–140, 1982.
2. Arey, L.B.: Developmental Anatomy. Philadelphia, W. B. Saunders Co., 1965, pp. 241–243.
3. Asp, A., Hasbargen, J., Blue, P., and Kidd, G.S.: Ectopic thyroid tissue on thallium technetium parathyroid scan. Arch. Intern. Med. 147:595–596, 1987.
4. Baughman, R.A.: Lingual thyroid and lingual thyroglossal tract remnants. Oral Surg. 34:781–798, 1972.
5. Bjorkman, U., Ekholm, R., et al.: Induced unidirectional transport of protein into the thyroid follicular lumen. Endocrinology 95:1506–1517, 1974.
6. Block, M.A., Wylie, J.A., et al.: Does benign thyroid tissue occur in the lateral part of the neck? Am. J. Surg. 112:476–481, 1966.
7. Bone, R.C., Biller, H.F., and Irwin, T.M.: Intralaryngotracheal thyroid. Ann. Otol. 81:424–428, 1972.
8. Brown, R.A., Al-Moussa, M., and Beck, J.S.: Histometry of normal thyroid in man. J. Clin. Pathol. 39:475–482, 1986.
9. Burke, B., Wick, M., et al.: Thyroid C cells in DiGeorge syndrome. Lab. Invest. 54:2P, 1986.
10. Burman, K.D., Adler, R.A., and Wartofsky, L.: Hemiagenesis of the thyroid gland. Am. J. Med. 58:143–146, 1975.
11. Buley, I.D., Gatter, K.C., et al.: Expression of intermediate filament proteins in normal and diseased thyroid glands. J. Clin. Pathol. 40:136–142, 1987.
12. Butler, J.J., Tulinius, H., et al.: Significance of thyroid tissue in lymph nodes associated with carcinoma of the head, neck or lung. Cancer 20:103–112, 1967.
13. Carpenter, G.R., and Emery, J.L.: Inclusions in the human thyroid. J. Anat. 122:77–89, 1976.
14. Chandrasoma, P., and Janssen, M.: A thyroglossal cyst lined by gastric epithelium. J.A.M.A. 247:1406, 1982.
15. Connors, J.M., Huffman, L.J., and Hedge, G.A.: Effects of thyrotropin on the vascular conductance of the thyroid gland. Endocrinology 122:921–929, 1988.
16. Curtis, L.E., and Sheahan, D.G.: Heterotopic tissues in the gallbladder. Arch. Pathol. 88:677–683, 1969.
17. De Andrade, M.A.: A review of 128 cases of post-mediastinal goiter. World J. Surg. 1:789–797, 1977.
18. DeLellis, R.A., Nunnemacher, G., and Wolfe, H.J.: C-cell hyperplasia: an ultrastructural analysis. Lab. Invest. 36:237–248, 1978.
19. de Sauza, F.M., and Smith, P.E.: Retrosternal goiter. J. Otolaryngol. 12:393–396, 1983.
20. Dockhorn-Dworniczak, B., Franke, W.W., et al.: Patterns of expression of cytoskeletal proteins in human thyroid gland and thyroid carcinomas. Differentiation 35:53–71, 1987.
21. Donegan, J.O., and Wood, M.D.: Intratracheal thyroid—a familial occurrence. Laryngoscope 95:6–8, 1985.
22. Eales, J.G.: The influence of nutritional state on thyroid function in various vertebrates. Amer. Zool. 28:351–362, 1988.
23. Eggo, M.C., Burrow, G.N., et al.: Iodination and the structure of human thyroglobulin. J. Clin. Endocrinol. Metab. 51:7–11, 1980.
24. Ericson, L.E., and Engstrom, G.: Quantitative electron microscopic studies on exocytosis and endocytosis in the thyroid follicle cell. Endocrinology 103:883–892, 1978.
25. Feind, C.: The Head and Neck. Chapter 5. In: Haagensen, C.D., Feind, C., et al. (eds.): The Lymphatics in Cancer. Philadelphia, W. B. Saunders Co., 1972, pp. 59–63.
26. Finkle, H.I., and Goldman, R.L.: Heterotopic cartilage in the thyroid. Arch. Pathol. 95:48–49, 1973.
27. Fisher, D.A., and Dussault, J.H.: Development of the Mammalian Thyroid Gland. In: Greer, M.A., and Solomon, D.H. (eds.): Handbook of Physiology. Section 7, Endocrinology, vol. III, The Thyroid. Washington, American Physiological Society, 1974, pp. 21–38.

28. Frantz, V.K., Forsythe, R., et al.: Lateral aberrant thyroids. Ann. Surg. *115:*161–183, 1942.
29. Gaby, M.: The role of thyroid dysgenesis and maldescent in the etiology of sporadic cretinism. J. Pediatr. *60:*830–835, 1962.
30. Gardner, W.R.: Unusual relationships between thyroid gland and skeletal muscle in infants. Cancer *6:*681–691, 1956.
31. Gavilan, J., and Gavilan, C.: Recurrent laryngeal nerve: identification during thyroid and parathyroid surgery. Arch. Otolaryngol. Head Neck Surg. *112:*1286–1288, 1986.
32. Gerard-Marchant, R.: Thyroid follicle inclusions in cervical lymph nodes. Arch. Pathol. *77:*637–643, 1964.
33. Gitlin, D., and Biasucci, A.: Ontogenesis of immunoreactive thyroglobulin in the human conceptus. J. Clin. Endocrinol. Metab. *29:*849–853, 1969.
34. Gould, V.E., Johannessen, J.V., and Sobrinho-Simoes, M.: The Thyroid Gland. *In:* Johannessen, J.V. (ed.): Electron Microscopy in Human Medicine, vol. 10, Endocrine Organs. New York, McGraw-Hill, 1981, pp. 29–107.
35. Guimaraes, S.B., Uceda, J.E., and Lynn, H.B.: Thyroglossal duct remnants in infants and children. Mayo Clin. Proc., *47:*117–120, 1972.
36. Gwinup, G., and Morton, M.E.: High-lying thyroid: cause of pseudogoiter. J. Clin. Endocrinol. Metab. *40:*37–42, 1975.
37. Haimoto, H., Hosoda, S., and Kato, K.: Differential distribution of immunoreactive S-100α and S-100β proteins in normal non-nervous human tissues. Lab. Invest. *57:*489–497, 1987.
38. Harach, H.R.: Solid cell nests of the human thyroid in early stages of postnatal life. Acta Anat. *127:*262–264, 1986.
39. Harach, H.R.: Solid cell nests of the thyroid. J. Pathol. *155:*191–200, 1988.
40. Harada, T., Nishikawa, Y., and Ito, K.: Aplasia of one thyroid lobe. Am. J. Surg. *124:*617–619, 1972.
41. Hardwick, D.F., Cormode, E.J., and Riddell, D.G.: Respiratory distress and neck mass in a neonate. J. Pediat. *89:*501–505, 1976.
42. Harrison, R.G.: The Ductless Glands. *In:* Romanes, G.J. (ed.): Cunningham's Textbook of Anatomy. London, Oxford University Press, 1964, pp. 529–551.
43. Hazard, J.B.: The C-cells (parafollicular cells) of the thyroid gland and medullary thyroid carcinoma. Am. J. Pathol. *88:*214–249, 1977.
44. Hegedus, L., Karstrup, S., and Rasmussen, N.: Evidence of cyclic alterations of thyroid size during the menstrual cycle in healthy women. Am. J. Obstet. Gynecol. *155:*142–145, 1986.
45. Hegedus, L., Perrild, H., et al.: The determination of thyroid volume by ultrasound and its relationship to body weight, age and sex in normal subjects. J. Clin. Endocrinol. Metab. *56:*260–263, 1983.
46. Heimann, P.: Ultrastructure of human thyroid. Acta Endocrinol. *53*, Suppl. *110:*5–102, 1966.
47. Howieson-Gibson, W.C., Peng, T.C., and Croker, B.P.: C-cell nodules in adult human thyroid: a common autopsy finding. Am. J. Clin. Pathol. *73:*347–350, 1980.
48. Hoyt, R.F., Hamilton, D.W., and Tashjian, A.H.: Distribution of thyroid, parathyroid and ultimobranchial hypocalcemic factors in birds. II. Morphology, histochemistry and hypocalcemic activity of pigeon thyroid glands. Anat. Rec. *176:*1–34, 1973.
49. Ibrahim, N.B.N., Milewski, P.J., et al.: Benign thyroid inclusions within cervical lymph nodes. Aust. N., Z. J. Surg. *51:*188–189, 1981.
50. Ide, M.: Immunoelectron microscopic localization of thyroglobulin in the human thyroid gland. Acta Pathol. Jpn. *34:*575–584, 1984.
51. Imada, M., Kurosimi, M., and Fujita, H.: Three dimensional imaging of blood vessels in thyroids from normal and levothyroxine sodium-treated rats. Arch. Histol. Jpn. *49:*359–367, 1986.
52. Imada, M., Kurosimi, M., and Fujita, H.: Three dimensional aspects of blood vessels in thyroids from normal, low iodine diet-treated, TSH-treated and PTU-treated rats. Cell Tissue Res. *245:*291–296, 1986.
53. Ingbar, S.H.: The Thyroid Gland. Chapter 21. *In:* Wilson, J.D., and Foster, D.W. (eds.): Williams Textbook of Endocrinology. 7th ed., Philadelphia, W. B. Saunders Company, 1985, pp. 682–815.
54. Ishimura, K., Senda, T., et al.: Immunocytochemical localization of calspectin (a nonerythroid spectrin-like protein) in thyroid glands of normal and TSH-treated rats. Histochemistry *86:*537–539, 1987.
55. Janzer, R.C., Weber, E., and Hedinger, C.: The relation between solid cell nests and C-cells of the thyroid gland. Cell Tissue Res. *197:*295–312, 1979.
56. Johnson, R.L., and Hartman, W.H.: The Thyroid. Chapter 45. *In:* Silverberg, S. (ed.): Principles and Practice of Surgical Pathology, vol. 2. New York, Wiley Medical Publishers, 1983, pp. 1415–1441.
57. Kabel, P.J., Voorbij, H.A.M., et al.: Intrathyroidal dendritic cells. J. Clin. Endocrinol. Metab. *65:*199–207, 1988.
58. Kantelip, B., Lusson, J.R., et al.: Intracardiac ectopic thyroid. Hum. Pathol. *17:*1293–1296, 1986.
59. Kerjaschki, D., Krisch, K., et al.: The structure of tight junctions in human thyroid tumors. Am. J. Pathol. *96:*207–226, 1979.
60. Kingsbury, B.F.: Ultimobranchial body and thyroid gland in the fetal calf. Am. J. Anat. *56:*445–479, 1935.

61. Kirby, M.L., and Bockman, D.E.: Neural crest and normal development: a new perspective. Anat. Rec. *209:*1–6, 1984.
62. Klopp, C.T., and Kirson, S.M.: Therapeutic problems with ectopic non-cancerous follicular thyroid tissue in the neck. Ann. Surg. *163:*653–664, 1966.
63. Larochelle, D., Arcand, P., et al.: Ectopic thyroid tissue—a review of the literature. J. Otolaryngol. *8:*523–530, 1979.
64. Leitz, H.: C-cells: Source of calcitonin. Curr. Topics Pathol. *55:*109–146, 1971.
65. LiVolsi, V.A.: Calcitonin: The hormone and its significance. Progr. Surg. Pathol. *1:*71–103, 1980.
66. LiVolsi, V.A., Perzin, K.H., and Savetsky, L.: Carcinoma arising in median ectopic thyroid (including thyroglossal duct tissue). Cancer *34:*1301–1315, 1974.
67. Melander, A., Ericson, L.D., et al.: Sympathetic innervation of the mouse thyroid and its significance in thyroid hormone secretion. Endocrinology *94:*959–966, 1974.
68. Melander, A., Westgren, U., et al.: Influence of histamine and 5-hydroxy-tryptamine-containing thyroid mast cells on thyroid blood flow and permeability in the rat. Endocrinology *97:*1130–1137, 1975.
69. Melnick, J.C., and Stemkowski, P.E.: Thyroid hemiagenesis (hockey stick sign): A review of the world literature and a report of four cases. J. Clin. Endocrinol. Metab. *52:*247–252, 1981.
70. Meyer, J.S., and Steinberg, L.S.: Microscopically benign thyroid follicles in cervical lymph nodes. Cancer *24:*302–311, 1969.
71. Millikan, J.S., Murr, P., et al.: A familial pattern of thyroglossal duct cysts. J.A.M.A. *244:*1714, 1980.
72. Moses, D.C., Thompson, N.W., et al.: Ectopic thyroid tissue in the neck. Cancer *38:*361–365, 1976.
73. Myers, E.N., and Pantangco, I.P.: Intratracheal thyroid. Laryngoscope *85:*1833–1840, 1975.
74. Neinas, F.W., Gorman, C.A., et al.: Lingual thyroid. Clinical characteristics of 15 cases. Ann. Intern. Med. *79:*205–210, 1973.
75. Nitsch, L., Tramontano, D., et al.: Morphological and functional polarity of an epithelial thyroid cell line. Europ. J. Cell Biol. *38:*57–66, 1985.
76. Norris, E.H.: The early morphogenesis of the human thyroid gland. Am. J. Anat. *24:*443–465, 1918.
77. Norris, E.H.: The parathyroid glands and the lateral thyroid in man: their morphogenesis, histogenesis, topographic anatomy and prenatal growth. Contrib. Embryol. Carneg. Inst. *159:*249–294, 1937.
78. Noyek, A.M., and Friedberg, J.: Thyroglossal duct and ectopic thyroid disorders. Otolaryngol. Clin. North Amer. *14:*187–201, 1981.
79. O'Morchoe, P.J., Han, Y., et al.: Lymphatic system of the thyroid gland in the rat. Lymphology *20:*10–19, 1987.
80. O'Toole, K., Fenoglio-Prieser, C., and Pushparaj, N.: Endocrine changes associated with the human aging process. III. Effect of age on the number of calcitonin immunoreactive cells in the thyroid gland. Hum. Pathol. *16:*991–1000, 1985.
81. Pankow, B.G., Michalak, J., and McGee, M.K.: Adult human thyroid weight. Health Physics *49:*1097–1103, 1985.
82. Piera, J., Garriga, J., et al.: Thyroid hemiagenesis. Am. J. Surg. *151:*419–421, 1986.
83. Pollice, L., and Caneso, G.: Struma cordis. Arch. Pathol. Lab. Med. *110:*452–453, 1986.
84. Prinz, R.A., Sandberg, L., and Chandhuri, P.K.: Androgen receptors in human thyroid tissue. Surgery *96:*996–1000, 1984.
85. Reaume, C.E., and Sofie, V.L.: Lingual thyroid. Oral Surg. *45:*841–845, 1978.
86. Reinhoff, W.F.: Gross and microscopic structure of thyroid gland in man. Contrib. Embryol. Carneg. Inst. *21:*99–123, 1930.
87. Richardson, G.M., and Assor, D.: Thyroid tissue within the larynx. Laryngoscope *81:*120–125, 1971.
88. Rahn, J.: An unusual heterotopia of thyroid gland tissue. Zbl. Allg. Pat. *99:*80–86, 1959.
89. Roth, L.: Inclusions of nonneoplastic thyroid tissue within cervical lymph nodes. Cancer *18:*105–111, 1965.
90. Rubenfeld, S., Joseph, U.A., et al.: Ectopic thyroid in the right carotid triangle. Arch. Otolaryngol. Head Neck Surg. *114:*913–915, 1988.
91. Shemin, R.J., Marsh, J.D., and Schoen, F.J.: Benign intracardiac thyroid mass causing right ventricular outflow tract obstruction. Am. J. Cardiol. *56:*828–829, 1985.
92. Shepard, T.H.: Onset of function in the human fetal thyroid: Biochemical and radioautographic studies from organ culture. J. Clin. Endocrinol. Metab. *27:*945–958, 1967.
93. Sinadinov, J., Savin, S., and Micic, J.V.: Some characteristics of soluble thyroid proteins in human fetus during morphogenesis of follicular structure. Exp. Clin. Endocrinol. *88:*346–354, 1986.
94. Sobrinho-Simoes, M., and Johannessen, J.V.: Scanning electron microscopy of the human thyroid. J. Submicro. Cytol. *13:*109–222, 1981.
95. Steinwald, O.P., Muehrcke, R.C., and Economou, S.G.: Surgical correction of complete lingual ectopia of the thyroid gland. Surg. Clin. North Amer. *50:*1177–1186, 1970.
96. Strickland, A.L., Macfie, J.A., et al.: Ectopic thyroid glands simulating thyroglossal duct cysts. J.A.M.A. *208:*307–310, 1969.
97. Sugiyama, S.: Histological studies of the human thyroid gland observed from the viewpoint of its postnatal development. Ergebn. Anat. Entwickl. Gesch. *39:*H3:7–72, 1967.

98. Sugiyama, S.: The embryology of the human thyroid gland including ultimobranchial body and others related. Ergebn. Anat. Entwickl. Gesch. *44:*H2:6–110, 1971.

99. Sugiyama, S., Taki, A., et al.: Histological studies of the human thyroid gland in middle and late prenatal life. Folia Anat. Jpn. *33:*75–84, 1959.

100. Tice, L.W., and Creveling, C.R.: Electron microscopic identification of adrenergic nerve endings on thyroid epithelial cells. Endocrinology *97:*1123–1129, 1975.

101. Toran-Allerand, C.D.: Normal development of the hypothalamic-pituitary-thyroid axis. Chapter 2. *In:* Ingbar, S.H., and Braverman, L.E. (eds.): Werner's The Thyroid. Philadelphia, J. B. Lippincott Co., 1986, pp. 7–23.

102. Uchiyama, Y., Murakami, G., and Ohno, Y.: The fine structure of nerve endings on rat thyroid follicular cells. Cell Tissue Res. *242:*457–460, 1985.

103. Van Herli, A.J., Vassart, G., and Dumont, J.E.: Control of thyroglobulin synthesis and secretion. N. Engl. J. Med. *301:*239–249, 1979.

104. Ward, R.: Relation of tumors of lateral aberrant thyroid tissue to malignant disease of the thyroid gland. Arch. Surg. *40:*606–645, 1940.

105. Weller, G.L.: Development of the thyroid, parathyroid and thymus glands in man. Contrib. Embryol. Carneg. Inst. No. *141:*93–140, 1933.

106. Wolfe, H.F., DeLellis, R.A., et al.: Distribution of calcitonin-containing cells in the normal neonatal human thyroid gland. J. Clin. Endocrinol. Metab. *41:*1076–1081, 1975.

107. Wolfe, H.F., Voelkel, E.F., and Tashjian, A.H.: Distribution of calcitonin-containing cells in the normal adult human thyroid gland. J. Clin. Endocrinol. Metab. *38:*688–694, 1974.

108. Yamaoka, Y.: Solid cell nests (SCN) in the human thyroid gland. Acta Pathol. Jpn. *23:*493–506, 1973.

THYROID FUNCTION, NORMAL AND ABNORMAL, AND ITS EVALUATION

2

In this chapter, a review of normal thyroid metabolism, hyper- and hypothyroidism and the principal etiologies of these functional abnormalities is presented. Since this monograph is devoted principally to morphologic aspects of thyroid pathology, detailed clinical and biochemical features of thyroid functional disorders are not presented.[55] However, an overview is given, since it is considered necessary to review the major features of these conditions in order to correlate morphologic changes with clinical findings.

THYROID METABOLISM: THE NORMAL STATE

Hormone Production

The function of the thyroid gland is to produce the hormones thyroxine (T_4) and triiodothyronine (T_3). In the normal state, the gland is influenced primarily by the pituitary hormone, thyroid stimulating hormone (thyrotropin, TSH), and secondarily by the hypothalamus; the latter secretes thyrotropin releasing hormone (TRH) and stimulates the pituitary, and thence the thyroid.[67, 96, 97, 126]

The second important regulator of thyroid function is iodine, since this element forms an integral part of the thyroid hormones.[43, 67]

The production of thyroid hormones entails a number of integrated steps.[43] These include:

1. Trapping and concentration of inorganic iodide; iodide is derived from the circulation (ingested iodide) or from recycled iodide arising during the hormone production process;

2. Oxidation of iodide to the organic form; this reaction involves thyroid peroxidase, which is located at the follicular apical cell membrane;

3. The organic iodide reacts with tyrosine via a peroxidase-mediated reaction within thyroglobulin to form mono- and di-iodothyrosine;

4. Coupling of mono- and di-iodothyronines to form the two thyroid hormones triiodothyronine (T_3) and thyroxine (T_4). In patients with hyperactive glands or damaged glands or in cases of iodine deficiency, relatively more T_3 is produced.[67]

These substances are incorporated and stored in thyroglobulin, i.e., the colloid.

Once formed, thyroid hormones are released by endocytosis of thyroglobulin into apical portions of the follicular epithelial cells. These droplets of thyroglobulin fuse with lysosomes and are hydrolyzed with consequent release of T_3 and T_4 into the blood stream. (Any mono- and di-iodinated tyrosines are deiodinated via a deiodinase enzyme, and iodide is restored into the intrathyroidal pool for re-use.)[21, 43]

The normal secretion rate from the thyroid of T_4 is 80 μg/day and of T_3, 5 μg/day.[67]

In the circulation, thyroid hormones circulate bound to plasma proteins: thyroxine binding globulin (TBG) and thyroxine binding prealbumin (TBPA). Although T_4 constitutes the major portion of circulating thyroid hormone, peripheral deiodination (at sites of activity in various organs) produces the more potent substance, T_3.[67]

The binding of T_4 and its relatively slow release from TBG account for the slow onset of action of the hormone. T_3, which is weakly bound to serum proteins, is rapidly released and acts quickly and transiently.[64, 73]

Metabolic inactivation of thyroid hormones results from deiodination in extrathyroidal tissues; released iodine is recycled through the thyroid gland.[43] In extrathyroidal tissues, T_4 may be deiodinated differently, producing not T_3 but reverse T_3. This substance is inactive as a hormone; radioimmunoassay studies show it is increased in hypothyroidism.[14]

Actions of Thyroid Hormones

The mode of action of thyroid hormones remains disputed.[67] It has been suggested that they act via induction of beta-adrenergic catecholamine receptors in peripheral tissues and activation of ATP-ase.[67, 94] By the latter reaction, thyroid hormones control oxygen consumption in mitochondria.

Thyroid hormones also bind to nuclear receptors and presumably stimulate gene transcription with increased production of specific proteins, i.e., growth factors, hormones, and enzymes. Hence, thyroid hormones regulate most body tissues by affecting enzymes involved in intermediary metabolism and affecting growth.[10, 43, 81–83, 94, 95, 111]

HYPOTHYROIDISM

Hypothyroidism results from a subnormal amount of circulating thyroid hormone. This disorder has numerous etiologies, some thyroidal, and others of extrathyroidal origin. (See Table 2–1.)

Biosynthetic Defects. Numerous "inborn errors" of thyroid metabolism have been described; in many instances, a few members of one family have been discovered to harbor a defect.[33, 62, 66] Although these cases may be insignificant in terms of patients affected, they provide new insights into the normal pathways of thyroid hormone production and metabolism. Lever et al. have summarized the known metabolic pathway errors in thyroid hormone production and secretion.[66] Virtually any step in the biosynthetic and/or release pathways can be affected:

1. Unresponsiveness of thyroid cell receptor to TSH[18]

2. Iodide transport defects[103]

3. Organification defect (peroxidase deficiency); some cases are associated with deafness (Pendred's syndrome)[43, 66]

Table 2–1. Hypothyroidism: Causes

1. **Primary Thyroid Causes**
   a. Biosynthetic defects—"inborn errors of metabolism"
   b. Developmental abnormalities
   c. Destruction of thyroid
      (i) Surgery
      (ii) Radiation
      (iii) Autoimmune thyroiditis
   d. Replacement of thyroid tissue
      (i) Neoplasms
      (ii) Fibrosis
   e. Drug effects—interference with hormone production and/or secretion
2. **Secondary Hypothyroidism**
   a. Pituitary destruction
      (i) Neoplasms
      (ii) Infarcts
      (iii) Trauma
   b. Isolated TSH deficiency
3. **"Tertiary" Hypothyroidism**
      Hypothalamic destruction
      (i) Neoplasms
      (ii) Granulomas
      (iii) Trauma
4. **Euthyroid "Sick" Syndrome**

4. Abnormalities of coupling-production of T_3 and T_4[35]
5. Defects in the structure of thyroglobulin[68]
6. Deiodinase abnormalities—intra- or extraglandular

In each of these categories, the patients are hypothyroid (often from birth), may have severe motor, growth, and mental retardation, and frequently have goiters. The marked decrease in thyroid hormone signals the pituitary to secrete TSH; TSH levels rise and drive the follicular cells to produce and secrete hormone. Since this is blocked by the inborn defect, the gland undergoes a remarkable degree of hyperplasia. The classic morphology of the enlarged hyperplastic thyroid is discussed in Chapter 9.

Other congenital abnormalities occur that affect hormone transport; thus, families with deficiency, excess, or abnormal structure of thyroid binding globulin or thyroid binding prealbumin have been described; such patients, usually discovered by routine testing of thyroid function, often do not show effects of hypothyroidism.[5, 11, 80, 84, 98, 102, 113, 122, 130]

Abnormalities of Development. Thyroid agenesis and other defects can, of course, lead to severe hypothyroidism since thyroid tissue would be absent.[76, 88] (See Chapter 1.)

Iodine and Drug Effects. Deficient amounts of iodine can produce goitrous hypothyroidism since the major component of the hormone is lacking.[74, 120] Certain drugs interfere with certain steps in the biosynthetic pathway—thiourea derivations affect iodination of tyrosine and coupling of iodothyrosines to T_3 and T_4. Iodine excess and lithium affect proteolysis and interfere with release of thyroid hormone into the circulation.[43, 120] Many iodine-containing radiologic contrast agents and therapeutic drugs contain iodine and can lead to hypothyroidism.[43] The antiarrhythmic drug amiodarone, which contains large quantities of iodine, can cause hypothyroidism.[43, 71]

Thyroid Destruction. Obviously a thyroid that has been removed, destroyed, or replaced cannot function appropriately and hypothyroidism results.[125]

1. Chronic thyroiditis, usually of autoimmune etiology, produces slow deterio-

ration of the gland with follicular atrophy, cellular metaplasia, fibrosis, and lymphocytic infiltration.[6, 60, 104, 119, 123]

2. Infiltrative diseases such as primary or metastatic tumors, amyloid or fibrosis (as in scleroderma) may replace sufficient amounts of the thyroid to produce hypofunction.[41]

3. Surgical and/or radiotherapeutic (radioiodine) ablation, usually for hyperthyroidism, may result in hypofunction. Following surgical removal, a finite percentage of patients may become hypothyroid, but after several years a plateau is reached; in the population treated with radioiodine, the risk of developing hypothyroidism continues without leveling off.[39, 69]

Secondary Hypothyroidism from TSH Deficiency. The thyroid itself is normal, but the pituitary is not functioning adequately. This may result from pituitary replacement by tumor, infarction, or surgical extirpation.[7, 30, 108] Some patients with so-called "central" hypothyroidism have secretion of abnormal TSH;[29] in an unusual case reported by Dickstein and Barzilai, a pituitary adenoma produced biologically inactive TSH, leading to hypothyroidism.[22] Isolated TSH deficiency has also been reported as causing central hypothyroidism.[26, 77]

"Tertiary" Hypothyroidism. This results from hypothalamic lesions (tumor, granuloma, or hamartoma), which result in decreased TRH and a consequent decline in TSH and ultimately thyroid hormones.[29, 30, 43, 96]

So-called Euthyroid "Sick" Syndrome. This is found in severely ill patients (sepsis, etc.) who appear chemically hypothyroid, but are not so.[17] The mechanisms for this phenomenon are not worked out, but probably reflect nutritional and metabolic disturbances which affect cellular receptor and enzyme systems needed for appropriate thyroid hormone function.[9, 12, 43, 79, 93, 116]

The clinical manifestations of hypothyroidism vary between children and adults. In congenital forms of the disease, mental and growth retardation, hypothermia, constipation, dry skin, and somnolence are found. In the adult, hypothyroidism is accompanied by subcutaneous deposition of "myxedema" fluid, edema fluid rich in mucopolysaccharides. Thus the face is puffy, the tongue enlarges, joints and muscles become stiff, and there is pericardial effusion. The low metabolic rate is often accompanied by hypothermia, cold intolerance, bradycardia, somnolence, and constipation.[43, 67]

HYPERTHYROIDISM

Hyperthyroidism (thyrotoxicosis) results from excess circulation of (and therefore tissue and organ exposure to) thyroid hormones.

Excess production of thyroid hormones can occur either as a result of oversecretion of stimulatory hormones (TSH; TRH) or mimickers thereof; or it may be caused by substances that mimic the stimulating actions of these hormones (immunoglobulins).[38, 44]

The causes of hyperthyroidism are varied and include those discussed below. (See also Table 2–2.) (See also Chapter 9 for detailed discussion.)

Diffuse Toxic Goiter (Graves' Disease). This is the most common cause of hyperthyroidism,[42, 43, 55, 110] comprising 70 to 80 percent of cases. It affects predominantly young women who manifest diffuse thyroid enlargement, ophthalmopathy, and hyperthyroid symptoms and signs (see below). Currently classified among the autoimmune thyroid disorders, Graves' disease is characterized by the presence of circulating groups of thyroid-stimulating antibodies (thyroid-receptor antibodies). These immunoglobulins apparently bind to TSH receptors on the follicular

Table 2–2. Hyperthyroidism: Causes*

Diffuse toxic goiter (Graves' disease)
Toxic nodular goiter
Toxic adenoma
Thyroid carcinoma
Thyroiditis
Subacute
Painless
Drug-associated
Factitious hyperthyroidism
Struma ovarii
Central hyperthyroidism; excess TSH
Pituitary tumor
Pituitary resistance to thyroid hormone
Excess TRH?
Trophoblastic disease

*See also Table 9–3 (Chapter 9).

epithelial cells, "fool" the cells into thinking TSH is present, and consequently the thyroid cells are stimulated to grow and to produce thyroid hormones. (Probably different subsets of immunoglobulins cause growth stimulation and hypersecretion.) The thyroid hormones present in excess feed back to the pituitary-hypothalamic system and cause decreased to unmeasurable secretion of TSH and TRH. Hence, the immunoglobulins interfere with the normal hypothalamic-pituitary-thyroid feedback axis.[25, 42, 43]

Toxic Nodular Goiter. This is seen chiefly in middle-aged to elderly patients, and consists of focal (?multifocal) areas of hyperfunctioning thyroid tissue in an otherwise multinodular goiter. The disease accounts for 5 to 15 percent of hyperthyroidism.[110] It develops gradually in patients with prior nontoxic goiter; presumably one or a few regions of alternating hyperplastic and involuting thyroid tissue become autonomous.[36, 114] Autoimmune factors may play a role in the pathogenesis of this disorder.[43, 44, 114]

Toxic Nodule (Toxic Adenoma). This comprises about 5 to 10 percent of hyperthyroidism cases.[110] Also seen chiefly in older adult women, a solitary autonomous follicular nodule may produce hyperthyroidism. Such lesions can best be classified pathologically as encapsulated "adenoma."[48] Thyroid tissue surrounding the adenoma usually appears atrophic. In a significant proportion of patients with toxic adenoma, the predominant hormone secreted is T_3—so-called T_3 toxicosis.[43, 56]

Thyroid Carcinoma. The overwhelming majority of well-differentiated thyroid carcinomas can produce thyroglobulin, and take up iodide. However, in most tumors the neoplastic cells are less able to function than normal surrounding thyroid. In one large series of patients with thyroid cancer, the few cases of associated hyperthyroidism were due to concomitant Graves' disease or toxic adenomas.[72] Very rare cases of hyperfunctioning thyroid cancers have been recorded;[19, 32] most of these are follicular carcinomas.

Rare cases of rapidly growing thyroid carcinomas or lymphoma have produced hyperthyroidism; the presumed mechanism resembles that seen in subacute thyroiditis, i.e., rapid destruction of thyroid follicles with release of large amounts of stored thyroid hormone.[92, 106, 117]

Struma Ovarii. Thyroid tissue associated with teratomas of the ovary usually is asymptomatic from a functional standpoint. Rarely, however, hyperthyroidism may be produced by excess thyroid hormone secreted by this ectopic tissue. It is important to remember, however, that most patients with hyperthyroidism and struma ovarii have goiters in the neck; the hyperthyroidism is more likely caused by the latter, although the ovarian thyroid hormone secretion may add to the excess circulating hormone concentration.[43, 110] (See Chapter 16.)

Thyroiditides. Subacute thyroiditis can be associated with hyperthyroidism in the initial phase of the disease, since follicular destruction is followed by subsequent release of stored hormone. (See Chapter 4.)

Painless thyroiditis with hyperthyroidism, originally classified as a form of subacute thyroiditis, is now considered an autoimmune disease.[31] It is relatively common (about 20 percent of hyperthyroidism), occurs equally in both sexes, is of relatively acute onset (often in the postpartum period), and although spontaneous remissions occur, a substantial number of these patients progress to hypothyroidism.[2, 3, 110, 115] (See also Chapter 5.)

Iatrogenic or Drug-Induced Hyperthyroidism. Administration of thyroid hormone supplements, if excessive, can lead to hyperthyroidism.[70]

Iodine supplementation, particularly in patients with large goiters or in individuals suffering iodine deficiency (as in endemic goiter regions), can lead to hyperthyroidism (Jod-Basedow disease).[34, 89, 121]

Trophoblastic Disease. Hydatidiform mole and choriocarcinoma can cause hyperthyroidism.[54] Overt signs of thyroid overfunction are less common than chemical abnormalities of elevated T_3 and T_4.[54, 78, 87] (See Chapter 9.)

Excess TSH. "Secondary" hyperthyroidism may result from increased circulating TSH.[75] Many, but not all, of these patients harbor pituitary adenomas which produce TSH.[37, 49, 107]

A small subgroup of patients do not have pituitary tumors, but have inappropriate feedback response to thyroid hormone—the syndrome of pituitary resistance to thyroid hormone.[37, 61, 109]

Another subset of patients shows both pituitary and peripheral end organ resistance to thyroid hormone. Such patients have goiters and increased T_4, T_3, and often TSH, but they are clinically euthyroid. This combined resistance syndrome is often familial.[4, 13, 129]

Ectopic Production of TSH by Nonendocrine Tumors. This is theoretically a possible cause of hyperthyroidism. Unequivocally documented cases of this entity remain to be described, however.

The clinical manifestations of hyperthyroidism are myriad since thyroid hormones affect virtually every organ system in the body. Classically, hyperthyroid patients show hyperactivity, nervousness, tachycardia, and intolerance to heat. Weight loss due to hypermetabolism may occur. Diarrhea due to increased intestinal transit time is common. The severity of the hyperthyroidism varies from mild to life-threatening (thyroid storm).

Between the endpoints of overt hypothyroidism and hyperthyroidism, a variety of symptom complexes may be found. The reader is referred to clinical texts for descriptions of these entities.[55]

TESTING THYROID FUNCTION

Testing of thyroid function has evolved over decades from measurements of basal metabolic rate, used as a crude assessment of oxygen consumption and caloric expenditure, to refined radioimmunologic measurements of minute quantities of circulating hormones.

The limitations of tests such as basal metabolic rate are numerous and include patient factors, technician ability, and the influence of many nonthyroidal diseases.[8, 14, 27, 52, 63, 65, 101, 124] The huge number of tests to measure thyroid function indicates that no single test is completely adequate or reliable.

Methods for evaluating thyroid function* have been divided by Cavalieri[14] into (a) those which measure effects of thyroid hormone such as basal metabolic rate; (b) those measuring thyroid iodine metabolism; (c) those which measure circulating thyroid hormones; and (d) those which assess feedback and control mechanisms.[65, 91] The following discussion will review specific tests in the latter three categories.

Thyroid Iodine Metabolism Measurement

Radionuclide Uptake. Radioactive iodine injected into an individual will be preferentially trapped by the thyroid gland. Measurement of radioactivity over the thyroid over several time intervals (30 minutes, 6 hours, 24 hours) allows an estimation of the ability of the thyroid to trap iodine, organify it, and accumulate isotope, presumably producing T_4 and T_3.[51, 100]

This very useful test can be influenced by isotope, equipment, and technique used[46, 101] as well as by drugs taken by the patient, particularly those containing iodine.[14]

To avoid a significant degree of radiation exposure in adults, but especially in testing children, radioactive 99m-technetium in the form of the pertechnetate ion can be used. This substance, because it is similar in charge and size to iodide, can substitute in uptake tests; it offers the advantage of low radiation exposure.[40, 53]

A number of conditions influence uptake of the radioisotopes: hence increased uptake is found in hyperthyroidism, iodine deficiency states, trophoblastic disease, and some inborn errors of thyroid metabolism. Decreased uptake is identified in hypothyroidism, primary and central, the active phase of subacute thyroiditis, and states of iodine excess.[14]

Perchlorate Test. If organification is impaired (congenital dyshormonogenesis syndromes, autoimmune thyroiditis, or drugs that interfere with the organification step), iodide accumulates in the gland and can be identified by administration of perchlorate (which inhibits the iodide-concentrating mechanism). The test involves giving an oral dose of radioiodide followed two hours later by perchlorate salt. If organification is delayed, the radionuclide will exist as nonorganified iodide and will be displaced by perchlorate—"discharged" out of the thyroid. If a significant portion of the administered radioiodide (5 percent or more) is discharged, the test is considered positive.[14, 59]

Measurement of Circulating Thyroid Hormones[127]

Since measurement of thyroid hormones, circulating bound to proteins, was an almost impossible task before the advent of radioimmunoassays, indirect assessments were devised. The thyroid's unique relationship to iodine allowed for the

---

*Additional tests are utilized commonly to assess nodular thyroid disease, including isotope scans, echography, computerized tomography, magnetic resonance imaging, and minimally invasive procedures such as fine needle aspiration and large bore needle biopsy. These latter techniques and their diagnostic utility will be discussed in Chapter 17; in the present chapter, tests used to assess thyroid *function* will be reviewed. Assays for antithyroid antibodies in autoimmune thyroid diseases are discussed in reference 25.

development of many tests based on measurement of iodine. The myriad of assays and their modifications indicate that none was very good.[50] The tests, briefly mentioned here primarily for historical reasons, included protein-bound iodine (PBI) and butanol extractable iodine (BEI).[45] Since these tests revolved around iodine concentrations and since a variety of altered physiologic or pathologic (nonthyroidal) states can affect iodine, the tests were considered accurate 75 percent of the time; they are now obsolete.

Competitive protein-binding assays that can utilize radiolabeled antibodies (radioimmunoassay) or endogenous binding proteins[14, 28, 85, 86] form the basis of most modern measurements of circulating thyroid hormone. These tests involve the separation of thyroid hormone from its binding proteins, and addition of radiolabeled tracer hormone and a standard amount of thyroxine-binding globulin (or specific antibody to T_4 or T_3). Bound T_4 (or T_3) is separated from free T_4 (or T_3) and the ratio of bound to free radioactivity is compared with a standard curve.[58] Newer methods employing enzyme immunoassay and capable of adapting to multichannel serum analyzers are becoming popular.[59] These competitive binding assays bypass disadvantages associated with indirect iodide measurements.[14, 15]

Free T_4 and Free T_3. Radioimmunoassay methods for measuring free (unbound to serum proteins) thyroid hormones are available and have replaced the tedious equilibrium dialysis techniques.[16, 23, 112] Normal values include free T_4 of 2.0 ng/dl and free T_3 of 0.33 ng/dl.[14] These hormones are elevated in 95 to 100 percent of hyperthyroid patients; T_4 is decreased in all hypothyroid individuals whereas T_3 may be normal in about 30 percent.

T_3 Uptake Test. If thyroxine binding globulin is normal in structure and amount, some of the binding sites will be unoccupied by thyroid hormone in the euthyroid individual. In this test, a known amount of radiolabeled T_3 is added to the serum sample and placed on a resin (agarose, dextran, etc.). After a designated time period, the adsorbing material is separated from the serum and the amount of labeled T_3 by the adsorber (uptake) is measured. In hyperthyroidism, when most TBG sites are occupied, the fractional uptake of labeled hormone to resin is increased; the opposite situation holds for hypothyroidism.[14, 45, 47] Factors that affect TBG (congenitally abnormal TBG's, estrogen administration, etc.) may affect the results of this test.[14]

Tests of Feedback Mechanisms

Measurement of TSH by radioimmunoassay has become a useful diagnostic tool.[90] Normal range is approximately 0.5 to 50 mU/L.[14] Elevated levels of this hormone are often found in hypothyroid states; TSH levels rise early in hypothyroidism and this test is exquisitely sensitive as the initial indicator of hypofunction. Methods that discriminate low levels of TSH from normal have only recently become available.[1, 118]

The TRH Stimulation Test.[99] TRH, the tripeptide hypothalamic hormone, can be injected to test the integrity of the hypothalamic-pituitary axis. This test may be helpful in the distinction of primary from secondary hypothyroidism. If a hypothyroid patient with a nonelevated TSH level shows a brisk rise in TSH after TRH administration, the pituitary is intact; on the other hand, if the TSH response is blunted, the result suggests an intrinsic pituitary abnormality as the cause of hypothyroidism.[14, 57, 59]

This brief review of the major useful tests of thyroid function is not all-inclusive; the reader is referred to texts and reviews on this subject.[14, 55, 59, 105, 128] Cost effectiveness of individual tests and/or combinations of tests also must be considered.[24]

For evaluation of suspected hypothyroidism,[15, 20, 24] the following scheme may be useful:

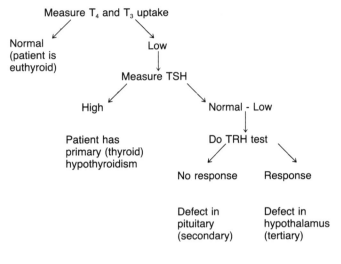

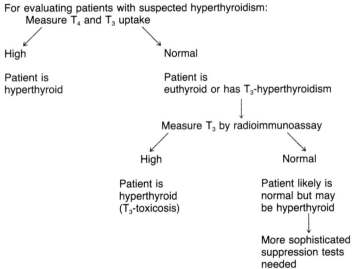

REFERENCES

1. Alexander, W.D., Kerr, D.J., and Ferguson, M.M.: First-line test of thyroid function. Lancet 2:647–648, 1984.
2. Amino, N., Miyai, K., et al.: Transient postpartum hypothyroidism: fourteen cases with autoimmune thyroiditis. Ann. Intern. Med. 87:155–159, 1977.
3. Amino, N., Mori, H., et al.: High prevalence of transient postpartum thyrotoxicosis and hypothyroidism. N. Engl. J. Med. 306:849–852, 1982.
4. Bantle, J.P., Seeling, S., et al.: Resistance to thyroid hormones. Arch. Intern. Med. 142:1867–1871, 1982.

5. Barlow, J.W., Csicsmann, J.M., et al.: Familial euthyroid thyroxine excess: Characterization of abnormal intermediate affinity thyroxine-binding to albumin. J. Clin. Endocrinol. Metab. *55:*244–250, 1982.
6. Bastenie, P.E., Neve, P., et al.: Clinical and pathological significance of asymptomatic atrophic thyroiditis. Lancet *1:*915–918, 1976.
7. Beck-Peccoz, P., Amr, S., et al.: Decreased receptor binding of biologically inactive thyrotropin in central hypothyroidism. N. Engl. J. Med. *312:*1085–1090, 1985.
8. Becker, D.V., Metabolic Indices. *In:* Werner, S.C., and Ingbar, S.H. (eds.): The Thyroid: A Fundamental and Clinical Text. Hagerstown, MD, Harper & Row, 1978, pp. 347–363.
9. Bermudez, F., Surks, M.I., and Oppenheimer, J.H.: High incidence of decreased serum triiodothyronine concentration in patients with nonthyroidal disease. J. Clin. Endocrinol. Metab. *41:*27–40, 1975.
10. Bernal, J., Liewandahl, K., and Lamberg, B.A.: Thyroid hormone receptors in fetal and hormone resistant tissues. Scand. J. Clin. Lab. Invest. *45:*577–583, 1985.
11. Borst, G.C., Eil, C., and Burman, K.D.: Euthyroid hyperthyroxinemia. Ann. Intern. Med. *98:*366–378, 1983.
12. Brent, G.A., Hershman, J.M., and Braunstein, G.D.: Patients with severe nonthyroidal illness and serum thyrotropin concentrations in the hypothyroid range. Am. J. Med. *81:*463–466, 1986.
13. Brooks, M.H., Barbato, A.L., et al.: Familial thyroid hormone resistance. Am. J. Med. *71:*414–421, 1981.
14. Cavalieri, R.R.: Laboratory Evaluation of Thyroid Status. *In:* Green, W.L. (ed.): The Thyroid. New York, Elsevier, 1977, pp. 107–155.
15. Chertow, B.S., Motto, G.S., and Shah, J.H.: A biochemical profile of abnormalities in hypothyroidism. Am. J. Clin. Pathol. *61:*785–788, 1974.
16. Chopra, I.J.: A radioimmunoassay for measurement of thyroxine in unextracted serum. J. Clin. Endocrinol. Metab. *34:*938–947, 1972.
17. Chopra, I.J., Solomon, D.H., et al.: Misleadingly low free thyroxine index and usefulness of reverse tri-iodothyronine measurement in nonthyroidal illnesses. Ann. Intern. Med. *90:*905–912, 1979.
18. Codaccioni, J.L., Carayon, P., et al.: Congenital hypothyroidism associated with thyrotropin unresponsiveness and thyroid cell membrane alterations. J. Clin. Endocrinol. Metab. *50:*932–937, 1980.
19. Cooper, D.S., Ridgeway, E.C., and Maloof, F.: Unusual types of hyperthyroidism. Clin. Endocrinol. Metab. *7:*199–220, 1978.
20. Corns, C.M., and Miller, A.L.: Evaluation of strategy for testing thyroid function applied to hypothyroidism. J. Clin. Pathol. *39:*293–296, 1986.
21. Deiss, W.P., and Peake, R.L.: The mechanism of thyroid hormone secretion. Ann. Intern. Med. *69:*881–890, 1968.
22. Dickstein, G., and Barzilai, D.: Hypothyroidism secondary to biologically inactive thyroid-stimulating hormone secretion by a pituitary chromophobe adenoma. Arch. Intern. Med. *142:*1544–1545, 1982.
23. dos Remedios, L.V., Weber, P.M., et al.: Detecting unsuspected thyroid dysfunction by the free thyroxine index. Arch. Intern. Med. *140:*1045–1049, 1980.
24. Drake, J.R., Miller, D.K., and Evans, R.G.: Cost effectiveness of thyroid function tests. Arch. Intern. Med. *142:*1810–1812, 1982.
25. Dumont, J.E., Roger, P.P., and Ludgate, M.: Assays for thyroid growth immunoglobulins and their clinical implications: methods, concepts and misconceptions. Endocrinol. Rev. *8:*448–452, 1987.
26. Emerson, C.H.: Central hypothyroidism and hyperthyroidism. Med. Clin. N. Amer. *69:*1019–1034, 1985.
27. Ericsson, U.B., and Thorell, J.I.: A prospective critical evaluation of in vitro thyroid function tests. Acta Med. Scand. *220:*47–56, 1986.
28. Evered, D.C., Vice, P.A., et al.: Assessment of thyroid hormone assays. J. Clin. Pathol. *29:*1054–1059, 1976.
29. Faglia, G., Beck-Peccoz, P., et al.: Excess of B subunit of thyrotropin (TSH) in patients with idiopathic central hypothyroidism due to secretion of TSH with reduced biological activity. J. Clin. Endocrinol. Metab. *56:*908–914, 1983.
30. Faglia, G., Bitensky, L., et al.: Thyrotropin secretion in patients with central hypothyroidism: Evidence for reduced biological activity of immunoreactive thyrotropin. J. Clin. Endocrinol. Metab. *48:*989–998, 1979.
31. Farid, N.R., Howe, B.S., and Walfish, P.G.: Increased frequency of HLA-DR$_3$ and 5 in the syndromes of painless thyroiditis with transient thyrotoxicosis: Evidence for an autoimmune etiology. Clin. Endocrinol. *19:*699–704, 1983.
32. Federman, D.D.: Hyperthyroidism due to functioning metastatic carcinoma of the thyroid. Medicine *43:*267–274, 1964.
33. Fisher, D.A., and Klein, A.H.: Thyroid development and disorders of thyroid function in the newborn. N. Engl. J. Med. *304:*702–712, 1981.
34. Fradkin, J.E., and Wolff, J.: Iodide-induced thyrotoxicosis. Medicine *62:*1–20, 1983.

35. Gattereau, A., Bernard, B., et al.: Congenital goiter in four euthyroid siblings with glandular and circulating iodoproteins and defective iodothyronine synthesis. J. Clin. Endocrinol. Metab. *37:*118–128, 1973.
36. Gemsenjager, E., Staub, J.J., et al.: Preclinical hyperthyroidism in multinodular goiter. J. Clin. Endocrinol. Metab. *43:*810–816, 1976.
37. Gharib, H., Carpenter, P.C., et al.: The spectrum of inappropriate pituitary thyrotropin secretion associated with hyperthyroidism. Mayo Clin. Proc. *57:*556–563, 1982.
38. Ginsberg, J., and von Westrap, C.: Clinical applications of assays for thyrotropin receptor antibodies in Graves' disease. Canad. Med. Assoc. J. *134:*1141–1147, 1986.
39. Glennon, J.A., Gordon, E., and Sawin, C.T.: Hypothyroidism after low dose 131-I treatment of hyperthyroidism. Ann. Intern. Med. 76:721–723, 1972.
40. Goolden, A.W.G., Glass, H.E., and Williams, E.D.: Use of 99-Tc for the routine assessment of thyroid function. Br. Med. J. *4:*396–399, 1971.
41. Gordon, M.B., Klein, I., et al.: Thyroid disease in progressive systemic sclerosis. Ann. Intern. Med. *95:*431–435, 1981.
42. Gossage, A.A.R., and Munro, D.S.: The pathogenesis of Graves' disease. Clin. Endocrinol. Metab. *14:*299–330, 1985.
43. Green, W.L.: Physiology of the Thyroid Gland and Its Hormones. Chap. 1. *In:* Green, W.L. (ed.): The Thyroid. New York, Elsevier, 1987, pp. 1–46.
44. Grubeck-Loebenstein, B., Derfler, K., et al.: Immunologic features of nonimmunogenic hyperthyroidism. J. Clin. Endocrinol. Metab. *60:*150–155, 1985.
45. Gruhn, J.G., Barsano, C.P., and Kumar, Y.: The development of thyroid function tests. Arch. Pathol. Lab. Med. *111:*84–100, 1987.
46. Halpern, S., Alazraki, N., et al.: 131-I thyroid uptakes: Capsule vs. liquid. J. Nucl. Med. *14:*507–510, 1973.
47. Hamada, S., Nakagawa, T., et al.: Reevaluation of thyroxine binding and free thyroxine in human serum by paper electrophoresis and equilibrium dialysis, and a new free thyroxine index. J. Clin. Endocrinol. Metab. *31:*166–179, 1970.
48. Hamburger, J.I.: Evolution of toxicity in solitary nontoxic autonomously functioning thyroid nodules. J. Clin. Metab. Endocrinol. *50:*1089–1093, 1980.
49. Hamilton, C.R., Adams, L.C., and Maloof, F.: Hyperthyroidism due to thyrotropin-producing pituitary chromophobe adenoma. N. Engl. J. Med. *283:*1077–1080, 1970.
50. Havard, C.W.H.: Which tests of thyroid function. Br. Med. J. *1:*553–556, 1974.
51. Havard, C.W.H., and Boss, M.: In vivo tests of thyroid function. Br. Med. J. *3:*678–681, 1974.
52. Hay, I.D., and Klee, G.G.: Thyroid dysfunction. Endocrinol. Metab. Clin. N. Amer. *17:*473–509, 1988.
53. Hays, M.T., and Wesselossky, B.: Simultaneous measurement of thyroidal trapping (99TcO$_4$-) and binding (131-I): Clinical and experimental studies in man. J. Nucl. Med. *14:*785–792, 1973.
54. Hershman, J.M., and Higgins, H.P.: Hydatidiform mole—a cause of clinical hyperthyroidism. N. Engl. J. Med. *284:*573–577, 1971.
55. Ingbar, S.H., and Braverman, L.E. (eds.): Werner's The Thyroid, 5th ed. Philadelphia, J. B. Lippincott Co., 1986.
56. Ivy, H.K., Wahner, H.W., and Gorman, C.A.: Triiodothyronine (T$_3$) toxicosis. Arch. Intern. Med. *128:*529–534, 1971.
57. Jackson, I.M.D.: Thyrotropin releasing hormone. N. Engl. J. Med. *306:*145–155, 1982.
58. Kaplan, L.A., Chen, I.W., et al.: Evaluation and comparison of radio-, fluorescence and enzyme-linked immunoassay for serum thyroxine. Clin. Biochem. *14:*182–188, 1981.
59. Kaplan, M.M.: Clinical and laboratory assessment of thyroid abnormalities. Med. Clin. N. Amer. *69:*863–880, 1985.
60. Kidd, A., Okita, N., et al.: Immunologic aspects of Graves' and Hashimoto's diseases. Metabolism *29:*80–99, 1980.
61. Kourides, I.A., Pekonen, F., and Weintraub, B.D.: Absence of thyroid-binding immunoglobulins in patients with thyrotropin-mediated hyperthyroidism. J. Clin. Endocrinol. Metab. *51:*271–274, 1980.
62. Koutras, D.A., Souvatzoglou, A., et al.: Iodide organification defect in iodine deficient endemic goiter. J. Clin. Endocrinol. Metab. *47:*610–614, 1978.
63. Ladenson, P.W.: Diseases of the thyroid gland. Clin. Endocrinol. Metab. *14:*145–173, 1985.
64. Larsen, P.R.: Triiodothyronine: Review of recent studies on its physiology and pathophysiology in man. Metabolism *21:*1073–1092, 1972.
65. Larsen, P.R., Alexander, N.M., et al.: Revised nomenclature for tests of thyroid hormones and thyroid-related proteins in serum. Arch. Pathol. Lab. Med. *111:*1141–1145, 1987.
66. Lever, E.G., Medeiros-Neto, G.A., and DeGroot, L.J.: Inherited disorders of thyroid metabolism. Endocrinol. Rev. *4:*213–239, 1983.
67. Liddle, G.W., and Liddle, R.A.: Endocrinology. Chap. 7. *In:* Smith, L.H., and Thier, S.O. (eds.): Pathophysiology. Philadelphia, W. B. Saunders Company, 1981, pp. 653–754.
68. Lissitzky, S., Bismuth, J., et al.: Congenital goiter with impaired thyroglobulin synthesis. J. Clin. Endocrinol. Metab. *36:*17–29, 1973.
69. Malone, J.F., and Cullen, M.J.: Two mechanisms for hypothyroidism after 131-I therapy. Lancet *2:*73–75, 1976.

70. Mariotti, S., Martino, E., et al.: Low serum thyroglobulin as a clue to the diagnosis of thyrotoxicosis factitia. N. Engl. J. Med. *307*:410–412, 1982.
71. Martino, E., Safran, N., et al.: Environmental iodine intake and thyroid dysfunction during chronic amiodarone therapy. Ann. Intern. Med. *101*:28–34, 1984.
72. Mazzaferri, E.L., Young, R.L., et al.: Papillary thyroid carcinoma: The impact of therapy on 576 patients. Medicine *56*:171–196, 1977.
73. McGuire, R.A., and Hays, M.T.: A kinetic model of human thyroid hormones and their conversion products. J. Clin. Endocrinol. Metab. *53*:852–862, 1981.
74. Mehta, P.S., Mehta, S.J., and Vorherr, H.: Congenital iodide goiter and hypothyroidism: A review. Obst. Gynecol. Survey *38*:237–247, 1983.
75. Mihailovic, V., Feller, M.S., et al.: Hyperthyroidism due to excess thyrotropin secretion: follow-up studies. J. Clin. Endocrinol. Metab. *50*:1135–1138, 1980.
76. Millikan, J.S., Murr, P., et al.: A familial pattern of thyroglossal duct cysts. J.A.M.A. *244*:1714, 1980.
77. Miyai, K., Azukizawa, M., and Kumahara, Y.: Familial isolated thyrotropin deficiency with cretinism. N. Engl. J. Med. *285*:1043–1048, 1971.
78. Miyai, K., Tanizawa, O., et al.: Pituitary thyroid function in trophoblastic disease. J. Clin. Endocrinol. Metab. *42*:254–259, 1976.
79. Morley, J.E., Slag, M.F., et al.: The interpretation of thyroid function tests in hospitalized patients. J.A.M.A. *249*:2377–2379, 1983.
80. Moses, A.C., Lawlor, J., et al.: Familial euthyroid hyperthyroxinemia resulting from increased thyroxine binding to thyroxine binding prealbumin. N. Engl. J. Med. *306*:966–969, 1982.
81. Muller, M.J., and Seitz, H.J.: Thyroid hormone action on intermediary metabolism. I. Respiration, thermogenesis and carbohydrate metabolism. Klin. Wochenschr. *62*:11–18, 1984.
82. Muller, M.J., and Seitz, H.J.: Thyroid hormone action on intermediary metabolism. II. Lipid metabolism in hypo- and hyperthyroidism. Klin. Wochenschr. *62*:49–55, 1984.
83. Muller, M.J., and Seitz, H.J.: Thyroid hormone action on intermediary metabolism. III. Protein metabolism in hyper- and hypothyroidism. Klin. Wochenschr. *62*:97–102, 1984.
84. Murata, Y., Takamatsu, J., and Refetoff, S.: Inherited abnormality of thyroxine-binding globulin with no demonstrable thyroxine-binding activity and high serum levels of denatured thyroxine binding globulin. N. Engl. J. Med. *314*:694–699, 1986.
85. Murphy, B.E.P.: In vitro tests of thyroid function. Semin. Nucl. Med. *1*:301–315, 1971.
86. Murphy, B.E.P., and Pattee, C.J.: Determination of thyroxine utilizing the property of protein-binding. J. Clin. Endocrinol. Metab. *24*:187–196, 1964.
87. Nagataki, S., Mizuno, M., et al.: Thyroid function in molar pregnancy. J. Clin. Endocrinol. Metab. *44*:254–263, 1977.
88. Neinas, F.W., Gorman, C.A., et al.: Lingual thyroid. Ann. Intern. Med. *79*:205–210, 1973.
89. Ober, K.P., and Hennessy, J.F.: Jodbasedow and thyrotoxic periodic paralysis. Arch. Intern. Med. *141*:1225–1227, 1981.
90. Odell, W.B., Wilbur, J.F., and Utiger, R.D.: Studies of thyrotropin physiology by means of radioimmunoassay. Rec. Progr. Horm. Res. *23*:47–85, 1967.
91. Oliver, J.W., and Held, J.P.: Thyrotropin stimulation test. J. Am. Vet. Med. Assoc. *187*:931–934, 1985.
92. Oppenheim, A., Miller, M., et al.: Anaplastic thyroid cancer presenting with hyperthyroidism. Am. J. Med. *75*:702–704, 1983.
93. Oppenheimer, J.H.: Thyroid function tests in nonthyroidal disease. J. Chronic Dis. *35*:697–701, 1982.
94. Oppenheimer, J.H.: Thyroid hormone action at the nuclear level. Ann. Intern. Med. *102*:374–384, 1985.
95. Oppenheimer, J.H., and Samuels, H.H.: Molecular Basis of Thyroid Hormone Action. New York, Academic Press, 1983.
96. Pittman, J.A.: Thyrotropin-releasing hormone. Adv. Intern. Med. *19*:303–325, 1974.
97. Pittman, J.A., Haigler, E.D., et al.: Hypothalamic hypothyroidism. N. Engl. J. Med. *285*:844–845, 1971.
98. Refetoff, S., Robin, N.I., and Alper, C.A.: Study of four new kindreds with inherited thyroxine-binding globulin abnormalities. J. Clin. Invest. *51*:848–867, 1972.
99. Ridgway, E.C.: Thyrotropin radioimmunoassays: birth, life and demise. Mayo Clin. Proc. *63*:1028–1034, 1988.
100. Robertson, J.S., Verhasselt, M., and Wahner, H.W.: Use of 123-I thyroid uptakes by incomplete dissolution of capsule filler. J. Nucl. Med. *15*:770–774, 1974.
101. Rosenberg, I.N.: Evaluation of thyroid function. N. Engl. J. Med. *286*:924–927, 1972.
102. Ruiz, M., Rajatanavin, R., et al.: Familial dysalbuminemic hyperthyroxinemia. N. Engl. J. Med. *306*:635–639, 1982.
103. Saito, K., Yamamoto, K., et al.: Goitrous hypothyroidism due to iodide-trapping defect. J. Clin. Endocrinol. Metab. *53*:1267–1272, 1981.
104. Sawin, C.T., Chopra, D., et al.: The aging thyroid. J.A.M.A. *242*:247–250, 1979.
105. Seth, J., and Beckett, G.: Diagnosis of hyperthyroidism: The newer biochemical tests. Clin. Endocrinol. Metab. *14*:373–396, 1985.
106. Shimaoka, K., Vanherle, A.J., and Dindogau, A.: Thyrotoxicosis secondary to involvement of the thyroid gland with malignant lymphoma. J. Clin. Endocrinol. Metab. *43*:64–68, 1976.

107. Smith, C.E., Smallridge, R.C., et al.: Hyperthyroidism due to a thyrotropin secreting pituitary adenoma. Arch. Intern. Med. *142*:1709–1711, 1982.
108. Snyder, P.J., Jacobs, L.S., et al.: Assessment of thyrotrophin and prolactin secretion in 100 patients. Ann. Intern. Med. *81*:751–757, 1974.
109. Spanheimer, R.G., Bar, R.S., and Hayford, J.C.: Hyperthyroidism caused by inappropriate thyrotropin hypersecretion. Arch. Intern. Med. *142*:1283–1286, 1982.
110. Spaulding, S.W., and Lippes, H.: Hyperthyroidism. Med. Clin. North Amer. *69*:937–951, 1985.
111. Sterling, K.: Thyroid hormone action at the cell level. N. Engl. J. Med. *300*:117–123; 173–177, 1979.
112. Sterling, K., and Hegedus, A.: Measurement of free thyroxine concentration in human serum. J. Clin. Invest. *41*:1031–1040, 1962.
113. Stockigt, J.R., Topliss, D.J., et al.: Familial euthyroid thyroxine excess: An appropriate response to abnormal thyroxine binding associated with albumin. J. Clin. Endocrinol. Metab. *53*:353–359, 1981.
114. Studer, H., Peter, H.J., and Gerber, H.: Toxic nodular goitre. Clin. Endocrinol. Metab. *14*:351–372, 1985.
115. Taylor, H.C., and Sheeler, L.R.: Recurrence and heterogeneity in painless thyrotoxic lymphocytic thyroiditis. J.A.M.A. *248*:1085–1088, 1982.
116. Tibaldi, J.M., and Surks, M.I.: Effects of nonthyroidal illness on thyroid function. Med. Clin. North Amer. *69*:899–911, 1985.
117. Trokoudes, K.M., Rosen, I.B., et al.: Carcinomatous pseudothyroiditis. Canad. Med. Assoc. J. *119*:896–898, 1978.
118. Tseng, Y.-C., Burman, K.D., et al.: A rapid, sensitive enzyme-linked immunoassay for human thyrotropin. Clin. Chem. *31*:1131–1134, 1985.
119. Tunbridge, W.M.G., Evered, D.C., et al.: The spectrum of thyroid disease in a community. Clin. Endocrinol. *7*:481–493, 1977.
120. Vagenakis, A.G., and Braverman, L.E.: Adverse effects of iodides on thyroid function. Med. Clin. North Amer. *59*:1075–1088, 1975.
121. Vidor, G.I., Stewart, J.C., et al.: Pathogenesis of iodine-induced thyrotoxicosis. J. Clin. Endocrinol. Metab. *37*:901–909, 1973.
122. Viscardi, R.M., Shea, M., et al.: Hyperthyroxinemia in newborns due to excess thyroxine-binding globulin. N. Engl. J. Med. *309*:897–899, 1983.
123. Volpe, R.: The role of autoimmunity in hypoendocrine and hyperendocrine function. Ann. Intern. Med. *87*:86–99, 1977.
124. Volpe, R.: Diagnosis of thyroid diseases. Canad. Med. Assoc. J. *110*:1001–1002, 1974.
125. Watanakunakorn, C., Hodges, R.E., and Evans, T.C.: Myxedema. Arch. Intern. Med. *116*:183–190, 1965.
126. Wilber, J.F.: Thyrotropin releasing hormone: secretion and actions. Ann. Rev. Med. *24*:353–364, 1973.
127. Wilke, T.J.: Estimation of free thyroid hormone concentrations in the clinical laboratory. Clin. Chem. *32*:585–592, 1986.
128. Wong, E.T., and Steffes, M.W.: A fundamental approach to the diagnosis of diseases of the thyroid gland. Clin. Lab. Med. *4*:655–670, 1984.
129. Wortsman, J., Premachandra, B.N., et al.: Familial resistance to thyroid hormone associated with decreased transport across the plasma membrane. Ann. Intern. Med. *98*:904–909, 1983.
130. Young, R.A., Stoffer, S.S., and Braverman, L.E.: Familial dysalbuminemic hyperthyroxinemia associated with primary thyroid disease. Am. J. Med. *82*:221–223, 1987.

ACUTE INFLAMMATION IN THE THYROID

3

Acute inflammatory reactions in the thyroid gland can be conveniently divided into those associated with infection, trauma, radiation, or tumor necrosis. In this chapter, acute infectious thyroiditis is discussed; inflammation associated with trauma and radiation is briefly mentioned; tumor necrosis is considered in greater detail in the individual chapters on neoplasms.

ACUTE THYROIDITIS

Introduction

Acute inflammation of the thyroid gland is defined as that process in which there is an inflammatory reaction dominated by the presence of polymorphonuclear leukocytes. Focal areas of necrosis frequently accompany the reaction. Most of the diseases characterized by this histologic picture are linked to primary infection of the thyroid itself.[7] The terms acute infectious thyroiditis and acute suppurative thyroiditis are therefore often applied to describe this group of disorders.

The incidence of acute thyroiditis is difficult to determine since the terminology has been confused in the literature. Some authors have included cases of subacute thyroiditis in series describing the acute form.[59] In many cases, microbiological data are missing or incomplete. Hence, etiologic, epidemiologic, and prognostic data are hard to evaluate from many reported series.[23]

Acute infectious thyroiditis is a rare but often severe disease, tending to occur in young malnourished children, elderly debilitated adults, or immunocompromised individuals.[23, 26] Most cases are associated with an infection elsewhere in the patient (e.g., pharyngitis, tonsillitis) or with generalized sepsis.[7, 23, 26, 46, 71] Acute thyroiditis may follow major cervical trauma when an open wound may provide a portal of entry for microorganisms.[8, 23]

Clinical Features

Clinically, affected patients present with fever, chills, malaise, and a painful swollen neck. The pain, which may be referred to the ear or the jaw, may be accentuated by moving the neck. Hoarseness, dyspnea, or dysphagia may occur.[3, 7, 23, 26] Usually the thyroid is diffusely enlarged, although in some cases swelling of one lobe will predominate.[4, 7, 23, 36, 71] On physical examination, the thyroid may feel hot and fluctuant. Abscess formation may occur;[22, 41] this is more common if the infection takes place in a nodular gland.[7] Thyroid function tests are usually normal, although mild degrees of hyper- or even hypothyroidism during the course of the illness have been described.[23, 26, 71]

Pathologic Findings and Microbiology

Grossly, the thyroid in acute infectious thyroiditis may appear normal or may be focally or diffusely softened. Occasionally, purulent foci will be noted. Microscopically, the changes are those of acute inflammation including microabscess formation, necrosis, vascular damage, and sometimes the presence of bacteria (Figs. 3–1, 3–2). In the increasingly common situation, with the increase in organ transplantation and with the advent of aggressive systemic chemotherapy of neoplastic disease, fungal organisms are identified in the thyroid tissue. Although one might expect the presence of granulomatous inflammation in the latter situation (and, indeed, this is occasionally found; see Chapter 4), in the author's experience, more often fungal thyroiditis has been associated with an acute purulent reaction (Figs. 3–3 to 3–6).

The acute inflammatory reaction may be explained in most instances by the fact that individuals susceptible to fungal thyroiditis are those who are immunocompromised. In some cases, the inflammatory response is meager or absent and only

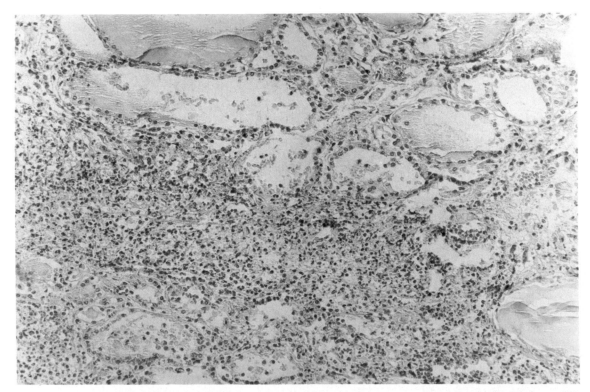

Figure 3–1. Acute thyroiditis—note follicular destruction, acute inflammatory cells, and necrotic debris. × 100, H & E.

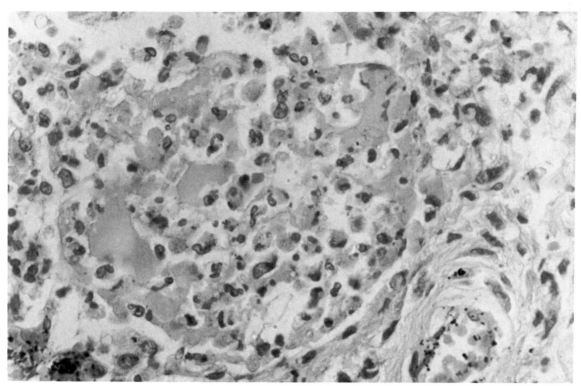

Figure 3–2. Inflammatory cells amid extruded colloid from destroyed follicles. Small black dots in lower right and lower left are clumps of *Staphylococcus aureus* × 250, H & E.

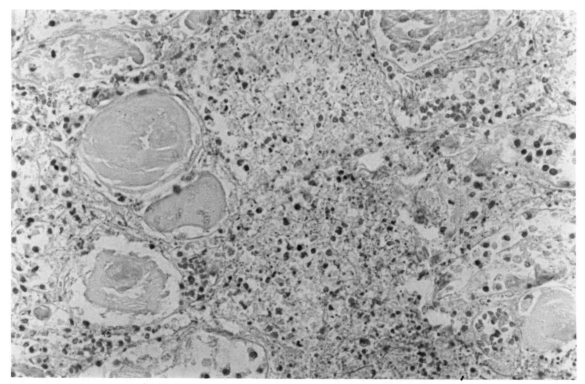

Figure 3–3. Focus of necrosis with leukocytic debris is seen in this thyroid from a 70-year-old woman who died of sepsis following chemotherapy for lymphoma. Note degenerating thyroid follicles on left. × 200, H & E.

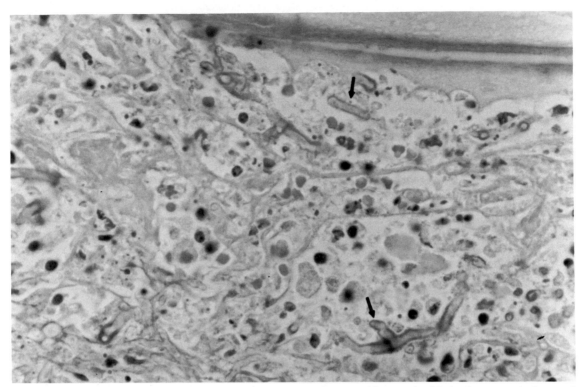

Figure 3–4. Higher power view of gland in Figure 3–3 shows, amid necrotic debris, fragmented elongated organisms (arrows) suggestive of fungus. × 400, H & E.

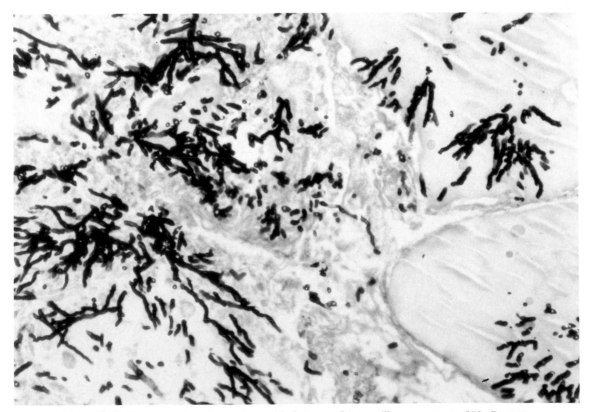

Figure 3–5. Numerous fungal organisms with features of Aspergillus are seen. × 250, Grocott.

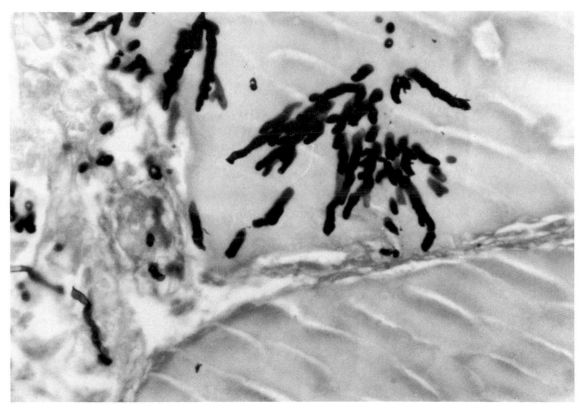

Figure 3–6. Higher power view of Aspergillus in and near colloid. The organisms were numerous in vessel walls also. × 400, Grocott.

abundant organisms are seen. Immunosuppression may result in reduced numbers of macrophages, decreased white blood cell counts, and low or abnormal antibody production.[5, 45, 48] Hence, immunocompromised patients may be incapable of mounting the "expected" inflammatory reaction to fungal infection. In addition, certain organisms, e.g., Aspergillus sp., exhibit a marked propensity to invade blood vessels. The resultant thrombosis and subsequent infarction and tissue necrosis add to the acute inflammatory histologic picture.[45, 72]

A variety of microorganisms may cause acute thyroiditis. Those most frequently identified as causing acute bacterial thyroiditis are Gram-positive cocci such as Staphylococcus, Streptococcus, and Pneumococcus.[7, 19, 23, 26, 66] Gram-negative and mixed infections with aerobes and anaerobes may also occur, especially following direct major trauma to the neck.[1, 2, 4, 7, 9, 14, 24, 26, 47, 53, 55, 65, 68, 69, 71] Walfish et al.[67] reported a case of mixed infection of the thyroid resulting from a carcinomatous esophago-thyroidal fistula. Candida, Aspergillus, Cryptococcus, Actinomyces, Coccidioidomyces, and unusual organisms (e.g., *Pseudoallescheria boydii*) have been reported in immunocompromised hosts.[11, 12, 20, 28, 35, 38, 40, 51, 60] Rare instances of tuberculous, luetic, and parasitic infections of the thyroid have been described.[17, 18, 30, 33, 34, 42, 50, 52, 56, 57] An apparently unique case of thyroid cysticercosis has been reported from Thailand.[36]

Viral infection of the thyroid is considered unusual. Hypothyroidism, and very rarely hyperthyroidism, has been reported in children with congenital rubella syndrome.[6, 10, 21, 44, 49, 54, 73, 74] In one such patient, rubella virus antigen was identified in thyroid tissue, which histologically showed changes of chronic lymphocytic thyroiditis. No virus was isolated by culture, however.[74] Menser et al. suggest that the diabetes seen in congenital rubella syndrome is produced by viral infection of the pancreatic islets.[44] Whether or not abnormal function results from actual viral infection and consequent morphologic changes in the thyroid or other endocrine organs, or whether functional disturbances result from autoimmune responses to viral antigens remains to be determined.[44, 74] Recently, cytomegalovirus infection (CMV) of the thyroid has been documented, especially in patients with acquired immunodeficiency syndrome[15] (Fig. 3–7). In these cases, CMV inclusions are found in nonthyroidal organs, and other infections, especially fungal, are present. In the thyroid, CMV is found in the follicular epithelial and not in endothelial cells. No reaction is present to the inclusions seen.[15]

Some authors have suggested that subacute thyroiditis is caused by a virus;[70] however, proof of this by culture or ultrastructural analysis is still disputed. (See discussion in Chapter 4.)

Pneumocystis carinii thyroiditis has been reported rarely in immunosuppressed patients with overwhelming infection.[16]

Pathogenesis

What is the pathogenesis of thyroid infection? Infection of the thyroid is apparently rare, despite the rich vascular and lymphatic network of the gland. Abe et al.[1] suggested that the rich iodine content of the thyroid may not provide favorable conditions for growth of organisms. These authors also believe that the thyroid's complete encapsulation may prevent direct extension from infections in nearby cervical structures.[1]

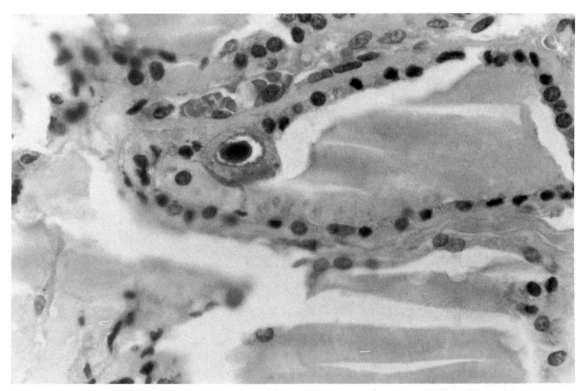

Figure 3–7. Cytomegalovirus inclusion in follicular epithelium occurring in a patient with acquired immune deficiency syndrome (AIDS). Note lack of inflammatory reaction. × 600, H & E.

To produce infectious thyroiditis experimentally, direct intraglandular inoculation with organisms is required.[23] In man, the routes of infection to the thyroid include: (a) hematogenous spread from a distant focus of infection; (b) direct extension from a focus in the head or neck, such as tonsils, pharynx, or infected thyroglossal duct cyst; or (c) direct trauma to the neck, serving as a route of entry for organisms.[7, 23, 24, 46, 64, 66, 67] Takai et al.[61] have described a syndrome of acute suppurative thyroiditis associated with left pyriform sinus fistula. This disorder is characterized clinically by onset in childhood, left lobe involvement, and recurrent thyroiditis. These authors ascribed the thyroiditis to bacterial infection of this sinus, which spreads along a congenital fistulous tract either into the thyroid directly or more commonly into the perithyroidal space, secondarily invading the gland. Occasional cases present in adults.[31] Removal of the fistula results in cure.[46, 61]

Diagnosis, Treatment, Outcome

The diagnosis and therapy of acute infectious thyroiditis depend upon the demonstration of the offending organisms and the institution of appropriate antimicrobial and/or antifungal therapy. Needle biopsy of the thyroid can yield material for bacteriologic studies.[32]

Many patients with bacterial thyroiditis recover: thyroid function usually returns to normal. Rare cases of recurrence have been reported.[2, 63] If suppuration and abscess formation occur, surgical drainage may be required.[7, 26, 62] In the preantibiotic era, such complications were associated with a guarded prognosis and a 25 percent mortality rate. Mortality from bacterial thyroiditis is very rare in modern times.[7, 23, 26, 66]

Fungal thyroiditis is often an incidental autopsy finding in patients dying of systemic fungemia. In those cases in which it is diagnosed in life, the fungal thyroiditis is frequently associated with infection in other organs. Systemic antifungal therapy may be successful in eradicating the infection.[20, 35, 38, 51]

TRAUMATIC THYROIDITIS

Direct severe trauma to the neck, such as bullet wounds, or severe blows with soft tissue and skin disruption, can serve as a source of bacterial infection of the thyroid.[7, 8, 23]

Trauma to the gland of a milder nature, i.e., palpation, produces a peculiar granulomatous reaction (described in Chapter 4).

Currently, the surgical pathologist is not infrequently faced with evaluation of a thyroid specimen removed after less severe trauma of an iatrogenic nature: aspiration or needle biopsy. Depending upon the strength and enthusiasm of the person performing the biopsy, varying degrees of hemorrhage, inflammation, and vascular and fibroblastic proliferation may be seen. In some cases, actual necrosis of thyroid tissue (nodule or portion thereof) may occur with associated acute inflammation.[27] In such cases, the diagnosis of the inflammatory lesion is not difficult, especially if the history is supportive; in the author's experience, definition of the original underlying lesion may occasionally be difficult or even impossible.

RADIATION-ASSOCIATED THYROIDITIS

Experimental studies describing the acute pathologic reaction of the thyroid to radiation have been reported.[25, 39, 43] Acute changes occurring in the first few weeks after therapy include follicular disruption, epithelial "desquamation," hyperemia, vascular stasis, neutrophilic infiltration, cellular necrosis, and edema; subsequently, vascular damage with thrombosis, hemorrhage, and further gland destruction take place.[39, 43] Holten recently reported the effects of external radiation (therapeutic doses for head and neck cancer) in humans.[25] In this controlled study, patients were evaluated by thyroid function tests and aspiration cytology. Acutely, i.e., within two days to two months after fractionated doses of radiation were delivered to the thyroid, functional changes were noted. These included decreases in radioiodine uptake and serum thyroxine levels; low levels of antithyroid antibodies were found in 4 to 27 percent of patients. Aspiration cytology samples showed vacuolated follicular cells, and large numbers of macrophages. However, no significant differences between controls and radiated glands could be identified. Acutely, external radiation produces little if any morphologic change in the thyroid even though mild functional abnormalities can be detected.[25]

Droese et al.[13] studied seven patients treated with [131]-iodine. In needle aspiration cytology samples, cytoplasmic vacuolization and minimal degenerative cellular changes were identified in only three cases. The mild changes seen do not necessarily occur uniformly in the gland and are not seen in all patients treated with radiation. Differences may result from variations in radiation dose, type of radiation (external source or radioiodine), nodularity of the gland, gland size, and poorly understood host response factors.[37, 58]

Changes that occur months to years after large doses of external radiation or therapeutic radioiodine include a grossly small and fibrotic gland, often associated with hypothyroidism.[29, 37] (See Chapter 6.)

REFERENCES

1. Abe, K., Taguchi, T., et al.: Acute suppurative thyroiditis in children. J. Pediatr. *94*:912–914, 1979.
2. Abe, K., Taguchi, T., et al.: Recurrent acute suppurative thyroiditis. Am. J. Dis. Child. *132*:990–991, 1978.
3. Adler, M.E., Jordan, G., and Walter, R.M.: Acute suppurative thyroiditis. West. J. Med. *128*:165–168, 1978.
4. Alsever, R.N., Stiver, H.G., et al.: Hemophilus influenza pericarditis and empyema with thyroiditis in an adult. J.A.M.A. *230*:1426–1427, 1974.
5. Armstrong, D., Young, L.S., et al.: Infectious complications of neoplastic disease. Med. Clin. North Amer. *55*:729–745, 1971.
6. AvRuskin, T.W., Brakin, M., and Juan, C.: Congenital rubella and myxedema. Pediatrics *69*:495–496, 1982.
7. Berger, S.A., Zonszein, J., et al.: Infectious diseases of the thyroid gland. Rev. Infect. Dis. *5*:108–122, 1983.
8. Bishop, H.M., and Durman, D.C.: Traumatic rupture of the thyroid gland. Am. J. Surg. *75*:524–525, 1948.
9. Bussman, Y.C., Wong, M.C., et al.: Suppurative thyroiditis with gas formation due to mixed anaerobic infection. J. Pediatr. *90*:321–322, 1977.
10. Comas, A.P., and Betances, R.E.: Congenital rubella and acquired hypothyroidism secondary to Hashimoto thyroiditis. J. Pediatr. *88*:1065–1066, 1976.
11. Dan, M., Garcia, A., and von Westrap, C.: Primary actinomycosis of the thyroid mimicking carcinoma. J. Otolaryngol. *13*:109–112, 1984.
12. DeMent, S.H., Smith, R.R.L., et al.: Pulmonary, cardiac and thyroid involvement in disseminated *Pseudoallescheria boydii*. Arch. Pathol. Lab. Med. *108*:859–861, 1984.
13. Droese, M., Kempken, K., et al.: Cytologic changes in aspiration biopsy smears from various conditions of the thyroid treated with radioiodine. Verh. Dtsch. Ges. Pathol. *57*:336–338, 1973.
14. Elias, A.N., Kyaw, T., et al.: Acute suppurative thyroiditis. J. Otolaryngol. *14*:17–19, 1985.
15. Frank, T.S., LiVolsi, V.A., and Connor, A.M.: Cytomegalovirus infection of the thyroid in immunocompromised adults. Yale J. Biol. Med. *60*:1–8, 1987.
16. Gallant, J.E., Enriquez, R.E., et al.: Pneumocystis carinii thyroiditis. Am. J. Med. *84*:303–306, 1988.

17. Goldfarb, H., Schifrin, D., and Graig, F.A.: Thyroiditis caused by tuberculous abscess of the thyroid gland. Am. J. Med. *38:*825–828, 1965.
18. Gutman, L.T., Handwerger, S., et al.: Thyroiditis due to *Mycobacterium chelonei.* Am. Rev. Respir. Dis. *110:*807–809, 1974.
19. Hagan, A.D., Goffinet, J., and Davis, J.W.: Acute streptococcal thyroiditis. J. A. M. A. *202:*842–843, 1967.
20. Halazun, J.F., Anast, C.S., and Lukens, J.N.: Thyrotoxicosis associated with *Aspergillus thyroiditis* in chronic granulomatous disease. J. Pediatr. *80:*106–108, 1972.
21. Hanid, T.K.: Hypothyroidism in congenital rubella. Lancet *2:*854, 1976.
22. Hawbaker, E.L.: Thyroid abscess. Am. Surg. *37:*290–292, 1971.
23. Hazard, J.B.: Thyroiditis: a review. Am. J. Clin. Pathol. *15:*289–298, 1955.
24. Himsworth, R.L., and Kark, A.E.: Studies on a case of suppurative thyroiditis. Acta Endocrinol. *85:*55–63, 1977.
25. Holten, I.: Acute response of the thyroid to external radiation. Acta Pathol. Microbiol. Scand. *91*(Suppl. 283):9–111, 1983.
26. Hurley, J.R.: Thyroiditis. Disease-A-Month, December, 1977.
27. Jones, J.D., Pittman, D.L., and Sanders, L.R.: Necrosis of thyroid nodules after fine needle aspiration. Acta Cytol. *29:*29–32, 1985.
28. Kakuda, K., Kanokogi, M., et al.: Acute mycotic thyroiditis. Acta Pathol. Jpn. *33:*147–151, 1983.
29. Kennedy, J.S., and Thompson, J.A.: The changes in the thyroid gland after irradiation with I-131 or partial thyroidectomy for thyrotoxicosis. J. Pathol. *112:*65–72, 1974.
30. Klassen, K.P., and Curtis, G.M.: Tuberculous abscess of the thyroid gland. Surgery *17:*552–559, 1945.
31. Kodama, T., Ito, Y., et al.: Acute suppurative thyroiditis in appearance of unusual neck mass. Endocrinol. Jpn. *34:*427–430, 1987.
32. Kohler, P.O., Floyd, W.L., and Wynn, J.: Indications for thyroid needle biopsy: suppurative thyroiditis. South. Med. J. *59:*182–184, 1966.
33. Laird, S.M.: Gumma of the thyroid gland. Br. J. Vener. Dis. *21:*162–165, 1945.
34. Laohapand, T., Ratanarapee, S., et al.: Tuberculous thyroiditis. J. Med. Assoc. Thai. *64:*256–260, 1981.
35. Leers, W.D., Dussault, J., et al.: Suppurative thyroiditis: an unusual case caused by *Actinomyces naeslundii.* Can. Med. Assoc. J. *101:*714–717, 1969.
36. Leelachaikul, P., and Chuahirun, S.: Cysticercosis of the thyroid gland in severe cerebral cysticercosis: Report of a case. J. Med. Assoc. Thai. *60:*405–410, 1977.
37. Lindsay, S., Dailey, M.E., and Jones, M.E.: Histologic effects of various types of ionizing radiation on normal and hyperplastic human thyroid glands. J. Clin. Endocrinol. Metab. *14:*1179–1193, 1954.
38. Loeb, J.M., Livermore, B.M., and Wofsy, D.: Coccidioidomycosis of the thyroid. Ann. Intern. Med. *91:*409–411, 1979.
39. Lu, S.T., Michaelson, S.M., and Quinlan, W.J.: Sequential pathophysiologic effects of ionizing radiation on the Beagle thyroid gland. J. Natl. Cancer Inst. *51:*419–441, 1973.
40. Machac, J., Nejatheim, M., and Goldsmith, S.J.: Gallium-67 citrate uptake in cryptococcal thyroiditis in a homosexual male. J. Nucl. Med. All. Sci. *29:*283–285, 1985.
41. Mann, C.H.: Thyroid abscess in a 3-1/2 year old child. Arch. Otolaryngol. *103:*299–300, 1977.
42. Markowicz, H., and Shanon, E.: Tuberculosis of the thyroid gland. Ann. Otol. Rhinol. Laryngol. *67:*223–226, 1958.
43. McClellan, R.O., Clarke, W.J., et al.: Comparative effects of I-131 and X-irradiation on sheep thyroids. Health Physics *9:*1363–1368, 1963.
44. Menser, M.A., Forrest, J.M., and Bransby, R.D.: Rubella infection and diabetes mellitus. Lancet *1:*57–60, 1978.
45. Meyer, R.D., Young, L.S., et al.: Aspergillosis complicating neoplastic disease. Am. J. Med. *54:*6–15, 1973.
46. Miyauchi, A., Matsuzuka, F., et al.: Piriform sinus fistula: a route of infection in acute suppurative thyroiditis. Arch. Surg. *116:*66–69, 1981.
47. Negi, S.C., Gupta, M.K., et al.: A case of Salmonella thyroiditis. Indian J. Pathol. Microbiol. *17:*295–298, 1984.
48. Neu, H.C.: The role of cellular and humoral factors in infections. Clin. Hematol. *5:*449–465, 1976.
49. Nieburg, P.I., and Gardner, L.I.: Thyroiditis and congenital rubella syndrome. J. Pediatr. *89:*156, 1976.
50. Olin, R., LeBien, W.E., and Leigh, J.E.: Acute suppurative thyroiditis. Report of two cases including one caused by *Mycobacterium intracellulare.* Minn. Med. *56:*586–588, 1973.
51. Robinson, M.F., Forgan-Smith, W.R., and Craswell, P.W.: *Candida* thyroiditis treated with 5-fluorocytosine. Aust. N. Z. J. Med. *5:*472–474, 1975.
52. Sachs, M.K., Dickinson, G., and Amazon, K.: Tuberculous adenitis of the thyroid mimicking subacute thyroiditis. Am. J. Med. Sci. *85:*573–575, 1988.
53. Saksouk, F., and Salti, I.S.: Acute suppurative thyroiditis caused by *Escherichia coli.* Br. Med. J. *2:*23–24, 1977.

54. Salisbury, S., and Embil, J.A.: Graves' disease following congenital cytomegalovirus infection. J. Pediatr. *92*:954–955, 1978.

55. Sharma, R.K., and Rapkin, R.H.: Acute suppurative thyroiditis caused by *Bacteroides melaninogenicus.* J.A.M.A. *119*:1470, 1974.

56. Shaw, H.M.: A case of hydatid disease of the thyroid gland. Med. J. Aust. N. Z. *2*:413–415, 1946.

57. Skalkeas, G.D., and Sechas, M.N.: Echinococcosis of the thyroid gland. J.A.M.A. *200*:188–189, 1967.

58. Straus, F.H., and Spitalnik, P.F.: Histologic parenchymal changes in the human thyroid after low dose childhood irradiation. *In:* DeGroot, L.G. (ed.): Radiation Associated Thyroid Carcinoma. New York, Grune & Stratton, 1977, p. 183.

59. Swann, N.H.: Acute thyroiditis. Five cases associated with adenovirus infection. Metabolism *13*:908–910, 1964.

60. Szporn, A.H., Tepper, S., and Watson, C.W.: Disseminated cryptococcosis presenting as thyroiditis. Acta Cytol. *29*:449–453, 1985.

61. Takai, S.I.K., Miyauchi, A., et al.: Internal fistula as a route of infection in acute suppurative thyroiditis. Lancet *1*:751–752, 1979.

62. Thomas, C.G.: Acute Suppurative Thyroiditis: Surgical Treatment. *In:* Werner, S.C., and Ingbar, S.H. (eds.): The Thyroid. New York, Harper and Row, 1971, p. 852.

63. Tovi, F., Gatot, A., et al.: Recurrent suppurative thyroiditis due to fourth branchial pouch sinus. Int. J. Pediat. Otorhinolaryngol. *9*:89–96, 1985.

64. Tucker, H.M., and Skolnick, M.L.: Fourth branchial cleft (pharyngeal pouch) remnant. Trans. Am. Acad. Ophthalmol. Otol. 77:368–371, 1973.

65. Van Heerden, J.A., and O'Connell, P.: Acute suppurative thyroiditis due to *Salmonella enteritidis.* Va. Med. Mon. *98*:556–557, 1971.

66. Volpe, R.: Acute suppurative thyroiditis. *In:* Werner, S.C., and Ingbar, S.H. (eds.): The Thyroid. New York, Harper and Row, 1971, p. 849.

67. Walfish, P.G., Chan, H.Y.C., et al.: Esophageal carcinoma masquerading as recurrent acute suppurative thyroiditis. Arch. Intern. Med. *145*:346–347, 1985.

68. Walter, R.M., and McMonagle, J.R.: *Salmonella* thyroiditis, apathetic thyrotoxicosis and follicular carcinoma in a Laotian woman. Cancer 50:2493–2495, 1982.

69. Weissel, M., Wolf, A., and Linkesch, W.: Acute suppurative thyroiditis caused by *Pseudomonas aeruginosa.* Br. Med. J. *2*:580, 1977.

70. Werner, J., and Gelderblom, H.: Isolation of foamy viruses from patients with de Quervain thyroiditis. Lancet 2:258–259, 1979.

71. Womack, N.A.: Thyroiditis. Surgery *16*:770–782, 1944.

72. Young, R.C., Bennett, J.E., et al.: Aspergillosis: the spectrum of disease in 98 patients. Medicine *49*:147–173, 1970.

73. Ziring, P.R., Fedun, B.A., and Cooper, L.Z.: Thyrotoxicosis in congenital rubella. J. Pediatr. *87*:1002, 1975.

74. Ziring, P.R., Gallo, G., et al.: Chronic lymphocytic thyroiditis: Identification of rubella virus antigen in the thyroid of a child with congenital rubella. J. Pediatr. *90*:419–420, 1977.

4

GRANULOMAS IN THE THYROID

Granulomatous inflammation, including well-formed granulomas, can be seen in the thyroid in several conditions that affect the gland; these are listed in Table 4–1.

GRANULOMATOUS THYROIDITIS

Introduction and Epidemiology

Granulomatous thyroiditis is a disease that has been given a variety of names: pseudotuberculous thyroiditis, giant cell thyroiditis, nonsuppurative thyroiditis, subacute thyroiditis, and deQuervain's thyroiditis. The term subacute thyroiditis is a clinical one, predominantly used by endocrinologists, whereas pathologists prefer the descriptive term granulomatous thyroiditis, emphasizing its characteristic histologic appearance.[3, 15, 30, 32, 49, 55, 91, 92, 94, 107, 108]

The incidence of this disease is not known since it may be confused clinically and pathologically with other types of thyroiditis, and because mild cases may never be diagnosed. It is estimated that classic subacute thyroiditis represents from 0.05 to 3 percent of all thyroid disorders.[37, 49, 79, 83, 91, 92, 94]

Granulomatous thyroiditis, a disease of adults, predominantly women, has a sex ratio of 2:1 to 6:1.[3, 23, 30, 32, 49, 79, 91, 92, 94, 107] The studies of Nyulassy et al.[61] indicate a genetic predisposition to the development of this disease: 70 percent of individuals with subacute thyroiditis had HLA subtype Bw35, whereas this was found in only 9 percent of the control population. These results were confirmed recently by Goto et al.[29] and Benker et al.[5]

Table 4–1. Granulomatous Conditions Affecting the Thyroid

- Granulomatous thyroiditis
- "Palpation" thyroiditis
- Histiocytic reaction near hemorrhage in goiter, tumors, etc.
- Infection (tuberculosis, fungus)
- Sarcoidosis
- Vasculitides
- Foreign body reaction

Etiology

Granulomatous thyroiditis is believed to represent the response of the thyroid to systemic viral infection; some authors suggest that it represents actual viral infection of the gland. Karlsson et al.[42] and Totterman et al.[89] studying lymphocytes from patients' serum and thyroid aspirates, identified greater T-cell concentrations in the thyroid than in the sera of affected patients. These authors suggested that their findings support a viral etiology for granulomatous thyroiditis.[89] Wall et al. tested seven patients with subacute thyroiditis and found evidence of lymphocyte transformation in five individuals when exposed to human thyroid extract.[97] Wall et al. felt that since this abnormality was reversible upon recovery, it was a temporary T-cell defect; this differed from the permanent abnormalities identified in patients with autoimmune thyroid disease, chronic lymphocytic thyroiditis, and Graves' disease.[97] Although mild increases in antithyroid antibody titers may be found in patients with this disease, these abnormalities usually resolve with resolution of the clinical symptoms and are not believed to be causative or pathogenetic agents in it; rather they may represent epiphenomena secondary to thyroid damage.[6, 61, 82, 91–93, 95]

A viral causation for this disorder can be supported by both clinical and epidemiologic studies. Subacute thyroiditis is preceded by an upper respiratory tract infection in 50 to 90 percent of patients. Fever and other systemic manifestations suggest an infectious origin. There is no elevation of white blood cell count, which would be expected in bacterial infection, thus favoring viral etiology. In addition, antibiotics appear to have no effect on the course of the disease. Complete recovery is the rule, even without therapy.[33]

However, the most convincing evidence for viral causation is gleaned from epidemiologic studies that show that specific viruses are associated with "epidemics" of subacute thyroiditis. Eylan et al. isolated mumps virus from the thyroids of 2 of 11 patients with subacute thyroiditis in a mumps epidemic in Israel.[18] Complement fixing antibodies to mumps were identified in most of these patients as well. Greene[30] summarized reports of subacute thyroiditis associated infections with many viruses, including mumps, measles, influenza, Coxsackie, mononucleosis, and adenovirus.[15, 18, 20, 27, 37, 84, 91–93] In further support of the viral etiology theory, Volpe et al. noted elevated complement fixing antibodies to different viruses in 50 percent of 72 patients with subacute thyroiditis.[93] The viruses implicated in this study were influenza, Coxsackie, adenovirus and mumps.

In 1976, Stancekova et al. isolated a previously unknown virus in the serum, urine and thyroid of 5 of 28 individuals with subacute thyroiditis.[78] The cytopathic agent, termed MGI virus, when grown in rat lung cultures, produced changes identical to those seen in the thyroids of affected individuals. In addition, these patients' sera contained antibodies to this agent as demonstrated by immunofluorescence. By ultrastructural analysis, the organisms appeared as rod-shaped and oval viral forms; Stancekova et al. suggested that the MGI virus belonged to the pilomyxovirus group.[78] Werner and Gelderblom supported the work of the earlier investigators.[102] In tissue culture studies, Werner and Gelderblom noted that viral replication was associated with cytopathic lesions consisting of multinucleated giant cells and extensive cytoplasmic vacuolization. No inclusion bodies were identified. In their electron microscopic studies, the authors found the virus particles either as virions budding from plasma membranes of infected cells or lying extracellularly. The envelope of the virions was studded with prominent surface projections and the envelope was separated from a central core of about 50 nanometers in diameter. Aggregates of the core structure were seen within the cytoplasm of some of the infected cells.[102]

Several recent studies have shown no morphologic effects of viral infection in mouse thyroids;[44, 77] these interesting animal data suggest viral infection may alter the cell immunologically, perhaps inciting or initiating autoimmune disease but not evoking the granulomatous response of subacute thyroiditis. Hence, actual viral infection of the thyroid may not be present in the latter disease.

Clinical Features

Clinically, subacute thyroiditis is considered a systemic illness, with milder cases showing minimal symptoms whereas more severely affected patients show fever, malaise, weakness, elevation of sedimentation rate, and abnormal thyroid function.[21, 33, 39, 46, 47, 86, 92, 94, 101, 111] *Pain*, present in classic cases, may be localized to the neck or the thyroid or referred to the jaw, face, or chest. The course of subacute thyroiditis has been divided into phases: hyperthyroid, hypothyroid, and recovery.[46, 50, 62, 101, 111] Symptoms, laboratory values, and echography reflect the phase of the disease.[8, 33] Thus, in the hyperthyroid phase, thyroid hormone levels may be elevated as stored hormone is extruded from destroyed follicles, but radioiodine uptake is low.[21, 46, 56, 63, 86, 98, 101, 111] Once enough of the gland is destroyed and there is no iodine uptake and no hormone production, a phase of hypothyroidism ensues.[3, 21, 37, 39, 46, 62, 79, 86, 91, 98, 101, 111] During this time, suppressor T-cell elevation is noted;[42] antithyroid antibodies might be identified in the serum.[6, 82, 93, 109] This resolves with recovery.[33]

Recovery after weeks or months is the rule and documented recurrence or progression to permanent hypothyroidism is unusual (<5 percent of cases).[4, 33, 36, 52] An unusual case of subacute thyroiditis progressing to hyperthyroidism or Graves' disease has been reported by Werner.[103] There is no *proven* relationship between subacute thyroiditis and other thyroiditides, however.

Although most investigators believe that there is no autoimmune disorder underlying subacute thyroiditis, Ahmann and Burman cite some unsettling studies in this regard.[1] Some patients recover from the episode of thyroiditis, but continue to manifest long-term immunologic abnormalities. Further studies are needed to evaluate these findings.

Painless subacute thyroiditis has been estimated to constitute as many as 40 percent of all cases of subacute thyroiditis (Table 4–2), although the true incidence of this disease is unknown since patients with painless thyroiditis without goiter or with minimal symptoms do not seek medical attention.[81] One form of painless subacute thyroiditis is seen in patients who present with a dominant mass in one lobe of the thyroid; they will therefore be diagnosed only at surgery or by needle core biopsy.[91, 92] The clinical symptomatology of pain which would be a clue to the diagnosis is absent in these cases. Rotenberg et al. recently described another type of painless subacute thyroiditis that simulated malignancy.[66] In their 13 patients, prolonged fever and weight loss were noted; 10 had slight thyromegaly, but none had painful thyroids or thyrotoxicosis. Elevated sedimentation rates and low radioiodine uptake were characteristic. Needle biopsies performed in 10 of the 13 patients showed classic granulomatous thyroiditis.[7, 66]

Table 4–2. "Painless" Subacute Thyroiditis: Types

1. Dominant mass lesion
2. Systemic illness simulating malignancy
3. Silent thyrotoxic thyroiditis*

*Probably not subacute, but autoimmune disease.

On the other hand, a few cases have been reported in which the clinical signs and symptoms suggested subacute thyroiditis with painful goiter and fever. Biopsy of such glands disclosed malignant tumors, ranging from papillary to anaplastic carcinomas, and even metastatic carcinoma.[65, 100] This clinicopathologic entity has been variously called carcinomatous pseudothyroiditis and malignant pseudothyroiditis.[11, 65, 66, 90]

Painless thyroiditis with hyperthyroidism, which was originally included as a subtype of subacute disease, has many features suggestive of autoimmune disease.[2, 7, 13, 14, 16, 17, 19, 22, 25, 26, 28, 38, 54, 58–60, 74, 75, 76, 85–87, 104–106] This disorder, also described by a plethora of terms (Table 4–3), is characterized by hyperthyroidism, significant titers of antithyroglobulin antibodies, histologic features of lymphocytic infiltration of the gland without granulomas, and absence of goiter, neck pain, or fever. This disorder has been recognized commonly in the postpartum period, can manifest remission and re-exacerbation and may progress to hypothyroidism. (See also Chapter 5.) At least an occasional case of painless thyroiditis may represent subacute disease. Sanders et al. described such a case, which appears well documented.[69]

By contrast, Zimmerman et al. have reported painful goiters in patients with laboratory and histologic evidence of chronic lymphocytic thyroiditis.[112] The cause of pain is unknown but *painful* chronic lymphocytic thyroiditis represents another clinicopathologic entity and yet another permutation in the ever-growing and confusing list of thyroiditides. Until causes and hence biologic relationships are defined, the literature on the thyroiditides will remain largely descriptive and empirical.

Pathology

The pathologic picture of subacute thyroiditis is characterized by asymmetrical or uneven involvement of the gland. The gland is firm, but not rock-hard. On cut section, an irregular white-tan lesion or several small poorly demarcated nodules are noted; the white nodules range from several millimeters to a few centimeters in size, may appear tumor-like and simulate carcinoma.[3, 32, 49, 55, 94, 107, 108]

Microscopically (Figs. 4–1 to 4–6), the picture varies with the phase of the disease. Initially, there is alteration of the follicular epithelium with "desquamation" and degeneration followed by colloid depletion. At this point, apparent leakage of stored hormone and thyroglobulin occur, with these gaining access to the circulation. (Elevation of thyroid hormone levels in blood and possible clinical hyperthyroidism can be seen; antithyroglobulin antibodies can be identified in some patients.) An inflammatory response follows and is composed initially of polymorphonuclear leukocytes; the presence of microabscesses may be noted in about half the cases.[3, 32, 49, 55, 94, 107]

Table 4–3. Painless Thyroiditis with Hyperthyroidism: Synonyms*

1. Silent thyrotoxic thyroiditis
2. Lymphocytic thyroiditis with spontaneously resolving hyperthyroidism
3. Silent thyroiditis
4. Transient painless thyroiditis with hyperthyroidism
5. Postpartum thyroiditis
6. Subacute autoimmune thyroiditis
7. Hyperthyroiditis
8. Silent subacute thyroiditis
9. Atypical subacute thyroiditis

*Since virtually every author who writes about this entity varies the name a bit, this list should not be considered all-inclusive.

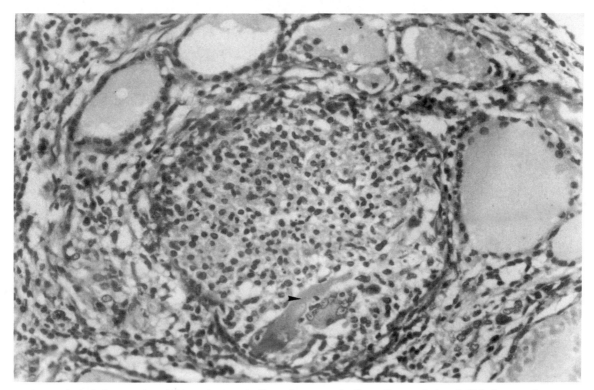

Figure 4–1. Subacute thyroiditis, microscopically early stage. Outline of pre-existing follicle is seen in center. Arrowhead shows tiny amount of residual colloid abutting upon multinucleated giant cell. Most of the expanded follicular area is occupied by lymphocytes and histiocytes, with a few polymorphonuclear leukocytes intermixed. Inflammatory cells "spill out" into surrounding relatively intact follicles. × 200, H & E.

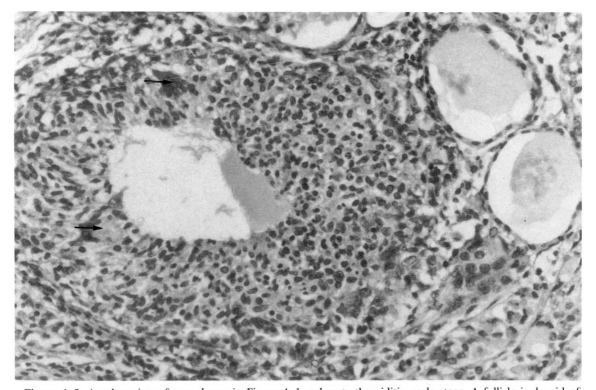

Figure 4–2. Another view of case shown in Figure 4–1: subacute thyroiditis, early stage. A follicle is devoid of epithelium and a residual wisp of colloid is encircled by spindled histiocytes, lymphocytes, and focally polymorphonuclear leukocytes. Note also occasional giant cells in the infiltrate *(arrows)*. Note also inflammation extending to neighboring follicles (especially on right of photograph). × 200, H & E.

51

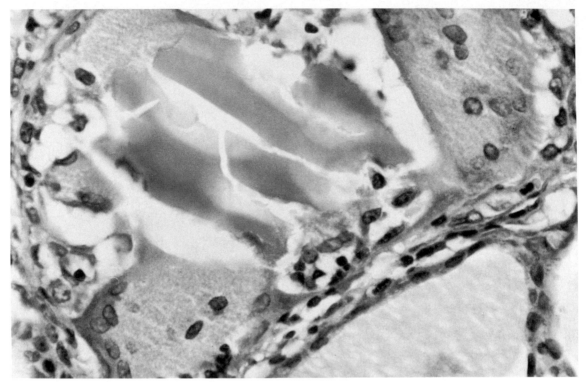

Figure 4–3. In this example of subacute thyroiditis, colloid is fractured in the affected follicle, and epithelial cells have disappeared and are replaced by macrophagic giant cells. × 500, H & E.

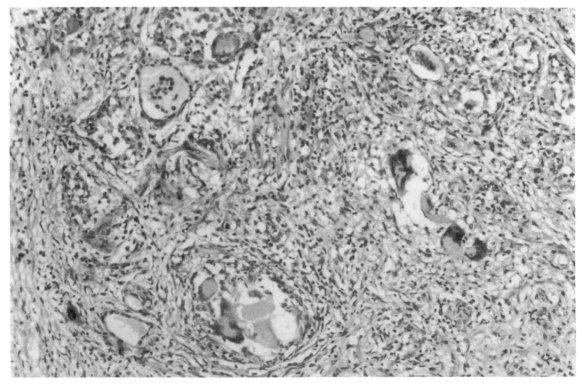

Figure 4–4. Low-power view shows panorama of fully developed, classic subacute thyroiditis. Scattered identifiable follicles can be seen (left side of photograph), and numerous multinucleated giant cells are present. The histiocytic and lymphoplasmacytic inflammatory reaction encircles dying follicles and "granulomas." Increase in interstitial connective tissue is also seen. × 100, H & E.

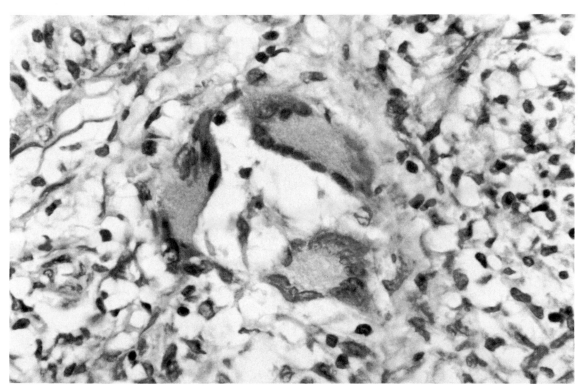

Figure 4–5. Subacute thyroiditis. Three multinucleated giant cells occupy remains of a dead follicle. Inflammatory cells surround this "granuloma." Neither colloid nor epithelium can be identified; it is difficult from this picture to define this tissue as thyroid. × 400, H & E.

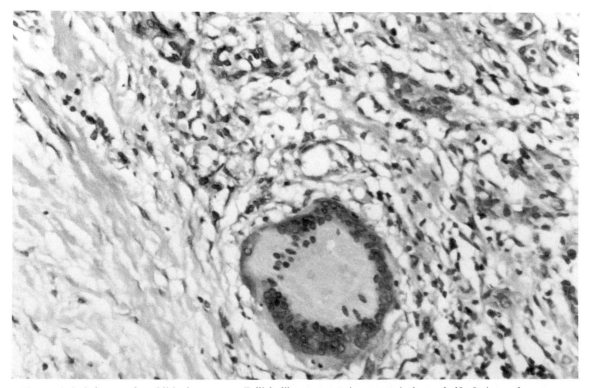

Figure 4–6. Subacute thyroiditis, later stage. Follicle-like structure is present in lower half of picture but appears replaced by a huge giant cell with myriads of nuclei. Surrounding lymphohistiocytic reaction contains increased fibrous tissue. × 300, H & E.

As the disease progresses, lymphocytes, plasma cells, and histiocytes become the major components of the inflammatory response. The follicular epithelium may disappear and be replaced by a rim of histiocytes and giant cells. Disruption and duplication of follicular basement membrane also occurs.[55] Foreign body giant cells form around remnants of colloid after the follicles have degenerated completely. Periodic acid-Schiff (PAS) stains can demonstrate PAS-positive colloid in these giant cells.

Subsequently and simultaneously, fibrosis occurs, which may be found in interfollicular or interlobular areas. Woolner et al. emphasized the characteristic central fibrotic reaction and follicular destruction found histologically.[107, 108] Finally, regeneration of follicles from the edges of these areas occurs: complete histologic and clinical recovery usually takes place,[3, 32, 49, 94, 107, 108] although focal fibrosis may remain in about 50 percent of cases.[75]

The diagnosis of subacute thyroiditis may be documented by core needle biopsy or cytology.[66, 69] (See also Chapter 18.) It must be remembered that lymphocytes make up a part of subacute thyroiditis, and their presence alone should not lead to a diagnosis of chronic lymphocytic thyroiditis; it must similarly be recalled that occasional giant cells may be noted in chronic lymphocytic thyroiditis and their presence alone should not lead to a diagnosis of subacute disease.[45, 55]

The origin of the giant cell in subacute thyroiditis has produced much speculation in the literature. Virtually every investigator agrees that many (if not all) of the giant cells represent macrophages or histiocytes, some of which have coalesced. Thus, they resemble the epithelioid histiocytes found in tuberculous and fungal granulomas.[3, 49, 55, 57, 94, 107, 108] These cells can phagocytize PAS-positive colloid material, further suggesting their histiocytic origin;[49] ultrastructurally and immunohistochemically they appear to be nonepithelial in nature.[3, 55, 57, 64] Some authors, however, consider some of the giant cells to represent altered follicular epithelial cells that are displaying the cytopathic effect of viral infection.[72, 73, 78] In support of this theory, these authors cite ultrastructural studies showing epithelial characteristics to some of the cells. In addition, their electron microscopic studies show viral particles in the cytoplasm of some of the cells in question. Whether or not the giant cells can represent either histiocytes or altered follicular cells remains unclear, although the body of evidence strongly supports the former.[57]

PALPATION THYROIDITIS (MULTIFOCAL GRANULOMATOUS FOLLICULITIS)

Palpation thyroiditis represents a histologic finding rather than a true lesion of the thyroid. Found in most surgically resected thyroids (85 to 95 percent), this entity probably represents the thyroid's final common pathway of response to minor trauma.

The term coined by Carney et al., who first described this entity, is "multifocal granulomatous folliculitis."[12] This phrase aptly encompasses the histologic features of this "lesion": (Figs. 4–7 to 4–12)

- multiple isolated follicles or small groups of follicles (three to five, rarely more) are involved;
- the follicles involved show partial or circumferential loss of epithelium;
- replacement of the lost epithelium by inflammatory cells, predominantly macrophages, but also lymphocytes and plasma cells. The dominance of the histiocyte in the inflammatory response gives a granulomatous character to the "lesion."

- Hemorrhage or iron deposition may be found occasionally; rarely, necrosis is seen. The changes may occur in a follicle, near a follicle, or in a perifollicular location.

What evidence exists for this entity's being related to or caused by trauma? From both clinical (Table 4–4) and experimental data, the evidence is abundant. Studies of clinical material disclose that palpation thyroiditis can be found in 85 to 95 percent of surgically resected thyroids. Most of these are found in glands or lobes removed for nodules. By comparison, only about 10 to 40 percent of glands from autopsies of patients dying in hospital contain palpation thyroiditis. In addition, it is virtually never found in autopsies of patients who died at home or in forensic autopsies.

These facts led the original authors, Carney et al.,[12] and others to conclude that the only major difference among these groups of patients was the greater likelihood of the in-hospital and surgical patients to have had neck examinations when compared with outpatients or "non-patients." Such neck examinations would include palpation of the thyroid; patients who were scheduled to have thyroid surgery would also be more likely to undergo more vigorous and perhaps more numerous thyroid examinations. Recently, Blum and Schloss described "martial arts thyroiditis," which resulted from trauma to the neck in individuals practicing Oriental defense techniques.[9] It probably reflects an exaggerated form of palpation thyroiditis.

These clinical observations were confirmed by experimental work performed by Carney et al.[12] Using dog thyroids, the authors vigorously palpated one lobe only, leaving the unpalpated lobe to serve as control. The experiments disclosed that only the palpated lobes contained the "lesion" and, furthermore, that the

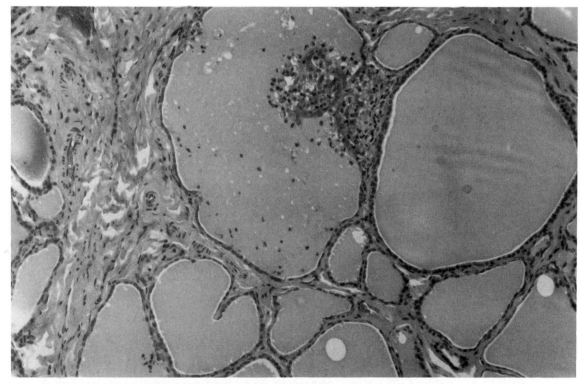

Figure 4–7. Palpation thyroiditis. Partial involvement of follicle with histiocytes, lymphocytes, and plasma cells, and a few follicular epithelial cells, disrupting orderly anatomy of this follicle. × 100, H & E.

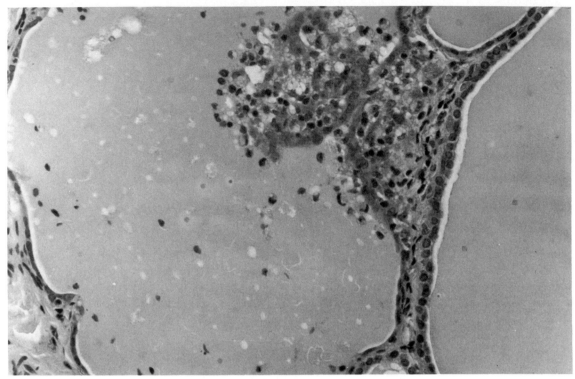

Figure 4–8. Higher power view of Figure 4–7—some histiocytes appear vacuolated and a few inflammatory cells intrude into subjacent stroma. × 300, H & E.

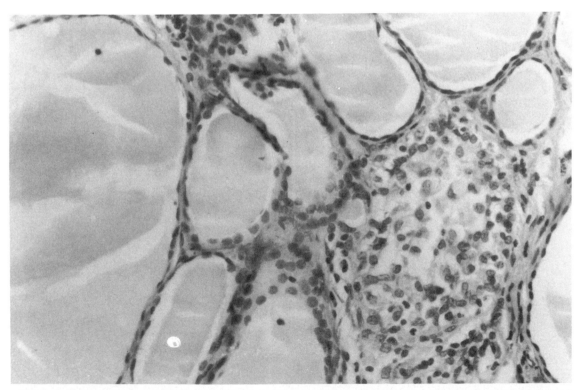

Figure 4–9. Palpation thyroiditis. Isolated follicle (perhaps two) looks different from surrounding normal thyroid. Macrophages with occasional giant cells are seen. Much of the colloid has disappeared; however, a rim of follicular epithelium is noted at edge of most of this follicle. Minimal extension of inflammatory cells is seen in immediately adjacent stroma. × 100, H & E.

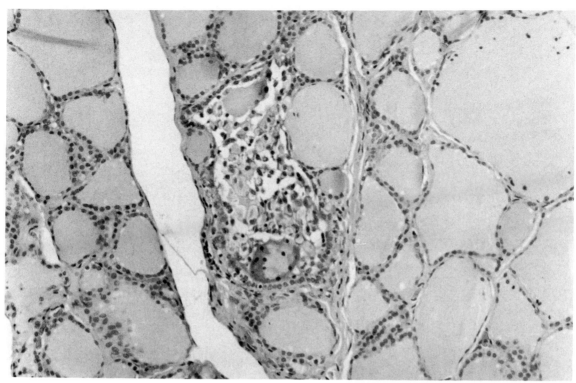

Figure 4–10. Another case of palpation thyroiditis is shown. A follicle is replaced by histiocytes and a few lymphocytes as well. Note lack of extension of inflammation into neighboring follicles. Compare with Figures 4–1 and 4–2. × 200, H & E.

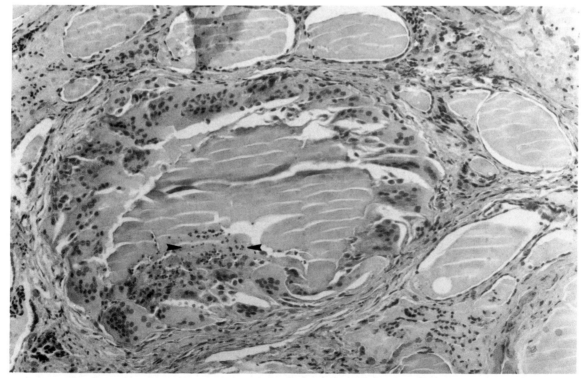

Figure 4–11. An unusual finding in palpation thyroiditis is illustrated here—focal necrosis. This expanded follicle is lined by multinucleated giant cells surrounding residual colloid. At one focus *(arrowheads)*, nuclear dust, polymorphonuclear leukocytes, and necrosis are seen. × 100, H & E.

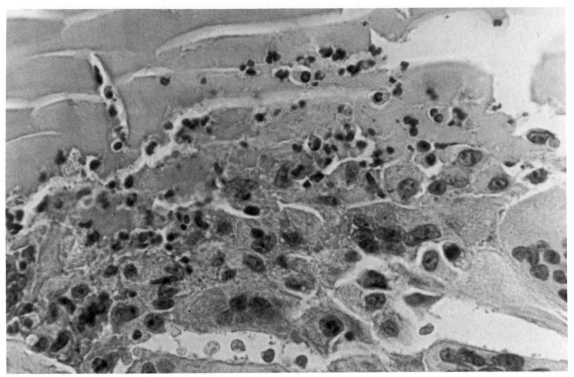

Figure 4–12. Higher power of Figure 4–11 shows area indicated by arrow. Note polymorphonuclear leukocytes and nuclear debris here abutting on colloid. Stains for organisms were negative. This thyroid lobe resulted from completion thyroidectomy performed for papillary carcinoma in opposite lobe, which had been removed one week before. No tumor was identified in this side. Other foci of more typical palpation thyroiditis without necrosis were seen, however. × 400, H & E.

number of foci correlated directly with the vigor of the "palpation." These experiments eliminated toxins, microbial factors, or other etiologic entities except palpation, since any other etiologic cause which could be proposed should affect both thyroid lobes.

It is believed that these histologic changes spontaneously regress and that no significant clinical sequelae result. Buergi et al. measured serum thyroglobulin levels in 24 patients (12 normals, 12 with goiters) one hour and 24 hours after vigorous palpation of the gland.[10] They found no significant alteration in thyroglobulin level and concluded that palpation of the thyroid has no significant clinical effect. Lever et al. also noted no change in thyroglobulin levels following external manual palpation of the thyroid;[48] however, transient increases in serum thyroglobulin were found in patients undergoing aspiration biopsy.

Although the term "palpation thyroiditis" was introduced by the Mayo Clinic group in 1975,[12] a similar morphologic finding had been described 20 years earlier

Table 4–4. Palpation Thyroiditis

	Found in:	
	Carney et al. (Percent)	LiVolsi* (Percent)
Surgically resected glands	95	85
Autopsy (in-patients)	40	10
Forensic autopsies	—	0
Autopsy (nonhospital deaths)	0	—

*Unpublished results on about 150 cases.

as "colloidophagy."[34, 35] This was defined as a histiocytic response to extruded colloid. Carney et al. believed that colloidophagy differs from palpation thyroiditis because follicular epithelium is destroyed in the latter.[12] In addition, colloidophagy was found more often in goiter and chronic thyroiditis.[35]

HISTIOCYTIC REACTION TO HEMORRHAGE

In adenomatous nodules, occasionally in neoplasms, and in nodular goiters, hemorrhage and an associated inflammatory response are seen. The current practice of needle aspiration of nodules has increased the incidence of this phenomenon. A macrophage reaction near areas of hemorrhage and inflammation is usual. Often the histiocytes contain cytoplasmic iron. These areas are usually focal in a gland showing another lesion (nodule, tumor, etc.) and should not present diagnostic problems for the pathologist.

Foreign body giant cells can be seen in common thyroid lesions: around hemorrhage and cholesterol debris in nodular goiter, in papillary carcinomas and in chronic lymphocytic thyroiditis. In the author's experience, giant cells are seen in the latter two conditions much more frequently in fine needle aspirates than in histologic preparations. However, after finding them quite often in cytology samples, the author has noticed these giant cells much more frequently in tissue sections of papillary cancer and chronic thyroiditis. The finding of giant cells in an aspiration cytology sample may raise the diagnostic differential of subacute thyroiditis versus chronic lymphocytic thyroiditis. However, in chronic thyroiditis, giant cells are few, and numerous lymphocytes and oncocytes are found. The pattern in subacute thyroiditis is usually one of acute inflammatory cells and mononuclear as well as multinucleated histiocytes. (See Chapter 18.)

FUNGAL THYROIDITIS

This entity, described in Chapter 3, represents fungal infection of the gland.[40] Although it would be expected that fungal infection would produce granulomatous reactions in the thyroid, most instances show an acute necrotizing reaction or no reaction at all. Since the patients with fungal thyroiditis frequently are immunosuppressed, the appropriate reaction may be lacking. Loeb et al. described three patients with coccidioidomycosis of the thyroid whose clinical symptoms resembled subacute thyroiditis;[51] histologic examination disclosed acute and chronic inflammation with fibrosis. Granulomas were not described or illustrated in these cases; however, numerous organisms were found. Recent reports illustrate that sometimes granulomata do arise in response to thyroid fungal infection.[40] (See Chapter 3.)

TUBERCULOUS THYROIDITIS

Tuberculous infection of the thyroid produces caseating granulomata similar to the reaction in other viscera.[31, 43, 53, 67, 68] However, tuberculous infection of the gland is extremely rare, even in patients with overwhelming miliary tuberculosis.[68] Most cases of this disease recently reported have been found in areas of the world where tuberculosis is widespread, and malnutrition and poor health care standards exist.

SARCOIDOSIS

Sarcoidosis can involve the thyroid. Interstitial noncaseating granulomata have been described in the thyroid in an estimated 1 to 4.2 percent of patients with systemic sarcoidosis.[41, 71, 88, 96] (The latter figure seems high and leads this author to wonder if some of these cases did not represent palpation thyroiditis.)

GRANULOMATOUS VASCULITIS

Vessels in the thyroid may be involved in systemic vasculitides. In some of these, the granulomatous character of the vasculitis may cause confusion with other granulomatous lesions affecting the gland. Usually the angiocentric nature of the process is easily recognized, however. Figures 4–13 to 4–15 illustrate the thyroid gland from a patient who died of systemic hypersensitivity vasculitis as a reaction to Dilantin (phenytoin).[24, 110]

FOREIGN MATERIAL

Foreign material may occasionally find its way to the thyroid via a lymphatic route. In such patients, one can occasionally see a true foreign body reaction in the gland. Such a case, illustrated in Chapter 7, involved a patient who had Polytef (Teflon) implants for vocal cord paralysis. Polarizable crystalline material is noted in the centers of the granulomas composed of histiocytes and lymphocytes. Many

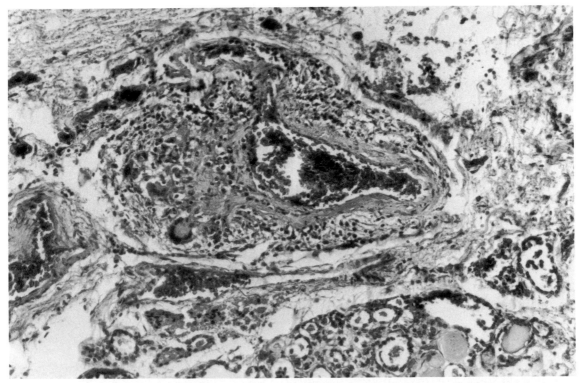

Figure 4–13. Hypersensitivity vasculitis in reaction to phenytoin; see text. Granulomatous inflammatory response with giant cells surrounding this medium-sized artery in the thyroid. × 100, H & E.

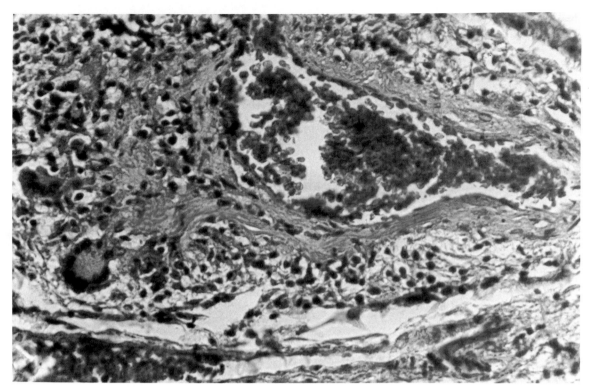

Figure 4–14. Higher power of Figure 14–13. × 300, H & E.

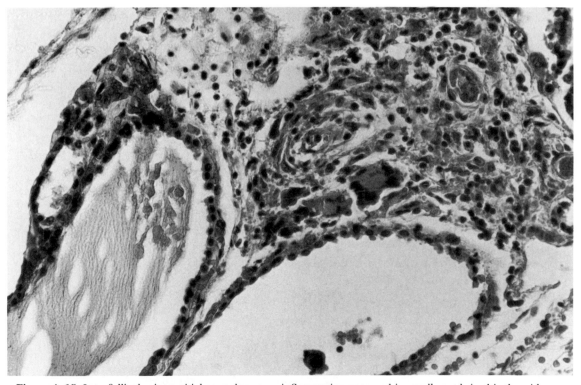

Figure 4–15. Interfollicular interstitial granulomatous inflammation near and in small vessels in this thyroid; same case as in Figures 4–13 and 4–14. × 300, H & E.

Table 4–5. Granulomas in the Thyroid

	Clinical Features	Gross Pathology	Microscopy	Etiology	Significance
Subacute thyroiditis	Adult age; usually women; systemic illness (fever, etc.); local or regional *pain*; goiter often; sometimes thyroid dysfunction.	Mass lesion multiple irregular tan— rarely soft, often firm.	Initial microabscesses followed by lymphocytic & histiocytic "granulomatous" reaction around destroyed or degenerating follicles; fibrosis centrally in foci.	Probably viral— many species.	Phases: hyperthyroidism, hypothyroidism— recovery. Rarely permanent residua.
Variants Painless thyroiditis with hyperthyroidism I	Usually young females; some postpartum; goiter clinically or chemically hyperthyroid; may recur.	?	Virtually all cases diagnosed clinically or by cytology or core biopsy only. Usually lymphocytic infiltration, mild fibrosis; ± follicular cell metaplasia; resembles autoimmune thyroiditis.	?	May remit and recur; some progress to hypothyroidism.
Painless thyroiditis with hyperthyroidism II	Similar to classic form except without pain.		Probably quite rare.		
Painless thyroiditis simulating malignancy	Fever, weight loss; painless goiter; no hyperthyroidism, but low radioiodine uptake.	?	By needle biopsy—"classic granulomatous thyroiditis."	?	Mistaken for systemic malignancy; patients should be treated for subacute thyroiditis and recover.
Chronic lymphocytic thyroiditis (painful)	As autoimmune thyroiditis per lab data; *painful* goiter.	?	"Chronic lymphocytic thyroiditis."	?	Significance is that of autoimmune thyroiditis.
Malignant (carcinomatous) pseudothyroiditis	Adult patients with enlarged painful goiters and fever; occasionally hyperthyroid.	Mass lesions found.	Carcinomas (often papillary) but others also.	Presumed destruction of gland by invading tumor may simulate effect of inflammatory destruction in classic subacute thyroiditis.	Prognosis is that of malignant tumor and hence treatment needs to be directed to that.
Palpation thyroiditis	Usually found in patients who have surgically resected glands, often for nodules.	None.	One to five follicles involved by histiocytic and lymphoplasmacytic inflammation encircling preexisting follicle. Rare necrosis; giant cells less common than in subacute disease.	Minor trauma to gland with follicular disruption.	None known; should not be mistaken for a disease.

Table 4–5. Granulomas in the Thyroid *Continued*

	Clinical Features	Gross Pathology	Microscopy	Etiology	Significance
Histiocytic reaction with round hemorrhage	Usually patient with nodule(s) representing nodular goiter or neoplasm. Hemorrhage may be spontaneous or biopsy-associated.	May see gross hemorrhage or cystic areas, usually near or in nodule(s).	Histiocytes often hemosiderin-laden and accompanying chronic inflammatory cells are seen in vicinity of the hemorrhage. Depending on stage of the lesion, varying degrees of fibrous and granulation tissue may be present.	Reaction to hemorrhage.	That of underlying nodule.
Fungal thyroiditis	Usually immunosup-pressed patient.	May see areas of softening and necrosis.	May see no signs or necrotizing inflammation with easily found organisms; rarely, thyroid granulomas are seen.	Fungal infection usually reflection of systemic fungemia.	Prognosis poor—usually postmortem finding.
Tuberculous thyroiditis	Usually reported from underdeveloped countries where tuberculosis is common. Often patients have significant debilitating infection.	May see miliary tubercles.	Caseating granulomas; mycobacteria on special stains.	Tuberculous infection of gland.	Equals that of systemic (? miliary) tuberculosis.
Sarcoidosis of thyroid	Most cases reported have evidence of pulmonary and/ or systemic sarcoidosis.	?	Noncaseating "tight" granulomas.	?	Equals that of sarcoid involvement of other organs.
Granulomatous vasculitis	Systemic illness; may be related to hypersensitivity to drug.	? Small foci of necrosis related to vascular damage.	Angiocentric granulomatous reaction; depending on type of vasculitis and vessel size, may find vessel necrosis and destruction.	Immunologic (? hypersen-sitivity) reaction attacking vessels in many organs.	Part of a systemic vasculitis.
Foreign material	History may indicate prior surgery, trauma, instillation or injection of material into neck or gland.	?	Identify foreign crystals, cotton, etc.; polarizing lens may help.	Reaction to foreign substance.	History of surgery or injection in neck may be obtained.

giant cells containing the crystals can be seen. Similar histologic reactions have been reported in the larynx and cervical soft tissues in patients who had undergone Teflon implantation of the vocal cord.[70, 80, 99]

One case report indicates thyroid enlargement secondary to the Teflon implant procedure;[70] histologic documentation of foreign body reaction to refractile particles is presented. By energy-dispersion x-ray analysis, fluorine, a component of Teflon, was identified. Whether the foreign particles represented excessive injected material or whether they migrated beyond the larynx via lymphatic or vascular channels is unknown. It can be theorized that in patients with vocal cord palsy caused by injury or tumor involvement of the laryngeal nerve, lymphatic blockade or disruption may alter lymph channels so as to allow migration of the foreign material into cervical soft tissues and rarely to the thyroid.

SUMMARY

This chapter has reviewed those thyroid lesions that show a granulomatous histology (see Table 4–5). By far the most common of these are reaction to hemorrhage in goiter and palpation thyroiditis. The most important disease entity in this category of disease is granulomatous or subacute thyroiditis. The multitude of variants and variations of subacute thyroiditis have been discussed.

REFERENCES

1. Ahmann, A. J., and Burman, K. D.: The role of T lymphocytes in autoimmune thyroiditis disease. Endocrinol. Metab. Clin. N. Amer. 16:287–326, 1987.
2. Amino, N., Mujai, K., et al.: Transient hypothyroidism after delivery in autoimmune thyroiditis. J. Clin. Endocrinol. Metab. 42:296–301, 1976.
3. Bastenie, P. A., Bonnyns, M., and Neve, P.: Subacute and chronic granulomatous thyroiditis. In: Bastenie, P. A., and Ermans, A. M. (eds.): Thyroiditis and Thyroid Function, Clinical, Morphological and Physiological Studies. Oxford, Pergamon Press, 1972, pp. 69–97.
4. Bauman, A., and Friedman, A.: Recurrent subacute thyroiditis: A report of three cases. N. Y. State J. Med. 83:987–988, 1983.
5. Benker, G., Olbricht, T., et al.: The sonographic and functional sequelae of de Quervain's subacute thyroiditis. Acta Endocrinol. 117:435–441, 1988.
6. Bliddal, H., Bech, K., et al.: Humoral autoimmune manifestation in subacute thyroiditis. Allergy 40:599–604, 1985.
7. Blonde, L., Witkin, M., and Harris, R.: Painless subacute thyroiditis simulating Graves' disease. West. J. Med. 125:75–78, 1976.
8. Blum, M., Passalaqua, A. M., et al.: Thyroid echography of subacute thyroiditis. Radiology 125:795–788, 1977.
9. Blum, M., and Schloss, M. F.: Martial-arts thyroiditis. N. Engl. J. Med. 311:199–200, 1984.
10. Buergi, U., Gebel, F., et al.: Serum thyroglobulin before and after palpation of the thyroid. N. Engl. J. Med. 308:777, 1983.
11. Burch, W. M.: Thyroid malignancy masquerading as thyroiditis. No. Carolina Med. J. 45:560–562, 1984.
12. Carney, J. A., Moore, S. B., et al.: Palpation thyroiditis (multifocal granulomatous thyroiditis). Am. J. Clin. Pathol. 64:639–647, 1975.
13. Check, J., and Avellino, J.: Painless thyroiditis and transient thyrotoxicosis after Graves' disease. J.A.M.A. 244:1361, 1980.
14. Dahlberg, P. A., and Jansson, R.: Different aetiologies in postpartum thyroiditis? Acta Endocrinol. 104:195–200, 1983.
15. DePauw, B. E., and deRooy, H. A. M.: DeQuervain's subacute thyroiditis: A report of 14 cases and a review of the literature. Neth. J. Med. 18:70–78, 1975.
16. Dorfman, S., Cooperman, M., et al.: Painless thyroiditis and transient hyperthyroidism without goiter. Ann. Intern. Med. 86:24–28, 1977.
17. Dorfman, S. G., Young, R. L., and Nusynowitz, M. L.: Thyroiditis and thyrotoxicosis. J.A.M.A. 240:1520–1521, 1978.
18. Eylan, E., Zmucky, R., and Sheba, C.: Mumps virus and subacute thyroiditis—evidence of a causal association. Lancet 1:1062–1063, 1957.

19. Fein, H., Goldman, J., and Weintraub, B.: Postpartum lymphocytic thyroiditis in American women: A spectrum of thyroid dysfunction. Am. J. Obstet. Gynecol. *138*:504–510, 1980.
20. Fennell, J. S., and Tomkin, G. H.: Sub-acute thyroiditis and hepatitis in a case of infectious mononucleosis. Postgrad. Med. J. *54*:351–352, 1978.
21. Fragu, P., Rougier, P., et al.: Evolution of thyroid I-127 stores measured by X-ray fluorescence in subacute thyroiditis. J. Clin. Endocrinol. Metab. *54*:162–166, 1982.
22. Fui, S. N. T., and Jefferys, D. B.: Subacute autoimmune thyroiditis simulating deQuervain's thyroiditis. Lancet *1*:622, 1979.
23. Furszyfer, J., McConahey, W. M., et al.: Subacute (granulomatous) thyroiditis in Olmsted County, Minnesota. Mayo Clin. Proc. *45*:396–404, 1970.
24. Gaffey, C. M., Chun, B., et al.: Phenytoin-induced systemic granulomatous vasculitis. Arch. Pathol. Lab. Med. *110*:131–135, 1986.
25. Ginsberg, J., and Walfish, P.: Post-partum transient thyrotoxicosis with painless thyroiditis. Lancet *1*:1125–1128, 1977.
26. Gluck, F. B., Nusynowitz, M. L., and Plymate, S.: Chronic lymphocytic thyroiditis, thyrotoxicosis and low radioactive iodine uptake: report of four cases. N. Engl. J. Med. *293*:624–628, 1975.
27. Goldman, J., Bochna, A. J., and Becker, F. O.: St. Louis encephalitis and subacute thyroiditis. Ann. Intern. Med. *87*:250, 1977.
28. Gorman, C., Duick, D., et al.: Transient hyperthyroidism in patients with lymphocytic thyroiditis. Mayo Clin. Proc. *53*:359–365, 1978.
29. Goto, H., Uno, H., et al.: Genetic analysis of subacute (deQuervain's) thyroiditis. Tissue Antigens *26*:110–113, 1985.
30. Greene, J. N.: Subacute thyroiditis. Am. J. Med. *51*:97–108, 1971.
31. Gutman, L. T., Handwerger, S., et al.: Thyroiditis due to Myocobacterium chelonei. Am. Rev. Resp. Dis. *110*:1807–1809, 1974.
32. Hazard, J. B.: Thyroiditis: a review. Am. J. Clin. Pathol. *25*:289–298, 1955.
33. Hay, I. D.: Thyroiditis: a clinical update. Mayo Clin. Proc. *60*:836–843, 1985.
34. Hellwig, C. A.: Colloidophagy in the human thyroid gland. Science *113*:725–726, 1951.
35. Hellwig, C. A.: Colloidophagy in the thyroid gland. Arch. Pathol. *58*:151–152, 1954.
36. Hnilica, P., and Nyulassy, S.: Plasma cells in aspirates of goitre and overt permanent hypothyroidism following subacute thyroiditis. Endocrinol. Exp. *19*:221–226, 1985.
37. Hurley, J. R.: Thyroiditis. Disease-a-Month. Dec., 1977.
38. Inada, M., Nishikawa, M., et al.: Transient thyrotoxicosis associated with painless thyroiditis and low radioactive iodine uptake. Arch. Intern. Med. *139*:597–599, 1979.
39. Izumi, M., and Larsen, P. R.: Correlation of sequential changes in serum thyroglobin, triiodothyronine, and thyroxine in patients with Graves' disease and subacute thyroiditis. Metabolism *27*:449–460, 1978.
40. Kakudo, K., Kanokogi, M., et al.: Acute mycotic thyroiditis. Acta Pathol. Jpn. *33*:147–151, 1983.
41. Karlish, A. J., and MacGregor, G. A.: Sarcoidosis, thyroiditis and Addison's disease. Lancet *2*:330–333, 1970.
42. Karlsson, F. A., Totterman, T. H., and Jansson, R.: Subacute thyroiditis: activated HLA-DR and interferon-gamma expressing T cytotoxic/suppressor cells in thyroid tissue and peripheral blood. Clin. Endocrinol. *25*:487–493, 1986.
43. Klassen, K. P., and Curtis, G. M.: Tuberculous abscess of the thyroid gland. Surgery *17*:552–559, 1945.
44. Klavinskis, L. S., Notkins, A. L., and Oldstone, M. B. A.: Persistent viral infection of the thyroid gland: Alteration of thyroid function in the absence of tissue injury. Endocrinology *122*:567–575, 1988.
45. Knecht, H., and Hedinger, C. E.: Ultrastructural findings in Hashimoto's thyroiditis and focal lymphocytic thyroiditis with reference to giant cell formation. Histopathology *6*:511–538, 1982.
46. Larsen, P. R.: Serum triiodothyronine, thyroxine and thyrotropin during hyperthyroid, hypothyroid and recovery phases of subacute nonsuppurative thyroiditis. Metabolism *23*:467–471, 1974.
47. Lebacq, E. G., Therasse, G., et al.: Subacute thyroiditis. Eleven cases with histological confirmation and thyrotrophic response to thyrotrophin releasing hormone. Acta Endocrinol. *81*:707–715, 1976.
48. Lever, E. G., Refetoff, S., et al.: The influence of percutaneous fine needle aspiration on serum thyroglobulin. J. Clin. Endocrinol. Metab. *56*:26–29, 1983.
49. Lindsay, S., and Dailey, M. E.: Granulomatous or giant cell thyroiditis. Surg. Gynecol. Obstet. *98*:197–212, 1954.
50. Lio, S., Pontecorvi, A., et al.: Transitory subclinical and permanent hypothyroidism in the course of subacute thyroiditis (deQuervain). Acta Endocrinol. *106*:67–70, 1984.
51. Loeb, J. M., Livermore, B. M., and Wofsy, D.: Coccidioidomycosis of the thyroid. Ann. Intern. Med. *91*:409–412, 1979.
52. Madeddu, G., Casu, A., et al.: Serum thyroglobulin levels in the diagnosis and follow-up of subacute "painful" thyroiditis. Arch. Intern. Med. *145*:243–247, 1985.
53. Markowicz, H., and Shanon, E.: Tuberculosis of the thyroid gland. Ann. Otol. Rhinol. Laryngol. *67*:223–226, 1958.
54. McConnon, J. K.: Thirty-five cases of transient hyperthyroidism. Canad. Med. Assoc. J. *130*:1159–1161, 1984.

55. Meachim, G., and Young, M. H.: DeQuervain's subacute granulomatous thyroiditis: histological identification and incidence. J. Clin. Pathol. *16*:189–199, 1963.

56. Milutinov, P. S., Han, R., and Nastic-Miric, D.: Relative diagnostic potency of various laboratory findings in the acute stage of subacute nonsuppurative thyroiditis. Radiobiol. Radiother. *25*:279–282, 1984.

57. Mizukami, Y., Michigishi, T., et al.: Immunohistochemical and ultrastructural study of subacute thyroiditis, with special reference to multinucleated giant cells. Hum. Pathol. *18*:929–935, 1987.

58. Morrison, J., and Caplan, R. H.: Typical and atypical ('silent') subacute thyroiditis in a wife and husband. Arch. Intern. Med. *138*:45–48, 1978.

59. Nikolai, T., Coombs, G., and McKenzie, A.: Lymphocytic thyroiditis with spontaneously resolving hyperthyroidism and subacute thyroiditis. Arch. Intern. Med. *141*:1455–1458, 1981.

60. Nikolai, T., Coombs, G., et al.: Treatment of lymphocytic thyroiditis with spontaneously resolving hyperthyroidism (silent thyroiditis). Arch. Intern. Med. *142*:2281–2283, 1982.

61. Nyulassy, S., Hnilica, P., et al.: Subacute (deQuervain's) thyroiditis: Association with HLA-Bw35 antigen and abnormalities of the complement system, immunoglobulins and other serum proteins. J. Clin. Endocrinol. Metab. *45*:270–274, 1977.

62. Radfar, N., Kenny, F. M., and Larsen, P. R.: Subacute thyroiditis in a lateral thyroid gland: evaluation of the pituitary-thyroid axis during the acute destructive and the recovery phases. J. Pediatr. *87*:34–37, 1975.

63. Rapoport, B., Block, M. B., et al.: Depletion of thyroid iodine during subacute thyroiditis. J. Clin. Endocrinol. Metab. *36*:610–611, 1973.

64. Reidbord, H. E., and Fischer, E. R.: Ultrastructural features of subacute granulomatous thyroiditis and Hashimoto's disease. Am. J. Clin. Pathol. *59*:327–337, 1973.

65. Rosen, I. B., Strawbridge, H. G., et al.: Malignant pseudothyroiditis: a new clinical entity. Am. J. Surg. *136*:445–449, 1978.

66. Rotenberg, Z., Weinberger, I., et al.: Euthyroid atypical subacute thyroiditis simulating systemic or malignant disease. Arch. Intern. Med. *146*:105–107, 1986.

67. Rundle, F. F.: Granulomatous diseases of the thyroid gland. *In*: Joll's Diseases of the Thyroid Gland. London, William Heinemann, Ltd., 1951, pp. 325–333.

68. Sachs, M. K., Dickinson, G., and Amazon, K.: Tuberculous adenitis of the thyroid mimicking subacute thyroiditis. Am. J. Med. *85*:573–575, 1988.

69. Sanders, L. R., Moreno, A. J., et al.: Painless giant cell thyroiditis diagnosed by fine needle aspiration and associated with intense thyroidal uptake of gallium. Am. J. Med. *80*:971–975, 1986.

70. Sanfilippo, F., and Shelburne, J.: Analysis of a Polytef granuloma mimicking a cold thyroid nodule 17 months after laryngeal injection. Ultrastruct. Pathol. *1*:471–475, 1980.

71. Sasaki, H., Harada, T., et al.: Concomitant association of thyroid sarcoidosis and Hashimoto's thyroiditis. Am. J. Med. Sci. *294*:441–443, 1987.

72. Satoh, M.: Virus-like particles in the follicular epithelium of the thyroid from a patient with subacute thyroiditis (deQuervain). Acta Pathol. Jpn. *25*:499–501, 1975.

73. Satoh, M.: Ultrastructure of the giant cell in deQuervain's subacute thyroiditis. Acta Pathol. Jpn. *26*:133–137, 1976.

74. Schneeberg, N. G.: Silent thyroiditis. Arch. Intern. Med. *143*:2214, 1983.

75. Schnyder, B., and Hedinger, C.: Die Fibrosierungstendenz bei subakuter thyreoditis de Quervain. Schweiz. Med. Wschr. *116*:1093–1097, 1986.

76. Singer, P., and Gorsky, J.: Familial postpartum transient hyperthyroidism. Arch. Intern. Med. *145*:240–242, 1985.

77. Srinivasappa, J., Garzelli, C., et al.: Virus-induced thyroiditis. Endocrinology *122*:563–566, 1988.

78. Stancekova, M., Stancek, D., et al.: Morphological, cytological and biological observations on viruses isolated from patients with subacute thyroiditis of deQuervain. Acta Virol. *20*:183–188, 1976.

79. Steinberg, F. U.: Subacute granulomatous thyroiditis: a review. Ann. Intern. Med. *52*:1014–1025, 1960.

80. Stephens, C. B., Arnold, G. E., and Stone, J. W.: Larynx injected with polytef paste. Arch. Otolaryngol. *102*:432–435, 1976.

81. Stonebridge, P. A.: Occult subacute thyroiditis with unusual features. Lancet *2*:727, 1985.

82. Strakosch, C. R., Joyner, D., and Wall, J. R.: Thyroid stimulating antibodies in patients with subacute thyroiditis. J. Clin. Endocrinol. Metab. *46*:345–348, 1978.

83. Sugrue, D., Loergan, M., and Drury, M. I.: DeQuervain's subacute granulomatous thyroiditis: five cases. Ir. Med. J. *73*:308–310, 1980.

84. Swann, N. H.: Acute thyroiditis. Five cases associated with adenovirus infection. Metabolism *13*:908–910, 1964.

85. Taylor, H., and Sheeler, L.: Recurrence and heterogeneity in painless thyrotoxic lymphocytic thyroiditis. J.A.M.A. *248*:1085–1088, 1982.

86. Teixeira, V. L., Romaldini, J. H., et al.: Thyroid function during the spontaneous course of subacute thyroiditis. J. Nucl. Med. *26*:457–460, 1985.

87. Thompson, C., and Farid, N.: Post-partum thyroiditis and goitrous (Hashimoto's) thyroiditis are associated with HLA-DR4. Immunology Letters *11*:301–303, 1985.

88. Thompson, W. D., McGrouther, D. A., and Stockdell, G.: Thyrotoxicosis with sarcoid-like granulomata. J. Pathol. *111*:289–291, 1973.
89. Totterman, T. H., Gordin, A., et al.: Accumulation of thyroid antigen-reactive T-lymphocytes in the gland of patients with subacute thyroiditis. Clin. Exp. Immunol. *32*:153–158, 1978.
90. Trokoudes, K. M., Rosen, I. B., et al.: Carcinomatous pseudothyroiditis: a problem in differential diagnosis. Canad. Med. Assoc. J. *119*:896–898, 1978.
91. Volpe, R.: Thyroiditis: Current views of pathogenesis. Med. Clin. North Amer. *59*:1163–1175, 1975.
92. Volpe, R.: Subacute (deQuervain's) thyroiditis. Clin. Endocrinol. Metab. *8*:81–95, 1979.
93. Volpe, R., Row, V. V., and Ezrin, C.: Circulating viral and thyroid antibodies in subacute thyroiditis. J. Clin. Endocrinol. Metab. *27*:1275–1281, 1967.
94. Volpe, R.: The pathology of thyroiditis. Hum. Pathol. *9*:429–438, 1978.
95. Volpe, R.: Etiology, pathogenesis and clinical aspects of thyroiditis. Pathol. Annu. *13*(Part 2):399–413, 1978.
96. von Knorring, J., and Selroos, O.: Sarcoidosis with thyroid involvement, polymyalgia rheumatica and breast carcinoma. Scand. J. Rheumatol. *5*:77–80, 1976.
97. Wall, J. R., Fang, S.-L., Ingbar, S. H., and Braverman, L. E.: Lymphocyte transformation in response to human thyroid extract in patients with subacute thyroiditis. J. Clin. Endocrinol. Metab. *43*:587–590, 1976.
98. Wall, J. R., Strakosch, C. R., et al.: Nature of thyrotropin displacement activity in subacute thyroiditis. J. Clin. Endocrinol. Metab. *54*:349–353, 1982.
99. Walsh, F. M., and Castelli, J. B.: Polytef granuloma clinically simulating carcinoma of the thyroid. Arch. Otolaryngol. *101*:262–263, 1975.
100. Watts, N. B., and Sewell, C. W.: Carcinomatous involvement of thyroid presenting as subacute thyroiditis. Am. J. Med. Sci. *296*:126–128, 1988.
101. Weihl, A. C., Daniels, G. H., et al.: Thyroid function tests during the early phase of subacute thyroiditis. J. Clin. Endocrinol. Metab. *44*:1107–1114, 1977.
102. Werner, J., and Gelderblom, H.: Isolation of foamy virus from patients with deQuervain thyroiditis. Lancet *2*:258–259, 1979.
103. Werner, S. C.: Graves' disease following acute (subacute) thyroiditis. Arch. Intern. Med. *139*:1313–1315, 1979.
104. Woolf, P. D.: Painless thyroiditis as a cause of hyperthyroidism. Arch. Intern. Med. *138*:26–27, 1978.
105. Woolf, P. D.: Transient painless thyroiditis with hyperthyroidism: a variant of lymphocytic thyroiditis. Endocrine Rev. *1*:411–420, 1980.
106. Woolf, P., and Daly, R.: Thyrotoxicosis with painless thyroiditis. Am. J. Med. *60*:73–79, 1976.
107. Woolner, L. B., McConahey, W. B., and Beahrs, O. H.: Granulomatous thyroiditis (deQuervain's thyroiditis). J. Clin. Endocrinol. Metab. *17*:1202–1221, 1957.
108. Woolner, L. B.: Thyroiditis: classification and clinicopathologic correlation. *In*: Hazard, J. B., and Smith, D. E. (eds.): The Thyroid. Baltimore, Williams and Wilkins, 1964, p. 123.
109. Yamamoto, M., Sakurada, T., et al.: Thyroid function and antimicrosomal antibody during the course of silent thyroiditis. Endocrinol. Jpn. *34*:357–363, 1987.
110. Yermakov, V. M., Hitti, I. F., and Sutton, A. L.: Necrotizing vasculitis associated with diphenylhydantoin: two fatal cases. Hum. Pathol. *13*:182–184, 1983.
111. Yoshida, K., Sakurada, T., et al.: Serum free thyroxine and triiodothyroxine concentrations in subacute thyroiditis. J. Clin. Endocrinol. Metab. *55*:185–188, 1982.
112. Zimmerman, R. S., Brennan, M. D., et al.: Hashimoto's thyroiditis: An uncommon cause of painful thyroid unresponsive to corticosteroid therapy. Ann. Intern. Med. *104*:355–357, 1986.

5

LYMPHOCYTES IN THE THYROID

This chapter will review those lesions of the thyroid that manifest lymphoid and/or lymphoplasmacytic infiltration of the gland. (See Table 5–1.) As a preface to the morphologic descriptions of these entities, a brief overview of the autoimmune phenomenon in general and in the thyroid is given. (It is beyond the scope of this monograph to delve into the large body of knowledge regarding autoimmunity and its relationship to human diseases; the field of immunology is rapidly expanding and new research often disproves current theories. Hence what follows below is a short review of what is undisputed or at least still seems plausible.*)

In the discussions in this chapter, the eponyms Hashimoto's disease and Graves' disease are used interchangeably with chronic lymphocytic thyroiditis and diffuse toxic goiter with hyperthyroidism, respectively. The author is aware of dispute regarding the histologic requirements for a diagnosis of Hashimoto's disease, with some pathologists insisting on the full-blown morphologic picture of lymphoid infiltration, oxyphilia, and follicular atrophy whereas others use the term in more general fashion. The author is also aware of discrepancies regarding the crediting of the descriptions of hyperthyroidism to Graves or others and that in the European literature other eponyms are used. In addition, the diagnoses of Graves' ophthalmopathy without hyperthyroidism and of euthyroid Graves' disease are acknowledged. This chapter will address the descriptions of these disorders predominantly from the morphologic viewpoint and classic cases will be discussed.

AUTOIMMUNITY (See also Chapter 9)

Both hormonal and cell-mediated immunity function together to maintain immunologic defenses against invasion by foreign antigens. Normally, self-antigens are not involved in an immunologic reaction. In autoimmune disease, however, there is breakdown of the unresponsiveness in self-tolerance.[7, 57, 58, 191, 239, 268]

The cells involved in autoimmune disorders include both members of the lymphocytic series and components of the "monocyte-macrophage system." Cells in the latter category, including macrophages and dendritic cells,[142] are responsible for clearing, processing and presentation of antigen to cells of lymphocytic lineage.[142, 268, 294] Classic immune mechanisms can be conveniently divided into

---

*The author is indebted to Dr. Chester Andrzejewski, Jr., for his assistance and input in this section.

Table 5–1. Lymphocytes in the Thyroid

1. Chronic lymphocytic thyroiditides
   (a) Classic form—oxyphilic and nonoxyphilic
   (b) Fibrous variant
   (c) Atrophic variant
   (d) Hyperplastic epithelial variant (juvenile form)
   (e) Painless thyroiditis
   (f) "Hashitoxicosis"
   (g) Lymphoma-like variant
   (h) Focal "nonspecific" thyroiditis
2. Diffuse toxic goiter—Graves' disease
3. Nodular goiter, toxic
4. Nodular goiter, nontoxic
5. Drug-associated thyroiditis
6. Radiation-associated thyroiditis
7. Peri-tumor thyroiditis
8. Subacute granulomatous thyroiditis
9. Riedel's disease
10. Healing phases of acute thyroiditis; posttraumatic or postsurgical thyroid injury
11. Developmental rests—thymus, ? branchial cleft; ultimobranchial body rests
12. Malignant lymphoma

Modified with permission from LiVolsi, V.A., and LoGerfo, P.: *Thyroiditis*. Boca Raton, FL, CRC Press, copyright 1981.

cellular and humoral aspects. Cellular immunity principally involves lymphocytes of the thymus-dependent lineage (T cells). Various subpopulations of T cells (T helper, T suppressor, T cytotoxic) have been identified based on both functional and cell-surface marker studies. The various subpopulations of T cells modulate both cellular and humoral immune processes, including antibody production by B cells, "delayed type" hypersensitivity responses, and cellular cytotoxicity against foreign tissue grafts or virus-infected cells.[3–6, 15, 25] In contrast, humoral immunity resides with the "bursa-derived" B lymphocytes and functionally manifests itself by the production and secretion of immunoglobulins.[268, 294]

Antibody production and secretion can be correlated with well-recognized stages in the maturation and differentiation of B cells. Cytoplasmic immunoglobulin synthesis precedes surface immunoglobulin expression and is usually seen early in B cell development. Secretion of antibody is correlated with the development of the B cell to the plasma cell stage.

Although much knowledge has accumulated concerning the pathogenesis of autoimmune diseases, the etiology of these disorders remains undefined. The initiation of autoreactivity may involve modifications of self antigens by viruses, other organisms, or chemical agents. This generation of "modified self" may trigger disturbances in the immunoregulatory circuits which may in turn affect the threshold of unresponsiveness of B and T cells in the body and lead to an auto-aggressive state.[26, 27, 30, 32, 33, 49, 50, 53, 61, 64, 125, 149] Clearly the development of an autoantibody is not the sole factor in the progression to autoimmune disease since normal individuals have been shown to have a variety of autoantibodies present,[223, 268] yet they do not suffer disease.

In addition to theories of "altered self," other hypotheses concerning the development of autoimmunity revolve around disruptions of the immunologic network. Although evidence from animal models and humans exists demonstrating intrinsic B cell defects and/or T cell dysfunction, it is probably the interplay of disturbances in both humoral and cellular compartments that leads to autoimmune diseases' initiation and continuing progression. Family and genetic studies have shown that in autoimmune thyroid diseases both genetic and environmental factors appear to play a role.[1, 69, 100, 179, 200, 205, 223, 230, 231, 243, 248, 258, 286]

Considerable evidence has accumulated over the past several decades of the role of organ-specific autoimmunity in chronic lymphocytic thyroiditis (Hashimoto's thyroiditis) and diffuse toxic goiter with hyperthyroidism (Graves' disease).[36, 128, 194, 219, 223] Clinical and pathologic evidence has been cited in support of the autoimmune factors in the cause of these disorders and of the interrelationships.[169] Thus,

a. Autoimmune thyroid disorders are often found in several members of the same family, suggesting a genetic predisposition.[51, 80, 81, 84, 88, 90, 179, 231, 232, 258] Some studies show nonrandom distribution of certain HLA subtypes.[80, 82, 176, 182, 205, 231, 232, 254, 256, 260, 266]

b. Several autoimmune or purported autoimmune diseases may be found in the same individual.[52, 76, 87, 94, 167, 168, 198, 241, 274, 281, 294]

c. Sometimes hyperthyroidism or Graves' disease develops following hypothyroidism and vice versa, indicating a relationship between these disorders.[39, 41, 55, 79, 85, 99, 104, 120, 121, 243, 246, 292, 305]

d. Circulating antithyroid antibodies against various thyroid components are demonstrated.[30, 31, 100, 135, 145, 159, 221, 223, 227, 235, 257, 258, 265, 268, 313]

e. Lymphocytic infiltration of the thyroid is present.[79, 85, 110, 120, 291]

However, definite clinical and morphologic differences are found between diffuse toxic goiter and chronic lymphocytic thyroiditis. Although there is overlap, most patients with Graves' disease are hyperthyroid and many of those with thyroiditis are clinically or preclinically hypothyroid.[223, 258, 290, 291] Glandular hyperplasia is the most common histologic manifestation of Graves' disease, whereas the gland is destroyed or atrophic in chronic thyroiditis.[85, 120, 194, 223]

At the two ends of the spectrum of autoimmune thyroid disease, different types of immunopathogenetic mechanisms may be at work. Antibodies generated by lymphocyte subsets not within the gland may act on the thyroid (humoral immunity in diffuse toxic goiter). Immunocytes in the thyroid itself can also affect the gland either by local secretion of antibodies or by recruitment of cells that can by their actions or secretions produce gland injury (cell-mediated immunity in chronic lymphocytic thyroiditis with hypothyroidism).[223, 258]

Volpe and his coworkers[258, 286, 290, 291] postulate that autoimmune thyroid disease is a reflection of an *inherited defect* in immune surveillance probably of antigen-specific suppressor T cell function which allows for a specific randomly mutating clone of helper T cells to produce α-interferon and induce self-reactive antibody-producing B cells. The interferon causes HLA-DR antigen expression on thyroid epithelial cells,[172, 289] implying that the epithelium can act *directly* as antigen-presenting cells[37, 62, 63, 65, 74, 105, 131, 133, 155, 156, 172–174, 176, 186, 218, 270, 288, 289] Thyrocyte HLA-DR expression may prove important in presenting thyroid antigen secondarily, amplifying the signal and continuing to stimulate and activate T lymphocytes. Thus, chronicity would ensue. However, in individuals in whom there is no disturbance in autoimmune regulation such as in cases of subacute thyroiditis, the presence of HLA-DR expression in thyroid cells is transient, is not a self-perpetuating phenomenon, and autoantibodies in subacute thyroiditis disappear with recovery.[147] It has been shown that in the circulation of normal individuals, B cells capable of binding thyroglobulin or microsomal antigen can be noted in the circulation.[193, 195] The role of autoantibodies may aggravate thyroid destruction, since, in humans, activated thyroid B cells are abundant in the gland.[110, 119, 136, 258, 271, 277, 289, 297, 312]

Autoimmune Thyroiditis

Since the discovery by Roitt et al. in 1956[229] of anti-thyroglobulin antibodies in serum from patients with Hashimoto's thyroiditis, many autoantibodies directed against thyroid-related antigens have been identified. These include antibodies to TSH receptor, thyroid growth-stimulating antibodies, thyroid growth-blocking antibodies, antimicrosomal antibodies, antithyroglobulin antibodies of various types, antibodies to second colloid antigen, antithyroxine, and anti-T_3 and anti-TSH antibodies.[68, 69, 100, 204, 223, 258, 286]

In addition, in autoimmune thyroid disorders, autoantibodies to nonthyroid antigens can also be found, including antibodies to gastric parietal cells, adrenal cells, and smooth muscle.[69, 258, 286] (Antibodies to the bacterium *Yersinia enterocolitica* are also encountered;[298, 299] these may not be related to thyroid autoimmunity but may reflect merely an epiphenomenon.[289])

In classic autoimmune thyroiditis, the histologic features show intrathyroidal infiltration with lymphocytes and plasma cells, and the formation of reactive follicular centers with destruction of normal thyroid follicles and fibrosis (see below). This damage may be explained by several mechanisms: (a) a cytotoxic effect of antibody,[228] (b) immune complex deposition on the follicular basement membrane,[47, 143, 217, 300, 311] or (c) antibody-dependent cell-mediated cytotoxicity.[234]

The differences between goitrous and atrophic thyroiditis may be due to the fact that in the former new thyroid acini may grow rapidly enough to outstrip the tendency of the cytotoxic autoimmune reaction to destroy the older thyroid follicles. The possibility that certain growth factors are also produced or stimulated by the antibodies present should be considered. Antithyroid and antimicrosomal antibodies are found in about 70 percent of the population of Hashimoto's thyroiditis and in most patients with atrophic idiopathic myxedema.[20, 69, 70, 157, 204, 228, 238, 276] Autopsy studies have shown a good correlation between the presence of lymphocytic infiltration and these antibodies.[69, 163]

It has been shown in experimental autoimmune thyroiditis that susceptibility to this disorder in the mouse is linked to the H2 complex.[1, 14, 155, 182, 232] The thyroid antigen, thyroglobulin, is the presumed initiating antigen which turns on T cells in *susceptible* mice. These T cells are autoreactive in that they recognize thyroglobulin and proliferate *in vitro* in response to it. In patients with Hashimoto's thyroiditis, T cells may proliferate in response to stimulation *in vitro* with human thyroglobulin.[213] In man, it appears that the triggering of autoreactive helper T cells can occur in the peripheral lymphoid system as well as in the thyroid. The peripheral sensitization leads to a cascade of the T cell network with expansion and differentiation of different subsets of T cells. The thyroglobulin-specific effector T cells are then retained in the thyroid. Lymphokine production, including interferons and chemotactic factors, leads to HLA-DR expression on thyrocytes and to recruitment of other T cells and macrophages which may continue the process and contribute to the chronic nature of Hashimoto's disease.[180, 202, 204, 212, 213, 263, 272, 273]

Hyperthyroidism: Graves' Disease

At the other end of the spectrum, in classic hyperthyroidism (Graves' disease), the normal thyroid function predicated via a hypothalamic pituitary-thyroid axis and directly controlled by pituitary-derived TSH is bypassed.

Adams and Purves[2] identified a nonthyrotropin humoral factor that stimulated thyroid function in Graves' disease; subsequently this factor was shown to be an immunoglobulin known as LATS—*long acting thyroid stimulator*.[43, 160, 192, 196, 211, 310] Some authors doubted LATS was the "cause" of hyperthyroidism;[244] however, further studies clarified the situation. It is now believed a family of immunoglobulins that possess thyroid growth and/or function stimulatory activity is responsible for the hyperthyroidism in diffuse toxic goiter.[23, 100, 252, 258, 283] This family of immunoglobulins is now variously called thyroid stimulating immunoglobulins (TSIgs) or thyrotropin-receptor antibodies (TR Abs).[100, 258] In patients with Graves' hyperthyroidism, TSH receptor antibodies produced by the patient's lymphocytes "fool" the TSH receptor on thyroid follicular epithelial cells into thinking that there is excess TSH around, and stimulation of growth and function occurs. TSH from the pituitary is thus suppressed. TSH receptor antibodies, depending on the method of measurement, can be found in 57 to 100 percent of patients with untreated Graves' disease.[100, 258, 286]

Extraction of T cells grown from thyroid glands of patients with autoimmune thyroid disease have shown direct sensitization to thyroid follicular cells. In addition to the organ-specific defect in suppressor T lymphocytes, resulting from genetic variations, variations in nonspecific suppressor T lymphocyte function induced by changes within the environment, such as viral infection, would add to the thyroid-specific defect. Hyperthyroidism would result and this would have an adverse effect on generalized suppressor T lymphocyte function and may be a self-perpetuating factor in Graves' disease.[258, 271, 286, 291] Drug therapy for Graves' disease results in a marked decline in the number of activated T helper cells and a transient increase in activated T suppressor cells.[40, 83, 161, 258] This may, therefore, reduce thyroid autoantibody production by the B cells infiltrating the gland.[17]

AUTOIMMUNE THYROIDITIS: CLINICAL ASPECTS

The clinical presentation and therapeutic aspects of thyroiditis can be found in classic textbooks of medicine. The thyroiditic syndromes vary widely.[22] A brief review of the major aspects will be given here; the morphologic aspects will be stressed below.

Classic Hashimoto's thyroiditis is clinically found more commonly in women than men (average ratio quoted is 20:1) and may be associated with euthyroidism or occasionally hyperthyroidism;[70, 223] however, this form of thyroid disease is the lesion most often seen in patients with overt hypothyroidism.[66] In most cases, clinical evidence of a goiter is found; laboratory data support a frankly or subclinical hypothyroid state and antithyroid (antithyroglobulin and/or antimicrosomal) antibodies are present. If not found at diagnosis, hypothyroidism tends to develop during follow-up; goiter may persist or, rarely, thyroid atrophy may ensue.[70, 98, 116, 275, 282]

The fibrous or fibrosing variant of this disease is discussed in detail in Chapter 7. In comparison to the classic subtype, the fibrous variant occurs more commonly in men (ratio, female:male, is 5:1) and is usually associated with large symptomatic goiter and often with severe hypothyroidism. Antithyroid antibody titers are significantly elevated.[70, 148]

Fibrous atrophy of the thyroid (which may be the end result of classic lymphocytic thyroiditis in some patients, but not all) is the thyroid lesion of idiopathic myxedema. Overwhelmingly a disease of women, this disorder is associated with severe hypothyroidism and elevated antithyroid antibody titers but no goiter.[12, 19, 20, 22, 70, 141, 148, 223, 240]

The so-called juvenile variant of lymphocytic thyroiditis shows significant clinical differences from the other forms.[69, 158, 166, 181, 308] Affecting children, teenagers, and young adults, this disease may be associated with small goiters, minimally elevated antibody titers, and remitting and recurrent *hyper*thyroidism.[42, 237, 276]

There are clinical and histologic similarities between this form and so-called "painless thyroiditis with hyperthyroidism," which probably belongs within this group of disorders.[72, 75, 77, 90, 117, 127, 189, 203, 207, 208, 215] In this disease, young patients, chiefly women, are affected, often with episodic hyperthyroidism (curiously clustered around puerperium or postpartum periods);[75, 86, 96, 134, 137, 138, 226, 250, 264, 269, 280, 284, 307] the disorder in many cases is transient, but may recur and eventuate into hypothyroidism.[264, 293] Initially classified in the spectrum of subacute thyroiditis without pain (hence the name), biopsy results,[189] antibody data, and follow-up studies now firmly establish this thyroiditis among the autoimmune group.[10, 11, 97, 126, 132, 209, 267, 293, 306]

PATHOLOGY OF AUTOIMMUNE THYROID DISEASE

The presence of lymphoid cells in the substance of the thyroid parenchyma probably always reflects an abnormal immunologic state; the exceptions to this rule include developmental anomalies such as ectopic thymic tissue or lymphocytes associated with rests of ultimobranchial body. (See Chapter 1.)

Although lymphocytes can be found in the inflammatory infiltrates of granulomatous thyroiditis, nodular nontoxic goiter, or healing phases of other inflammatory conditions (e.g., post-trauma), the presence of lymphocytes in the thyroid is classically associated with chronic thyroiditis and diffuse toxic goiter—the two ends of the spectrum of autoimmune thyroid disease.

In 1912, Hashimoto described four patients with a thyroid disease that bears his name.[114] The thyroids were described grossly as symmetrically enlarged and firm. Microscopically, the follicular epithelium ranged from hyperplastic to atrophic; the follicles were dilated or atrophic, and the gland was infiltrated by lymphocytes, both within the lobules and in the interstitium. Germinal centers were present, as was fibrosis, which ranged from mild to prominent. In Hashimoto's original description, two striking features were emphasized: eosinophilic change in the follicular epithelium (now known as oncocytes, oxyphils or Hürthle cells) and a shrinkage of colloid, which exhibited altered staining characteristics, with an intense eosinophilia.

Confusion has been noted in the literature between "classic" Hashimoto's disease and Riedel's disease on the one hand[148] and between "classic" Hashimoto's thyroiditis and nonspecific thyroiditis on the other. The first of these issues is discussed in Chapter 6. The interrelationships among the classic form of chronic thyroiditis, its variants, and "nonspecific" thyroiditis is problematic. Since the initiating event and/or cause of any of these disorders is unknown, attempts at relating one to the other remain speculative at best. However, the morphologic and immunopathologic overlap between "nonspecific" lymphocytic thyroiditis and "classic" Hashimoto's disease suggest that they represent a spectrum of "autoimmune" injury to the thyroid, i.e., the differences are quantitative rather than qualitative.[70, 223, 308]

Classification Schemes

The classifications of chronic thyroiditis are as numerous as the authors who write about them.[70, 118, 309] (See Table 5–2.)

The present author prefers the Doniach and Roitt classification,[70] since it (a) best correlates morphologic, laboratory, and clinical findings; (b) includes Graves'

Table 5–2. Classification Schemes of Lymphocytic Thyroiditis

Hazard[118]	Woolner et al.[308, 309]	Doniach and Roitt[70]

1. Struma lymphomatosa (Hashimoto's struma)
  A. lymphoid predominant
  B. fibrous variant
  C. fibrolymphoid variant
2. Lymphocytic thyroiditis
3. Chronic thyroiditis, unspecified type
	1. Diffuse thyroiditis
	  A. with pronounced epithelial destruction and fibrosis
	  B. with oxyphilic epithelium
	  C. with variable oxyphilia
	  D. lymphoid type
	2. Thyroiditis with hyperplastic epithelium
	3. Focal thyroiditis
		1. Diffuse
		  A. Goitrous (Hashimoto type)
		    i) hypercellular variants
		      a) primarily oxyphilic
		      b) primarily nonoxyphilic
		  B. Non-goitrous
		    i) severe atrophic type (idiopathic myxedema)
		    ii) mild atrophic type
		2. Multifocal
		  A. Thyrotoxicosis (Graves')
		  B. Peritumor (usually papillary cancer)
		  C. Colloid goiter

disease and "Hashitoxicosis" as part of the spectrum; and (c) includes focal "nonspecific" thyroiditis in the group. In addition, the changes that are seen in the thyroid following radiation injury or use of certain pharmacologic agents resemble lymphocytic thyroiditis (see below) and are included in our classification of lymphoid thyroiditis for completeness. (See Table 5–1.) The lymphoid infiltrate in nodular nontoxic goiter may reflect "immune reactions" as well.

Autoimmune Thyroiditis: Morphology

Classic Form[21, 70, 101, 109, 118, 140, 171, 184, 255, 285, 308, 309]

Gross Anatomy (Figs. 5–1 and 5–2). The gland is usually moderately enlarged from two to four times normal size; weights range from 25 to 250 grams but most fall into the 40- to 100-gram range. Typically, the enlargement is symmetric; the pyramidal lobe may appear prominent. Although the gland may be adherent to surrounding tissues, the adhesions are easily dissected and the thyroid capsule is thin. The gland is firm but not hard. On cut section, the normal thyroid lobulation is accentuated and individual lobules bulge and are delimited by increased interlobular fibrous tissue. The normal red-brown color of the thyroid is replaced by a tan-yellow appearance attributed to the abundant lymphoid tissue; Bastenie and Ermans describe the Hashimoto's gland as similar to a hypertrophied thymus.[21] In most cases, the process is a diffuse one, distinguishing the lesion from carcinoma; rarely, a clinical and gross nodule may dominate.[29]

Microscopic Appearance. At scanning power, the gross lobulation of the gland is recapitulated. The thyroid follicles are small and atrophic; colloid may be absent or present focally. The colloid appears dense and stains deep pink with eosin. Although not present in every case, metaplasia of follicular cells is found in many; this change ranges from pale pink staining cells with abundant cytoplasm to classic oxyphil cells with pink granular cytoplasm (Fig. 5–3). Occasionally, clear cell metaplasia may be noted focally. These follicular cells, variously called oxyphils, oncocytes, or Askanazy or Hürthle cells, frequently contain large bizarre nuclei with prominent nucleoli. Occasionally epidermoid or squamous metaplasia of the follicular epithelium may be seen; this feature is much more commonly encountered in the fibrous variant, however.[107, 148]

The most characteristic microscopic feature is lymphoplasmacytic infiltration, consisting of lymphocytes, immunoblasts, and plasma cells in the stroma between

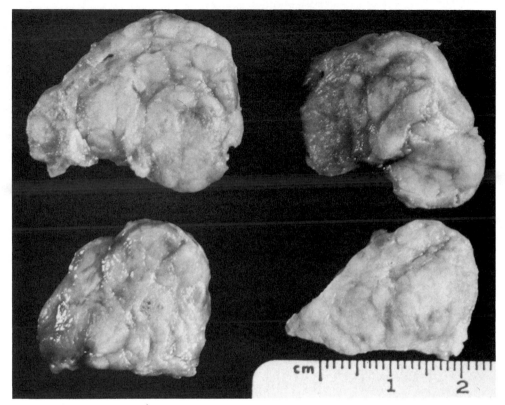

Figure 5–1. Gross appearance of classic Hashimoto's thyroiditis. Note pale color, markedly accentuated lobulation, and diffuse involvement of the gland.

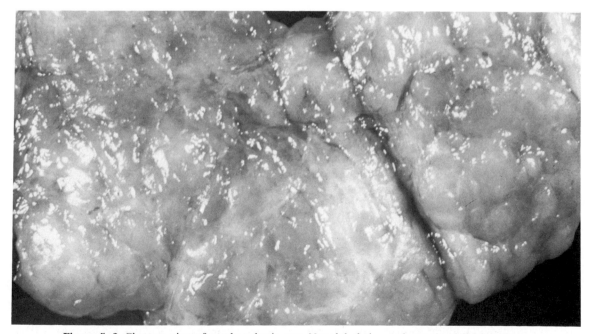

Figure 5–2. Close-up view of another classic case. Note lobulation and strands of fibrous tissue.

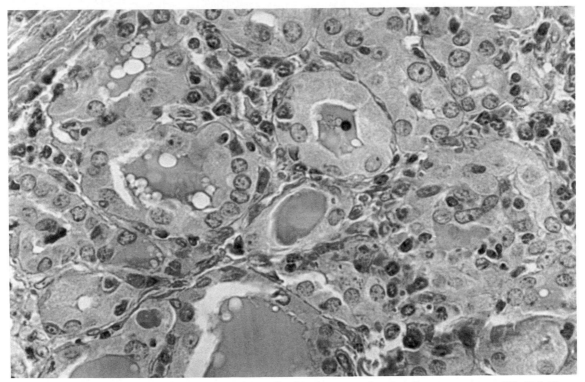

Figure 5–3. Small follicles with dense colloid are lined by large cytoplasmic cells—oncocytes. × 300, H & E.

follicles and occasionally overrunning the atrophic follicles (Figs. 5–4 and 5–5). Frequently these lymphoid cells are arranged into well-developed follicular centers, with central macrophages noted. Variable degrees of fibrosis, chiefly interlobular in location, are seen.

Occasionally, within the follicles a multinucleated giant cell is noted,[152] but the number of these cells is never as great as in subacute thyroiditis; in addition, the histiocytic granulomatous appearance of the latter is absent. (See Chapter 4.) Rarely, stromal fat can be noted.[108]

Ultrastructure. Bastenie and Ermans have reported on the electron microscopic appearance of the Hashimoto's thyroid.[21] They divide the epithelial cells into three types:

1. Hyperplastic cells, which show normal mitochondria, dilated endoplasmic reticulum, well-developed Golgi complexes, and colloid droplets; these elements are recognized more commonly in hyperplastic lesions, including those of juvenile thyroiditis.

2. Hürthle cells (Askanazy cells, oncocytes or oxyphilic cells), which demonstrate poorly developed Golgi complexes, decreased endoplasmic reticulum, and characteristically increased numbers of large mitochondria.[21, 225]

3. Colloid cells, which contain a large homogeneous area (? colloid) and appear to be end-stage cells.

Several electron microscopic studies have documented the presence of the spectrum of lymphocytes in this disease: thus transformed B cells, plasma cells, and immunoblasts are found. Bastenie and Ermans[21] and others[110, 150, 206, 225, 311] demonstrated lymphocytes penetrating into and/or between epithelial cells in Hashimoto's disorder; this does not occur in normal thyroids. Kalderon et al. noted follicular basement membrane deposits in eight cases of Hashimoto's that they examined ultrastructurally;[143] these authors felt these represented immune

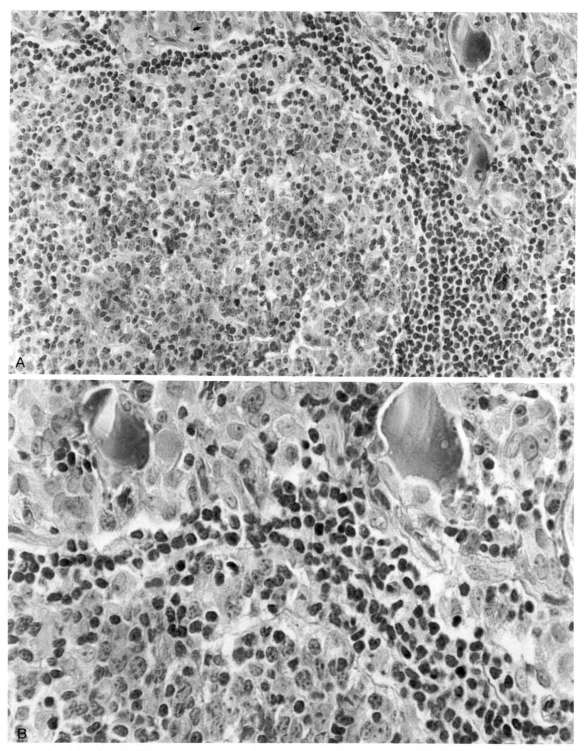

Figure 5–4. *A*, A very large follicular center with prominent spectrum of lymphoid cells is shown. "Mantle" of small lymphocytes encroaches upon atrophic follicles at upper right. × 250, H & E. *B*, At higher power, lymphoid cells are seen in and around follicles. × 400, H & E.

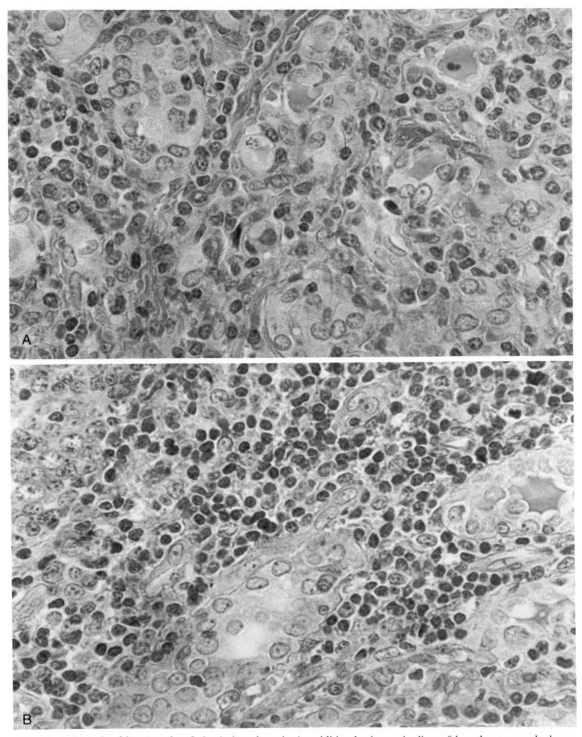

Figure 5–5. *A,* In this example of classic lymphocytic thyroiditis, the intermingling of lymphocytes and plasma cells within the follicular epithelium is seen. × 300, H & E. *B,* Similar field from another case. × 300, H & E.

complex deposits. Immunoglobulins and complement have been identified in the basement membrane of the follicle.[43, 217] Follicular basement membrane abnormalities, including rupture and duplication, are described.[150, 152, 178, 187, 206, 217, 245, 311]

The nature of the intrathyroidal lymphoid cells has been studied by many investigators.[34, 198, 301] The proportion of B and T cells within the thyroid differs from that in the peripheral blood: hence, T/B cell ratio in blood is normal (70 to 80 percent/20 percent), whereas in the thyroid the ratio is about 40 to 45 percent/50 percent.[272, 273] In addition, intrathyroidal B cells are predominantly of the IgG-kappa subclass.[107, 153, 311] Intrathyroidal secretion of autoantibodies appears likely.[48, 193, 194] Stuart identified fuchsinophilic material within follicular centers in Hashimoto's disease and considered it immunoglobulin.[261]

Immunologic studies have demonstrated that in autoimmune thyroiditis there is no generalized defect in T lymphocyte function.[151, 273, 277] T lymphocytes within the thyroid in patients with chronic lymphocytic thyroiditis are predominantly of suppressor type, whereas the peripheral blood of these patients contains mostly helper T cells. In addition, the suppressor T cells demonstrated cytolytic activity *in vitro*, suggesting that these cells may determine in part the tissue damage seen in this disease,[67] although these studies await further confirmation.[234]

Fibrous Variant

The fibrous or fibrosing variant of Hashimoto's thyroiditis, discussed in Chapter 7, constitutes 10 to 13 percent of cases, and often affects elderly patients who present with symptomatic goiters and hypothyroidism.[107, 148] Pathologically, the thyroid architecture is destroyed with severe follicular atrophy, dense keloid-like fibrosis, and prominent squamous or epidermoid metaplasia of the follicular epithelium.

Fibrous Atrophy

The gland of idiopathic myxedema is tiny, often 2 to 5 grams and usually barely identifiable as thyroid grossly or microscopically. Destruction of the thyroid parenchyma and replacement by fibrosis, and lymphocytic infiltrate are prominent. "Squamous" metaplasia of follicles is seen as well, although this change may reflect not a true metaplasia but hyperplasia of ultimobranchial body rests. (See Chapter 7.) The relationship between the fibrous variant of Hashimoto's thyroiditis characterized by a large goiter and fibrous atrophy remains unclear.[148] Both affect elderly individuals (fibrous atrophy more commonly is seen in women), who manifest severe hypothyroidism; antithyroid antibody titers are markedly elevated in both. Histologically, considerable similarities also exist (follicular atrophy, fibrosis, "squamous" metaplasia). Whether the ratios of different functional classes of immunoglobulins alone can produce the noted differences between the two disorders remains to be defined.[69, 70]

Juvenile Form

The so-called juvenile form of lymphocytic thyroiditis differs from the other types pathologically since follicular atrophy and oxyphilic metaplasia are focal or absent. Indeed, hyperplastic epithelial changes may be seen and in some patients, frank hyperthyroidism can be noted.[70, 97, 98, 118, 222, 308] The disease may remit, recur, or eventuate in hypothyroidism.

The similarity of the histologic changes to "Hashitoxicosis" is noteworthy (see below).[85, 122, 181, 237]

Painless Thyroiditis with Hyperthyroidism

Although initially considered a form of subacute thyroiditis, clinical, immunologic, and pathologic studies have firmly placed this disorder in the autoimmune group.[54, 59, 77, 86, 96, 117, 134, 137, 138, 199, 226, 250, 264, 269, 280, 284, 307] Virtually all morphologic studies have been based on needle biopsies of affected glands.[97, 126, 199, 236, 293, 306] Initially, it was felt that since lymphocytes are a component of granulomatous thyroiditis and since giant cells may be missed due to sampling problems, these patients still might be suffering from a form of granulomatous thyroiditis. (Needle biopsies of patients with clinically characteristic granulomatous thyroiditis often demonstrate granulomatous inflammation with giant cells.) However, over the past decade biopsies have been performed on many patients with painless thyroiditis, and the histologic appearance is uniformly that of lymphocytic infiltration of the thyroid with focal oxyphilic epithelial changes and/or focal epithelial hyperplasia.[126, 209, 236]

The most systematic study published on the morphology of the thyroid in this disorder is that of Mizukami et al.[199] Twenty-six biopsies from 23 patients were analyzed; all show follicular disruption and lymphocytic thyroiditis; stromal fibrous and oxyphilic changes were rare. Subset analysis of the intrathyroidal lymphocytes showed similarities to Hashimoto's thyroiditis.[77] In this study, three patients underwent repeat biopsy after clinical recovery; histologic resolution of the lesion was seen.

Hence, the morphologic evidence supports clinical, immunologic, and follow-up data for categorizing "painless thyroiditis" in the spectrum of autoimmune disorders. Ultimate prognosis appears to vary; chronicity and permanent hypothyroidism may occur but are unusual.

Other Variants

"Hashitoxicosis" or "Hyperthyroiditis." In 1971, Fatourecki et al. described patients with hyperthyroidism and pathological features of Hashimoto's disease.[85] Since that time the term Hashitoxicosis or hyperthyroiditis has been employed to refer to this disorder. The Mayo Clinic authors[85] defined three subsets:

- Group 1 included nine individuals, ages 38 to 65 (male:female—2:7) who had clinical and laboratory evidence of classic Graves' disease. On examination of their resected glands the histologic changes of Hashimoto's thyroiditis were recognized: lymphoid infiltration, oxyphilic epithelium, and follicular atrophy.
- Group 2 was composed of five subjects (ages 14 to 54, male:female—1:4) who showed clinical Graves' disease but whose thyroids demonstrated lymphocytic infiltration and focal epithelial hyperplasia. Hürthle cells were found rarely.
- Group 3 included ten women (ages 15 to 63) with clinical Graves' disease and pathologic evidence of both epithelial hyperplasia and marked lymphoid infiltration.

Certainly some of these patients would fall within the juvenile thyroiditis group (group 2) and/or the "painless thyroiditis" category (groups 1 and 3). These patients form a peculiar subgroup of those with autoimmune thyroid disease and lend support to Volpe's theory of a relationship between Graves' and Hashimoto's diseases.[291]

Lymphoma-like Thyroiditis. Woolner et al.[308, 309] described this variant of Hashimoto's which can produce difficulty for the histopathologist, since the lymphocytic infiltrate may mimic malignant lymphoma. This variant constitutes less than 1 percent of cases and affects primarily elderly women.[123] The presence of thyroid follicles and the reactive nature of the lymphoid centers, with a pleomorphic cell population of various types of lymphocytes and macrophages, serves to distinguish this lesion from true malignant lymphoma.[124] (See also Chapter 14.)

Focal "Nonspecific" Thyroiditis. Lymphocytic infiltration of the thyroid is found more frequently at autopsy and in surgical specimens since the addition of iodide to the water supplies of the United States about 60 years ago.[110–112, 163, 296] Iodide (iodine) may act as a hapten that combines with a protein, then acts as an antigen and evokes an immune response localized to the thyroid gland.

Do these lymphocytic infiltrates share the definition of autoimmune thyroiditis?[19] Clinically, this focal lesion is seen in older patients, without symptoms; low levels of antithyroid antibodies are found.[163, 247, 303] The incidence of this lesion parallels that of antithyroid antibodies in the general population.[69, 123, 163, 223, 238] Nodules resembling nodular or adenomatous goiter may be noted.[19]

Pathologically, no gross lesions are seen except if nodules are present. Microscopically, focal aggregates of lymphocytes are seen; occasionally germinal center formation is noted, and (rarely) oncocytes are present. The infiltrates occupy fibrous septa of the gland and spare any adenomatous nodules that may be present (Fig. 5–6). Follicular atrophy is rare.[163, 303]

Postmortem studies indicate an incidence of focal lymphocytic thyroiditis of about 15 to 20 percent,[163] but this may be higher depending on the population.[112] Women are affected more often than men. Kurashima and Hirokawa believe that focal lymphocytic infiltration of the thyroid represents an immunologic disorder associated with aging.[163] The female predominance may indicate a role for specific hormonal factors as well.

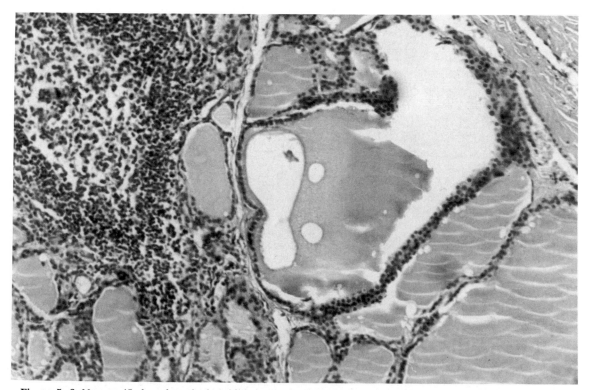

Figure 5–6. Nonspecific lymphocytic thyroiditis is seen in thyroid lobe removed for benign adenomatous follicular nodule; note lymphoid aggregate and early germinal center formation at left. × 150, H & E.

Other Entities with Lymphocytes in the Thyroid

Considered Autoimmune

Diffuse Toxic Goiter. Lymphoid infiltration, sometimes associated with follicular center formation, are often seen in patients with classic hyperthyroid Graves' disease.[100, 223] Usually the lymphoid cells are strewn in the interfollicular stroma and do not encroach on the follicles themselves (Figs. 5–7 and 5–8). The follicles show marked epithelial hyperplasia (unless presurgical iodide treatment has been administered). Plasma cells are rare in Graves' as contrasted to Hashimoto's disease.[272] Fibrosis is unusual, as is oxyphilia unless the Graves' disease is of long standing. (See also Chapters 8 and 9.)

Toxic Nodular Goiter. In glands with hyperfunctioning follicular nodules ("adenomas") lymphocytic collections can be seen, usually outside the capsule of the nodule. The immunopathogenetic mechanisms in this disorder or group of disorders are less well defined than those in classic Graves' disease.[102, 262] (See Chapter 9.)

Of Questionable Autoimmune Etiology

Nontoxic Nodular Goiter. Focal lymphocytic infiltration, usually without follicular center formation, is seen often in areas of hemorrhage and repair in nodular goiter. Whether these lymphocytes represent an immunologic response is unclear; abnormalities of T and B cell ratios and function have not been identified.[136]

Radiation-Associated Thyroiditis. Lymphocytic infiltration, fibrosis, follicular atrophy, and oxyphilic metaplasia can all be found in thyroids that have received low-dose external radiation. The morphologic picture resembles that of autoimmune thyroiditis and may represent reaction (autoimmunity) to release of thyroid antigens owing to the radiodestructive effects. (See Chapter 6.)

Drug-Associated Thyroiditis. Many drugs may alter thyroid function or, at least, interfere with laboratory thyroid function tests, but few have been implicated in the production of thyroiditis. Hence, "chemical hypothyroidism" has been associated with long-term use of such common drugs as thiazides, sulfonamides, and sulfonylureas.[44, 197] Drugs that may interfere with thyroid function tests include oral contraceptives, salicylates, steroids, and iodine-containing compounds such as radiographic dyes. Patients taking such medications may be euthyroid but laboratory tests will be abnormal. The histopathologic changes in the thyroids of these patients must be minimal or nonexistent since normal thyroid function is restored following discontinuance of the drug.

When considering drugs that may actually affect thyroid function and/or morphology, i.e., induce thyroiditis, the question that always must be considered is whether the drug is disclosing a preexisting subclinical thyroid disease.

However, several factors need to be considered. That use of a particular drug may change the incidence of lymphocytic thyroiditis cannot be assumed without substantial proof. Many environmental, therapeutic, and nutritional alterations have taken place over the last half-century; a particular drug may be the scapegoat. In addition, increased background radiation, widespread use of various agents (for medicinal or other purposes), and the addition of preservatives to food—these are but a few of the possibilities that need to be considered when related to changes in thyroid histopathology. Increasingly common use of biopsy and cytologic examination of the thyroid gland might also influence incidence rates.

However, the answer to the question of whether an etiologic relationship exists between an ingested drug and thyroiditis appears to be affirmative. The magnitude of this problem remains unknown.

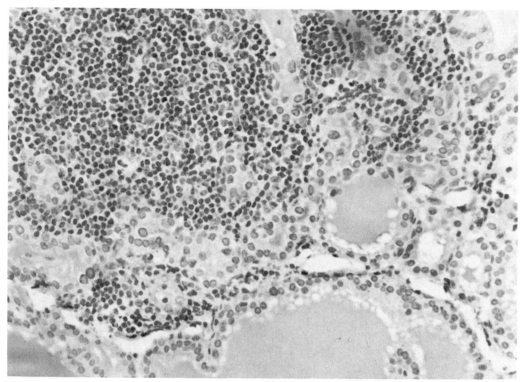

Figure 5–7. Lymphoid cells infiltrate stroma in hyperthyroidism; note hyperplasia of epithelium and scalloping of colloid (lower half). Diffuse toxic goiter. × 200, H & E.

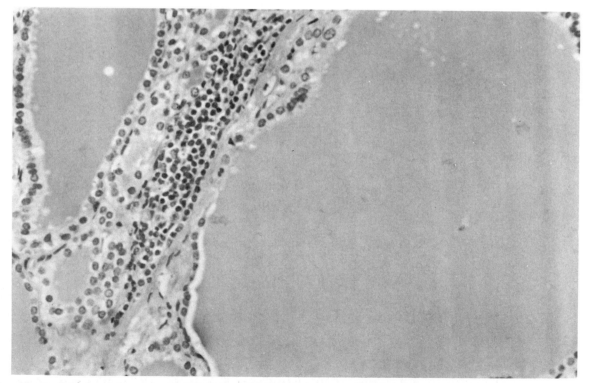

Figure 5–8. In another case, hyperplastic epithelium is seen in dilated follicle. Note lymphocytes in stroma "hugging" the follicle. Diffuse toxic goiter, partially treated with iodide. × 150, H & E.

The following discussion will describe the reported thyroiditis-associated drug reactions: lithium, phenytoin (diphenylhydantoin), iodides, and amiodarone. The list is certainly not all-inclusive, but does include those drugs most often implicated in the development of clinical thyroiditis.

Lithium. Lithium salts have been used for many years as therapy for manic and hypomanic states. The mode of action of lithium is as yet unclear,[251] but most hypotheses have suggested an effect of the lithium ion on cell membranes.

In experimental situations, lithium can interfere with accumulation of iodine, with iodination and release of iodinated tyrosine, and possibly with the actions of thyroid-stimulating hormone.[18, 28]

Goiter develops commonly in patients treated for prolonged periods with lithium salts;[165, 233, 249] hypothyroidism occurs in 3 to 12 percent of such cases. Perrild et al. described two patients without goiter who became irreversibly myxedematous following prolonged lithium carbonate intake.[216] Although histologic evidence was lacking, these authors postulated that fibrosis of the thyroid may occur. The present author has studied two patients with lithium-associated thyroiditis. Lymphocytic infiltration, focal follicular atrophy and mild degrees of stromal fibrosis were seen. The histologic picture was consistent with that seen in autoimmune thyroiditis. Baldessanni and Lipinski noted that most patients, when initially exposed to lithium ion, develop transiently decreased free thyroxine.[18] A small number of patients develop goiter, a few develop hypothyroidism, and rarely both occur. Occasional patients manifest hyperthyroidism.[190, 242] Most patients with thyroid dysfunction demonstrate antithyroid antibodies.[46, 139, 190] Which individuals will develop thyroid abnormalities cannot be predicted; women are more frequently affected than men.[18]

Why are certain individuals affected? Is it a genetic tendency perhaps related to HLA subtype? Is there a direct toxic effect of lithium on the thyroid? Do some individuals have an underlying subclinical thyroid abnormality?[45, 46] The answers are unknown at the present time.

Diphenylhydantoin (phenytoin) has been used to treat epileptic disorders for over 50 years. Side effects include metabolic and endocrine dysfunctions and idiosyncratic reactions.[95, 106] Phenytoin has been shown to compete with thyroxine for thyroxine-binding globulin binding sites.[214] It also decreases T_4 production.[78, 201]

Kuiper described a young woman who developed lymphocytic thyroiditis while taking diphenylhydantoin.[162] This patient developed a skin rash and fever three weeks after beginning therapy; the drug was withdrawn. She was rechallenged with the therapy; fever and the skin rash recurred. Lymphadenopathy, thyroidomegaly, lymphocytosis, neutropenia, and eosinophilia were noted. Thyroid function tests included elevated protein-bound iodine and thyroxine resin uptake but antibodies to thyroid cells and thyroglobulin were not identified. Biopsy demonstrated lymphocytic infiltration, follicular atrophy, and slight fibrosis, suggestive of Hashimoto's thyroiditis. Following cessation of diphenylhydantoin, the patient recovered; thyroid size and function tests reverted to normal. However, two years later the patient's serum demonstrated cytotoxic antibodies to thyroid epithelial cell fractions.

Kuiper considered the drug to be related to the thyroiditis.[162] Although the temporal associations are impressive, no proof of reversion of thyroid histology is given; the pre-drug status of the thyroid was not ascertained.

Diphenylhydantoin-induced thyroiditis is an example of an idiosyncratic reaction. That this drug can produce changes in the immune system has been adequately documented.[71, 93] Hypersensitivity reactions and lymphoproliferative disorders described as pseudolymphoma, immunoblastic lymphadenopathy, and immunoblastic sarcomas have been reported. The occurrence of these phenomena cannot be predicted.

In immunoblastic lymphadenopathy,[71, 177] the postulated mechanism includes a hyperimmune proliferation of B cells resulting from impaired suppressor T cell regulation, i.e., an autoimmune reaction. Hence it is possible that in Kuiper's patient and other patients reported[164, 210] a similar sequence of events took place, i.e., diphenylhydantoin evoked an "autoimmune" reaction, with the thyroid as the target organ. The development and persistence of thyroid cytotoxic antibody support this possibility.

Iodide. The incidence of lymphocytic thyroiditis has been increasing since the 1930's. Several authors postulate that the addition of iodide to the diet (e.g., iodized salt and flour), which occurred around 1925 to 1930 in the United States, might somehow be causative.[24] Volpe noted that the incidence of clinically overt lymphocytic thyroiditis (Hashimoto's thyroiditis) has risen tenfold since 1935;[287] the increase of the occult form is unknown. A report from Japan also links iodine ingestion to the development of thyroiditis; in a study of 10,000 children (ages 6 to 18), the incidence of biopsy-proven lymphocytic thyroiditis was 5.3 per 1000 in a high-iodine area compared to 1.4 per 1000 in a low-iodine zone.[129]

Braverman et al. found patients with Hashimoto's disease more susceptible to iodine-induced hypothyroidism than controls.[38] Volpe suggests that the patients with chronic lymphocytic thyroiditis show extreme sensitivity to iodine;[287] the latter may unmask the thyroiditis, rather than cause it.

The addition of iodine as iodate to bread in Tasmania produced overt hyperthyroidism in individuals with a latent form of thyrotoxicosis. Eighty percent of these patients developed thyroid autoantibodies.[56] Hyperthyroidism may result when iodide is added to the diet of patients with endemic or sporadic goiter.[56, 278] In these studies, the effect of the iodine has been superimposed upon an abnormal (at least physiologically) gland, either one that is iodine-deficient or one in which autonomous nodules are present.

Patients with chronic lymphocytic thyroiditis or treated Graves' disease show exquisite sensitivity to iodine, and hypothyroidism occurs readily with small doses. Wolff notes that subjects with minor disturbances of thyroid function tend to be more sensitive to iodine.[304]

Amiodarone. The antiarrythmic drug, amiodarone, is structurally an iodinated benzofuran derivative which has been linked to a variety of toxic side effects, including pulmonary toxicity.[183, 220] Pathologic changes include the finding of foamy inclusions in lung macrophages, lymph nodes, skin, leukocytes, and Kupffer cells in the liver. Ultrastructural studies have disclosed abnormal lysosomal inclusions of whorled lamellar bodies.[60] Dake et al. consider the amiodarone toxicity as an acquired systemic lysosomal storage disease.[60] Discontinuation of the drug often reverses the toxic reaction.

Thyroid functional abnormalities have been recognized in patients taking amiodarone.[8, 9, 35, 91, 92, 103, 115, 144, 185, 188, 220, 302] These derangements range from myxedema to frank hyperthyroidism; Alves et al. reported a 32 percent incidence of hypothyroidism and 23 percent of hyperthyroidism in 104 patients on chronic amiodarone treatment.[8] The mechanism of these effects include elevated thyronine (T_4) with or without elevated thyrotropin (TSH), normal T_4 but elevated TSH, or decreased T_4 levels.[35] It has been suggested that the iodinated drug interferes in an as yet unknown manner with thyroid hormone metabolism, production, or degradation.[35] However, Rabinowe et al. recently defined abnormalities in T lymphocyte function in hyperthyroid patients taking amiodarone.[220] Six of their 10 patients had significant titers of antithyroid (antimicrosomal and/or antithyroglobulin) antibodies. These authors suggest that in susceptible individuals, amiodarone induces an organ-specific, i.e., thyroid-specific, autoimmune reaction and leads to hyperthyroidism.

Smyrk et al. describe the pathologic findings in hyperthyroid patients on amiodarone.[253] Antithyroid antibodies were not present. The histologic changes included follicular damage and disruption, epithelial cell vacuolization, and macrophagic and lymphocytic reaction to degeneration follicles. By electron microscopy, a few lysosomes in the vacuolated cells showed the characteristic lamellar configuration previously described in the lung.[60, 183] The Mayo Clinic group postulated that the hyperthyroidism was produced by release of stored colloid from destroyed follicles, akin to the hyperthyroidism of granulomatous thyroiditis. Of interest is that Alves et al. indicated that in their hyperthyroid group of patients radioiodine uptake was low,[8] again resembling the result in granulomatous thyroiditis.

The mechanism(s) of hyper- and hypothyroidism may vary in these patients—some being related to pharmacologic mechanisms of interference with thyroid hormone metabolism, some "autoimmune," and some via thyroid destruction.

Peritumor Thyroiditis. The histologic finding of chronic thyroiditis in patients with thyroid carcinoma, chiefly papillary or mixed papillary-follicular type, has produced confusion regarding both the significance of this thyroiditis and the potential of chronic thyroiditis in general as a premalignant lesion.

The histopathologist encounters scattered lymphocytic and even mixed lymphocytic-plasmacytic infiltrates at the periphery of a thyroid neoplasm frequently. Especially in the vicinity of the infiltrative edges of the most common thyroid carcinoma, papillary cancer, this lymphoid infiltrate is found in the majority of cases.[21, 69, 70, 259, 309] (See Chapter 8.) Some authors have considered thyroiditis as a preneoplastic or predisposing condition and have advocated surgery for it. Others consider surgical intervention important if a patient with known thyroiditis develops a mass.[113, 170] Of course, cytologic evaluation of such a mass may be diagnostic and either prevent the need for surgery or allow for planning operative strategy.[16, 224]

The incidence of coexistent tumor thyroiditis and papillary cancer is unknown; since both are common thyroid lesions, their coexistence may be only fortuitous. However, when one recognizes the thyroiditis changes solely in the vicinity of the tumor with sparing of the noninvolved gland, speculation arises regarding an interrelationship. Volpe suggests the lymphoid infiltrate results from a "local antigenic perturbation" to altered antigen on the tumor cells.[289]

Rarely, a thyroid cancer may be associated with an extensive thyroiditis. Thus, the histopathology of full-blown, classic Hashimoto's disease with lymphoplasmacytic infiltrates, the formation of germinal centers, and follicular atrophy with Hürthle cell metaplasia may be found in a gland also containing a neoplasm. Indeed, the lymphoid infiltrate may become intimately admixed with the tumor, so that it involves even the fibrovascular cores of tumor papillae as well as the peripheral edge of the tumor, and even the entire gland.

It is florid cases of tumor-associated thyroiditis that have produced controversy regarding the premalignant potential of Hashimoto's disease. (See Chapter 14 for discussion of thyroiditis and lymphoma.)

Hypothyroidism Associated with Interleukin-2 (IL2) and Lymphokine-Activated Killer (LAK) Cell Treatment. Atkins et al. described hypothyroidism occurring in several patients receiving IL2 and LAK cell therapy for advanced cancers.[13] Chemical evidence of hypothyroidism with elevated antimicrosomal antibody titers was found. These authors postulated that the hypothyroidism may have been caused by unmasking subclinical autoimmune thyroiditis; the hypothyroidism appeared associated with a favorable tumor response in these patients.

Non-Autoimmune Thyroid Lesions with Lymphocytes

Subacute Granulomatous Thyroiditis. (See Chapter 4.) Lymphocytes can be a prominent morphologic component of granulomatous thyroiditis, especially in some stages of the disease. However, immunopathologic analysis indicates intrathyroidal ratios of lymphocytes similar to those in normal peripheral blood.[130, 271, 295]

Riedel's Disease. Lymphocytes and plasma cells are a frequent component of the fibrous proliferation of Riedel's disease. The immunopathologic differences between the infiltrating cells in this condition and Hashimoto's disease are discussed in Chapter 7.

Healing Phases of Acute Thyroiditis, Post-traumatic or Surgical Injury. The inflammatory process accompanying healing can contain lymphocytes. The associated inflammatory cells of various types and granulation tissue serve to distinguish these processes. Of course, knowledge of the clinical circumstances is also useful.

Ultimobranchial Body Rest. Embryologic remnants of the fifth branchial pouch may be seen in the lateral portions of the gland. The epithelial nests may sometimes be associated with mature small lymphocytes. (See Chapter 1.)

Thymus/Thymoma. Occasionally, during embryologic development, remnants of thymus (epithelium and lymphocytes) can be contained within the thyroid. (See Chapter 1.) Very rare instances of cervical thymoma clinically presenting as a thyroid nodule are recorded. (See Chapter 15.)

Probable Branchial Cleft Remnants. Louis et al. reported two patients with Hashimoto's thyroiditis in which gross cysts were present.[175] These cysts were lined focally by respiratory epithelium and contained abundant lymphoid tissue in their walls. The authors postulated a developmental origin for the cysts.

Malignant Lymphoma. Malignant lymphoma of any histologic type and immunophenotype may arise primarily in the thyroid.[124] In most if not all cases, the lymphoma arises on an immunologically abnormal gland, i.e., one affected by chronic lymphocytic thyroiditis.

Patients with systemic malignant lymphoma may have thyroid involvement; usually the gland is otherwise histologically normal. These neoplasms are discussed in Chapter 14.

Autoimmune Thyroid Disease: In Search of a Reason

The spectrum of autoimmune thyroid disease ranges from severe myxedema to life-threatening hyperthyroidism, from severe thyroid atrophy to huge goiters. The age range of affected patients is from childhood to very old. Why is the spectrum of autoimmune disease so broad?

Recent research has begun to provide some clues to explain the wide range of symptom complexes. Studies on the function of immunoglobulins present in autoimmune thyroid disease have indicated that subgroups of these immunoglobulins (Igs) affect different aspects of the thyrotropin receptor.[73, 89, 146, 154, 279] Thus, some Igs stimulate growth, or function; others are blocking factors, suppressing growth and/or function. Hence, the myriad clinical syndromes may be produced by differing ratios of the antibody subgroups; i.e., in hyperthyroid Graves' disease the predominant Igs would stimulate both growth and function, whereas in atrophic thyroiditis, blocking effects would be noted.

This explanation seems too simplistic, and probably is, to explain this complex group of diseases; it is presented here as at least a point from which to begin understanding these disorders.

This chapter has reviewed those lesions of the thyroid gland whose morphologic expressions include the presence of lymphocytes. A brief overview of autoimmunity specifically applied to the thyroid is included.

REFERENCES

1. Adams, D.D., and Knight, J.G.: H gene theory of inherited autoimmune disease. Lancet *1:*396–398, 1980.
2. Adams, D.D., and Purves, H.D.: The role of thyrotropin in hyperthyroidism and exophthalmos. Metabolism *6:*26–35, 1957.
3. Ahmann, A.J., and Burman, K.D.: The role of T lymphocytes in autoimmune thyroid disease. Endocrinol. Metab. Clin. N. Amer. *16:*287–326, 1987.
4. Aho, K., Gordin, A., et al.: Development of thyroid autoimmunity. Acta Endocrinol. *108:*61–64, 1985.
5. Aichinger, G., Fill, H., and Wick, G.: In-situ immune complexes, lymphocyte subpopulations, and HLA-DR-positive epithelial cells in Hashimoto thyroiditis. Lab. Invest. *52:*132–140, 1985.
6. Allison, A.C.: Self-tolerance and autoimmunity in the thyroid. N. Engl. J. Med. *295:*821–827, 1976.
7. Allison, A.C.: Autoimmune disease: concepts of pathogenesis and control. *In:* Talal, N. (ed.): Autoimmunity. New York, Academic Press, 1977, pp. 91–139.
8. Alves, L.E., Rose, E.P., and Cahill, T.B.: Amiodarone and the thyroid. Ann. Intern. Med. *102:*412, 1985.
9. Amico, J.A., Richardson, V., et al.: Clinical and chemical assessment of thyroid function during therapy with amiodarone. Arch. Intern. Med. *144:*487–490, 1984.
10. Amino, N., Miyai, K., et al.: Transient postpartum hypothyroidism: fourteen cases with autoimmune thyroiditis. Ann. Intern. Med. *87:*155–159, 1977.
11. Amino, N., Mori, H., et al.: High prevalence of transient postpartum thyrotoxicosis and hypothyroidism. N. Engl. J. Med. *306:*849–852, 1982.
12. Arikawa, K., Ichikawa, Y., et al.: Blocking type antithyrotropin receptor antibody in patients with nongoitrous hypothyroidism: Its incidence and characteristics of action. J. Clin. Endocrinol. Metab. *60:*953–959, 1985.
13. Atkins, M.B., Mier, J.W., et al.: Hypothyroidism after treatment with interleukin-2 and lymphokine-activated killer cells. N. Engl. J. Med. *318:*1557–1563, 1988.
14. Bagchi, N., Brown, T.R., et al.: Induction of autoimmune thyroiditis in chickens by dietary iodine. Science *230:*325–327, 1985.
15. Bagnasco, M., Ferrini, S., et al.: Clonal analysis of T lymphocytes infiltrating the thyroid gland in Hashimoto's thyroiditis. Int. Arch. Allergy Appl. Immunol. *82:*141–146, 1987.
16. Baker, B.A., Gharib, H., and Markowitz, H.: Correlation of thyroid antibodies and cytologic features in suspected autoimmune thyroid disease. Am. J. Med. *74:*941–944, 1983.
17. Baker, J.R., Saunders, N.B., et al.: Seronegative Hashimoto thyroiditis with thyroid autoantibody production localized to the thyroid. Ann. Intern. Med. *108:*26–30, 1988.
18. Baldessanni, R.J., and Lipinski, J.F.: Lithium salts: 1970–1975. Ann. Intern. Med. *83:*527–533, 1975.
19. Bastenie, P.A., Bonnyns, M., and Vanhaelst, L.: Grades of subclinical hypothyroidism in asymptomatic autoimmune thyroiditis revealed by the thyrotropin-releasing hormone test. J. Clin. Endocrinol. Metab. *51:*163–166, 1980.
20. Bastenie, P.A., Bonnyns, M., and Vanhaelst, L.: Natural history of primary myxedema. Am. J. Med. *79:*91–100, 1985.
21. Bastenie, P.A., and Ermans, A.M.: Thyroiditis and Thyroid Function: Clinical, Morphological and Physiopathological Studies. Oxford, Pergamon Press, 1972.
22. Bech, K., Bliddal, H., et al.: Heterogeneity of autoimmune thyroiditis. Allergy *39:*239–247, 1984.
23. Bech, K., and Madsen, S.N.: Thyroid adenylate cyclase stimulating immunoglobulins in thyroid diseases. Clin. Endocrinol. *11:*47–58, 1979.
24. Bcierwaltes, W.H.: Iodine and lymphocytic thyroiditis. Bull. All India Inst. Med. Sci. *3:*145–151, 1969.
25. Bendtzen, K.: Immune hormones (cytokines); pathogenic role in autoimmune rheumatic and endocrine diseases. Autoimmunity *2:*177–189, 1989.
26. Benveniste, P., Row, V.V., and Volpe, R.: Studies on the immunoregulation of thyroid autoantibody production in vitro. Clin. Exp. Immunol. *61:*274–282, 1985.
27. Benveniste, P., Wenzel, B.E., et al.: Spontaneous secretion of thyroid autoantibodies by cultured peripheral blood lymphocytes from patients with Hashimoto's thyroiditis detected by micro-ELISA techniques. Clin. Exp. Immunol. *58:*273–282, 1984.

28. Berens, S.C., Bernstein, R.S., et al.: Antithyroid effects of lithium. J. Clin. Invest. *49:*1357–1367, 1970.
29. Bialas, P., Marks, S., et al.: Hashimoto's thyroiditis presenting as a solitary functioning thyroid nodule. J. Clin. Endocrinol. Metab. *43:*1365–1369, 1976.
30. Bigos, S.T., Hindson, D., and McCallum, J.: Serum thyroid-stimulating hormone and antimicrosomal antibodies as a screen for autoimmune thyroid disease. J. Lab. Clin. Med. *93:*1035–1040, 1979.
31. Biorklund, A., and Soderstrom, N.: Human autoimmune thyroiditis. Acta Otolaryngol. *82:*204–207, 1976.
32. Bliddal, H., Bech, K., et al.: Thyroid-stimulating immunoglobulins in Hashimoto's thyroiditis measured by radioreceptor assay and adenylate cyclase stimulation and their relationship to HLA-D alleles. J. Clin. Endocrinol. Metab. *55:*995–998, 1982.
33. Bogner, U., Schleusner, H., and Wall, J.R.: Antibody-dependent cell mediated cytotoxicity against human thyroid cells in Hashimoto's thyroiditis but not Graves' disease. J. Clin. Endocrinol. Metab. *59:*734–738, 1984.
34. Bonnyns, M., Bentin, J., et al.: Heterogeneity of immunoregulatory T cells in human thyroid autoimmunity: influence of thyroid status. Clin. Exp. Immunol. *52:*629–634, 1983.
35. Borowski, G.D., Garofano, C.D., et al.: Effect of long-term amiodarone therapy on thyroid hormone levels and thyroid function. Am. J. Med. *78:*443–450, 1985.
36. Bottazzo, G.F., and Doniach, D.: Autoimmune thyroid disease. Annu. Rev. Med. *37:*353–359, 1986.
37. Bottazzo, G.F., Pujol-Borrell, R., et al.: Role of aberrant HLA-DR expression and antigen presentation in induction of endocrine autoimmunity. Lancet *2:*1115–1118, 1983.
38. Braverman, L.E., Ingbar, S.H., et al.: Enhanced susceptibility to iodine myxedema in patients with Hashimoto's disease. J. Clin. Endocrinol. Metab. *32:*515–521, 1971.
39. Bremner, W.J., and Griep, R.J.: Graves thyrotoxicosis following primary thyroid failure. J.A.M.A. *235:*1361, 1976.
40. Brody, J., and Greenberg, S.: Lymphocyte dysfunction in thyrotoxicosis. J. Clin. Endocrinol. Metab. *35:*574–579, 1972.
41. Brown, J., Solomon, D.H., et al.: Autoimmune thyroid diseases—Graves' and Hashimoto's. Ann. Intern. Med. *88:*379–391, 1978.
42. Buckingham, B.A., Costin, G., et al.: Pathologic and immune factors in thyroid disease. J. Pediat. *91:*728–733, 1977.
43. Burke, G.: The cell membrane: a common site of action of thyrotropin (TSH) and long-acting thyroid stimulator (LATS). Metabolism *18:*720–729, 1969.
44. Burke, G., Silverstein, G.E., and Sorkin, A.I.: Effect of long-term sulfonylurea therapy on thyroid function in man. Metabolism *16:*651–657, 1967.
45. Burman, K.D., Demond, R.C., et al.: Sensitivity to lithium in treated Graves' disease: effects on serum T_4, T_3 and reverse T_3. J. Clin. Endocrinol. Metab. *43:*606–613, 1976.
46. Calabrese, J.R., Gulledge, A.D., et al.: Autoimmune thyroiditis in manic-depressive patients treated with lithium. Am. J. Psychiatry *142:*1318–1321, 1985.
47. Calder, E.A., Penhale, W.J., et al.: Evidence for circulating immune complexes in thyroid disease. Br. Med. J. *2:*30–31, 1974.
48. Canonica, G.W., Bagnasco, M., et al.: Why thyroid is major site of thyroid auto-antibody synthesis in autoimmune thyroid disease. Lancet *1:*1163, 1983.
49. Canonica, G.W., Caria, M., et al.: Proliferation of T8-positive cytolytic T lymphocytes in response to thyroglobulin in human autoimmune thyroiditis: analysis of cell interactions and culture requirements. Clin. Immunol. Immunopathol. *36:*40–48, 1985.
50. Canonica, G.W., Cosulich, M.E., et al.: Thyroglobulin-induced T-cell *in vitro* proliferation in Hashimoto's thyroiditis: identification of the responsive subset and effect of monoclonal antibodies directed to Ia antigens. Clin. Immunol. Immunopathol. *32:*132–141, 1984.
51. Carey, C., Skosey, C., et al.: Thyroid abnormalities in children of parents who have Graves' disease: possible pre-Graves' disease. Metabolism *29:*369–376, 1980.
52. Carpenter, C.C.J., Solomon, N., et al.: Schmidt's syndrome (thyroid and adrenal insufficiency): a review of the literature and a report of fifteen new cases including ten instances of coexistent diabetes mellitus. Medicine *43:*153–180, 1964.
53. Chan, J.Y.C., and Walfish, P.G.: Activated (Ia^+) T-lymphocytes and their subsets in autoimmune thyroid diseases: analysis by dual laser flow microfluorocytometry. J. Clin. Endocrinol. Metab. *62:*403–409, 1986.
54. Check, J.H., and Avellino, J.: Painless thyroiditis and transient thyrotoxicosis after Graves' disease. J.A.M.A. *244:*1361, 1980.
55. Christy, J.H., and Morse, R.S.: Hypothyroid Graves' disease. Am. J. Med. *62:*291–296, 1977.
56. Connolly, R.J., Vidor, G.I., and Stewart, J.C.: Increase in thyrotoxicosis in endemic goiter area after iodation of bread. Lancet *1:*500–502, 1970.
57. Cooke, A., Rayner, D., and Lydyard, P.: Autoimmune disorders. Immunol. Today *7:*325–327, 1986.
58. Cunningham-Rundles, S.: Approaches to the study of human immunoregulation. Immunol. Today *6:*251–254, 1985.
59. Dahlberg, P.A., and Jansson, R.: Different aetiologies in post-partum thyroiditis? Acta Endocrinol. *104:*195–200, 1983.

60. Dake, M.D., Madison, J.M., et al.: Electron microscopic demonstration of lysosomal inclusion bodies in lung, liver, lymph nodes and blood leukocytes of patients with amiodarone pulmonary toxicity. Am. J. Med. *78:*506–512, 1985.

61. Damante, G., Foti, D., et al.: Desensitization of the thyroid cyclic AMP response to thyroid stimulating immunoglobulin: comparison with TSH. Metabolism *36:*768–773, 1987.

62. Davies, T.F.: Cocultures of human thyroid monolayer cells and autologous T cells: impact of HLA Class II antigen expression. J. Clin. Endocrinol. Metab. *61:*418–422, 1985.

63. Davies, T.F., and Piccinini, L.A.: Intrathyroidal MHC Class II antigen expression and thyroid autoimmunity. Endocrinol. Metab. Clin. N. Amer. *16:*247–268, 1987.

64. Davies, T.F., Weber, C.M., et al.: Restricted hereterogeneity and T cell dependence of human thyroid autoantibody immunoglobulin G subclasses. J. Clin. Endocrinol. Metab. *62:*945–949, 1986.

65. DeBernardo, E., and Davies, T.F.: Antigen presentation in human autoimmune thyroid disease. Exp. Cell Biol. *54:*155–162, 1986.

66. Deboel, S., Bonnyns, M., et al.: Thyroid hormone reserve in asymptomatic autoimmune thyroiditis. Acta Endocrinol. *114:*336–339, 1987.

67. DelPrete, G.F., Maggi, E., et al.: Cytolytic T lymphocytes with natural killer activity in thyroid infiltrates of patients with Hashimoto's thyroiditis: analysis at clonal level. J. Clin. Endocrinol. Metab. *62:*52–57, 1986.

68. Doniach, D.: How thyroid autoimmunity was discovered: reminiscences of an autoimmunologist. *In:* Walfish, P.G., Wall, J.R., and Volpe, R. (eds.): Autoimmunity and the Thyroid. Orlando, Academic Press, 1985, pp. 1–8.

69. Doniach, D., Bottazzo, G.F., and Russell, R.C.G.: Goitrous autoimmune thyroiditis (Hashimoto's disease). Clin. Endocrinol. Metab. *8:*63–80, 1979.

70. Doniach, D., and Roitt, I.M.: Autoimmune thyroid disease. *In:* Miescher, P.A., and Muller-Eberhard, H.J. (eds.): Textbook of Immunopathology. New York, Grune and Stratton, 1976, pp. 715–735.

71. Dorfman, R.F., and Warnke, R.: Lymphadenopathy simulating malignant lymphoma. Hum. Pathol. *5:*519–534, 1974.

72. Dorfman, S.G., Cooperman, M.T., et al.: Painless thyroiditis and transient hyperthyroidism without goiter. Ann. Intern. Med. *86:*24–28, 1977.

73. Drexhage, H.A., Bottazzo, G.F., and Doniach, D.: Evidence for thyroid growth-stimulating immunoglobulins in some goitrous thyroid diseases. Lancet *2:*287–292, 1980.

74. Ebner, A.A., Stein, M.E., et al.: Murine thyroid follicular epithelial cells can be induced to express Class II (Ia) gene products but fail to present antigen *in vivo.* Cell Immunol. *104:*154–168, 1987.

75. Eckel, R.H., and Green, W.L.: Postpartum thyrotoxicosis in a patient with Graves' disease. J.A.M.A. *243:*1454–1456, 1980.

76. Edmonds, M., Lamki, L., et al.: Autoimmune thyroiditis, adrenalitis and oophoritis. Am. J. Med. *54:*782–787, 1973.

77. Elliot, I., Gupta, M., et al.: Immunologic studies in two patients with persistent lymphocytic thyroiditis, thyrotoxicosis and low radioactive iodine uptake. Am. J. Med. *77:*347–354, 1984.

78. Faber, J., Lumholtz, I.B., et al.: The effects of phenytoin (diphenylhydantoin) on the extrathyroidal turnover of thyroxine, 3, 5, 3′-triiodothyronine, 3, 3′, 5′-triiodothyronine and 3′, 5′-diiodothyronine in man. J. Clin. Endocrinol. Metab. *61:*1093–1099, 1985.

79. Falk, S.A., Birken, E.A., and Ronquillo, A.H.: Graves' disease associated with histologic Hashimoto's thyroiditis. Otolaryngol. Head Neck Surg. *93:*86–91, 1985.

80. Farid, N.R.: Immunogenetics of autoimmune thyroid disorders. Endocrinol. Metab. Clin. N. Amer. *16:*229–245, 1987.

81. Farid, N.R., Barnard, J.M., et al.: Thyroid autoimmune disease in a large Newfoundland family: The influence of HLA. J. Clin. Endocrinol. Metab. *45:*1165–1172, 1977.

82. Farid, N.R., Howe, B.S., and Walfish, P.G.: Increased frequency of HLA-DR3 and 5 in the syndromes of painless thyroiditis with transient thyrotoxicosis: evidence for an autoimmune etiology. Clin. Endocrinol. *19:*699–704, 1983.

83. Farid, N.R., Munro, R.E., et al.: Rosette inhibition test for the demonstration of thymus-dependent lymphocyte sensitization in Graves's disease and Hashimoto's thyroiditis. N. Engl. J. Med. *289:*1111–1117, 1973.

84. Farid, N.R., Sampson, L., et al.: A study of human leucocyte D locus related antigens in Graves' disease. J. Clin. Invest. *63:*108–113, 1979.

85. Fatourechi, V., McConahey, W.M., and Woolner, L.B.: Hyperthyroidism associated with histologic Hashimoto's thyroiditis. Mayo Clin. Proc. *46:*682–689, 1971.

86. Fein, H.G., Goldman, J.M., and Weintraub, B.D.: Postpartum lymphocytic thyroiditis in American women: A spectrum of thyroid dysfunction. Am. J. Obstet. Gynecol. *138:*504–510, 1980.

87. Feldt-Rasmussen, U., Bech, K., et al.: Autoantibodies, immune complexes and HLA-D in thyrogastric autoimmunity. Tissue Antigens *22:*342–347, 1983.

88. Fialkow, P.J., Zavala, C., and Nielsen, R.: Thyroid autoimmunity: increased frequency in relatives of insulin-dependent diabetes patients. Ann. Intern. Med. *83:*170–176, 1975.

89. Fine, R.M.: Autoimmune thyroid disease—antibodies that promote growth. Intl. J. Dermatol. *23:*314–315, 1984.

90. Fisher, D.A., Pandian, M.R., and Carlton, E.: Autoimmune thyroid diseases: An expanding spectrum. Pediatr. Clin. N. Amer. *34*:907–918, 1987.
91. Fragu, P., Schlumberger, M., et al.: Effects of amiodarone therapy in thyroid iodine content as measured by X-ray fluorescence. J. Clin. Endocrinol. Metab. *66*:762–769, 1988.
92. Gammage, M.D., and Franklyn, J.A.: Amiodarone and the thyroid. Quart. J. Med. *238*:83–86, 1987.
93. Gams, R.A., Neal, J.A., and Conrad, F.G.: Hydantoin-induced pseudo-pseudolymphoma. Ann. Intern. Med. *69*:557–561, 1968.
94. Genant, H.K., Hoagland, H.C., and Randall, R.V.: Addison's disease and hypothyroidism (Schmidt's syndrome). Metabolism *16*:189–194, 1967.
95. Gharib, H., and Munoz, J.M.: Endocrine manifestations of diphenylhydantoin therapy. Metabolism *23*:515–524, 1974.
96. Ginsberg, J., and Walfish, P.G.: Postpartum transient thyrotoxicosis with painless thyroiditis. Lancet *1*:1125–1127, 1977.
97. Gluck, F.B., Nusynowitz, M.L., and Plymate, S.: Chronic lymphocytic thyroiditis, thyrotoxicosis and low radioactive iodine uptake. N. Engl. J. Med. *293*:624–628, 1975.
98. Gordin, A., and Lamberg, B.A.: Natural course of symptomless autoimmune thyroiditis. Lancet *2*:1234–1238, 1975.
99. Gorman, C.A., Duick, D.S., et al.: Transient hyperthyroidism in patients with lymphocytic thyroiditis. Mayo Clin. Proc. *53*:359–365, 1978.
100. Gossage, A.A.R., and Munro, D.S.: The pathogenesis of Graves' disease. Clin. Endocrinol. Metab. *14*:299–330, 1985.
101. Graham, A., and McCullagh, E.P.: Atrophy and fibrosis associated with lymphoid tissue in the thyroid. Arch. Surg. *22*:548–567, 1931.
102. Grubeck-Loebenstein, D., Derfler, K., et al.: Immunological features of nonimmunogenic hyperthyroidism. J. Clin. Endocrinol. Metab. *60*:150–155, 1985.
103. Gudbjornsson, B., Kristinsson, A., et al.: Painful autoimmune thyroiditis occurring on amiodarone therapy. Acta Med. Scand. *221*:219–220, 1987.
104. Hamilton, C.R., and Maloof, F.: Unusual types of hyperthyroidism. Medicine *52*:195–215, 1973.
105. Hanafusa, T., Pujol-Borrel, R., et al.: Aberrant expression of HLA-DR antigen on thyrocytes in Graves' disease: relevance to autoimmunity. Lancet *2*:1111–1115, 1983.
106. Hansen, J.M., Skovsted, L., et al.: The effect of diphenylhydantoin on thyroid function. J. Clin. Endocrinol. Metab. *39*:785–789, 1974.
107. Harach, H.R., and Williams, E.D.: Fibrous thyroiditis—an immunopathological study. Histopathology *7*:739–751, 1983.
108. Harcout-Webster, J.N., and Stuart, A.E.: Fat in thyroiditis. J. Pathol. *86*:240–242, 1963.
109. Harland, W.A., Frantz, V.K.: Clinicopathologic study of 261 surgical cases of so-called "thyroiditis." J. Clin. Endocrinol. Metab. *11*:1433–1437, 1956.
110. Harris, M.: The cellular infiltrate in Hashimoto's disease and focal lymphocytic thyroiditis. J. Clin. Pathol. *22*:326–333, 1969.
111. Harris, M., and Palmer, M.K.: The structure of the human thyroid in relation to aging and focal thyroiditis. J. Pathol. *130*:99–104, 1980.
112. Harris, M., Summerell, J.M., and Swan, A.V.: The prevalence of focal thyroiditis in Jamaican adults. J. Pathol. *110*:309–317, 1973.
113. Harrison, T.S., Dagher, F.J., and Jaber, R.: Pathological dilemmas in the operative recognition of chronic thyroiditis. Surg. Clin. N. Amer. *50*:1067–1073, 1970.
114. Hashimoto, H.: Zur Kenntniss der lymphatosen Veranderung der Schilddruse (Struma lymphomatosa). Arch. f. klin. Chir. *97*:219–248, 1912.
115. Hawthorne, G.C., Campbell, N.P.S., et al.: Amiodarone-induced hypothyroidism. Arch. Intern. Med. *145*:1016–1019, 1985.
116. Hayashi, Y., Tamai, H., et al.: A long term clinical, immunological and histological follow-up study of patients with goitrous chronic lymphocytic thyroiditis. J. Clin. Endocrinol. Metab. *61*:1172–1178, 1985.
117. Hayslip, C.C., Baker, J.R., et al.: Natural killer cell activity and serum autoantibodies in women with postpartum thyroiditis. J. Clin. Endocrinol. Metab. *66*:1089–1093, 1988.
118. Hazard, J.B.: Thyroiditis: a review. Part II. Am. J. Clin. Pathol. *25*:399–426, 1955.
119. Hiromatsu, Y., Fukazawa, H., and Wall, J.B.: Cytotoxic mechanisms in autoimmune thyroid disorders and thyroid associated ophthalmopathy. Endocrinol. Metab. Clin. N. Amer. *16*:269–286, 1987.
120. Hiroto, Y., Tamai, H., et al.: Thyroid function and histology in forty-five patients with hyperthyroid Graves' disease in clinical remission more than ten years after thionamide drug treatment. J. Clin. Endocrinol. Metab. *62*:165–169, 1986.
121. Hochstein, M.A., Nair, V., and Nevins, M.: Hypothyroidism followed by hyperthyroidism. J.A.M.A. *237*:2222, 1977.
122. Hollingsworth, D.R., Butcher, L.K., and White, S.D.: Kentucky Appalachian goiter without iodine deficiency: evidence for evanescent thyroiditis. Am. J. Dis. Child. *131*:866–869, 1977.
123. Hurley, J.R.: Thyroiditis. Disease-a-Month, 1977 (December).
124. Hyjek, E., and Isaacson, P.G.: Primary B cell lymphoma of the thyroid and its relationship to Hashimoto's thyroiditis. Hum. Pathol. *19*:1315–1326, 1988.

125. Iitaka, M., Aguayo, J.F., et al.: Studies of the effect of suppressor T lymphocytes on the induction of antithyroid microsomal antibody-secreting cells in autoimmune thyroid disease. J. Clin. Endocrinol. Metab. *66:*708–714, 1988.

126. Inada, M., Nishikawa, M., et al.: Reversible changes of the histological abnormalities of the thyroid in patients with painless thyroiditis. J. Clin. Endocrinol. Metab. *52:*431–435, 1981.

127. Inada, M., Nishikawa, M., et al.: Transient thyrotoxicosis associated with painless thyroiditis and low radioactive iodine uptake. Arch. Intern. Med. *139:*597–599, 1979.

128. Ingbar, S.H.: The role of antibodies and other humoral factors in the pathogenesis of Graves' disease. *In:* Drexhage, H.A., and Wiersinga, W.M. (eds.): The Thyroid and Autoimmunity. Amsterdam, Elsevier Science Publishers, 1986, pp. 3–14.

129. Inoue, M., Taketani, N., et al.: High incidence of chronic lymphocytic thyroiditis in apparently healthy school children: epidemiological and clinical study. Endocrinol. Jpn. *22:*483–489, 1975.

130. Iwatani, Y., Amino, N., et al.: T lymphocyte subsets in autoimmune thyroid diseases and subacute thyroiditis detected with monoclonal antibodies. J. Clin. Endocrinol. Metab. *56:*251–254, 1982.

131. Iwatani, Y., Gerstein, H.C., et al.: Thyrocyte HLA-DR expression and interferon-gamma production in autoimmune thyroid disease. J. Clin. Endocrinol. Metab. *63:*695–708, 1986.

132. Jackson, I.M.D.: "Hyper-thyroiditis"—a diagnostic pitfall. N. Engl. J. Med. *293:*661–662, 1975.

133. Jackson, R.A., Haynes, B.F., et al.: Ia$^+$ T cells in new onset Graves' disease. J. Clin. Endocrinol. Metab. *59:*187–190, 1984.

134. Jansson, R., Bernander, S., et al.: Autoimmune thyroid dysfunction in the postpartum period. J. Clin. Endocrinol. Metab. *58:*681–687, 1984.

135. Jansson, R., Karlsson, A., and Dahlberg, P.A.: Thyroxine, methimazole and thyroid microsomal autoantibody titres in hypothyroid Hashimoto's thyroiditis. Br. Med. J. *290:*11–13, 1985.

136. Jansson, R., Karlsson, A., and Forsum, U.: Intrathyroidal HLA-DR expression and T lymphocyte phenotypes in Graves' thyrotoxicosis, Hashimoto's thyroiditis and nodular colloid goitre. Clin. Exp. Immunol. *58:*264–272, 1984.

137. Jansson, R., Safwenberg, J., and Dahlberg, P.A.: Influence of the HLA-DR4 antigen and iodine status on the development of autoimmune postpartum thyroiditis. J. Clin. Endocrinol. Metab. *60:*168–173, 1985.

138. Jansson, R., Totterman, T.H., et al.: Intrathyroidal and circulating lymphocyte subsets in different stages of autoimmune postpartum thyroiditis. J. Clin. Endocrinol. Metab. *58:*942–946, 1984.

139. Jefferson, J.W.: Lithium-carbonate induced hypothyroidism. J.A.M.A. *242:*271–272, 1979.

140. Joll, C.A.: The pathology, diagnosis and treatment of Hashimoto's disease (struma lymphomatosa). Br. J. Surg. *27:*351–389, 1939.

141. Jonckheer, M., Vanhaelst, L., et al.: Atrophic autoimmune thyroiditis: relationship between the clinical state and intrathyroidal iodine as measured *in vivo* in man. J. Clin. Endocrinol. Metab. *53:*476–479, 1981.

142. Kabel, P.J., Voorbj, H.A.M., et al.: Intra-thyroidal dendritic cells. J. Clin. Endocrinol. Metab. *65:*19–20, 1988.

143. Kalderon, A.E., Bogaars, H.A., and Diamond, I.: Ultrastructural alterations of the follicular basement membrane in Hashimoto's thyroiditis. Am. J. Med. *55:*485–491, 1973.

144. Kaptein, E.M., Egodage, P.M., et al.: Amiodarone alters thyroxine transfer and distribution in humans. Metabolism *37:*1107–1113, 1988.

145. Karlsson, F.A., Wibell, L., and Wide, L.: Hypothyroidism due to thyroid-hormone binding antibodies. N. Engl. J. Med. *296:*1146–1148, 1977.

146. Karlsson, F.A., Dahlberg, P.A., and Ritzen, E.M.: Thyroid blocking antibodies in thyroiditis. Acta Med. Scand. *215:*461–466, 1984.

147. Karlsson, F.A., Totterman, T.H., and Jansson, R.: Subacute thyroiditis: activated HLA-DR and interferon gamma expressing T cytotoxic suppressor cells in thyroid tissue and peripheral blood. Clin. Endocrinol. *25:*487–493, 1986.

148. Katz, S.M., and Vickery, A.L.: The fibrous variant of Hashimoto's thyroiditis. Hum. Pathol. *5:*161–170, 1974.

149. Kaulfersch, W., Baker, J.R., et al.: Immunoglobulin and T cell antigen receptor gene arrangements indicate that the immune response in autoimmune thyroid disease is polyclonal. J. Clin. Endocrinol. Metab. *66:*958–963, 1988.

150. Ketelbant-Balasse, P., and Neve, P.: Ultrastructural study of the thyroid in adult hypothyroidism. Virch. Arch. A. Path. Anat. Histol. *362:*195–205, 1974.

151. Kidd, A., Okita, N., et al.: Immunologic aspects of Graves' and Hashimoto's diseases. Metabolism *29:*80–99, 1980.

152. Knecht, H., and Hedinger, C.E.: Ultrastructural findings in Hashimoto's thyroiditis and focal lymphocytic thyroiditis with reference to giant cell formation. Histopathology *6:*511–538, 1982.

153. Knecht, H., Saremaslani, P., and Hedinger, C.: Immunohistological findings in Hashimoto's thyroiditis, focal lymphocytic thyroiditis and thyroiditis of de Quervain. Virch. Arch. A. Path. Anat. *393:*215–231, 1981.

154. Kohn, L.D., Alvarez, F., et al.: Monoclonal antibody studies defining origin and properties of autoantibodies in Graves' disease. *In:* Schwartz, R.S., and Rose, N.R. (eds.): Autoimmunity. Experimental and Clinical Aspects. New York, New York Academy of Science, 1986, pp. 157–173.

155. Kolb, H., Toyka, K.V., and Gleichmann, E.: Histocompatibility antigens and clinical reactivity in autoimmunity. Immunol. Today *8:*3–6, 1987.

156. Kong, Y.M., Bagnasco, M., and Canonica, G.W.: How do T cells mediate autoimmune thyroiditis? Immunol. Today 7:337–339, 1986.
157. Konishi, J., Iida, Y., et al.: Primary myxedema with thyrotrophin-binding inhibitor immunoglobulins. Ann. Intern. Med. 103:26–31, 1985.
158. Kontiainen, S., Lautenschlager, I., et al.: Cells infiltrating the thyroid in juvenile autoimmune thyroiditis. Clin. Exp. Immunol. 67:89–94, 1987.
159. Kraiem, Z., Lahat, N., et al.: Thyrotrophin receptor-blocking antibodies. Clin. Endocrinol. 27:409–421, 1987.
160. Kriss, J.P., Pleshakov, V., and Chien, J.R.: Isolation and identification of the long acting thyroid stimulator and its relation to hyperthyroidism and circumscribed pretibial myxedema. J. Clin. Endocrinol. Metab. 24:1005–1028, 1964.
161. Kromer, G., Schauenstein, K., and Wick, G.: Is autoimmunity a side-effect of interleukin 2 production? Immunol. Today 7:199–200, 1986.
162. Kuiper, J.J.: Lymphocytic thyroiditis possibly induced by diphenylhydantoin. J.A.M.A. 210:2370–2372, 1969.
163. Kurashima, C., and Hirokawa, K.: Focal lymphocytic infiltration of thyroids in elderly people. Survey Synth. Pathol. Res. 4:457–466, 1985.
164. Kushnir, M., Weinstein, R., et al.: Hypothyroidism and phenytoin intoxication. Ann. Intern. Med. 102:341–342, 1985.
165. Lauridsen, U.B., Kirkegaard, C., and Nerup, J.: Lithium and pituitary-thyroid axis in normal subjects. J. Clin. Endocrinol. Metab. 39:383–385, 1974.
166. Lautenschlager, I., Maenpaa, J., et al.: Thyroid infiltrating cells in juvenile autoimmune thyroiditis: a follow-up of 1 year. Clin. Immunol. Immunopathol. 49:143–148, 1988.
167. Lechuga-Gomez, E.E., Meyerson, J., et al.: Polyglandular autoimmune syndrome type II. Canad. Med. Assoc. J. 138:632–634, 1988.
168. Leshin, M.: Polyglandular autoimmune syndromes. Am. J. Med. Sci. 290:77–88, 1985.
169. Levine, S.N.: Current concepts of thyroiditis. Arch. Intern. Med. 143:1952–1956, 1983.
170. Lindem, M.C., and Clark, J.H.: Indications for surgery in thyroiditis. Am. J. Surg. 118:829–831, 1969.
171. Lindsay, S., Dailey, M.E., et al.: Chronic thyroiditis: a clinical and pathological study of 354 patients. J. Clin. Endocrinol. Metab. 12:1578–1600, 1952.
172. Lloyd, R.V., Johnson, T.L., et al.: Detection of HLA-DR antigens paraffin-embedded thyroid epithelial cells with a monoclonal antibody. Am. J. Pathol. 120:106–111, 1985.
173. Londei, M., Bottazzo, G.F., and Feldman, M.: Human T-cell clones from autoimmune thyroid glands: specific recognition of autologous thyroid cells. Science 228:85–89, 1985.
174. Londei, M., Lamb, J.R., et al.: Epithelial cells expressing aberrant MHC Class II determinants can present antigen to cloned human T-cells. Nature 312:639–641, 1984.
175. Louis, D.N., Vickery, A.L., et al.: Multiple branchial cleft-like cysts in Hashimoto's thyroiditis. Am. J. Surg. Pathol. 13:45–49, 1989.
176. Lucas-Martin, A., Foz-Sala, M., et al.: Occurrence of thyrocyte HLA Class II expression in a wide variety of thyroid diseases: Relationship with lymphocytic infiltration and thyroid autoantibodies. J. Clin. Endocrinol. Metab. 66:367–375, 1988.
177. Lukes, R.J., and Tindle, B.H.: Immunoblastic lymphadenopathy. N. Engl. J. Med. 292:1–5, 1975.
178. Lupulescu, A., and Petrovici, A.: Ultrastructure of the Thyroid Gland. Baltimore, Williams and Wilkins Co., 1968.
179. Lynch, H.T., Matoole, J.J., et al.: Iatrogenic hypothyroidism in a patient with Turner's syndrome. Am. J. Med. Sci. 250:542–546, 1965.
180. Madec, A.M., Allannic, H., et al.: T lymphocyte subsets at various stages of hyperthyroid Graves' disease. J. Clin. Endocrinol. Metab. 62:117–121, 1986.
181. Maenpaa, J., Raatikka, M., et al.: Natural course of juvenile autoimmune thyroiditis. J. Pediatr. 107:898–904, 1985.
182. Maron, R., and Cohen, I.R.: Mutation at H-2K locus influences susceptibility to autoimmune thyroiditis. Nature 279:715–716, 1979.
183. Marchlinski, F.E., Gansler, T.S., et al.: Amiodarone pulmonary toxicity. Ann. Intern. Med. 97:839–845, 1982.
184. Marshall, S.F., Meissner, W.A., and Smith, D.C.: Chronic thyroiditis. N. Engl. J. Med. 238:758–766, 1948.
185. Martino, E., Aghini-Lombardi, F., et al.: Amiodarone-induced hypothyroidism. Clin. Endocrinol. 26:227–237, 1987.
186. Matsunaga, M., Eguchi, K., et al.: Class II histocompatibility complex antigen expression and cellular interactions in thyroid glands of Graves' disease. J. Clin. Endocrinol. Metab. 62:723–728, 1986.
187. Matsuta, M.: Immunohistochemical and electron microscopic studies on Hashimoto's thyroiditis. Acta Pathol. Jpn. 32:41–56, 1982.
188. Mazonson, P.D., Williams, M.L., et al.: Myxedema coma during long-term amiodarone therapy. Am. J. Med. 77:751–754, 1984.
189. McConnon, J.K.: Thirty-five cases of transient hyperthyroidism. Canad. Med. Assoc. J. 130:1159–1161, 1984.

190. McDermott, M.T., Burman, K.D., et al.: Lithium-associated thyrotoxicosis. Am. J. Med. *80:*1245–1248, 1986.

191. McDevitt, H.O.: The molecular basis of autoimmunity. Clin. Res. *34:*163–175, 1986.

192. McKenzie, J.M.: Does LATS cause hyperthyroidism in Graves' disease? Metabolism *21:*883–894, 1972.

193. McLachlan, S.M., Dickinson, A., et al.: Enrichment and depletion of thyroglobulin autoantibody synthesizing lymphocytes. Clin. Exp. Immunol. *53:*397–405, 1983.

194. McLachlan, S.M., Jansson, R., et al.: Hypothyroidism and autoimmune thyroid destruction: a role for thyroid autoantibodies? *In:* Drexhage, H.A. and Wiersinga, W.W. (eds.): The Thyroid and Autoimmunity. Amsterdam, Elsevier, 1986, pp. 99–105.

195. McLachlan, S.M., Proud, G., et al.: Functional analysis of T and B cells from blood and thyroid tissue in Hashimoto's disease. Clin. Exp. Immunol. *59:*585–592, 1985.

196. Meek, J.-C., Jones, A.E., et al.: Characterization of the long-acting thyroid stimulator of Graves' disease. Proc. Natl. Acad. Sci. *52:*342–349, 1964.

197. Mehbod, H., Swartz, C.D., and Brest, A.N.: The effect of prolonged thiazide administration on thyroid function. Arch. Intern. Med. *119:*283–285, 1967.

198. Misaki, T., Konishi, J., et al.: Immunological phenotyping of thyroid infiltrating lymphocytes in Graves' disease and Hashimoto's thyroiditis. Clin. Exp. Immunol. *60:*104–110, 1985.

199. Mizukami, Y., Michigishi, T., et al.: Silent thyroiditis: a histologic and immunohistochemical study. Hum. Pathol. *19:*423–431, 1988.

200. Moens, H., Farid, N.R.: Hashimoto's thyroiditis is associated with HLA-DRw3. N. Engl. J. Med. *299:*133–134, 1978.

201. Molholm-Hansen, J., Skovsted, L., et al.: The effects of diphenylhydantoin on thyroid function. J. Clin. Endocrinol. Metab. *39:*785–789, 1974.

202. Mori, H., Hamada, N., and DeGroot, L.J.: Studies on thyroglobulin-specific suppressor T cell function in autoimmune thyroid disease. J. Clin. Endocrinol. Metab. *61:*306–312, 1985.

203. Morrison, J., and Caplan, R.H.: Typical and atypical ('silent') subacute thyroiditis in a wife and husband. Arch. Intern. Med. *138:*45–48, 1978.

204. Nakamura, R.M., and Binder, W.L.: Current concepts and diagnostic evaluation of autoimmune diseases. Arch. Pathol. Lab. Med. *112:*869–877, 1988.

205. Nakao, Y., Kishihara, M., et al.: HLA antigens in autoimmune thyroid diseases. Arch. Intern. Med. *138:*567–570, 1978.

206. Neve, P.: The ultrastructure of thyroid in chronic autoimmune thyroiditis. Virch. Arch. Abt. A. Path. Anat. *346:*302–317, 1969.

207. Nikolai, T.F., Coombs, G.J., and McKenzie, A.K.: Lymphocytic thyroiditis with spontaneously resolving hyperthyroidism and subacute thyroiditis. Long-term follow-up. Arch. Intern. Med. *141:*1455–1458, 1981.

208. Nikolai, T.F., Coombs, G.J., et al.: Treatment of lymphocytic thyroiditis with spontaneously resolving hyperthyroidism (silent thyroiditis). Arch. Intern. Med. *142:*2281–2283, 1982.

209. Nikolai, T.F., Turney, S.L., and Roberts, R.C.: Postpartum lymphocytic thyroiditis. Arch. Intern. Med. *147:*221–224, 1987.

210. Nishiyama, S., Matsukura, M., et al.: Reports of two cases of autoimmune thyroiditis while receiving anticonvulsant therapy. Eur. J. Pediatr. *140:*116–117, 1983.

211. Ochi, Y., and De Groot, L.J.: Long-acting thyroid stimulator of Graves's disease. N. Engl. J. Med. *278:*718–721, 1968.

212. Okita, N., How, J., et al.: Suppressor T lymphocyte dysfunction in Graves' disease. J. Clin. Endocrinol. Metab. *53:*1002–1007, 1981.

213. Okita, N., Kidd, A., et al.: Sensitization of T-lymphocytes in Graves' and Hashimoto's diseases. J. Clin. Endocrinol. Metab. *51:*316–320, 1980.

214. Oppenheimer, J.H., and Tavernetti, R.R.: Displacement of thyroxine from human thyroxine binding globulin by analogues of hydantoin. J. Clin. Invest. *41:*2213–2220, 1962.

215. Papapetrou, P.D., and Jackson, I.M.D.: Thyrotoxicosis due to "silent" thyroiditis. Lancet *1:*361–363, 1975.

216. Perrild, H., Madsen, A., and Hansen, R.: Irreversible myxedema after lithium carbonate. Br. Med. J. *1:*1108–1109, 1978.

217. Pfaltz, M., and Hedinger, C.E.: Abnormal basement membrane structures in autoimmune thyroid disease. Lab. Invest. *55:*531–539, 1986.

218. Piccinini, L.A., Goldsmith, N.K., et al.: Localization of HLA-DR α-chain messenger ribonucleic acid in normal and autoimmune human thyroid using *in-situ* hybridization. J. Clin. Endocrinol. Metab. *66:*1307–1315, 1988.

219. Pinchera, A., Fenzi, G., et al.: Autoimmune hypothyroidism. *In:* Drexhage, H.A., and Wiersinga, W.M. (eds.): Autoimmune Hypothyroidism in the Thyroid and Autoimmunity. Amsterdam, Elsevier Science Publishers, 1986, pp. 73–80.

220. Rabinowe, S.L., Larsen, P.R., et al.: Amiodarone therapy and autoimmune thyroid disease. Am. J. Med. *81:*53–57, 1986.

221. Raines, K.B., Baker, J.R., et al.: Antithyrotropin antibodies in the sera of Graves' disease patients. J. Clin. Endocrinol. Metab. *61:*217–222, 1985.

222. Rallison, M.L., Dobyns, B.M., et al.: Occurrence and natural history of chronic lymphocytic thyroiditis in childhood. J. Pediatr. *86:*675–682, 1975.

223. Rapoport, B.: Autoimmune mechanisms in thyroid disease. *In:* Green, W.L. (ed.): The Thyroid. New York, Elsevier, 1987, pp. 47–106.
224. Ravinsky, E., and Safneck, J.R.: Differentiation of Hashimoto's thyroiditis from thyroid neoplasms in fine needle aspirates. Acta Cytol. *32:*854–861, 1988.
225. Reidbord, H.E., and Fisher, E.R.: Ultrastructural features of subacute granulomatous thyroiditis and Hashimoto's disease. Am. J. Clin. Pathol. *59:*327–337, 1973.
226. Reith, P.E., and Kyner, J.: Postpartum thyroiditis: a common cause of thyrotoxicosis and/or hypothyroidism after pregnancy. Nebraska Med. J. *69:*356–359, 1984.
227. Roberts, I.M., Whittingham, S., and Mackay, I.R.: Tolerance to an autoantigen—thyroglobulin. Lancet *2:*936–940, 1973.
228. Roitt, I.M., and Doniach, D.: Human autoimmune thyroiditis. Serological studies. Lancet *2:*1027–1033, 1958.
229. Roitt, I.M., Doniach, D., et al.: Autoantibodies in Hashimoto's disease (lymphadenoid goiter). Lancet *2:*820–821, 1956.
230. Rose, N.R.: The thyroid gland as source and target of autoimmunity. Lab. Invest. *52:*117–119, 1985.
231. Rose, N.R., Bacon, L.D., et al.: Genetic regulation in autoimmune thyroiditis. *In:* Talal, N. (ed.): Autoimmunity. New York, Academic Press, 1977, pp. 63–87.
232. Rose, N.R., and Burek, C.L.: The genetics of thyroiditis as a prototype of human autoimmune disease. Ann. Allergy *54:*261–271, 1985.
233. Rosenbaum, A.H., Maruta, T., and Richelson, E.: Drugs that alter mood: lithium. Mayo Clin. Proc. *54:*401–407, 1979.
234. Sack, J., Baker, J.R., et al.: Killer cell activity and antibody-dependent cell mediated cytotoxity are normal in Hashimoto's disease. J. Clin. Endocrinol. Metab. *62:*1059–1064, 1986.
235. Salvi, M., Fukazawa, H., et al.: Role of autoantibodies in the pathogenesis and association of endocrine autoimmune diseases. Endocrine Rev. *9:*450–466, 1988.
236. Sasaki, H., Eimoto, T., et al.: Spontaneous remission of hypothyroidism in Hashimoto's (autoimmune) thyroiditis. Israel J. Med. Sci. *20:*625–629, 1984.
237. Sasaki, N., Tsuyusaki, T., et al.: Significant fluctuation of thyroid function in children with chronic lymphocytic thyroiditis. Endocrinol. Jpn. *30:*219–228, 1983.
238. Sawin, C.T., Bigos, S.T., et al.: The aging thyroid. Am. J. Med. *79:*591–595, 1985.
239. Schwartz, R.S., and Rose, N.R.: Autoimmunity: Experimental and Clinical Aspects. New York, New York Academy of Sciences, 1986.
240. Sclare, G.: The thyroid in myxedema. J. Pathol. Bacteriol. *85:*263–278, 1963.
241. Segal, B.M., and Weintraub, M.I.: Hashimoto's thyroiditis, myasthenia gravis, idiopathic thrombocytopenic purpura. Ann. Intern. Med. *85:*761–763, 1976.
242. Segal, R.L., Rosenblatt, S., and Eliasoph, I.: Endocrine exophthalmos during lithium therapy of manic-depressive disease. N. Engl. J. Med. *289:*136–138, 1973.
243. Selenkow, H.A., Wyman, P., and Allweiss, P.: Autoimmune thyroid disease: An integrated concept of Graves' and Hashimoto's diseases. Compr. Ther. *10:*48–56, 1984.
244. Sellers, E.A., Awad, A.G., and Schonbaum, E.: Long-acting thyroid stimulator in Graves' disease. Lancet *2:*335–338, 1970.
245. Shamsuddin, A.K.M., and Lane, R.A.: Ultrastructural pathology in Hashimoto's thyroiditis. Hum. Pathol. *12:*561–573, 1981.
246. Shane, L.L., Valensi, Q.J., et al.: Chronic thyroiditis: a potentially confusing clinical picture. Am. J. Med. Sci. *250:*532–541, 1965.
247. Sharpe, A.R., and Frable, W.J.: Thyroid function and thyroid microsomal antibody titre in focal autoimmune thyroiditis. Clin. Research *34:*180A, 1986.
248. Schoenfeld, Y., and Schwartz, R.S.: Immunologic and genetic factors in autoimmune disease. N. Engl. J. Med. *311:*1019–1029, 1984.
249. Shopsin, B., Shenkman, L., et al.: Iodine and lithium-induced hypothyroidism. Am. J. Med. *55:*695–699, 1973.
250. Singer, P.A., and Gorsky, J.E.: Familial postpartum transient hyperthyroidism. Arch. Intern. Med. *145:*240–242, 1985.
251. Singer, I., and Rotenberg, D.: Mechanisms of lithium action. N. Engl. J. Med. *289:*254–260, 1973.
252. Smith, B.R., and Hall, R.: Thyroid-stimulating immunoglobulins in Graves' disease. Lancet *2:*427–431, 1974.
253. Smyrk, T.C., Goellner, J.R., et al.: Pathology of the thyroid in amiodarone associated thyrotoxicosis. Am. J. Surg. Pathol. *11:*197–204, 1987.
254. Sridama, V., Hara, Y., et al.: HLA immunogenetic heterogeneity in Black American patients with Graves' disease. Arch. Intern. Med. *147:*229–231, 1987.
255. Statland, H., Wasserman, M.M., and Vickery, A.L.: Struma lymphomatosa (Hashimoto's struma): a review of 51 cases with discussion of endocrinologic aspects. Arch. Intern. Med. *88:*659–678, 1951.
256. Stenszky, V., Kozma, L., et al.: The genetics of Graves' disease: HLA and disease susceptibility. J. Clin. Endocrinol. Metab. *61:*735–740, 1985.
257. Strakosch, C.R., Joyner, D., and Wall, J.R.: Thyroid stimulating antibodies in patients with autoimmune disorders. J. Clin. Endocrinol. Metab. *47:*361–365, 1978.

258. Strakosch, C.R., Wenzel, B.E., et al.: Immunology of autoimmune thyroid diseases. N. Engl. J. Med. *307*:1499–1507, 1982.

259. Strauss, M., Laurian, N., and Antebi, E.: Coexistent carcinoma of the thyroid gland and Hashimoto's thyroiditis. Surg. Gynecol. Obstet. *157*:228–232, 1983.

260. Strominger, J.L.: Biology of the human histo-compatibility leukocyte antigen (HLA) system and a hypothesis regarding the generation of autoimmune diseases. J. Clin. Invest. *77*:1411–1415, 1986.

261. Stuart, A.E.: Fuchsinophilic material in the lymphoid follicles of Hashimoto's disease. J. Pathol. Bacteriol. *84*:249–250, 1963.

262. Studer, H., Peter, H.J., and Gerber, H.: Toxic nodular goitre. Clin. Endocrinol. Metab. *14*:351–372, 1985.

263. Sugenoya, A., Silverberg, J., et al.: Macrophage-lymphocyte interaction in Graves' disease and Hashimoto's thyroiditis. Acta Endocrinol. *91*:99–108, 1979.

264. Tachi, J., Amino, N., et al.: Long term follow-up and HLA association in patients with postpartum thyroiditis. J. Clin. Endocrinol. Metab. *66*:480–484, 1988.

265. Takasu, N., Naka, M., et al.: Two types of thyroid function-blocking antibodies in autoimmune atrophic thyroiditis and transient neonatal hypothyroidism due to maternal IgG. Clin. Endocrinol. *21*:345–355, 1984.

266. Tamai, H., Uno, H., et al.: Immunogenetics of Hashimoto's and Graves' diseases. J. Clin. Endocrinol. Metab. *60*:62–66, 1985.

267. Taylor, H.C., and Sheeler, L.R.: Recurrence and heterogeneity in painless thyrotoxic lymphocytic thyroiditis. J.A.M.A. *248*:1085–1088, 1982.

268. Theofilopoulos, A.N., and Dixon, F.J.: Autoimmune diseases: immunopathology and etiopathogenesis. Am. J. Pathol. *108*:321–365, 1982.

269. Thompson, C., and Farid, N.R.: Postpartum thyroiditis and goitrous (Hashimoto's) thyroiditis are associated with HLA-DR 4. Immunol. Letters *11*:301–303, 1985.

270. Todd, J.A., Acha-Orbea, H., et al.: A molecular basis for MHC Class II-associated autoimmunity. Science *240*:1003–1009, 1988.

271. Totterman, T.H.: Distribution of T-, B- and thyroglobulin-binding lymphocytes infiltrating the gland in Graves' disease, Hashimoto's thyroiditis, and de Quervain's thyroiditis. Clin. Immunol. Immunopathol. *10*:270–277, 1978.

272. Totterman, T.H., Andersson, L.C., and Hayry, P.: Evidence for thyroid antigen-reactive T lymphocytes infiltrating the thyroid gland in Graves' disease. Clin. Endocrinol. *11*:59–68, 1979.

273. Totterman, T.H., Maenpaa, J., et al.: Blood and thyroid infiltrating lymphocyte subclasses in juvenile autoimmune thyroiditis. Clin. Exp. Immunol. *30*:193–199, 1977.

274. Troutman, M.E., Efrusy, M.E., et al.: Simultaneous occurrence of adult celiac disease and lymphocytic thyroiditis. J. Clin. Gastroenterol. *3*:281–285, 1981.

275. Tunbridge, W.M.G., Brewis, M., et al.: Natural history of autoimmune thyroiditis. Br. Med. J. *282*:258–262, 1981.

276. Tung, K.S.K., Ramos, C.V., and Deodhar, S.D.: Antithyroid antibodies in juvenile lymphocytic thyroiditis. Am. J. Clin. Pathol. *61*:549–555, 1974.

277. Urbaniek, S.J., Penhale, W.J., and Irvine, W.J.: Circulating lymphocyte subpopulations in Hashimoto's thyroiditis. Clin. Exp. Immunol. *15*:345–354, 1973.

278. Vagenakis, A.G., Wang, C., et al.: Iodine-induced thyrotoxicosis in Boston. N. Engl. J. Med. *287*:523–527, 1972.

279. Valente, W.A., Vitti, P., et al.: Antibodies that promote thyroid growth: a distinct population of thyroid-stimulating autoantibodies. N. Engl. J. Med. *309*:1028–1034, 1983.

280. Vargas, M.T., Briones-Urbina, R., et al.: Antithyroid microsomal autoantibodies and HLA-DR 5 are associated with postpartum thyroid dysfunction: evidence supporting an autoimmune pathogenesis. J. Clin. Endocrinol. Metab. *67*:327–333, 1988.

281. Vazquez, A.M., and Kenny, F.M.: Ovarian failure and antiovarian antibodies in association with hypoparathyroidism, moniliasis, and Addison's and Hashimoto's diseases. Obstet. Gynecol. *41*:414–418, 1973.

282. Vickery, A.L., and Hamlin, E.: Struma lymphomatosa (Hashimoto's thyroiditis). N. Engl. J. Med. *264*:226–229, 1961.

283. Vitti, P., Chiovato, L., et al.: Thyroid-stimulating antibody mimics thyrotropin in its ability to desensitize the adenosine, 3', 5'-monophosphatase response to acute stimulation in continuously cultured rat thyroid cells. J. Clin. Endocrinol. Metab. *63*:454–458, 1986.

284. Vitug, A.C., and Goldman, J.M.: Silent (painless) thyroiditis: evidence of a geographic variation in frequency. Arch. Intern. Med. *145*:473–475, 1985.

285. Volpe, R.: The pathology of thyroiditis. Hum. Pathol. *9*:429–438, 1978.

286. Volpe, R.: The role of autoimmunity in hypoendocrine and hyperendocrine function: with special emphasis on autoimmune thyroid disease. Ann. Intern. Med. *87*:86–99, 1977.

287. Volpe, R.: Lymphocytic thyroiditis. *In:* Werner, S.C., and Ingbar, S.H. (eds.): The Thyroid. New York, Harper & Row, 1978, pp. 996–1003.

288. Volpe, R.: Immunoregulation in autoimmune thyroid disease. N. Engl. J. Med. *316*:44–45, 1987.

289. Volpe, R.: The immunoregulatory disturbance in autoimmune thyroid disease. Autoimmunity *2*:55–72, 1988.

290. Volpe, R., Edmonds, M., et al.: The pathogenesis of Graves' disease: a disorder of delayed hypersensitivity? Mayo Clin. Proc. *47:*824–834, 1972.
291. Volpe, R., Farid, N.R., et al.: The pathogenesis of Graves' disease and Hashimoto's thyroiditis. Clin. Endocrinol. *3:*239–261, 1976.
292. Wakakuri, N., Kubo, T., and Kitagawa, M.: Hyperthyroidism after primary hypothyroidism. Arch. Intern. Med. *145:*1527–1528, 1985.
293. Walfish, P.G., and Chan, J.Y.C.: Postpartum hyperthyroidism. Clin. Endocrinol. Metab. *14:*417–447, 1985.
294. Walfish, P.G., and Farid, N.R.: The immunogenetic basis of autoimmune thyroid disease. *In:* Walfish, P.G., Wall, J.R., and Volpe, R. (eds.): Autoimmunity and the Thyroid. Orlando, Academic Press, 1985, pp. 9–36.
295. Wall, J.R., Baur, R., et al.: Peripheral blood and intrathyroidal mononuclear cell populations in patients with autoimmune thyroid disorders enumerated using monoclonal antibodies. J. Clin. Endocrinol. Metab. *56:*164–169, 1983.
296. Weaver, D.K., Batsakis, J.G., and Nishiyama, R.H.: Relationship of iodine to "lymphocytic goiter." Arch. Surg. *98:*183–185, 1969.
297. Weetman, A.P., and McGregor, A.M.: Autoimmune thyroid disease: developments in our understanding. Endocrine Rev. *5:*309–355, 1984.
298. Weiss, M., Ingbar, S.H., et al.: Demonstration of a saturable binding site for thyrotropin in *Yersinia enterocolitica.* Science *219:*1331–1333, 1983.
299. Wenzel, B.E., Heesemann, J., et al.: Patients with autoimmune thyroid diseases have antibodies to plasmid encoded proteins of enteropathogenic Yersinia. J. Endocrinol. Invest. *11:*139–140, 1988.
300. Werner, S.C., Wegelius, O., et al.: Immunoglobulins (E, M, G) and complement in the connective tissues of the thyroid in Graves's disease. N. Engl. J. Med. *287:*421–425, 1972.
301. Wilkins, T.J., and Casey, C.: The distribution of immunoglobulin containing cells in human autoimmune thyroiditis. Acta Endocrinol. *106:*490–498, 1984.
302. Wiersinga, W.M., Touber, J.L., et al.: Uninhibited thyroidal uptake of radioiodine despite iodine excess in amiodarone-induced hypothyroidism. J. Clin. Endocrinol. Metab. *63:*485–491, 1986.
303. Williams, E.D., and Doniach, I.: The postmortem incidence of focal thyroiditis. J. Pathol. Bacteriol. *83:*255–264, 1962.
304. Wolff, J.: Iodide goiter and the pharmacologic effects of excess iodide. Am. J. Med. *47:*101–124, 1969.
305. Wood, L.C., and Ingbar, S.H.: Hypothyroidism as a late sequela in patients with Graves' disease treated with antithyroid agents. J. Clin. Invest. *64.*1429–1436, 1979.
306. Woolf, P.D.: Transient painless thyroiditis with hyperthyroidism: a variant of lymphocytic thyroiditis? Endocrinol. Rev. *1:*411–420, 1980.
307. Woolf, P.D., and Daly, R.: Thyrotoxicosis with painless thyroiditis. Am. J. Med. *60:*73–79, 1976.
308. Woolner, L.B.: Thyroiditis: classification and clinicopathologic correlation. *In:* Hazard, J.B., and Smith, D.E. (eds.): The Thyroid. Baltimore, Williams and Wilkins Co., 1964, pp. 123–142.
309. Woolner, L.B., McConahey, W.M., and Beahrs, O.H.: Struma lymphomatosa (Hashimoto's thyroiditis) and related disorders. J. Clin. Endocrinol. Metab. *19:*53–83, 1959.
310. Wu, S.Y., Reggio, R., et al.: Stimulation of thyroidal iodothyronine 5′-monodeiodinase by long acting thyroid stimulator (LATS). Acta Endocrinol. *114:*193–200, 1987.
311. Yagi, Y.: Electron microscopy and immunohistochemical studies in Hashimoto's thyroiditis. Acta Pathol. Jpn. *31:*611–622, 1981.
312. Yagi, Y., Sato, E., and Yagi, S.: Population of K-lymphocytes in various kinds of thyroid disease. Endocrinol. Jpn. *30:*113–119, 1983.
313. Zakarija, M., and McKenzie, J.M.: The spectrum and significance of autoantibodies reacting with the thyrotropin receptor. Endocrinol. Metab. Clin. N. Amer. *16:*343–363, 1987.

6

FIBROSIS IN THE THYROID

Fibrosis can occur in the thyroid in focal areas or diffusely throughout the gland. Table 6–1 lists those conditions in which fibrosis is seen pathologically in the gland. In some of these conditions, the fibrosis (usually diffuse throughout the organ) can interfere with gland function; hypothyroidism may result.

In some fibrous lesions, the mechanism of glandular destruction is immunologic (e.g., chronic lymphocytic thyroiditis); in others postinflammatory (e.g., radiation); and in others a vascular (ischemic) mechanism can be postulated (e.g., scleroderma) (Table 6–2).

THE THYROIDITIDES

Among the thyroiditis group, fibrosis is prominent in subacute and chronic forms.

Subacute Thyroiditis. As discussed in Chapter 4, subacute thyroiditis has associated fibrous areas in its later phases. As granulomatous inflammation subsides, central areas of fibrosis, occasionally resembling radial scars, are seen. Upon recovery and following regeneration of the follicles, fibrous scars shrink; functional abnormalities are unusual even in stressed patients;[62] the pathologic appearance of the thyroid is almost normal years after recovery.

Chronic Lymphocytic Thyroiditis. (See also Chapter 5.) This is often associated with interlobular and interfollicular fibrosis. Frequently the fibrous tissue is hidden by the extensive lymphoplasmacytic infiltrate—trichrome or reticulin stains may help in identifying the degree of connective tissue proliferation.

Table 6–1. Fibrous Lesions of the Thyroid

1. Thyroiditis
• subacute
• chronic lymphocytic (Hashimoto's) thyroiditis
• fibrous variant of Hashimoto's thyroiditis
• fibrous atrophy
2. Riedel's disease
3. Radiation thyroiditis
4. Amyloid in the thyroid
5. Nodular goiter
6. Trauma
7. Desmoplasia near tumors
8. Scleroderma

Modified with permission from LiVolsi, V. A., and LoGerfo, P.: *Thyroiditis.* Boca Raton, FL, CRC Press, copyright 1981.

Table 6–2. Thyroid Glandular Fibrosis: Suggested Mechanisms

Lesion	Mechanisms of Fibrosis
Thyroiditis	Immunologic
Riedel's disease	? Immunologic; replacement of normal tissue
Nodular goiter	Postinflammatory
Trauma	Postinflammatory
Tumors	Reactive desmoplasia; ?tumor growth factors
Radiation	Vascular (ischemic); ?postinflammatory
Amyloid	Vascular (ischemic) (partly); replacement of normal tissue
Scleroderma	?Immunologic; ?vascular (ischemic)

Fibrosing (Fibrous) Variant of Hashimoto's Thyroiditis. As indicated by its name, this is characterized by extensive fibrous proliferation. In Professor Hashimoto's original description of the disorder associated with his eponym,[27] one of the four patients he described had a gland that was extensively fibrotic. Between the publication in 1912 of Hashimoto's paper and the redefinition of this fibrosing variant in 1974 by Katz and Vickery,[35] the literature reflected confusion of this disorder and the lesion termed "Riedel's struma."[10] (See below.) (A pertinent exception to this statement is the work of Graham,[24] who in 1931 noted these two lesions were in fact different.)

The fibrosing variant of Hashimoto's thyroiditis constitutes about 10 to 13 percent of chronic lymphocytic thyroiditis. From the clinical viewpoint, the fibrosing variant occurs more frequently in older patients than ordinary forms of Hashimoto's thyroiditis. The disease often presents with large symptomatic goiter and severe hypothyroidism. Complaints of dysphagia or dyspnea in an older individual with a large thyroid may lead to a clinical diagnosis of anaplastic carcinoma. Laboratory evaluation indicates hypothyroidism; antithyroglobulin antibodies are present in very high titer.[35] This disorder often requires surgical treatment for relief of symptoms because of the size of the gland.

Although a few adhesions can be found, grossly the thyroid capsule is clearly demarcated from surrounding structures. (This feature should reassure the surgeon and pathologist that they are not dealing with Riedel's disease.[35, 41]) The thyroid, which is usually very large (weights of 200 grams are not rare), is pale yellow to tan and very firm; on section a vaguely lobular pattern with extensive fibrosis is seen (Fig. 6–1).

Histologically, the gland lobulation is noted at low power; this finding serves in distinguishing this lesion from carcinoma or from Riedel's disease. Broad fibrous bands separate residual zones of degenerating thyroid. The latter shows changes reminiscent of classic chronic lymphocytic thyroiditis, including follicular atrophy, oxyphil metaplasia and lymphoid infiltrate with germinal centers (Figs. 6–2 to 6–4). Inflammatory cells, usually plasma cells, are identified in the fibrous bands. Although found in other conditions, squamous metaplasia of the follicular epithelium is prominent in fibrosing Hashimoto's thyroiditis. Despite the term "squamous" metaplasia, keratin pearls are rarely found. Indeed, the present author finds that the metaplasia more closely resembles "morular" metaplasia of the endometrium or the postinflammatory epithelial changes of minor salivary glands found in necrotizing sialometaplasia. The metaplasia in fibrosing thyroiditis apparently results from a reaction of the damaged follicular epithelium from which the "squamous" cells arise.[26, 35] (Some authors[76] have suggested that this squamous change may be related to increase in solid cell nests rather than metaplasia of follicular epithelium—see Chapter 13.)

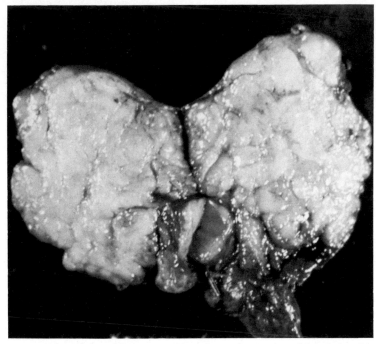

Figure 6–1. Fibrous Hashimoto's thyroiditis. Note pale color and accentuated lobular architecture of gland, and diffuse nature of the process.

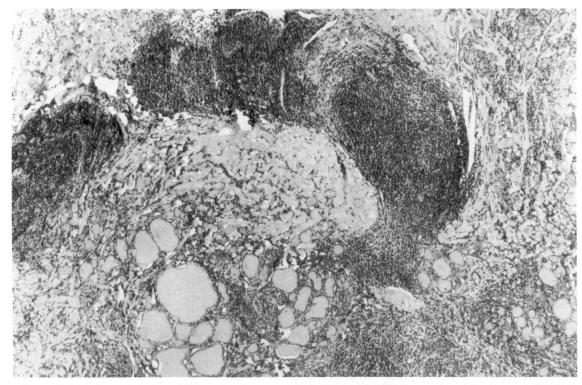

Figure 6–2. At low power, broad fibrous bands are seen intermixed with follicular centers and remnants of thyroid (lower left). × 50, H & E.

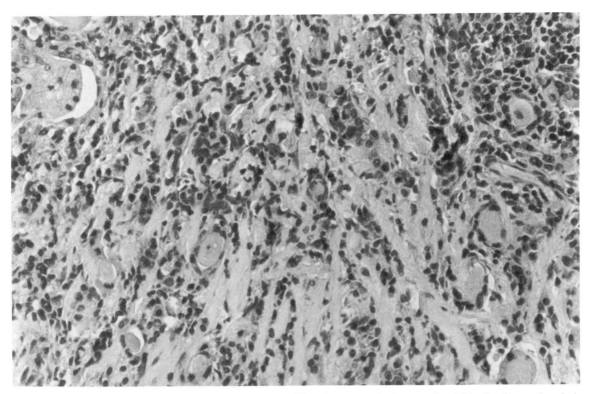

Figure 6–3. At higher power windswept appearance of lymphocytes and plasma cells within the fibrous bands is seen. Occasional atrophic follicles can be discerned. × 200, H & E.

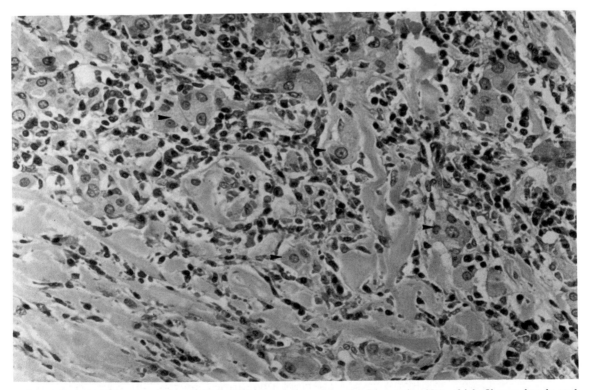

Figure 6–4. In this area, only residual atypical oncocytes *(arrowheads)* remain. Note thick fibrous bands and lymphocytes and plasma cells. × 250, H & E.

The relationship of the fibrous variant to other subtypes of chronic thyroiditis remains unclear. Katz and Vickery suggest from anecdotal data that there may be a progression from usual and mild forms of chronic lymphocytic thyroiditis to the fibrous type. These authors suggest also a relationship to fibrous atrophy of the thyroid; hence, there may exist divergent pathways of progression of lymphocytic thyroiditis as patients age—some go on to fibrous proliferation and others to atrophy.[35]

Fibrous Atrophy of the Thyroid. This describes the gland found in so-called idiopathic myxedema.[5, 64] Grossly, the thyroid is tiny with weights of 2 to 5 grams common (Fig. 6–5). It appears as a fibrotic mass of tissue totally unrecognizable as thyroid except for its location anterior to the trachea. Histologically, the gland in idiopathic myxedema shares many of the features of the fibrous variant of Hashimoto's disease, including follicular atrophy, oncocytic and squamous metaplasia, and infiltration of lymphocytes and plasma cells. The interfollicular zones are replaced by fibrosis (Fig. 6–6).

In both fibrous Hashimoto's disease and in idiopathic myxedema, interference with thyroid function and severe hypothyroidism result from the follicular destruction and replacement fibrosis.

RIEDEL'S DISEASE

Riedel's disease, also called *Riedel's struma,* has classically but probably incorrectly been included among the thyroiditides.[7, 10, 26, 29, 34, 35, 43, 44, 57, 58, 61, 66, 69, 79, 80] Indeed, this unusual lesion really is not a disorder *of* the thyroid but *involves* the thyroid. As the largest structure in the neck, the thyroid gland is the most obvious structure involved by the process and hence the word "struma" was attached to the disease. In the late 19th century, Riedel reported the clinical and pathological features of the disorder which bears his name.[57, 58] (This entity had been described earlier by Bowlby[7] and Semple.[66])

Clinically the disorder presented as goiter of recent rapid onset with associated dyspnea. At surgery, there was iron-hard "tumor" tissue infiltrating thyroid but also cervical soft tissues, trachea, blood vessels, and nerves. Microscopically, dense scar tissue and chronic inflammation were seen, although no evidence of infection was identified. It is of considerable interest that Riedel described an associated endarteritis which he attributed to inflammation.[57, 58] Although the clinical symptoms and surgical findings strongly suggested a neoplasm, Riedel noted that the lesion regressed, recurred, and regressed again over many years; he warned that this distinguished the entity from a true neoplasm.[57, 58]

Even though Hashimoto in 1912 admonished future authors that the disease he described differed from that reported by Riedel, and a classic paper on "invasive fibrous thyroiditis" by Woolner et al. appeared in 1957,[80] much confusion was found in the literature until the redefinition of fibrous Hashimoto's disease in 1974.[35] Thus, some authors considered Riedel's disease as an end-stage of Hashimoto's thyroiditis or subacute thyroiditis.[10] The incidence of this disease has hence been overestimated.[35, 80]

Riedel's disease or invasive fibrous thyroiditis is an extremely rare entity. In the Mayo Clinic series the incidence in 42,000 thyroidectomies was 0.05 percent.[80] It is a disease of adults and has an even sex distribution or a slight female dominance.[63] Recently, Schwaegerle et al.[63] reviewed the literature on Riedel's disease and added seven cases from their own material. They found a female preponderance (83 percent) and a mean age at diagnosis of 47.8 years. Thyroid

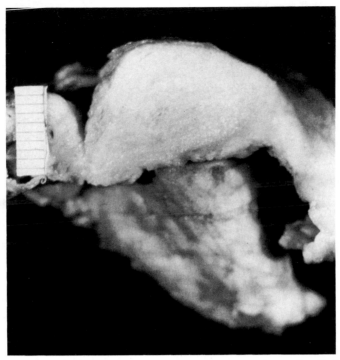

Figure 6–5. Markedly atrophic thyroid in patient with idiopathic myxedema who died of heart failure. Cross section is shown.

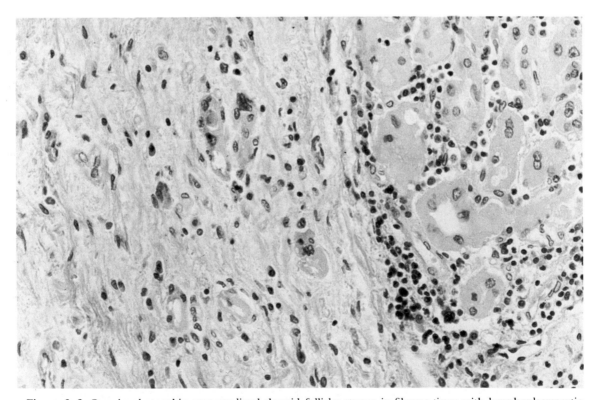

Figure 6–6. Occasional atrophic oncocyte-lined thyroid follicles strewn in fibrous tissue with lymphoplasmacytic infiltrate characterized the histology of the specimen shown in Figure 6–5. × 200, H & E.

function was noted to be normal in 64 percent; hypothyroidism occurred in 32 percent and hyperfunction in 4 percent.[63] The major symptom is a painless goiter, which may grow slowly or rapidly enlarge. Dyspnea is common and may progress to stridor, often out of proportion to the size of the mass. Occasionally vocal cord paralysis may occur.

The classic physical finding is described as a stony hard or woody mass fixed to surrounding structures;[11, 17, 26, 29, 34, 43, 44, 57, 58, 61, 69, 78, 80] hence the term "ligneous thyroiditis."[24] The involvement of the thyroid may be totally or predominantly one-sided or may be bilateral. Cervical lymphadenopathy may be noted; the hard, fixed gland and associated lymph node enlargement may lead to a strong clinical suspicion of carcinoma. When the lesion is confined to the neck no systemic abnormalities are found; however, in some patients the neck lesion represents part of a *systemic collagenosis;* hence, retroperitoneal, mediastinal, or retroorbital fibrosis as well as sclerosing cholangitis may occur. In the Schwaegerle et al. review,[63] 34 percent of patients with Riedel's disease reported after 1960 had other fibrosing lesions. In the latter situation, symptoms may be related to the fibrosing lesions in other body regions.[1, 3, 6, 11, 14, 17, 28, 29, 33, 39, 45, 51, 53, 55, 56, 61, 69, 73, 78, 79] Familial cases with multifocal involvement have been described.[11] In retroperitoneal fibrosis, a possible etiologic relationship to certain drugs such as methysergide has been suggested.[33, 39, 47] No such association is known for Riedel's disease.

The pathologic features of Riedel's disease are characteristic. Grossly, the fibrosis involves all or a part of the thyroid, may involve one or both lobes and is described as woody and very hard.[26, 35, 80] Extension of the fibrosis beyond the thyroid is characteristic and the surgeon may describe that there is no tissue plane. "Plaster from the platysma to the trachea" is an apt description.

Histologically, the involved portions of the gland are destroyed and replaced by fibrous tissue and associated lymphocytes and plasma cells.[26, 35, 80] The fibrous tissue extends into muscle, nerves, and fat, and entraps vessels (Figs. 6–7 to 6–10). In about 25 percent of cases the fibrous tissue also encases parathyroids.[10] There is an associated vasculitis (predominantly a phlebitis) with intimal proliferation, medial destruction, adventitial inflammation, and frequent thrombosis. These microscopic features are shared by retroperitoneal fibrosis and other fibrosing lesions.[28, 33, 45, 46, 47, 53, 79]

In 25 percent of cases of Riedel's disease, an adenoma is identified centrally in the fibrotic mass.[80] The relationship of the adenoma to the fibrous reaction is unknown, although some authors theorize that in these cases the fibrous tissue proliferation may be a reaction to the adenoma or its products.

Of particular importance are the features that by their absence separate Riedel's disease from the thyroiditides: lack of granulomatous reactions, absence of oncocytic change, lack of lobulation of the gland and lack of confinement of the histologic changes to the thyroid.[26, 35, 41, 80]

Recent studies by Harach and Williams[26] define immunopathologic distinctions between Hashimoto's thyroiditis and Riedel's disease. Quantitative studies of the immunoglobulin-containing cells showed that in fibrous Hashimoto's thyroiditis, cells containing kappa light chains outnumbered lambda-containing cells (64 percent versus 36 percent). In Riedel's disease lambda-containing cells constituted 71 percent of the test population. The heavy chain distribution in the plasma cell population varied also. In Hashimoto's thyroiditis IgG-containing cells predominated, whereas IgA cells made up 15 percent of the group; in contrast, IgA-containing plasma cells made up 47 percent of the immunocyte population in Riedel's cases. The significance of these differences with regard to pathogenesis of the Riedel's lesion is unknown; however, the immunologic evaluation supports

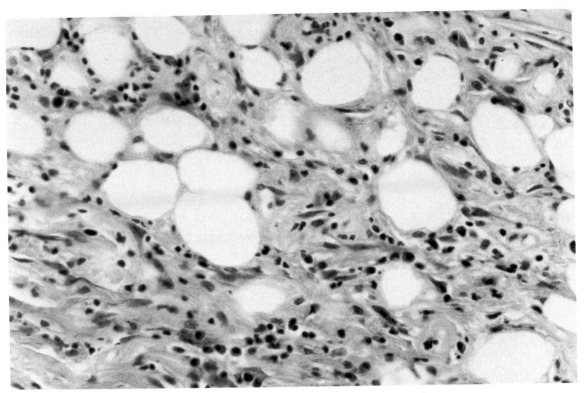

Figure 6–7. Riedel's disease is characterized by fibrous tissue, sometimes keloid-like, associated with inflammatory cells, infiltrating fat. × 200, H & E.

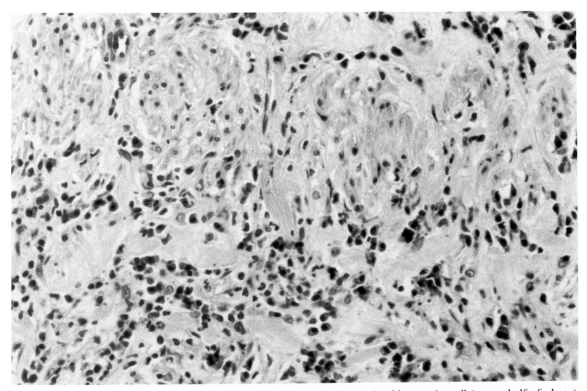

Figure 6–8. Another area from case shown in Figure 6–7; smooth muscle of large vein wall (upper half of photo) is infiltrated. × 200, H & E.

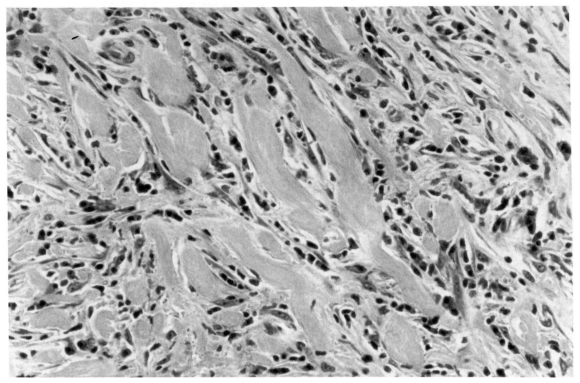

Figure 6–9. Keloid-like bands of fibrosis admixed with inflammatory cells in Riedel's lesion. × 300, H & E.

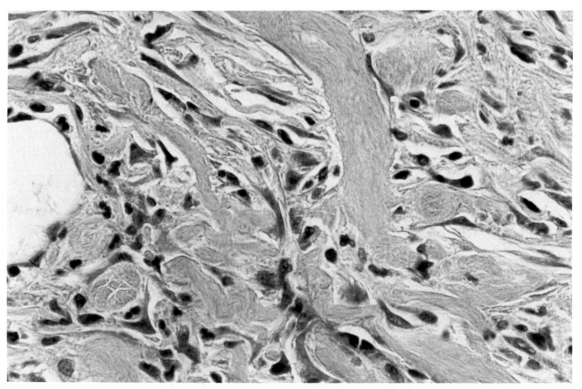

Figure 6–10. Higher power of Figure 6–9. × 400, H & E.

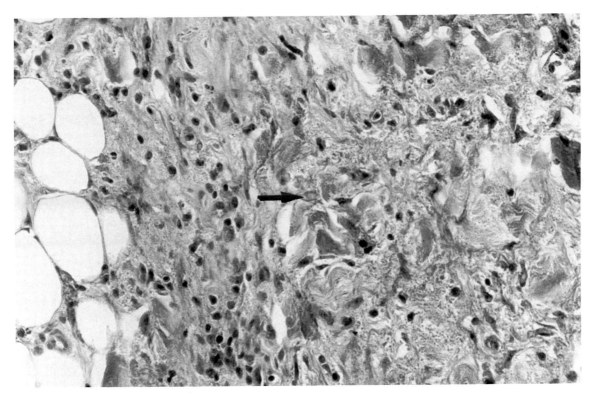

Figure 6–11. Fibrous tissue infiltrates fat. Note crystal at arrow. × 200, H & E.

the separation of the distinctive Riedel's lesion from the thyroiditides. Munro et al. recently reported similar immunologic findings,[48] i.e., a high proportion of IgA- and lambda-containing plasma cells in the inflammatory cells infiltrating retroperitoneal fibrosis, adding further evidence to an interrelationship between these collagen proliferations.

Schwaegerle et al. indicated that of 25 patients reported to have been evaluated, 16 had circulating antithyroid antibodies (67 percent).[63] Immunologic studies in their cases showed that the infiltrating inflammatory cells were a mixture of T and B cells; the distribution of helper and suppressor cells was similar to that of Hashimoto's thyroiditis. These authors suggested a possible autoimmune etiology for Riedel's disease, although they could not exclude the possibility that the autoantibodies present in these patients might represent an epiphenomenon, i.e., reaction to released antigens from destroyed thyroid tissue (similar to antibodies found in subacute thyroiditis—see Chapter 4).

In the author's own experience, a histologically characteristic lesion identical to Riedel's disease (but without vasculitis) was seen in an elderly woman with smoldering myeloma and crystalloglobulinemia. Crystals of precipitated immunoglobulin were identified in dense fibrous tissue in the neck and around the gallbladder. The relationship of the immunoglobulin deposits to the fibrosis is unclear; it seems too simplistic to assume a mechanical traumatic reaction to deposited crystals (Fig. 6–11).

RADIATION THYROIDITIS (See Tables 6–3 and 6–4.)

The major clinical consequence of radiation to the thyroid is the development of hypothyroidism. The incidence of this complication varies among individuals

Table 6–3. Radiation Effects on the Thyroid*

Finding	External**	Radioiodine
Fibrosis	+	+ +
Lymphocytic infiltration	+	±
Follicular atrophy	+	+ +
Oncocytic metaplasia	+	+ +
Squamous metaplasia	+	+
Vascular changes (sclerosis; ectasia; cuffing)	±	+ +
Nuclear atypism	±	+ +
Focal hyperplasia	+ +	−
Nodule formation		
Benign	+	±
Malignant	+	± ?***

*For acute effects, see Chapter 3.
**Changes and incidence of changes vary with dose.
***The incidence of neoplasms in glands treated for hyperthyroidism with radioiodine is not very great since glandular destruction is severe in many of these cases.

and is related to dose in cases of external radiation to the gland. When radioiodine is administered, the incidence of hypothyroidism increases with time and appears less dependent upon the dose received.[8, 13, 22, 42, 49, 67, 82]

The histologic effects of acute radiation on the thyroid have been discussed in Chapter 3. Hypothyroidism may appear relatively early following radiation.[8, 13, 22, 49, 67, 71, 82] Malone and Cullen described the two mechanisms of radiation-related hypothyroidism.[42] Early dysfunction appears dose-dependent, accounts for 5 to 40 percent of cases, and appears related to thyroid cell death. Late-onset hypothyroidism is non-dose-dependent and may be related to the presence of autoimmune factors, especially if these were present before the radiation was given. This late effect also appears related to preexisting thyroid nodularity, heterogeneous distribution of isotope, initial size of gland, and undefined "individual factors."[30, 42]

Pathologic changes that can occur months to years after administration of radioiodine include a grossly shrunken and fibrotic gland.[15, 20, 25, 36, 38, 40, 70] Histologically, fibrosis, follicular disruption, atrophy of follicles, oncocytic metaplasia, and nuclear abnormalities may be seen (Figs. 6–12 and 6–13). Squamous metaplasia of follicular epithelium also occurs; lymphocytic infiltration may be present.

Atypia, including nuclear enlargement and irregularity, is common in epithelial and stromal cells (Figs. 6–14 and 6–15).[36, 38, 40, 70] These nuclear anomalies resemble the nucleomegaly described in radiated tissues in general. However, nuclear changes alone are not pathognomonic for radiation effect in the thyroid. Kennedy and Thompson point out that such abnormal nuclei may be found in thyroid

Table 6–4. Radiation Effects on the Thyroid: Estimated Incidence

	(Percent)
Fibrosis	25
Lymphocytic infiltration	30
Follicular atrophy	@25
Oncocytic metaplasia	17–42
Squamous metaplasia	rare <5
Vascular changes	<5–@50
Nuclear atypism	<5–100
Focal hyperplasia	88
Nodule formation	
Benign	32–57
Malignant	26–59

See references 15, 20, 25, 36, 38, 40, 70, and 74.

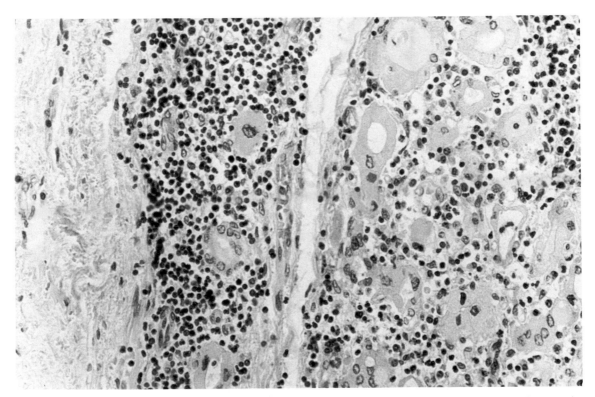

Figure 6–12. Postradiation effect in the thyroid. Marked follicular atrophy, oncocytic change with nuclear atypia, and lymphocytic infiltrates are seen. × 200, H & E.

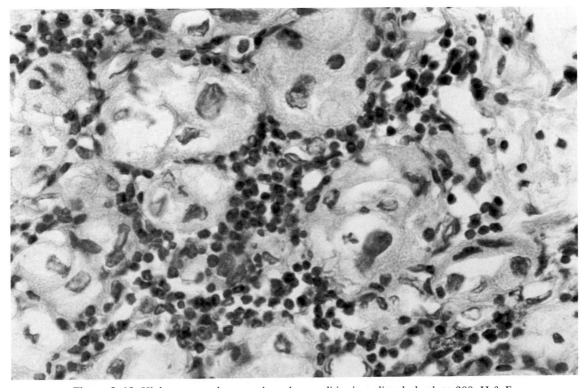

Figure 6–13. Higher power shows nuclear abnormalities in radiated gland. × 300, H & E.

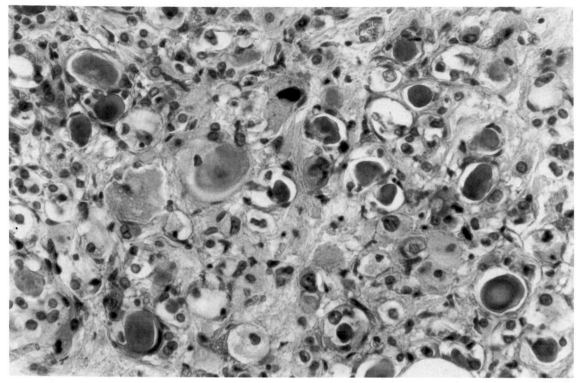

Figure 6–14. Following ^{131}I therapy, nuclear abnormalities in residual gland are more marked than after external radiation. × 200, H & E.

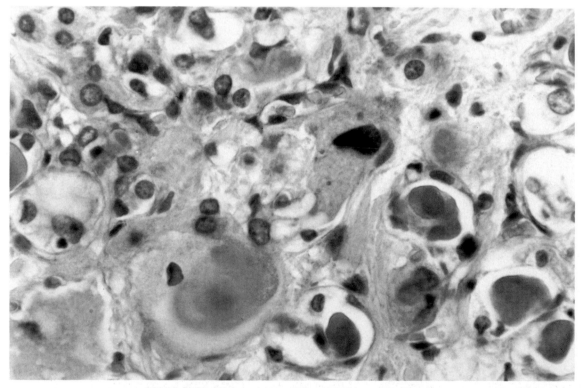

Figure 6–15. Higher power of Figure 6–14. × 300, H & E.

remnants following surgery in nonirradiated subjects.[36] Similar nuclear pleomorphism can be found in oncocytes in various forms of chronic thyroiditis and in the thyroids of patients with longstanding Graves' disease who have not received radiation.

One microscopic feature which is rarely seen in the absence of radiation, however, is the vascular change; this includes intimal thickening and sclerosis of arterial walls (endarteritis obliterans), often with inflammatory cell cuffing. This is a common histologic finding in radiated tissue generally.[36, 38, 40, 70]

Pathologic changes occur in the thyroid following external radiation in about 75 percent of cases. These changes include microscopic foci of follicular hyperplasia (88 percent), lymphocytic infiltration (67 percent), oncocytic metaplasia (42 percent), fibrosis (25 percent), and colloid and adenomatous nodules (51 percent).[36, 38, 74]

Occasionally, long-term follow-up studies of patients treated with external radiation for head and neck nonthyroidal tumors (especially Hodgkin's disease) show the development of hyperthyroidism.[31, 49] It is postulated in these cases that initial radiation damage leads to hypothyroidism, which in turn evokes a hypothalamic-pituitary response, increased thyrotropin levels, and secondary hyperplasia with hyperfunction.[31]

The development of thyroid nodules and carcinomas after radiation to the neck has elicited intensive study of a causal relationship between low-dose radiation and thyroid neoplasia.[4, 18, 19, 54, 59, 60, 65, 68, 72] This aspect of radiation-associated thyroid disease is discussed later in this monograph (Introduction to Part II and in Chapter 8).

AMYLOID IN THE THYROID

Amyloid in the thyroid occurs in three different settings. The most common of these is the amyloid in the stroma of medullary thyroid carcinoma (discussed in Chapter 10). Amyloid goiter[2, 32, 37] is a mass lesion composed of masses of amyloid associated with a foreign body giant cell response and with adipose tissue. This very rare condition may be unilateral or bilateral, is associated with systemic amyloidosis, and is basically a mass lesion producing a goiter.[37] This entity must be distinguished from amyloid-rich medullary carcinoma, in which the prognosis is that of the neoplasm. Careful search of sections of the lesions may be required to identify the epithelial cells of the tumor.

Amyloid deposition in the thyroid stroma and in glandular and periglandular blood vessels occurs in systemic amyloidosis and may be found in either primary or secondary forms of that disease. Goiter is not present, however. The amyloid deposits may be so extensive as to interfere with thyroid function and produce hypothyroidism.[37] Figure 6–16 illustrates the gland of a 37-year-old woman who died of "secondary" amyloidosis, having suffered for many years from tuberculosis. Widespread involvement of many organs was found. The thyroid was a firm, homogeneous mass, which histologically was difficult to recognize as thyroid. If the hyaline nature of the amyloid deposits is not recognized, the lesion may be considered as an unusual fibrous proliferation of the gland. Special stains for amyloid help to define the disorder.[21, 37] The type of amyloid seen in this case—most likely AA amyloid—would be expected to give a negative Congo red reaction following potassium permanganate treatment.[75, 81] The histopathologist may garner a clue as to the actual nature of the lesion by examination of the blood vessel walls, which are involved in amyloidosis and are relatively spared in fibrous thyroiditis.

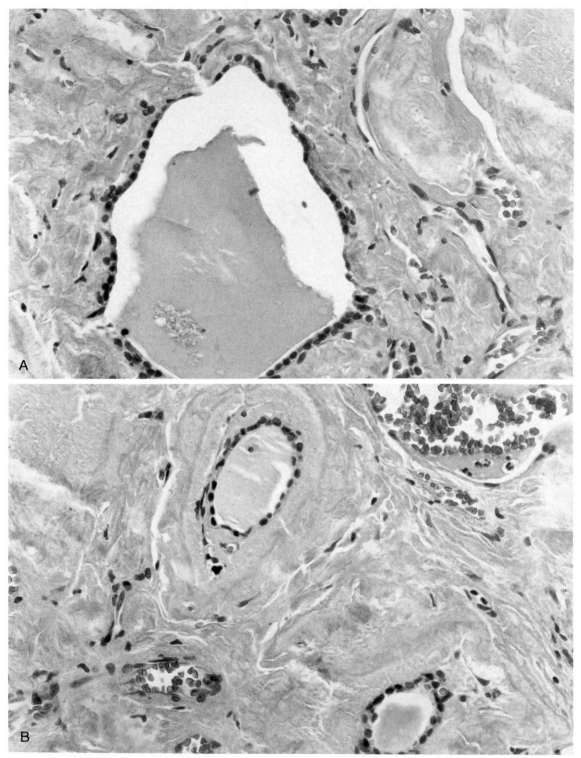

Figure 6–16. *A,* Amyloid "secondary type" involving thyroid. Note lone residual follicle in this section (left). Homogeneous material diffusely replaced thyroid tissue. × 200, H & E. *B,* Another area from the same case as Figure 6–16, *A.* Note amyloid "hugging" follicles. × 200, H & E.

TRAUMA

Fibrosis can be identified in the thyroid in areas of hemorrhage and inflammation in nodular goiter or following trauma (needle biopsy, surgery, etc.) (Fig. 6–17). These fibrous areas reflect the inflammatory process and are secondary to it. The presence of hemosiderin and macrophages and histologic features of goiter are helpful in diagnosing these lesions. (See also Chapter 9.)

Focal scars and areas of fibrosis are not uncommonly seen in thyroid nodules following needle biopsy. The mechanism of fibrosis here is similar to that in nodular goiter, although the size of the lesions may be much smaller.

Extensive fibrosis involving cervical soft tissue has been reported as a reaction to extruded thorium dioxide.[12]

DESMOPLASIA NEAR TUMORS

Desmoplasia in neoplasms of the thyroid is encountered frequently, most often in papillary carcinomas. The fibrous reaction may be found within the tumor itself but is more frequently noted at the invasive edges of the lesion. In the follicular variant of papillary carcinoma, this peripheral desmoplastic reaction may be a useful histologic hint to the differential diagnostic dilemma of follicular variant of papillary cancer versus true follicular carcinoma. (See also Chapters 8 and 9.) In the latter neoplasm, desmoplasia is unusual. In medullary carcinoma, fibrosis within the tumor (with or without associated amyloid) is common. A desmoplastic reaction at the infiltrative edge of the tumor may sometimes be seen, but in this author's experience is less often found than in papillary cancers.

SCLERODERMA

There are *systemic disorders* in which fibrosis of the thyroid occurs as a part of the basic disease; the thyroid is involved secondarily. The classic example of this type of fibrosis is *progressive systemic sclerosis (scleroderma)*.[16, 23] In the author's experience and that reported in the literature, some patients with scleroderma will experience some thyroid dysfunction (evident either clinically or by chemical evaluation via thyroid function tests);[23, 50, 77] the pathologic counterpart to these abnormalities is fibrosis, especially interfollicular in location (Fig. 6–18). The microscopic finding of fibrosis is seen in 14 to 24 percent of cases; 5 percent show evidence of chronic lymphocytic thyroiditis.[16, 23] Vascular sclerosis may also be found and may be etiologically related to the fibrosis seen;[9, 52] the possibility of an associated or superimposed immunologic mechanism for the thyroid fibrosis also must be considered. However, the degree of glandular sclerosis does not correlate directly with serologic evidence of autoimmune thyroiditis nor with the degree of thyroid dysfunction.[23] Rare cases of scleroderma associated with hyperthyroidism (Graves' disease) have been reported. In one study, HLA subtyping suggested a possible genetic predisposition to both diseases.[50] The possible interrelationships among the thyroid disorders and scleroderma need further study.

In summary, this chapter has reviewed those thyroid lesions characterized predominantly by fibrosis. Interrelationships, clinicopathologic features, and suggested etiologic mechanisms are reviewed.

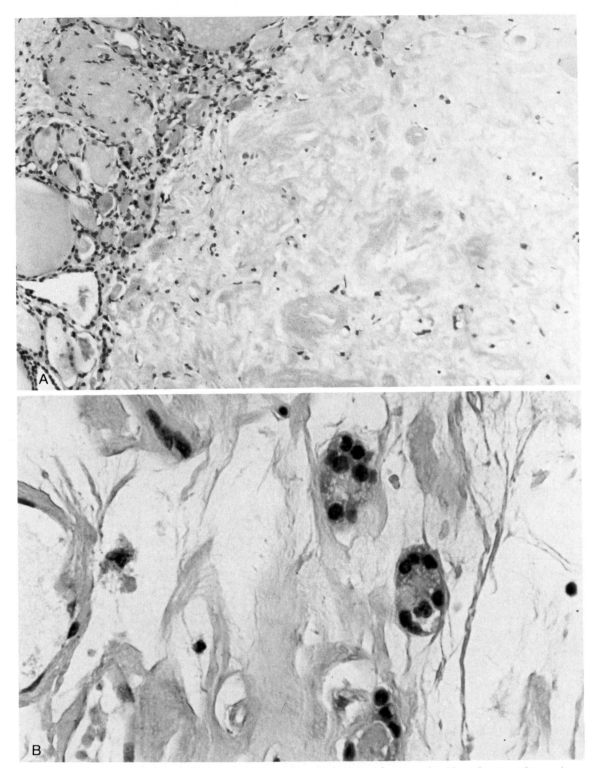

Figure 6–17. *A,* Area of dense fibrosis in nodular goiter. Such zones often contain siderophages and sometimes dystrophic calcification. × 100, H & E. *B,* At higher power, a few small follicles can be seen in fibrous tissue. × 300, H & E.

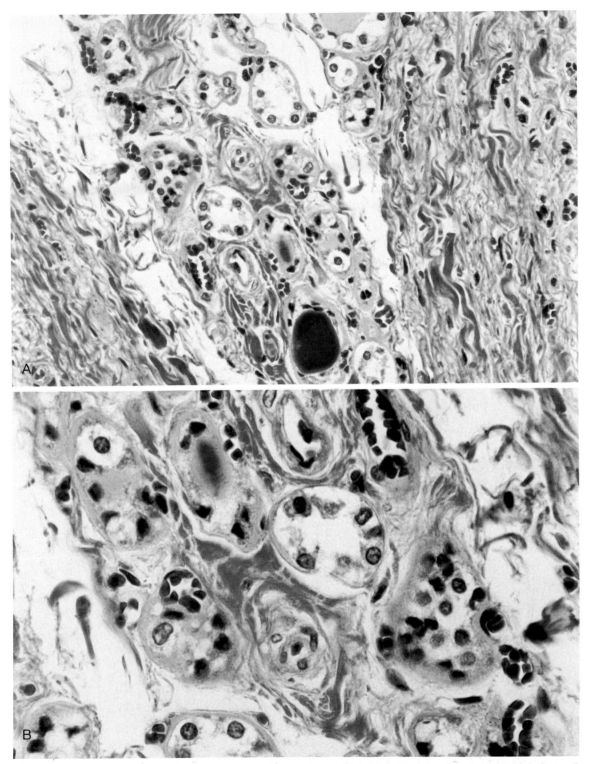

Figure 6–18. *A,* Scleroderma. In some patients with or without thyroid dysfunction, increased interlobular and interfollicular fibrosis is seen. × 200, H & E. *B,* Higher power shows interfollicular fibrosis. × 300, H & E.

REFERENCES

1. Amorosa, L.F., Shear, M.K., and Spiera, H.: Multifocal fibrosis involving thyroid, face and orbits. Arch. Intern. Med. 136:221–223, 1976.
2. Arean, V.M., and Klein, R.E.: Amyloid goiter; review of the literature and report of a case. Am. J. Clin. Pathol. 36:341–355, 1961.
3. Arnott, E.J., and Greaves, D.P.: Orbital involvement in Riedel's thyroiditis. Br. J. Ophthalmol. 49:1–5, 1965.
4. Auguste, L.J., and Sako, K.: Radiation and thyroid carcinoma: Radiotherapy, head and neck regions, thyroid carcinoma. Head and Neck Surg. 7:217–224, 1985.
5. Bastenie, P.A., Bonnyns, M., and Vanhaelst, L.: Natural history of myxedema. Am. J. Med. 79:91–100, 1985.
6. Bartholomew, L.G., Cain, J.C., et al.: Sclerosing cholangitis. Its possible association with Riedel's struma and fibrous retroperitonitis. N. Engl. J. Med. 269:8–12, 1963.
7. Bowlby, A.A.: Infiltrating fibroma (?sarcoma) of the thyroid gland. Trans. Pathol. Soc. Lond. 36:420–422, 1885.
8. Burke, G., and Silverstein, G.E.: Hypothyroidism after treatment with sodium iodide I-131. J.A.M.A. 210:1051–1058, 1969.
9. Campbell, P.M., and LeRoy, E.C.: Pathogenesis of systemic sclerosis: a vascular hypothesis. Sem. Arth. Rheum. 4:351–368, 1975.
10. Chopra, D., Wool, M.S., et al.: Riedel's struma associated with subacute thyroiditis, hypothyroidism, and hypoparathyroidism. J. Clin. Endocrinol. Metab. 46:869–871, 1978.
11. Comings, D.E., Skubi, K.B., et al.: Familial multifocal fibrosclerosis. Ann. Intern. Med. 66:884–892, 1967.
12. Conley, J., Janecka, I., and Harley, N.H.: Severe cervical fibrosis following thorium dioxide infection. N.Y. State J. Med. 78:292–294, 1978.
13. Constine, L.S., Donaldson, S.S., et al.: Thyroid dysfunction after radiotherapy in children with Hodgkin's disease. Cancer 55:878–883, 1984.
14. Coopersmith, N.H., and Appelman, H.D.: Multifocal fibrosclerosis with subcutaneous involvement. Am. J. Clin. Pathol. 55:369–376, 1971.
15. Curran, R.C., Eckert, H., and Wilson, G.M.: The thyroid gland after treatment of hyperthyroidism by partial thyroidectomy or iodine-131. J. Pathol. Bacteriol. 76:541–560, 1958.
16. D'Angelo, W.A., Fries, J.F., et al.: Pathologic observations in systemic sclerosis (scleroderma). Am. J. Med. 46:428–440, 1969.
17. Davies, D., and Furness, P.: Riedel's thyroiditis with multiple organ fibrosis. Thorax 39:959–960, 1984.
18. DeGroot, L.J., Reilly, M., et al.: Retrospective and prospective study of radiation-induced thyroid disease. Am. J. Med. 74:852–862, 1983.
19. Fjalling, M., Tisell, L.-E., et al.: Benign and malignant thyroid nodules after neck irradiation. Cancer 58:1219–1224, 1986.
20. Freedberg, A.S., Kurland, G.S., and Herrman, L.B.: The pathologic effects of I[131] on the normal thyroid gland of man. J. Clin. Endocrinol. 12:1315–1348, 1952.
21. Gharib, H., and Goellner, J.R.: Diagnosis of amyloidosis by fine-needle aspiration biopsy of the thyroid. N. Engl. J. Med. 305:586, 1981.
22. Glennon, J.A., Gordon, E.S., and Swain, C.T.: Hypothyroidism after low-dose 131-I treatment of hyperthyroidism. Ann. Intern. Med. 76:721–723, 1972.
23. Gordon, M.B., Klein, I., et al.: Thyroid disease in progressive systemic sclerosis: increased frequency of glandular fibrosis and hypothyroidism. Ann. Intern. Med. 95:431–435, 1981.
24. Graham, A.: Riedel's struma in contrast to struma lymphomatosa (Hashimoto). West. J. Surg. 39:681–689, 1931.
25. Hanson, G.A., Komorowski, R.A., et al.: Thyroid gland morphology in young adults: normal subjects versus those with prior low-dose neck irradiation in childhood. Surgery 94:984–988, 1983.
26. Harach, H.R., and Williams, E.D.: Fibrous thyroiditis—an immunopathological study. Histopathology 7:739–751, 1983.
27. Hashimoto, H.: Zur Kenntniss der lymphomatosen Veranderung der Schilddruse (Struma lymphomatosa). Arch. Klin. Chir. 97:219–248, 1912.
28. Hellstrom, H.R., and Perez-Stable, E.C.: Retroperitoneal fibrosis with disseminated vasculitis and intrahepatic sclerosing cholangitis. Am. J. Med. 46:184–187, 1966.
29. Hines, R.C., Scheuermann, H.A., et al.: Invasive fibrous (Riedel's) thyroiditis with bilateral fibrous parotitis. J.A.M.A. 213:869–871, 1970.
30. Hiraoka, T., Miller, R.C., et al.: Survival of human normal thyroid cells after X-ray irradiation. Int. J. Radiat. Biol. 47:299–307, 1985.
31. Jacobson, D.R., and Fleming, B.J.: Graves' disease with ophthalmopathy following radiotherapy for Hodgkin's disease. Am. J. Med. Sci. 288:217–220, 1984.
32. James, P.D.: Amyloid goitre. J. Clin. Pathol. 25:683–688, 1972.
33. Jones, J.H., Ross, E.J., et al.: Retroperitoneal fibrosis. Am. J. Med. 48:203–208, 1970.
34. Katsikas, D., Shorthouse, A.J., and Taylor, S.: Riedel's thyroiditis. Br. J. Surg. 63:929–931, 1976.

35. Katz, S.M., and Vickery, A.L.: The fibrous variant of Hashimoto's thyroiditis. Hum. Pathol. *5:*161–170, 1974.
36. Kennedy, J.S., and Thomson, J.A.: The changes in the thyroid gland after irradiation with [131]-I or partial thyroidectomy for thyrotoxicosis. J. Pathol. *112:*65–81, 1974.
37. Kennedy, J.S., Thomson, J.A., and Buchanan, W.M.: Amyloid in the thyroid. Quart. J. Med. *43:*127–143, 1974.
38. Komorowski, R.A., and Hanson, G.A.: Morphologic changes in the thyroid following low-dose childhood radiation. Arch. Pathol. Lab. Med. *101:*36–39, 1977.
39. Kurzel, R.B., Yoonesi, M., and Munabe, A.: Retroperitoneal fibrosis: A two decade experience and gynecologic manifestations. Int. J. Gynaecol. Obstet. *19:*271–280, 1981.
40. Lindsay, S., Dailey, M.E., and Jones, M.D.: Histologic effects of various types of ionizing radiation on normal and hyperplastic human thyroid glands. J. Clin. Endocrinol. Metab. *14:*1179–1219, 1954.
41. Lindsay, S., Dailey, M.E., et al.: Chronic thyroiditis: a clinical and pathologic study of 354 patients. J. Clin. Endocrinol. Metab. *12:*1578–1600, 1952.
42. Malone, J.F., and Cullen, M.J.: Two mechanisms for hypothyroidism after [131]-I therapy. Lancet *2:*73–75, 1976.
43. Meijer, S., and Hausman, R.: Occlusive phlebitis, a diagnostic feature in Riedel's thyroiditis. Virch. Arch. A Path. Anat. *377:*339–349, 1978.
44. Melato, M., and Mlac, M.: Riedel's thyroiditis and isolated thyroid amyloidosis. Pathologica *70:*30–37, 1978.
45. Meyer, S., and Hausman, R.: Occlusive phlebitis in multifocal fibrosclerosis. Am. J. Clin. Pathol. *65:*274–283, 1976.
46. Mitchinson, M.J.: The pathology of idiopathic retroperitoneal fibrosis. J. Clin. Pathol. *23:*681–689, 1970.
47. Mitchinson, M.J.: Retroperitoneal fibrosis revisited. Arch. Pathol. Lab. Med. *110:*784–786, 1986.
48. Munro, J.M., Van der Walt, J.D., and Cox, E.L.: A comparison of cytoplasmic immunoglobulins in retroperitoneal fibrosis and abdominal aortic aneurysms. Histopathology *10:*1163–1169, 1986.
49. Nelson, D.F., Reddy, K.V., et al.: Thyroid abnormalities following neck irradiation for Hodgkin's disease. Cancer *42:*2553–2562, 1978.
50. Nicholson, D., White, S., et al.: Progressive systemic sclerosis and Graves' disease. Arch. Intern. Med. *146:*2350–2352, 1986.
51. Nielsen, H.K.: Multifocal idiopathic fibrosclerosis. Acta Med. Scand. *208:*119–123, 1980.
52. Norton, W.L., and Nardo, J.M.: Vascular disease in progressive systemic sclerosis (scleroderma). Ann. Intern. Med. *73:*317–324, 1970.
53. Olsen, K.D., DeSanto, L.W., et al.: Tumefactive fibroinflammatory lesions of the head and neck. Laryngoscope *96:*940–944, 1986.
54. Pingitore, R., and Martino, E.: The histology of human radiation-related thyroid carcinoma. Pathologica *76:*107–112, 1984.
55. Rao, C.R., Ferguson, G.C., and Kyle, V.N.: Retroperitoneal fibrosis associated with Riedel's struma. Canad. Med. Assoc. J. *108:*1019–1021, 1973.
56. Raphael, H.A., Beahrs, D.H., et al.: Riedel's struma associated with fibrous mediastinitis. Mayo Clin. Proc. *41:*375, 382, 1966.
57. Riedel, B.M.C.L.: Die chronische, zur bildungeisenharter Tumoren fuhrende Entzundgung der Schilddruse. Verh. Deutsch. Gess. Chir. *225:*101–105, 1896.
58. Riedel, B.M.C.L.: Vorstellung eines Kranken mit chronischer Strumitis. Verh. Deutsch. Gess. Chir. *26:*127-129, 1897.
59. Schneider, A.B., Recant, W., et al.: Radiation-induced thyroid carcinoma. Ann. Intern. Med. *105:*405–412, 1986.
60. Schneider, A.B., Shore-Freedman, E., and Weinstein, R.A.: Radiation-induced thyroid and other head and neck tumors: occurrence of multiple tumors and analysis of risk factors. J. Clin. Endocrinol. Metab. *62:*107–112, 1986.
61. Schneider, R.J.: Orbital involvement in Riedel's struma. Canad. J. Ophthal. *11:*87–90, 1976.
62. Schnyder, B., and Hedinger, C.: Die Fibrosierungstendenz bei subakuter thyreoiditis de Quervain. Schweiz. med. Wschr. *116:*1093–1097, 1986.
63. Schwaegerle, S.M., Bauer, T.W., and Esselstyn, C.B.: Riedel's thyroiditis. Am. J. Clin. Pathol. *90:*715–722, 1988.
64. Sclare, G.: The thyroid in myxedema. J. Pathol. Bacteriol. *85:*263–278, 1963.
65. Segal, R.L., Cobin, R.H., et al.: Thyroid nodules in the irradiated patient—an indication for total thyroidectomy. J. Surg. Oncol. *28:*126–130, 1985.
66. Semple, P.: Fibroid enlargement of the thyroid body, with enlarged cervical glands. Trans. Pathol. Soc. Lond. *20:*397–399, 1869.
67. Shafer, R.B., Nuttall, F.Q., et al.: Thyroid function after radiation and surgery for head and neck cancer. Arch. Intern. Med. *135:*843–846, 1975.
68. Shore, R.E., Woodard, E., et al.: Thyroid tumors following thymus irradiation. J. Natl. Cancer Inst. *74:*1177–1184, 1985.
69. Spencer, M.G.: Riedel's thyroiditis discovered at tracheostomy. J. Laryngol. Otol. *99:*97–100, 1985.
70. Spitalnik, P.R., and Strauss, F.H.: Patterns of human thyroid parenchymal reaction following low-dose childhood irradiation. Cancer *41:*1098–1105, 1978.

71. Swelstad, J., Scanlon, E.F., et al.: Thyroid disease following irradiation for benign conditions. Arch. Surg. *112*:380–383, 1977.
72. Tiernan, A.M., Weiss, N.S., and Daling, J.R.: Incidence of thyroid cancer in women in relation to previous exposure to radiation therapy and history of thyroid disease. J. Natl. Cancer Inst. *73*:575–581, 1984.
73. Turner-Warwich, R., Nabarro, J.D., and Doniach, D.: Riedel's thyroiditis and retroperitoneal fibrosis. Proc. Royal Soc. Med. *59*:596–598, 1966.
74. Valdiserri, R.O., and Borochovitz, D.: Histologic changes in previously irradiated thyroid glands. Arch. Pathol. Lab. Med. *104*:150–152, 1980.
75. van Rijswijk, M.H., and van Heusden, C.W.G.J.: The potassium permanganate method. Am. J. Pathol. *97*:43–58, 1979.
76. Vollenweider, I., and Hedinger, C.: Solid cell nests (SCN) in Hashimoto's thyroiditis. Virch. Arch. Pathol. Anat. *412*:357–363, 1988.
77. Ward, J.A., Mendeloff, J., and Coberly, J.C.: Hyperthyroidism followed by scleroderma. J.A.M.A. *237*:1123, 1977.
78. Ward, M.J., and Davies, D.: Riedel's thyroiditis with invasion of the lungs. Thorax *36*:956–957, 1981.
79. Wold, L.E., and Weiland, L.H.: Tumefactive fibro-inflammatory lesions of the head and neck. Am. J. Surg. Pathol. *7*:477–482, 1983.
80. Woolner, L.B., McConahey, W.M., and Beahrs, O.H.: Invasive fibrous thyroiditis (Riedel's struma). J. Clin. Endocrinol. Metab. *17*:201–220, 1957.
81. Wright, J.R., Calkins, E., and Humphrey, R.L.: Potassium permanganate reaction in amyloidosis. Lab. Invest. *36*:274–281, 1977.
82. Zohar, Y., Tovim, R.B., et al.: Thyroid function following radiation and surgical therapy in head and neck malignancy. Head and Neck Surg. *6*:948–952, 1984.

7

PIGMENTS, CRYSTALS, AND INFILTRATIVE LESIONS OF THE THYROID

In this chapter, a series of unusual lesions affecting the thyroid will be described. These may be conveniently divided into the following areas:

1. Pigments in the thyroid
     iron
     lipofuscin
     minocycline-associated melanin
     ochronotic pigment
2. Crystals in the thyroid
     "birefringent" crystals; oxalate
     exogenous (Teflon)
3. Systemic and storage diseases affecting the thyroid

PIGMENTS IN THE THYROID

Iron. Iron can be found commonly in the thyroid. In nodular goiter, in the vicinity of neoplasms, and especially in the tracks of biopsy needles, areas of degeneration and hemorrhage are seen. Often in zones of fresh hemorrhage, red cells are found. However, as the process of resorption of the blood proceeds, hemosiderin accumulates. In some cases this is found free in the stroma, but more often it is seen within macrophages. As in other organs, the hemosiderin appears as coarse brown to brown-yellow pigment (Figs. 7–1 and 7–2). Special stains enhance the appearance of this pigment so that often much more hemosiderin is identified than noted on routine hematoxylin-eosin stain.

In some nodules, whether benign or malignant, iron pigment is found within the proliferating epithelial cells. In the author's experience, this phenomenon is particularly common in papillary carcinomas in which extensive areas of hemorrhage have occurred.

In disorders of iron metabolism, i.e., posttransfusional hemosiderosis and the primary hemochromatosis syndromes, iron pigment unassociated with obvious areas of hemorrhage or degeneration may be found in thyroid follicular cells or in stromal macrophages.[8, 37, 45] On rare occasions this iron deposition may be

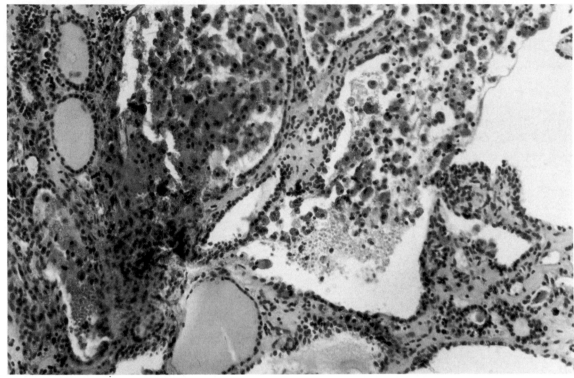

Figure 7–1. Area of hemorrhage and degeneration in nodular goiter. Note numerous macrophages. × 150, H & E.

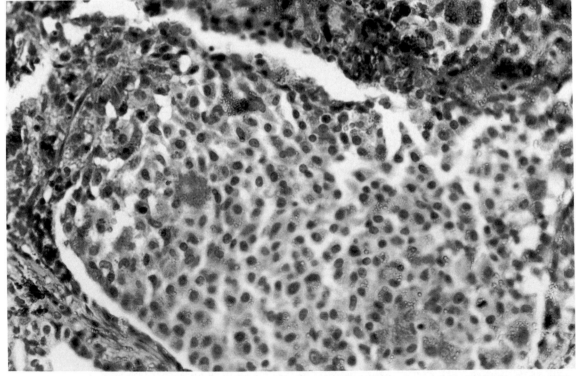

Figure 7–2. Higher power of Figure 7–1 shows macrophages with cytoplasmic granular hemosiderin. × 250, H & E.

sufficient to give the gland a grossly dark brown to rusty color. Microscopically, iron is seen as a golden brown granular pigment in the thyroid epithelium. Oliver identified iron in nine of 14 thyroids examined at autopsy of patients who had transfusional siderosis;[37] in only one of these did he identify increased thyroid fibrosis.

Clinically, thyroid dysfunction is unusual in iron storage disease; however, some patients may suffer secondary hypothyroidism because of pituitary impairment caused by iron overload.[15]

Lipofuscin Pigment. This can be found in the thyroid, as in most other organs.[20, 38] It is seen as yellow to light brown granular material scattered throughout the cytoplasm of follicular epithelial cells. It occurs in clusters of round to oblong bodies 1 to 3 micra in size. The nature of lipofuscin pigment is not known. Staining reactions (Table 7–1) indicate the presence of lipid and certain amino acids (histadine, tryptophan).[38] Apparently iron is not present, although in some tissues lipofuscin may be closely associated with hemosiderin.

Ultrastructural analyses indicate that lipofuscin granules have a polymorphic internal structure and are almost uniformly surrounded by a single membrane. Within the granules, vacuoles, presumably fat, are seen, as are laminated structures of variable size.[7] Histochemical studies show the presence of acid phosphatase and other enzymes, suggesting origin or at least association with lysosomes.[38] Theories as to the origin of lipofuscin include mitochondrial breakdown and/or environmental or nutritional factors accumulating in lysosomes. Borel and Reddy suggest that excess lipofuscin accumulation in thyroids of young patients dying of cystic fibrosis might be related to oxidation of lipids in thyroid epithelium caused by chronic vitamin E deficiency.[7]

Mahmoud et al. have shown experimentally that administration of a high iodide diet with thyroid hyperplasia (induced by low iodide diet and goitrogen) produced involution of the gland.[29] The involution was apparently mediated by a vasoconstriction; after 12 to 48 hours, necrosis and inflammation were abundant. Associated with necrosis, lipofuscin inclusions were noted in the thyroid epithelium. The acute appearance of lipofuscin suggests that the toxicity of iodide in iodide-deficient thyroid cells is mediated by lipid peroxidation, and lipofuscin results. The implication of these experiments in the human thyroid is unknown. Indeed, lipofuscins are considered a sign of senescence; Ohaki et al. found increase in

Table 7–1. Staining Reactions of Minocycline-Related Pigment*

Stain	Minocycline Pigment	Lipofuscin
H & E	Coarse granules, dark-brown to black	Small granules, yellow-brown
PAS	+/±	+
PAS-diastase	+/±	
Ziehl-Neelson	+	+
Fontana Masson	+/±	
Fontana Masson after bleaching	−/+	
Oil red O	+	
Osmium tetroxide (lipids)	+	
Birefringence	−	
Autofluorescence	−/±	+
Iron (Gomori; Turnbill blue)	−	
Sudan IV (lipids)	+	+
Nile blue sulfate for acidic and neutral lipids	−	
AFIP method for lipofuscin	−	+

*See references 1 and 17.

lipofuscin in the thyroid in older patients in their series of 500 autopsies.[36] In the thyroid, as in other organs, the functional and/or disease implications of lipofuscin, if any, remain unknown; the overwhelming majority of patients with thyroidal lipofuscin accumulation have no evidence of thyroid dysfunction.[7, 36]

Minocycline-Associated Pigment: The Black Thyroid. The presence of dark brown to black pigment in thyroid glands of animals given minocycline (a tetracycline derivative) was originally reported by Benitez et al.[4] Similar pigmentation had been noted in dogs following chronic administration of tetracycline itself.[11] Pigmentation of the skin in some patients has also been noted.[14]

Grossly, deposition of minocycline pigment is seen as brown-black to coal-black coloration of the gland. Histologically, a granular dust-like precipitate of black-brown pigment is noted in the apical portions of the follicular epithelial cells (Figs. 7–3, 7–4). In some animals, but not in man, the pigment is associated with evidence of thyroid epithelial hypertrophy or hyperplasia.[17]

Over the past decade, numerous case reports or small series of patients with black thyroid have been noted in the literature.[1, 3, 6, 23, 26, 33, 34, 39, 43, 50] Only rarely were abnormalities of thyroid function noted in these cases.[1] These patients had received minocycline for chronic conditions such as acne, bronchiectasis, or pyelonephritis. (See Table 7–2.)

What is the nature of minocycline-related pigment? As noted above, in man naturally occurring pigment in the thyroid (lipofuscin) accumulates with age[20, 33] without thyroid function changes. Different reports indicate variable results of staining reactions in different patients (Table 7–1). Are these caused by differences

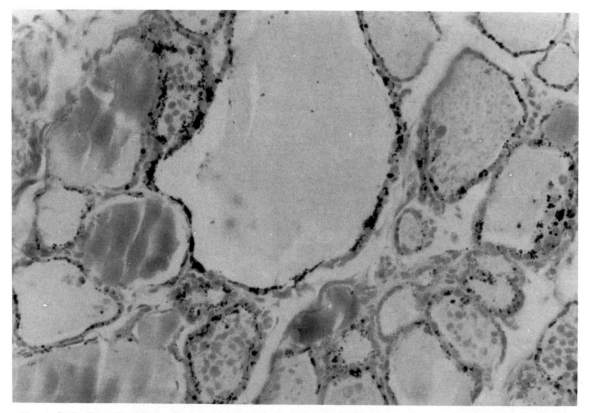

Figure 7–3. Granular black pigment predominantly found in follicular epithelial cells in patient on chronic minocycline therapy. × 100, H & E.

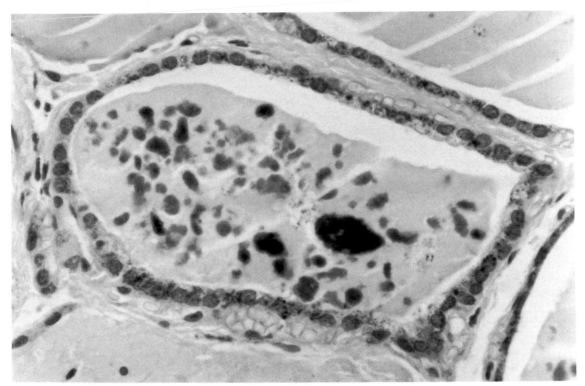

Figure 7–4. In this follicle, clumps of black pigment are seen in colloid as well as in epithelium. Same case as Figure 7–3. × 250, H & E.

in the nature of the pigment, different doses or durations of drug use, or individual variables?

Gordon et al. reported elegant studies on the minocycline pigment.[17] These authors used histochemistry, electron microscopy, and X-ray dispersion analysis to study the pigment; three experimental and clinical groups were examined: animals (rat, dog, monkey, guinea pig), human volunteers, and patients. Although some differences were identified among the three groups, Gordon et al. concluded that marked similarities exist between lipofuscin and minocycline pigment.[17]

Table 7–2. Minocycline-Related Thyroid Pigment: Clinical Features*

Male/female	10:9 (not available, 3)
Age	
Range	20–86 yrs.
Mean	46 yrs.
Basic disease	
Acne	7
Lung infection	3
Renal disease	1
Other (including incidental autopsy finding)**	7
Unknown	4
Duration of therapy	
Range	30 days–11 yrs.
Thyroid function	
Normal	8
Decreased	1
Increased	0
Not reported	13

*This table gives data on patients reported in the English literature through 1988.
**One patient reported by Landas et al.[26] had no definite history of minocycline usage.

Histochemical reactions, elemental analyses, and ultrastructural findings are similar.[17, 43] Thus, both lipofuscin and minocycline pigment fluoresce, and give positive reactions with PAS, lipid, and lipofuscin stains[17, 44] (Table 7–1); by electron microscopy both are found confined to lysosomes[17, 24] (Fig. 7–5). (It should be considered that the pigment noted in the two grossly dark cystic fibrosis thyroids by Borel and Reddy[7] might have been minocycline-related; such patients would probably have received many antibiotics for numerous pulmonary infections; no data on drug use are given, however.)

Gordon et al. concluded that minocycline pigment represents lipofuscin with a small amount of another as yet uncharacterized substance (? drug byproduct).[17] Saul et al. postulated that the pigment represented an oxidation degradation product of the drug itself or that the drug may alter tyrosine metabolism leading to pigment accumulation.[43] Alexander et al. suggest that "individual factors" need to be considered as well.[1] Lysosomal dysfunction could be caused by minocycline or possibly by other drugs. There is an intralysosomal accumulation of lipids producing a lipid-drug complex and impaired lysosomal function leading to pigmentation.[1, 25] Some authors found granular pigment in follicular cells more commonly in older than younger patients.[26, 33] These authors suggested the pigmentation is a normal aging process. Ohaki et al. agree but suggest that minocycline is needed to produce grossly black thyroid.[36]

Of interest is the finding in Saul et al.'s case wherein the adenomatous nodule in their case of black thyroid showed no pigment.[43] Conversely, in Reid's cases both the adenoma and the normal thyroid were pigmented,[39] and in the case

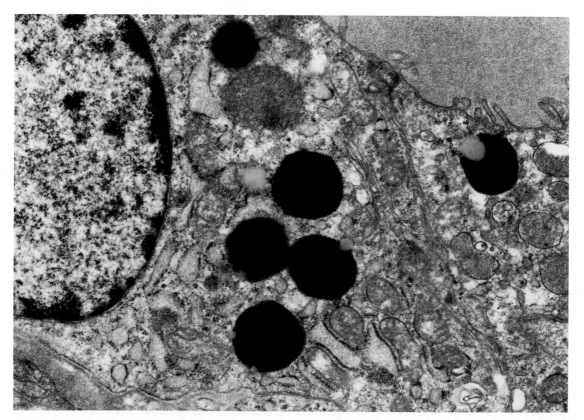

Figure 7–5. By electron microscopy, presence of dark masses of lysosomal-associated pigment is noted. × 30,000. (Photomicrograph courtesy of Dr. Renato V. Iozzo.)

reported by Wajda et al. the adenoma was black and the surrounding thyroid relatively nonpigmented.[48] Hence different areas (proliferative zones) in the same thyroid may react in different ways. In rats, Kurosumi and Fujita found no coloration if the minocycline-treated animals were given propylthiouracil or thyroxine;[24] black thyroid occurred if the rats were given thyrotropin. Hence, thyroid function may affect the occurrence of pigmentation, which may be related to some aspect of iodine metabolism.[24]

Finding "black thyroids" is unusual despite the availability and use of minocycline therapeutically for twenty years; hence, certain individual peculiarities must account for pigmentation.[17] The absence of thyroid functional changes in patients and human volunteers and the lack of pathologic evidence of thyroid hyperplasia or degeneration suggest that, despite its striking appearance, "black thyroid" pigment is innocuous. However, one patient reported by Alexander et al. did have significant hypothyroidism.[1]

Melanin. Melanin is found in the thyroid in two specific situations: metastatic malignant melanoma to the thyroid and melanin-producing medullary thyroid carcinoma. In each of these diseases, the pigment is found associated with tumor nodules and not dispersed in otherwise relatively normal-appearing follicular cells (e.g., minocycline pigment).

Metastatic melanoma can be found in the thyroid as a surgical lesion or at postmortem examination.[19, 22, 46] (See Chapter 16.)

Melanin production by medullary thyroid carcinoma is a rare but biologically intriguing event;[31, 32] this entity is discussed in Chapter 10.

Ochronotic Pigment. The present author is aware of one case of ochronosis in which dark brown-black pigment (nonstained by stains for iron) was found in the thyroid (personal communication: Dr. Scott H. Saul).

CRYSTALS IN THE THYROID

Birefringent crystalline material may be found commonly in colloid in normal or diseased glands. The scarcity of reports mentioning these crystals belies their frequency. Although described in the German literature in the late nineteenth and early twentieth century, it was only in 1954 that the study of Richter and McCarty on "anisotropic crystals" appeared in English.[41]

The crystals, seen in ordinary light, but more easily by polarized light (Fig. 7–6), are of different sizes and shapes, from elongated polyhedrons to irregular plaques.[41] These structures are always found within the colloid and are not seen in an intracellular or stromal location. The chemical and X-ray diffraction studies indicated that the crystals are composed of calcium oxalate.[41]

These authors examined almost 500 thyroids from autopsies and noted increasing frequency of crystals with age: 8 percent of glands from patients under 30 had them, whereas 54 percent of glands from patients over 60 did.[41] Crystals are identified only rarely, if at all, in hyperplastic glands (five of 45 diffuse toxic goiters[41]) and are variably seen in nontoxic nodular goiters.

The chemical nature of the crystals, their intracolloid location, and the age distribution suggested to Richter and McCarty that they may be caused by variations in colloid and in calcium concentrations in the gland, which may be altered by age and functional state.[41]

Few studies on the crystals have appeared.[40, 41] Reid et al. found them in 79 percent of autopsies of patients, and their number increased with age.[40] Gross noted a disproportionately large number of crystals in cases of subacute thyroid-

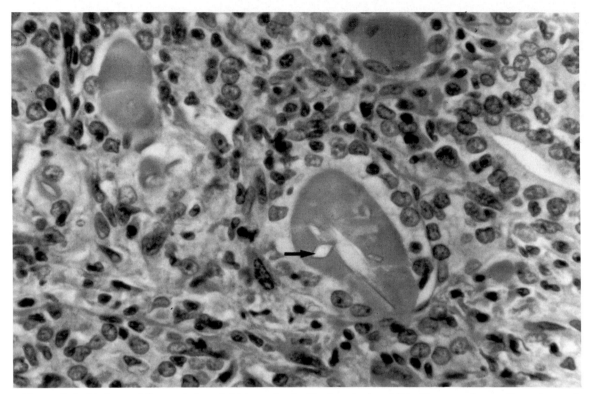

Figure 7–6. "Anisotropic" crystals in colloid in a gland with chronic thyroiditis. Note angular configuration and intracolloid localization (*arrow*). × 200, H & E.

itis.[18] Hence 14 of 14 cases of subacute thyroiditis, but only 4 of 29 thyroids with other types of nonneoplastic lesions (chronic thyroiditis, hyperplasia) contained crystals. In subacute thyroiditis the crystals are found in giant cells, in remnants of colloid, and free in the stroma of the gland. The crystals in this disorder probably reflect alterations in the physical (and ?chemical) state of the colloid; whether they play a role in inciting a granulomatous inflammatory reaction is not known.[18, 40]

MacMahon et al. evaluated the presence of thyroid crystals in a series of 500 autopsies.[28] These authors confirmed the findings of Richter and McCarty in that the crystals vary in size and shape, are always embedded in colloid, are noted more frequently in elderly subjects, and are rarely seen in areas of glandular hyperplasia.[41] MacMahon et al. found crystals in 40 percent of their 500 glands, and they were abundant in 29 percent.[28] These authors assumed that the frequency of finding these crystals in the thyroid and not in other organs may indicate a role for them in thyroid metabolism,[28] but no further analyses of this hypothesis have been found in the current literature.

Fayemi et al. have described oxalate crystals in 77 of 80 autopsies of patients who had received hemodialysis for renal failure.[13] In these cases, oxalate crystals were found predominantly in the colloid. These authors did examine 15 surgically resected thyroids (removed for a variety of thyroid diseases) and found oxalate crystals in these but with much less frequency than in their dialysis patients.[13] However, in the hemodialysis patients oxalate deposition in the kidneys and myocardium was prominent, suggesting a different clinical significance from that of the patient groups previously reported.[18, 41]

Cystine crystals are accumulated in the thyroid in cystinosis and lead to hypothyroidism (see below).

Exogenous "Crystals"

Teflon. In Chapter 4, I have alluded to the presence of Teflon (polytef) "crystals" or particles in the thyroid and cervical tissues. The clinical setting associated with this iatrogenic lesion is important to understand. In the neck (Fig. 7–7), Polytef (polytetrafluoroethylene) is injected into the larynges of patients with unilateral vocal cord paralysis of various etiologies, including neoplastic, traumatic, and idiopathic.[16, 30, 42, 47, 49] Polytef produces an inflammatory reaction, which allows for shifting of an abducted cord or restoration of an atrophic one; phonation improves dramatically.[16] The inflammatory reaction is predominantly granulomatous (foreign body type) (Fig. 7–7), with variable degrees of fibrosis; the latter depends on the duration of the presence of the material.[47]

The commonly injected material, in the form of polytef paste, contains numerous irregular and angular particles, ranging from 4 to 100 μm in size. Microscopically, these particles are nonstaining refractile and brightly birefringent when viewed under polarized light.[30] Migration of the Teflon particles into surrounding tissues and even to distant sites has been shown to occur in animals and in man.[30, 35]

In a few patients who have undergone vocal cord polytef injection, migration of the particles has been noted.[30, 42, 49] Whether this represents endolymphatic migration or simply a mechanical process is unclear. In at least two reported cases, "polytef granuloma" has simulated a thyroid nodule;[42, 49] in one of these actual

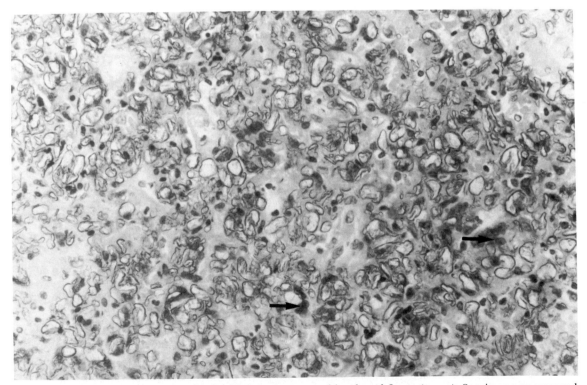

Figure 7–7. Polytef particles with reactive histiocytes, some multinucleated forms (*arrows*). Specimen was removed as cervical "node" in patient with history of vocal cord palsy. Similar lesions may rarely be seen in the thyroid. × 150, H & E.

thyroids infiltration occurred.[42] X-ray dispersion analysis performed in this latter case unequivocally identified the particulate material as polytef.[42]

STORAGE DISEASES AFFECTING THE THYROID

Glycogenosis. Pompe's disease (glycogenosis type IIA) is characterized morphologically by intralysosomal accumulation of normal glycogen in many tissues. Clinically, this rapidly fatal disease is associated with profound weakness, cardiomegaly, and eventually respiratory failure. The disease, inherited as an autosomal recessive trait, is associated with deficiency of the lysosomal enzyme acid alpha-1, 4-glucosidase.

Although the pathologic changes in the heart and nervous system in this disorder have been described extensively, only recently have the alterations in endocrine glands been addressed. Hui et al. reported the endocrine pathology in two infants with Pompe's disease;[21] although the glands were grossly normal, the authors described excess glycogen accumulation in adrenal cortex and thyroid gland (compared to controls). This presumably would correspond to the electron microscopic findings of intact lysosomes filled with glycogen; however, ultrastructural definition of this was masked by the granular colloid present in the follicular cells. The authors did note occasional parafollicular cells with glycogen-filled lysosomes, however.[21]

Lipidoses. This group of disorders connoted as "amaurotic family idiocy" comprises a number of autosomally recessive inherited diseases characterized by severe mental retardation. Infantile, late infantile, and juvenile forms have been described; a number of eponyms are appended to these diseases: Bielschowsky's disease, Batten's disease, or Batten-Spielmeyer-Vogt disease.[2, 10, 12]

Pathologically, neurons, autonomic ganglia, and other body cells are swollen by accumulation of large amounts of lipofuscin-like pigment.[2, 10] In the thyroids of some patients with these disorders, follicular epithelial cells contained yellow autofluorescent pigment granules with the histochemical staining reactions suggesting lipofuscin (see above). Electron microscopic examination of thyroid tissue from two cases of Batten's disease, however, showed characteristic osmiophilic curvilinear material in the cytoplasm of follicular cells.[2, 12] These findings had been previously seen in brain, muscle, and other tissues in patients with this disease. Interestingly, enzyme analyses have indicated deficiency of thyroid peroxidase levels in Batten's disease, and some patients are hypothyroid. Since it has been postulated that peroxidase abnormalities may be associated with lipofuscin accumulation (see above), and it remains unclear what lipofuscin is and how it is derived, and since in the lipidoses studied the structure and composition of the accumulated pigment material are not well characterized, it appears wise at present to refer to this pigment as lipofuscin-like.

Other Diseases. Dayan et al. examined thyroid tissue from patients with Tay-Sachs', Niemann-Pick, and Wolman's diseases, as well as cases of glycogen storage disease and metachromatic leukodystrophy.[10] In none of these was thyroid pigmentation or cytoplasmic inclusions recognized.

The present author is aware of a case of Gaucher's cells infiltrating thyroid stroma in a patient with longstanding Gaucher's disease.

Cystinosis. This inborn error of metabolism, inherited as an autosomal recessive trait, is characterized by widespread intracellular deposition of cystine.[9, 27] Although most clinical studies focused on the renal disease seen in this condition, Chan et al. recognized that many patients with cystinosis are clinically hypothyroid.[9] In seven of the eight thyroids they studied, Chan et al. identified follicular atrophy, shrunken colloid, and fibrosis. Associated with this are focal areas of papillary hyperplasia, widely dilated follicles, and focal acute inflammation. Older patients had severe thyroid atrophy. Although difficult or impossible to identify in fixed tissue, large numbers of cystine crystals were seen on frozen sections; these were within follicular epithelium, occasionally in colloid, and rarely in stromal macrophages.[9, 27] These crystals differ from the birefringent crystals noted by Richter and McCarty[41] and MacMahon et al.,[28] since the latter are common in "normal" glands, are almost always colloid-associated and not in epithelium, and are not destroyed by fixation and paraffin embedding (see above).

It has been postulated that the presence of cystine crystals produces gradual follicular atrophy, leading to hypothyroidism; whether by a mechanical, toxic, or other method is unknown.

The thyroid hypofunction is believed to be a primary thyroid disorder in cystinosis since hyperplasia of pituitary thyrotrophs was noted by Chan in some of her cases.[9] Although cystine deposits may be found in the stroma of other endocrine organs, no dysfunction results,[27] although further studies have indicated a possible associated pituitary functional defect.[5]

In summary, this chapter has described rare and unusual predominantly nonneoplastic thyroid lesions to serve as a review of pigments, crystals, and storage diseases affecting the gland.

REFERENCES

1. Alexander, C. B., Herrara, G. A., et al.: Black thyroid. Clinical manifestations, ultrastructural findings and possible mechanisms. Hum. Pathol. *16*:72–78, 1985.
2. Armstrong, D., van Wormer, D. E., et al.: Thyroid peroxidase deficiency in Batten-Spielmeyer-Vogt disease. Arch. Pathol. *99*:430–435, 1975.
3. Attwood, H. D., and Dennett, X.: A black thyroid and minocycline treatment. Br. Med. J. *2*:1109–1110, 1976.
4. Benitz, K. F., Roberts, G. K. S., and Yusa, A.: Morphologic effects of minocycline in laboratory animals. Toxicol. Appl. Pharmacol. *11*:150–170, 1967.
5. Bercu, B. B., Orloff, S., and Schulman, J. D.: Pituitary resistance to thyroid hormone in cystinosis. J. Clin. Endocrinol. Metab. *51*:1262–1268, 1980.
6. Billano, R. A., Ward, W. Q., and Little, W. P.: Minocycline and black thyroid. J.A.M.A. *249*:1887–1888, 1983.
7. Borel, D. M., and Reddy, J. K.: Excessive lipofuscin accumulation in the thyroid gland in mucoviscidosis. Arch. Pathol. *96*:269–271, 1973.
8. Cappell, D. F., Hutchison, H. E., and Jowett, M. D.: Transfusional siderosis: The effects of excessive iron deposits on the tissues. J. Pathol. Bacteriol. *74*:245–264, 1957.
9. Chan, A. M., Lynch, M. J. G., et al.: Hypothyroidism in cystinosis: a clinical, endocrinologic and histologic study involving sixteen patients with cystinosis. Am. J. Med. *48*:678–692, 1970.
10. Dayan, A. D., and Trickey, R. J.: Thyroid involvement in juvenile amaurotic idiocy (Batten's disease). Lancet *2*:296–297, 1970.
11. Deichmann, W. B., Bernal, E., et al.: The chronic oral toxicity of oxytetracycline HCl and tetracycline HCl in the rat, dog and pig. Indust. Med. Surg. *33*:787–806, 1964.
12. Dolman, C. L., and Chang, E.: Visceral lesions in amaurotic family idiocy with curvilinear bodies. Arch. Pathol. *97*:425–430, 1972.
13. Fayemi, A. O., Ali, M., and Braun, E. V.: Oxalosis in hemodialysis patients. Arch. Pathol. Lab. Med. *103*:58–62, 1979.
14. Fenske, N. A., Milns, J. L., and Greer, K. E.: Minocycline-induced pigmentation at sites of cutaneous inflammation. J.A.M.A. *244*:1103–1106, 1980.
15. Finch, S. C., and Finch, C. A.: Idiopathic hemochromatosis, an iron storage disease. Medicine *34*:381–430, 1955.
16. Goff, W. F.: Intracordal polytef (Teflon) injection. Arch. Otolaryngol. *97*:371–372, 1973.
17. Gordon, G., Sparano, B. M., et al.: Thyroid gland pigmentation and minocycline therapy. Am. J. Pathol. *117*:98–109, 1984.
18. Gross, S.: Granulomatous thyroiditis with anisotropic crystalline material. Arch. Pathol. *59*:412–417, 1955.

19. Harcourt-Webster, J. N.: Secondary neoplasm of the thyroid presenting as goitre. J. Clin. Pathol. *18*:282–287, 1965.
20. Heimann, P.: Ultrastructure of human thyroid. Acta Endocrinol. *53*:Suppl. *110*:1–102, 1966.
21. Hui, K. S., Williams, J. C., et al.: The endocrine glands in Pompe's disease. Arch. Pathol. Lab. Med. *109*:921–925, 1985.
22. Ivy, H. K.: Cancer metastatic to the thyroid: a diagnostic problem. Mayo Clin. Proc. *59*:856–859, 1984.
23. Kakudo, K., Yasoshima, H., et al.: Black thyroid in 3 autopsy patients on minocycline. Pathol. Clin. Med. *3*:525–529, 1985.
24. Kurosumi, M., and Fujita, H.: Fine structural aspects of the black thyroid induced by minocycline, and the effects of a low iodine diet, propylthiouracil, thyroxine tablet and TSH on the black discoloration of the rat thyroid. Virch. Arch. Cell Pathol. *48*:219–227, 1985.
25. Kurosumi, M., and Fujita, H.: Fine structural aspects of the fate of rat black thyroids induced by minocycline. Virch. Arch. Cell Pathol. *51*:207–213, 1986.
26. Landas, S. K., Schelper, R. L., et al.: Black thyroid syndrome: Exaggeration of a normal process? Am. J. Clin. Pathol. *85*:411–418, 1986.
27. Lucky, A. W., Howley, P. M., et al.: Endocrine studies in cystinosis: Compensated primary hypothyroidism. J. Pediatr. *91*:204–210, 1977.
28. MacMahon, H. E., Lee, H. Y., and Rivelis, C. F.: Birefringent crystals in human thyroid. Acta Endocrinol. *58*:172–176, 1968.
29. Mahmoud, I., Colin, I., et al.: Direct toxic effect of iodide in excess on iodine-deficient thyroid glands: Epithelial necrosis and inflammation associated with lipofuscin accumulation. Exp. Molec. Pathol. *44*:259–271, 1986.
30. Malizia, A. A., Reiman, H. M., et al.: Migration and granulomatous reaction after periurethral injection of Polytef (Teflon). J.A.M.A. *251*:3277–3281, 1984.
31. Marcus, J. N., Dise, C. A., and LiVolsi, V. A.: Melanin production in a medullary thyroid carcinoma. Cancer *49*:2518–2526, 1982.
32. Martins, M. I. B., Goncalves, V., and Trincao, R. D. C.: Un marcador histologico do carcinoma medular da tireoide. Arquivos Patolog. Geral. Anat. Patolog. Univ. Coinbra *17*:61–72, 1979.
33. Matsubara, F., Mizukami, Y., and Tanaka, Y.: Black thyroid: morphological, biochemical and geriatric studies on the brown granules in the thyroid follicular cells. Acta Pathol. Jpn. *32*:13–22, 1982.
34. Medeiros, L. J., Federman, M., et al.: Black thyroid associated with minocycline therapy. Arch. Pathol. Lab. Med. *108*:268–269, 1984.
35. Mittelman, R. E., and Marraccini, J. V.: Pulmonary Teflon granulomas following periurethral Teflon injection for urinary incontinence. Arch. Pathol. Lab. Med. *107*:611–612, 1983.
36. Ohaki, Y., Misugi, K., and Hasegawa, H.: "Black thyroid" associated with minocycline therapy. Acta Pathol. Jpn. *36*:1367–1375, 1986.
37. Oliver, R. A. M.: Siderosis following transfusions of blood. J. Pathol. Bacteriol. *77*:171–194, 1959.
38. Porta, E. A., and Hartroft, W. S.: Lipid pigments (lipofuscins). *In:* Wolman, M. (ed.): Pigments in Pathology. New York, Academic Press, 1969, pp. 191–235.
39. Reid, J. D.: The black thyroid associated with minocycline therapy. Am. J. Clin. Pathol. *79*:739–646, 1983.
40. Reid, J. D., Choi, C. H., and Oldroyd, N. O.: Calcium oxalate crystals in the thyroid: their identification, prevalence, origin and possible significance. Am. J. Clin. Pathol. *87*:443–454, 1987.
41. Richter, M. N., and McCarty, K. S.: Anisotropic crystals in the human thyroid gland. Am. J. Pathol. *30*:545–553, 1954.
42. Sanfilippo, F., and Shelburne, J.: Analysis of a Polytef granuloma mimicking a cold thyroid nodule 17 months after laryngeal injection. Ultrastruct. Pathol. *1*:471–475, 1980.
43. Saul, S. H., Dekker, A., et al.: The black thyroid: its relation to minocycline use in man. Arch. Pathol. Lab. Med. *107*:173–177, 1983.
44. Senba, M., Toda, Y., and Yamashita, H.: Black thyroid associated with minocycline therapy: histochemical and ultrastructural studies on the brown pigment. Isr. J. Med. Sci. *24*:51–53, 1988.
45. Sheldon, J. H.: Hemochromatosis. London, Oxford University Press, 1935.
46. Shimaoka, K., Sokal, J. E., and Pickren, J. W.: Metastatic neoplasms in the thyroid gland: pathological and clinical findings. Cancer *15*:557–565, 1962.
47. Stephens, C. B., Arnold, G. E., and Stone, J. W.: Larynx injected with polytef paste. Arch. Otolaryngol. *102*:432–435, 1976.
48. Wajda, K. J., Wilson, M. S., et al.: Fine needle aspiration cytologic findings in the black thyroid syndrome. Acta Cytol. *32*:862–865, 1988.
49. Walsh, F. M., and Castelli, J. B.: Polytef granuloma clinically simulating carcinoma of the thyroid. Arch. Otolaryngol. *101*:262–263, 1975.
50. White, S. W., and Besanceney, C.: Systemic pigmentation from tetracycline and minocycline therapy. Arch. Dermatol. *119*:1–2, 1983.

II

Thyroid Tumors

INTRODUCTION

Certain clinical and epidemiologic details of thyroid neoplasms are reviewed in this introductory section.

How important is thyroid cancer in the general population? As a cause of cancer mortality? Why does thyroid cancer elicit such great interest among internists, radiologists, surgeons, endocrinologists, pathologists, and oncologists? Why is there considerable public concern with this disease?

General Remarks

Despite its low incidence and generally low mortality rates, thyroid cancer elicits interest among physicians far beyond that to be expected.

Thyroid cancer is diagnosed in only 37 patients per one million population in the United States each year[1] and constitutes 1.3 percent of all malignancies,[1] yet it accounts for only 0.4 percent of cancer deaths.[11, 18] Thyroid cancer elicits great interest among a variety of physicians because it is included in the differential diagnosis of thyroid nodules in general; in the United States, it is estimated that 1 to 10 percent of the population will have nodular thyroids that are clinically evident; hence a large number of patients seek medical attention for this problem each year.[19, 21, 25] It is difficult to know how many of these nodules represent cancer, but the number must be very low; some studies indicate that 3 to 28 percent of excised solitary nodules represent cancer.[6, 15, 24] (These studies are surgical series published before the use of fine needle aspiration screening of nodules.) The one prospective study from the Framingham group indicated that in 5000 individuals followed over a 15-year period, 1.4 percent developed thyroid nodules, but that none of these behaved in a clinically malignant fashion.[31]

Thyroid cancer affects a wide age range of patients, from children to the elderly. The lesions are usually easily accessible to minimally invasive diagnostic and screening techniques—principally needle biopsy.

Thyroid cancer in general arouses interest among physicians and epidemiologists because of the geographic and dietary influences on the different histologic subtypes of the disease.[35] Animal models for several thyroid malignancies are available for epidemiologic, dietary, and genetic studies. In addition, the relationship of thyroid cancer to exposure to radiation has stimulated public and media awareness. Recent history discloses the public concern with nuclear power plant accidents and near disasters; one of these concerns is the development of thyroid cancer.

Classification of Thyroid Tumors. In general, the present author concurs with the latest WHO classification of thyroid tumors (second edition).[17] We concur with the recognition of the follicular variant of papillary carcinoma, the deletion of the entity "small cell carcinoma," and the conservative approach to acceptance of mixed follicular-parafollicular tumors. The following chapters adhere for the most part to this scheme and the philosophy it represents.

Epidemiologic Factors. Epidemiologic factors involved in cancer of the thyroid vary with the histologic type of tumor. Franssila and Saxen noted that pathologic classifications differ and different interpretations of certain thyroid tumors make epidemiologic and clinical studies difficult to interpret.[13] Williams has outlined certain factors that appear causally related to some thyroid cancers.[34]

Papillary Carcinoma. This is often found in patients with a history of neck irradiation, usually but not always administered in childhood.[3] In animal models of thyroid neoplasia, papillary tumors are found more commonly in animals given diets with iodine excess.

Follicular Carcinoma. The incidence of follicular carcinoma is high in endemic goiter areas of the world, i.e., among patients with iodine-deficient diets. In animal models also, iodine deficiency leads to the development of follicular cancers.

Anaplastic Carcinoma. Goiter predisposes to anaplastic carcinoma; the thyroid enlargement may be caused by nodular adenomatous change or a low-grade carcinoma. This suggests a *transformation* of a benign or low-grade lesion into a highly malignant one. In some studies, external radiation has been implicated in the development of anaplastic carcinoma; the possibility that radiation enhances this transformation process has been suggested.[20]

Medullary Thyroid Carcinoma. The genetic influences in the development of medullary thyroid carcinoma are well established; about 10 to 20 percent of patients with this tumor have the familial form of the disease.[23] In these patients, autosomal dominant mode of inheritance is known. Neoplasms and hyperplasias of other endocrine glands in the same patient or in relatives is common; in the affected thyroid the putative precursor lesion, C-cell hyperplasia, can be demonstrated.[36] However, the majority of patients (over 80 percent) with medullary thyroid cancer have the sporadic form of the disease. No predisposing factors for this lesion are known.

Malignant Lymphoma. Malignant lymphoma of the thyroid almost always arises in a gland affected by autoimmune thyroiditis. Such a development parallels that seen in other organ systems, such as the gastrointestinal tract, wherein an immunologically abnormal tissue undergoes malignant change.[10] However, malignant lymphoma of the thyroid is rare and thyroiditis is a common disorder; this suggests other as yet unknown factors may be at work.

Clinical Features

Certain clinical features provide helpful clues to raise the suspicion of cancer in a thyroid nodule.

Thyroid tumors present as enlargements of the gland, usually although not uniformly as *solitary* nodules. However, although most malignant tumors of the gland present as nodules, the overwhelming majority of nodules, even those that appear clinically as solitary ones, are indeed benign and may represent physiologic hyperplasias.

All thyroid disorders occur more commonly in females, and thyroid cancer is no exception. However, whereas the female:male ratio for certain thyroid diseases, e.g., Graves' disease, is 9:1, the ratio for thyroid cancer is about 2.5:1.[15] Hence, a thyroid nodule found in a *male* patient should raise a higher suspicion of carcinoma than that found in a woman.

Age is also an important variable. A single nodule in a child or in an elderly patient is more worrisome than a similar lesion found in a young or middle-aged adult.[19, 21]

Nonfunctioning nodules, that is, those that are cool or cold on radioiodine thyroid scan, should be considered suspicious. Whereas the great majority of cold nodules are benign, thyroid cancers virtually always are nonfunctional.[7, 26] Indeed, warm or hot, functional nodules should all be considered benign.[33]

A history of *irradiation* to the head and neck, especially if remote in time, i.e., greater than five years, raises the risk of cancer in a thyroid nodule.[12, 22, 28, 29] The exact degree of risk is not known since the number of individuals exposed to radiation in childhood or youth (i.e., the denominator) is unknown.

Therapy

The therapy of thyroid cancer has elicited considerable rancor and debate. Radical surgery advocates have battled in the literature (and elsewhere) the advocates of the conservative approach.

Is total thyroidectomy needed for papillary carcinoma? Should neck dissection be done? Will node picking suffice? Papillary carcinoma is the most common type of thyroid cancer but it is also the most indolent. Hence, in order to satisfactorily answer such questions, studies of huge numbers of patients treated in standard randomized fashion and followed for 20 to 30 years would be required. These are not forthcoming and may indeed be impossible to perform. Hence the answers come from retrospective series, and although many recent ones indicate that the conservative surgical approach for papillary cancer is adequate in most cases,[2, 5, 14, 27] the debate and the practice of many physicians continues unchanged.[9, 21, 30]

The data for follicular carcinoma therapy are less satisfactory, since many of the published series appear in the surgical literature, are retrospective, and rarely if ever contain pathologic review of the tumors. Thus, almost certainly included in these series of follicular carcinoma are follicular variants of papillary cancer, which have a biologic behavior different from that of true follicular cancer. Therapeutic data gathered from such material are virtually useless.

Therapy of anaplastic carcinoma is so often futile that any new approaches will be welcomed. Almost all reports indicate that radical approaches do little to improve miserable survival rates.[8, 20]

The therapy of familial medullary carcinoma is standard,[4] and appropriately includes total thyroidectomy since multifocal tumors and precursor hyperplasia are found in virtually every instance. Whether total thyroidectomy is the correct approach to sporadic forms of the tumor is unclear. Since any case that is apparently sporadic may represent the proband of familial disease and thus have multiple microscopic lesions, total thyroidectomy seems the correct therapeutic modality.

The most agreed upon therapy for a thyroid tumor is that for lymphoma of the thyroid; after careful staging of the disease, radiation and/or chemotherapy can palliate and perhaps cure the tumor.[10]

Diagnostic Approach

In the modern era, the development of and increasing experience with fine needle aspiration (FNA) biopsy cytology of thyroid nodules has changed the diagnostic and therapeutic approach to these lesions.[14, 21, 32] Thus, endocrinologists, surgeons, and even pathologists can perform biopsies on these nodules in the outpatient setting with minimal or no morbidity, and no mortality. Cost-efficient diagnosis is possible in many cases of papillary, medullary, and anaplastic cancers.[16, 32] For the much more common follicular lesions, FNA biopsy can provide a screening technique to guide the need for surgery. Hence, modern series indicate that the percentage of carcinomas in surgically removed thyroid nodules has risen dramatically, from 3 percent before the use of FNA to over 70 percent.[31] This connotes cost savings of significant proportion as well as decreased morbidity for the population with thyroid nodules.[16, 32]

The following chapters in this monograph will describe the gross and microscopic features of thyroid tumors and nodules—nonneoplastic, benign, and malignant. These will be discussed in the forum of pattern types—e.g., papillary, follicular.

REFERENCES

1. American Cancer Society: 1976 Cancer Facts and Figures. CA *26*:150–159, 1976.
2. Baroni, C. D., Manente, L., Maccallini, V., and DiMatteo, G.: Primary malignant tumors of the thyroid gland. Tumori *69*:205–213, 1983.
3. Becker, F. O., Economou, S. G., Southwick, H. W., and Eisenstein, R.: Adult thyroid cancer after head and neck irradiation in infancy and childhood. Ann. Intern. Med. *83*:347–351, 1975.
4. Block, M. A., Miller, J. M., and Horn, R. C.: Medullary carcinoma of the thyroid: Surgical implications. Arch. Surg. *96*:521–526, 1968.
5. Bocker, W., Schroder, S., and Dralle, H.: Minimal thyroid neoplasia. *In:* Grundmann, E., and Beck, L. (eds.): Minimal Neoplasia. Berlin, Springer-Verlag, 1988, pp. 131–138.
6. Brooks, J. R.: The solitary thyroid nodule. Am. J. Surg. *125*:477–481, 1973.
7. Burrow, G. N., Majtaba, Q., LiVolsi, V. A., and Cornog, J. L.: The incidence of carcinoma in solitary "cold" thyroid nodules. Yale J. Biol. Med. *51*:13–17, 1978.
8. Carcangiu, M. L., Steeper, T., Zampi, G., and Rosai, J.: Anaplastic thyroid carcinoma. Am. J. Clin. Pathol. *83*:135–158, 1985.
9. Clark, O. H.: Total thyroidectomy; The treatment of choice for patients with differentiated thyroid cancer. Ann. Surg. *196*:361–368, 1982.
10. Compagno, J., and Oertel, J. E.: Malignant lymphoma and other lymphoproliferative disorders of the thyroid gland. Am. J. Clin. Pathol. *74*:1–11, 1980.
11. DeGroot, L. J., and Stanbury, J. B.: The Thyroid and Its Diseases. New York, John Wiley & Sons, 1975.
12. Fjalling, M., Tissel, L. E., et al.: Benign and malignant thyroid nodules after neck irradiation. Cancer *58*:1219–1224, 1986.
13. Franssila, K. O., and Saxen, E.: Histologic classification as a problem in the epidemiology of thyroid cancer. *In:* Grundmann, E., and Tulinies, H. (eds.): The Epidemiology of Cancer and Lymphomas. Berlin, Springer-Verlag, 1972, pp. 47–55.
14. Griffin, J. E.: Management of thyroid nodules. Am. J. Med. Sci. *296*:336–347, 1988.
15. Haff, R. C., Schechter, B. C., et al.: Factors influencing the probability of malignancy in thyroid nodules. Am. J. Surg. *131*:707–709, 1976.
16. Hamberger, B., Gharib, H., et al.: Fine needle aspiration biopsy of thyroid nodules. Am. J. Med. *73*:381–384, 1982.
17. Hedinger, C., Williams, E. D., and Sobin, L. H.: WHO histological classification of thyroid tumor: a commentary on the second edition. Cancer *63*:908–911, 1989.
18. Heitz, P., Moser, H., and Staub, J.: Thyroid cancer. A study of 573 thyroid tumors and 161 autopsy cases observed over a thirty-year period. Cancer *37*:2329–2337, 1976.
19. Hoffman, G. L., Thompson, N. W., and Heffron, C.: The solitary thyroid nodule—a reassessment. Arch. Surg. *105*:379–384, 1972.
20. Kapp, D., LiVolsi, V. A., and Sanders, M. M.: Anaplastic carcinoma following well differentiated thyroid cancer: Etiological considerations. Yale J. Biol. Med. *55*:521–528, 1982.
21. Lawson, W., and Biller, H. F.: The solitary thyroid nodule. Am. J. Otolaryngol. *4*:43–73, 1983.
22. McTiernan, A. M., Weiss, N. S., and Daling, J. R.: Incidence of thyroid cancer in women in relation to previous exposure to radiation therapy and history of thyroid disease. J. Natl. Cancer Inst. *73*:575–581, 1984.
23. Melvin, K. E. W., Tashjian, A. H., and Miller, H. H.: Studies in familial medullary thyroid carcinoma. Rec. Progr. Horm. Res. *28*:399–470, 1972.
24. Messaris, G., Evangelou, G. N., and Tountas, C.: Incidence of carcinoma in cold nodules of the thyroid gland. Surgery *74*:447–451, 1973.
25. Mortensen, J. D., Woolner, L. B., and Bennett, W. A.: Gross and microscopic findings in clinically normal thyroid glands. J. Clin. Endocrinol. *15*:1270–1280, 1955.
26. Ochi, H., Sawa, H., et al.: Thallium-201-chloride thyroid scintigraphy to evaluate benign and/or malignant nodules. Cancer *50*:236–240, 1982.

27. Ontai, S., and Strachley, C. J.: The surgical treatment of well-differentiated carcinoma of the thyroid. Am. Surg. *51*:653–657, 1985.
28. Ron, E., Kleinerman, R. A., Boice, J. D., et al.: A population-based case-control study of thyroid cancer. J. N. C. I. *79*:1–12, 1987.
29. Schneider, A. B., Bekerman, C., et al.: Continuing occurrence of thyroid nodules after head and neck irradiation. Ann. Intern. Med. *94*:176–180, 1981.
30. Starnes, H. F., Brooks, D. C., et al.: Surgery for thyroid carcinoma. Cancer *55*:1376–1381, 1985.
31. Vander, J. B., Gaston, E. A., and Dawber, T. R.: The significance of nontoxic thyroid nodules. Ann. Intern. Med. *69*:537–540, 1968.
32. van Herle, A. J., Rich, P., et al.: The thyroid nodule. Ann. Intern. Med. *96*:221–232, 1982.
33. Vickery, A. L.: Thyroid papillary carcinoma. Pathological and philosophical controversies. Am. J. Surg. Pathol. *7*:777–807, 1983.
34. Williams, E. D.: Pathologic and natural history. *In:* Duncan, W. (ed): Thyroid Cancer. New York, Springer-Verlag, 1980, pp. 47–55.
35. Williams, E. D., Doniach, I., et al.: Thyroid cancer in an iodide rich area. Cancer *39*:215–222, 1977.
36. Wolfe, H. J., Melvin, K. E. W., et al.: C-cell hyperplasia preceding medullary thyroid carcinoma. N. Engl. J. Med. *289*:437–441, 1973.

8

PAPILLARY LESIONS OF THE THYROID

Papillary lesions of the thyroid constitute a group that may produce diagnostic difficulty; the lesions include papillary hyperplasia (often associated with hyper-function), papillary change in an adenoma or adenomatous follicular nodule, and, of course, papillary carcinoma (Table 8–1). This chapter will review the pathologic features of these lesions and discuss the distinctive features that differentiate the benign from the malignant ones. In discussing papillary cancer of the thyroid, the usual and rarer subtypes of this tumor and the prognostic implications of such lesions will be reviewed (Table 8–2).

PAPILLARY CARCINOMA

Papillary carcinoma of the thyroid is the most common malignant tumor of the gland in countries having iodine-sufficient or iodine-excess diets.[208] In this country, it makes up about 33 to 90 percent of thyroid cancer; the wide range of incidence may be attributed to two main reasons: (a) some pathologists subdivide papillary cancers into papillary, mixed papillary and follicular, and follicular variants; and (b) some pathologists classify predominantly follicular-patterned papillary cancers among follicular carcinomas.[130]

In my opinion the incidence for papillary cancer in the United States is somewhere in the range of 80 percent of thyroid malignancies. I include in this figure all papillary cancers, mixed papillary and follicular cancer, and follicular variant. Virtually all papillary cancers contain some follicular elements, although there is marked variation among lesions in this regard. In many so-called occult or incidental papillary cancers, the lesion is totally follicular. However, all these tumors share a certain biologic and clinical behavior that, in my opinion, warrants their being grouped together.[21, 52, 203, 212] The biology of this group of tumors is similar and quite distinct from pure follicular cancer; hence, solely one histologic criterion (the abundance of follicles) should not force a tumor into a category that defines its behavior!

Table 8–1. Papillary Lesions of the Thyroid

Papillary carcinoma
Papillary hyperplasia
Papillary hyperplastic nodule
Papillary variant of medullary carcinoma

Table 8–2. Papillary Carcinoma of Thyroid: Subtypes

Usual type	Clear cell variant
Follicular variant	Oxyphilic variant
Tall cell variant	Encapsulated variant
Columnar cell variant	Papillary carcinoma with lipomatous stroma
Diffuse sclerosis variant	(Mucoepidermoid carcinoma)
Solid variant	

Before discussing papillary carcinoma in general terms, I will define certain features that are important in the tumor's recognition and differentiation from other papillary lesions.

Papillae were best described by Kini.[105] This author compared neoplastic papillae in thyroid tumors to ears of corn: the central fibrovascular core is the equivalent of the cob and the lining cells are represented by a single layer of kernels (Fig. 8–1). A hyperplastic papilla on the other hand is similar but it lacks a central stromal core.

Thus, the neoplastic papilla contains a central core of fibrovascular (occasionally just fibrous) tissue lined by one or occasionally several layers of cells with crowded oval nuclei showing the characteristics described below. On the other hand, hyperplasia of thyroid follicles may sometimes exaggerate into papillary change; there is infolding of the lining epithelium composed of tall columnar cells with basal round and uniform nuclei. There is either no central core or there may be a core of edematous or myxomatous paucicellular stroma, often including small follicles (subfollicle formation). Vickery et al. note, however, that in extreme examples of hyperplasia true papillae can form.[203]

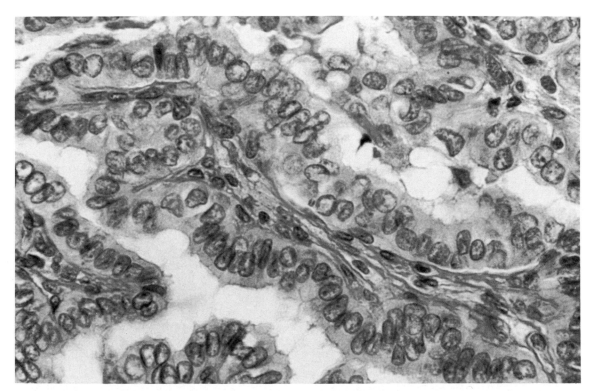

Figure 8–1. Classic papilla with fibrovascular core surrounded by a single layer of neoplastic cells. Note also large nuclei, clearing of some of them (lower right), and occasional grooves. × 400, H & E.

Psammoma bodies, which represent the "ghosts" of dead papillae or "tombstones" marking the place where papillae had been,[107] must be differentiated from dystrophic calcifications, which are common in many thyroid lesions. True psammoma bodies apparently are formed by focal areas of infarction of the tips of papillae; presumably the delicate vessels within the fibrous cores undergo thrombosis or damage as a result of minimal trauma. Certain as yet poorly understood biochemical mechanisms are then responsible for the attraction of calcium, which is deposited upon the dying infarcted cells. Progressive infarction of the papilla and ensuing calcium deposition lead to lamellation characteristic of the psammoma body[4, 50, 94, 107, 140] (Fig. 8–2, *A* and *B*). In some examples, residual neoplastic cells will be found intimately associated with the psammoma body. Psammoma bodies are usually found within the cores of papillae or in the tumor stroma, but not usually in the neoplastic follicles.

Rarely psammoma bodies are found in benign conditions in the thyroid, including Graves' disease[107, 142] and Hashimoto's thyroiditis;[42] however, this is so unusual that the presence of true psammoma bodies should be taken as a signal for diligent search for a papillary cancer in the gland.

The mimics of psammoma bodies include dystrophic calcification in areas of hemorrhage and fibrosis in goiter (Fig. 8–2, *C*); in addition, dense colloid, especially found in follicles in Hürthle cell lesions, can mimic calcifications and because of their rounded configuration can mimic psammoma bodies. However, lamellations are rarely seen in the dystrophic calcifications, which tend to be irregular and even jagged; dense colloid is extremely round in configuration but lacks lamellation.

The *nuclei* of papillary cancer of the thyroid are quite characteristic; they have been described as pale, clear, ground-glass, water-clear, empty, or Orphan Annie–eyed (Fig. 8–3). These nuclei are larger and more ovoid than normal follicular nuclei and contain hypodense chromatin as well as a prominent nuclear membrane. Rarely, the nucleolus can be seen in the center of the nucleus; more often, it is pressed against the thickened nuclear membrane where it may appear as a slight bulge. The reason for the peculiar appearance of the papillary cancer nucleus remains unknown; some theories have proved wrong—the nuclei are not hypodiploid; the clearing is not caused by cytoplasmic invagination.[21, 90, 115] Some authors prefer to consider the appearance as a useful artifact since the clearing is not usually found in frozen sections or fine needle aspirate samples of papillary cancer.[21, 38, 202, 203] However, it seems unlikely that one can attribute the clearing of the nucleus to artifact alone since it is so reproducible among many laboratories around the world and in many thousands of papillary cancers; perhaps, as Carcangiu et al. state, it is an artifact but has some basis in fact—perhaps peculiar physical and/or chemical properties of the chromatin.[21]

In addition, in papillary cancer these nuclei often appear crowded, overlapping one another (Fig. 8–4).

Ultrastructural studies of these nuclei have shown a finely dispersed chromatin, a highly folded nuclear membrane,[93, 95, 96, 184] and a paucity of nuclear pores (Fig. 8–5). Another feature noted by electron microscopic studies and found as a prominent diagnostic clue in cytologic preparations is the presence of intranuclear cytoplasmic invaginations;[38, 186] these are not specific for papillary cancer, since many other human tumors show this feature (melanoma being the most renowned example). These invaginations are not responsible for the clear appearance of the nucleus seen by light microscopy, however.

Another recently noted characteristic of the papillary cancer nucleus is the nuclear groove.[22, 177] These are quite prominent in some tumors (Fig. 8–3, *B*), but

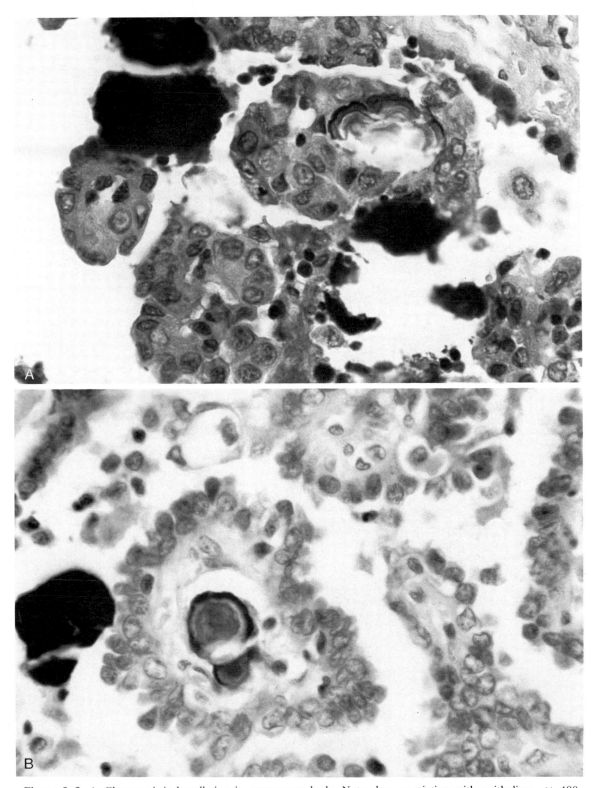

Figure 8–2. *A,* Characteristic lamellation in psammoma body. Note close association with epithelium. × 400, H & E. *B,* Note psammoma body within fibrous core of papilla. × 380, H & E.

Illustration continued on following page

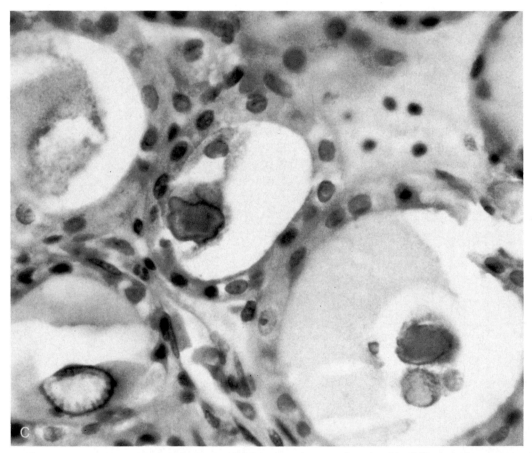

Figure 8–2 *Continued C,* Note intraluminal colloid-associated concretions in this follicular adenoma. × 300, H & E.

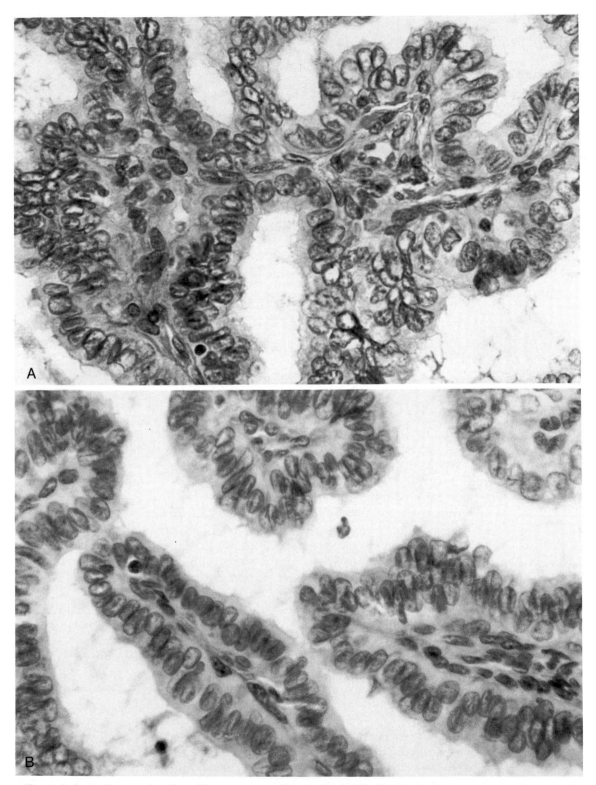

Figure 8–3. *A,* Clear nuclei of papillary cancer are illustrated. × 400, H & E. *B,* Grooves are prominent in this example. × 400, H & E.

Illustration continued on following page

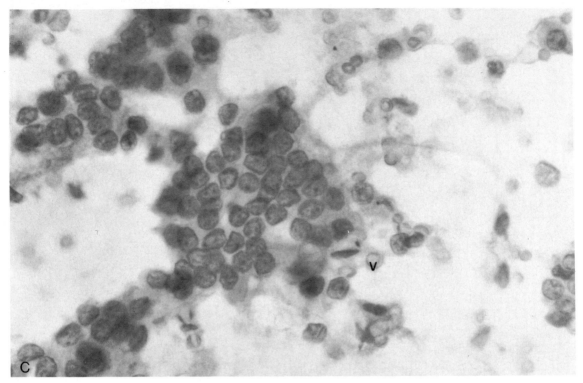

Figure 8–3 *Continued C,* In cytologic preparation, note grooves and occasional cytoplasmic invagination (*V*). × 500, Pap stain.

they had not gained wide attention in the literature until recently,[22] although they had been commented upon earlier as clefted nuclei.[72] Once described and illustrated in detail, however, it is easy to identify them in papillary tumors. Indeed, the grooves are as helpful and in some cases more useful in the diagnosis than the clear nucleus itself. Chan and Saw believed that these grooves represent the light microscopic equivalent of the ultrastructural nuclear infoldings.[22] In their paper, these authors mentioned finding occasional grooved nuclei in a few adenomas, and in one case each of Graves' disease and chronic thyroiditis; however, the nuclei in these conditions were found focally while in papillary cancer they were found in abundance in each case.[22] Cytopathologists have also recently described the utility of nuclear grooves in the cytodiagnosis of papillary thyroid cancer.[38, 177] Shurbaji et al. indicate that in their cytologic material nuclear grooves were found in 100 percent of papillary cancers, whereas they were seen in only 1.8 percent of benign follicular nodules.[177] In Deligeorgi-Politi's series, 34 of 37 papillary carcinomas showed nuclear grooves in fine needle aspirate samples; they were not seen in benign lesions.[38]

Two questions need to be addressed in discussing the nuclear features of papillary carcinoma: how often do they occur in thyroid papillary cancers and are they seen in any other conditions, including benign ones, in the thyroid? The occurrence of these characteristic nuclei has been estimated at between 55 and 88 percent of papillary thyroid cancers;[21, 68] in the present author's experience those papillary cancers that do not show the nuclei are readily recognizable as malignant tumors and often show well-developed papillary differentiation—e.g., the tall cell variant often does not have clear nuclei.

The more serious question seems to be whether these nuclei can be found in

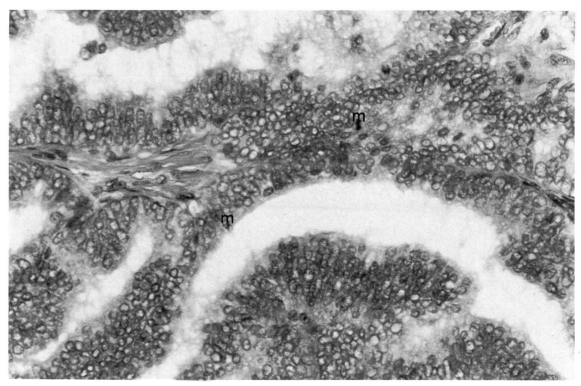

Figure 8–4. This example shows prominent overlapping, and rare mitoses (*m*). This case is also unusual in that the papillae are lined by multiple layers of epithelium. × 300, H & E.

other lesions in the thyroid, and the answer is, unfortunately, yes. However, although the clear nucleus can be found in Graves' disease and in chronic lymphocytic thyroiditis as well as in some follicular adenomas, in these conditions the nucleus is usually found only focally, and grooves or overlapping are usually absent.

The so-called pseudoclear nucleus described by Hapke and Dehner[68] needs to be distinguished from the clear one of papillary carcinoma. The former has dispersed but still visible chromatin, and its nuclear membrane is not thick. This nucleus can be found in a variety of thyroid lesions—hyperplasia, thyroiditis—and even in normal glands.

Features of Papillary Carcinoma. Thyroid carcinoma makes up about 1 percent of all cancers in the United States and has a mortality rate of about 0.2 percent.[179, 218] Most of these cancers are of the papillary type.

These common tumors tend to be biologically indolent with an excellent prognosis (>90 percent at 20 years).[6, 9, 26, 72, 78, 83, 113, 125, 134, 203, 211, 212] The tumors avidly invade lymphatics, leading to "multifocal" lesions and to regional node metastases. Distant metastases outside the neck are unusual (~5 to 7 percent of cases).[122–126, 170, 211, 212]

The usual type of papillary carcinoma has been the subject of numerous studies and reviews.[20, 21, 67, 72, 83, 113, 122–126, 152, 154, 202, 203, 211, 212] Large series have focused on certain pathologic and clinical features of these tumors that may impact on prognosis. However, since the outlook for most patients with this type of cancer is so good and disease-free survival is prolonged, large numbers of patients need to be studied, and the follow-up time should be at least 10 years in order to define

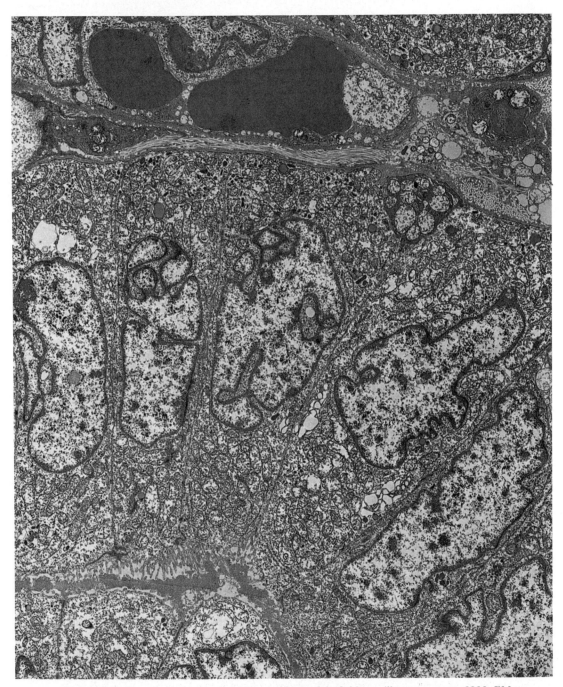

Figure 8–5. Prominent nuclear infolding in the nuclei of this papillary cancer. × 6000, EM.

meaningful prognostic indicators. The following discussion summarizes many of the available large series of papillary cancer and focuses predominantly on the pathologic features—some of which bear upon prognosis. (The discussion of the subtypes, which have somewhat different outlooks, is separate and appears later in this chapter.)

Clinical Parameters. Papillary carcinoma can occur at any age and has even been reported to develop in utero, diagnosed as a congenital tumor.[132] This neoplasm accounts for 80 percent of thyroid cancers in the prepubertal age group.[14, 46, 73, 101, 112, 116, 175, 189] Most tumors are diagnosed in patients in the third and fifth decades.[52–54, 122, 125, 130, 211, 212] Most studies indicate that older individuals, especially over the age of 45 to 50, seem to fare less well overall.[52–54, 72, 125, 211, 212]

Although the incidence between the sexes varies among different series, women seem to be affected more often than men in ratios of 2:1 to 4:1.[52, 72, 122, 125, 211, 212]

Etiologic Factors. The etiologic factors for papillary carcinoma are not well established. However, from animal studies it appears that iodine excess may predispose to its development.[220] In humans, it has been shown that with the addition of iodine in the diet in endemic goiter areas in Europe, the incidence of follicular cancer decreases and the percentage of papillary carcinoma rises.[35, 69, 79, 206, 208]

The role of external radiation in the development of papillary cancer has received wide general publicity as well as in the medical literature; it probably plays a role in the development of clinical papillary cancer,[10, 48, 66, 102, 144, 151, 153, 167, 210] although the extent of the risk cannot be known since the figures indicating the number of individuals potentially at risk (i.e., the number of people who received radiation to the neck as children) is unknown. Studies from Japan that have compared the incidence of small thyroid cancers at autopsy in patients who lived in the vicinity of Hiroshima and Nagasaki (and were exposed to radiation from the atomic bomb explosions) indicate an exceptionally high incidence of thyroid cancer (about 25 percent versus 16 percent) in these individuals as compared to other Japanese. However, clinically evident thyroid cancer is relatively rare in Japan.[104, 163–166]

Whether a history of external radiation in a patient who develops thyroid papillary cancer has implications for prognosis has been answered by a large study of Samaan et al., which compared nonradiated and radiated groups.[161] They found that the latter had more extensive disease at diagnosis (more nodal spread and bilaterality), but the prognosis is both groups was similar. It appears that treatment with I-131 does not increase the risk for the development of papillary cancer of the thyroid.[81]

Papillary cancer may be increasing in incidence in patients who survived therapy (radiation and/or chemotherapy) for childhood malignancies.[73, 167, 190, 199]

Familial papillary carcinoma has been described in twins;[43] one study found an association of papillary cancer and HLA-DR7.[187] The genetic implications of these studies await further information.

Whether or not benign thyroid lesions predispose to cancer remains disputed. Some series indicate that thyroids of patients with Graves' disease have a higher than expected incidence of papillary cancer;[47, 139, 176] other studies dispute this.[58, 133, 206] The debate is sharper when the question of the preneoplastic potential of chronic thyroiditis is raised. Many articles, especially in the surgical literature, seem to indicate that up to one-third of papillary cancers arise in the setting of thyroiditis. However, these studies tend to lack serologic proof of preexisting thyroiditis or even thyroid dysfunction. In addition follow-up studies of patients with documented thyroiditis seem to indicate that the tumor arising in a disproportionately frequent manner in these glands is malignant lymphoma, not papillary cancer. (See Chapters 5 and 14.)

It must be recalled that papillary cancer and thyroiditis are both common conditions, and the possibility of coincidental coexistence is more likely than that one predisposes to the other. In addition to lack of serologic evidence of thyroiditis, the studies indicating thyroiditis plays an etiologic role in cancer fail to document the pathologic features of the inflammatory lesion. It is noted again below that most papillary cancers show a lymphocytic infiltration at the invasive edges of the tumor; this probably reflects an immunologic response to the tumor[205] and not preexisting autoimmune thyroiditis.

Can papillary cancers arise in benign nodules or adenomas? The answer is, of course, "yes";[21, 183, 202, 203] however, this does not indicate that the nodule is premalignant. It may merely result from a malignant tumor's arising in this particular area of the gland instead of in a non-nodular zone; i.e., it is likely to be a random event of location and may not indicate a causal relationship.

Rare syndromes of papillary carcinoma associated with lesions in other organs have been described. Yasuda et al. described a patient with papillary thyroid cancer and bilateral adrenal pheochromocytomas and culled six additional similar cases from the literature.[217] Banik et al. reported an unusual case of a woman with multiple pituitary, adrenal, and pancreatic islet cell neoplasms as well as papillary cancer of the thyroid.[3]

The association of papillary carcinoma and parathyroid adenoma and/or hyperplasia has been described by several authors. Although a variety of mechanisms for this relationship have been suggested, the one most recently favored appears to be that both types of lesions are associated with a history of low dose external radiation to the neck.[117, 118, 146, 149]

Pathology of Papillary Carcinoma (Table 8–3)

The gross appearance of papillary thyroid cancer is quite variable[63, 72, 203, 211] (Figs. 8–6 and 8–7). This has led to classifications of the tumor based upon gross type. The two largest series to address this specific issue were published by Woolner et al.[211, 212] and Hawk and Hazard.[72] Table 8–4 compares these schemes.

The occult papillary cancer has been accepted by some and refuted by others since, if this is meant to be a clinically occult lesion, defining it by size (basically a pathology parameter) seems inappropriate. Hence Hawk and Hazard[72] and others[106, 202, 203] prefer the term "small papillary cancer" or "papillary microcarcinoma."[2, 12, 37, 72, 84, 85, 122–126, 133] The acceptance of this new term, of course, requires a definition: what is small? Most pathologists agree that a lesion that fits into this category should measure one centimeter;[59, 150] some authors consider the upper limit of size to be 1.5 centimeters. (However, lesions of this size should be clinically

Table 8–3. Papillary Carcinoma: Pathologic Features

Gross Types	Histologic Features
Small (occult; minute; minimal)	Papillae
Intrathyroidal	Follicles common
encapsulated	Desmoplasia
invasive	Lymphocytes
diffuse	Psammoma bodies
cystic	Nuclei (clear, overlapping, grooves)
Extrathyroidal (massive)	

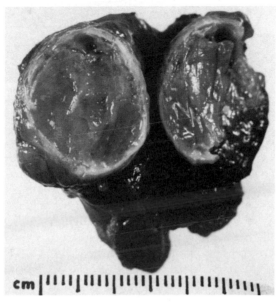

Figure 8–6. Grossly encapsulated papillary carcinoma. Note thick capsule.

detectable.) Vickery et al. pointed out that most of these tumors fall in the 4 to 7 millimeter range.[203]

How common are these lesions? The answer to this question depends upon geography, i.e., the population studied. (See Table 8–5.)

As if the definition of small papillary carcinoma were not problematic enough, a newer subclassification of these lesions has been proposed.[103, 133, 138, 213] These studies divide tumors into minute cancers (defined as under 5 millimeters in

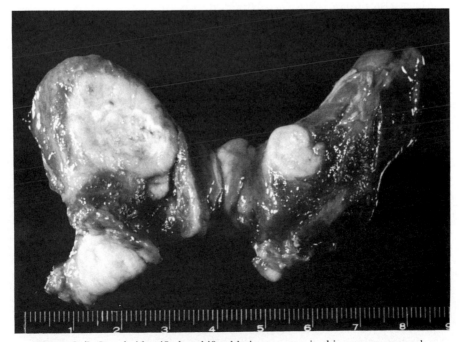

Figure 8–7. Grossly identified multifocal lesions as seen in this case are unusual.

Table 8–4. Papillary Carcinoma: Gross Subtypes

Woolner et al. (Mayo Clinic)[211, 212]	Hawk & Hazard (Cleveland)[72]
Occult	Small
Intrathyroidal	Intrathyroidal
	Diffuse
	Encapsulated
Extrathyroidal	Massive

diameter) and tiny (defined as between 5 and 10 millimeters in size). Such lesions found in surgical material were often incidental lesions in glands removed for adenomatous goiter (29 percent), thyroiditis (21 percent), adenoma (8.6 percent) or toxic goiter (5.3 percent). The authors admit that these frequencies are obviously biased by surgical selection.[213] In further studies of this problem, it has been suggested that minute carcinomas arise from a few follicles as a nonencapsulated lesion (often totally follicular in pattern), which may or may not be associated with sclerosis. Some progress to become encapsulated at least partially; the latter may progress further to clinically evident lesions. Those lesions that for unknown reasons remain sclerosing apparently remain clinically silent throughout the lifetime of the patient.[213–215]

The tiny cancers differ from the minute ones not only in size but also in other features. Kasai and Sakamoto found a higher incidence of extrathyroidal extent in the tiny lesions (10 percent versus 3 percent) and in nodal metastases (59 percent versus 13 percent).[103] These authors suggested more aggressive therapy for the tiny lesions.

Harach et al. noted in their autopsy study that 35.6 percent of patients subjected to autopsy in Finland had occult papillary carcinoma.[70] These authors suggested that tumors measuring under 5 millimeters be considered a "normal" finding and be left untreated. However, documented instances of lymph node metastases from lesions less than 0.5 centimeters are known.[11, 59] Distant spread, although very rare, is also documented.[143] (See Table 8–6.)

Only rarely do tumors in this size range found at autopsy have associated metastases.[162] (Siedal and Modan noted two patients who had lesions with lung metastases, however.[178]) From the clinical viewpoint, lesions of this size are often the "primary" in the thyroid of a patient who presented with nodal metastases.

Table 8–5. Incidence of Occult Thyroid Carcinoma (Microcarcinoma)*

Author (Reference)	Country	Percent
Fukunaga and Yatani (58)	Japan	28.4
	Poland	9
	Canada	6
	Colombia	5.6
Fransilla and Harach (55)	Finland	14
Siegal and Modan (178)	Israel	6.5
Sampson et al. (165)	Japan	17.9
Sampson et al. (166)	USA (Minnesota)	5.7
Komorowski and Hanson (109)	USA (Milwaukee)	3
Silverberg and Vidone (180)	USA (Connecticut)	2.7
Harach et al. (70)	Finland	35.6
Lang et al. (110)	Germany	6.2

*These data are representative studies only. They represent findings at autopsy, presumably in patients without clinical evidence of thyroid disease. The methodology of pathologic examination varies among the series with some using subserial blocking of the entire thyroid and others utilizing less rigorous examination.

Table 8–6. Well-documented Cases of Small Papillary Cancers (Papillary Microcarcinomas) with Distant Metastases

Histologic Type	Size	Metastases	Author (Ref.)
Papillary sclerosing	0.3 cm.	Femur	Young (219)
Papillary sclerosing	0.85 mm.	Vertebrae	Patchefsky (143)
Papillary sclerosing	2.4 mm.	Lung	Strate et al. (188)
Papillary sclerosing	6 mm.	Bone	Lloyd et al. (119)
Papillary	4 mm.	Pericardium	Jancic-Zguricas (91)

Are we to assume that these tumors are different? Or that the host is different? It seems a problem not to extrapolate from the latter scenario to all small incidentally found papillary cancers in surgical specimens; however, if the literature so far available is accurate, despite the presence of node metastases, the incidence of death from lesions in this size range is very, very rare; in these unusual cases, some other factors may be at work. Some of these cases have been reported in the older literature; however, in some it appears that aneuploid cell populations in the tumor may predict their unusually aggressive behavior.[75, 91, 98, 119, 143, 188]

The gross appearance of the small papillary carcinoma is that of a nonencapsulated sclerotic white-to-tan nodule often located in a subcapsular area of the gland. Histologically, the tumors may be totally follicular or (usually the lesions over 5 millimeters) papillary and follicular. Sclerosis may be recapitulated microscopically as well (Figs. 8–8 and 8–9); the lesions are nonencapsulated and often infiltrate the surrounding thyroid.

Since the small papillary cancer found in the thyroid in a patient presenting with nodal metastasis may be difficult to identify grossly because of its size,[120, 133, 150]

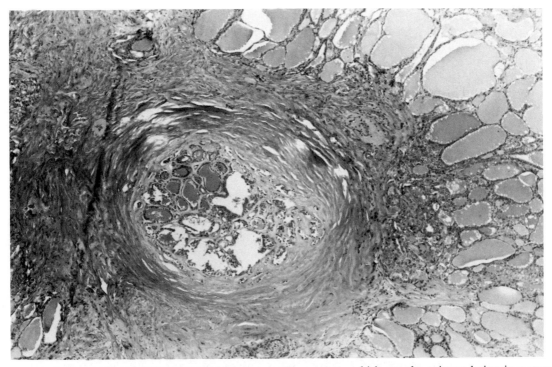

Figure 8–8. Low-power view shows small sclerosing papillary tumor, which was the primary lesion in a young woman who presented with cervical node metastasis. × 10, H & E.

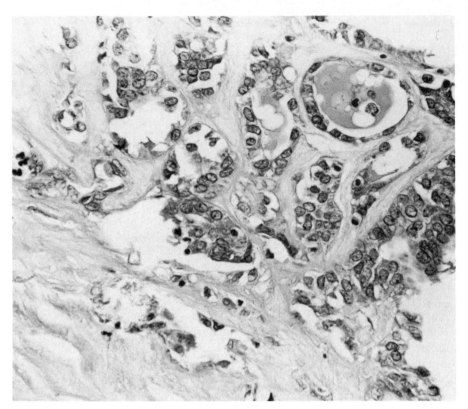

Figure 8–9. Higher power of the central part of the lesion in Figure 8–8 shows a follicular pattern to the tumor with marked sclerotic response; note large nuclei. × 150, H & E.

the older literature indicated that papillary cancer could on occasion arise from "developmental rests" in lymph nodes in the lateral neck—so-called lateral aberrant thyroid. (See also Chapters 1 and 16.) Brewer has stressed how this concept is in fact spurious.[13]

Most clinical papillary cancers (approximately 35 to 78 percent) are masses that are clinically palpable in the gland. The tumor may be located anywhere in the gland, even in the isthmus.[211, 212] These intrathyroidal lesions, which usually measure over 1.5 centimeters, may grossly appear as firm nonencapsulated or partly encapsulated lesions. Calcification may be present, and rarely this is so striking as to necessitate decalcification of the tissue in order to process it. Gross cystic changes may be present; however, in a papillary cancer there is always a portion of the cystic tumor that contains solid lesional tissue. (This differentiates the carcinoma from a benign cyst.[65, 157]) Occasionally gross papillations will be seen. Areas of hemorrhage may be present; sometimes, cholesterol clefts, as evidence of old hemorrhage, may be found.[52, 130, 202, 203, 211, 212] Necrosis is uncommon in the usual papillary cancer in the absence of prior needle biopsy and should alert the pathologist to the possibility of a more serious lesion.

Some papillary carcinomas (estimates range from 2 to 39 percent and the lower figure is probably closer to the true one), usually lesions of large size (5 centimeters or greater), will be found to extend grossly beyond the thyroid capsule and into cervical soft tissues. Many of these lesions conform to the "massive" category defined by Hawk and Hazard.[72] (See Table 8–4.)

Encapsulated papillary carcinoma makes up about 8 to 13 percent of the group[72, 173] and resembles an adenoma grossly.[45, 203] (See below.)

Microscopically, these papillary carcinomas share certain features. Thus many of them will contain predominant or focal papillary areas.[128, 130] A large number will contain follicular areas as well. Various series indicate that the percentage of tumors that are predominantly papillary ranges between 20 and 40 percent; the number that are predominantly follicular is between 15 and 35 percent, and the remainder are about equally mixed papillary and follicular[20, 21, 52–54, 72, 130, 154, 203, 211, 212] (Figs. 8–10 to 8–13).

The tumor cells are usually columnar and contain considerable amounts of amphophilic cytoplasm. The characteristic clear nuclei are found in over 80 percent of such lesions, intranuclear inclusions in about 80 to 85 percent, and nuclear grooves are seen in almost all the cases.

Mitoses are exceptional in usual papillary carcinoma[203] (Fig. 8–4). Lee et al. found a mean of 17 mitoses/100 high-power fields in their study of papillary tumors.[111] This correlates well with analysis of growth fraction by cytometric techniques and probably reflects the indolent biologic features of the tumor. In cases in which preoperative needle biopsy was done, however, mitoses may be seen in the vicinity of the needle track, reflecting reaction to hemorrhage and repair.

Psammoma bodies, which are so characteristic of this tumor, are unfortunately found in only about 40 to 50 percent of cases[21, 52, 129, 130, 154, 203, 211] (Figs. 8–2 and 8–14). However, their presence is a very good indication that the lesion is a papillary cancer. In addition, since psammoma bodies represent the ghosts of

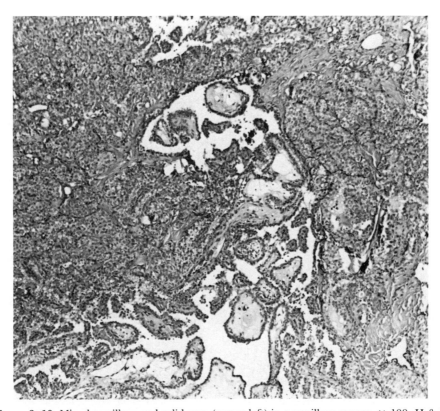

Figure 8–10. Mixed papillary and solid area (upper left) in a papillary cancer. × 100, H & E.

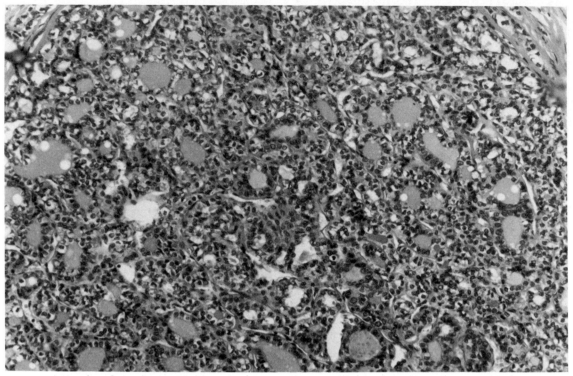

Figure 8–11. Follicular variant of papillary cancer. Note enlarged nuclei, and overlapping. × 100, H & E.

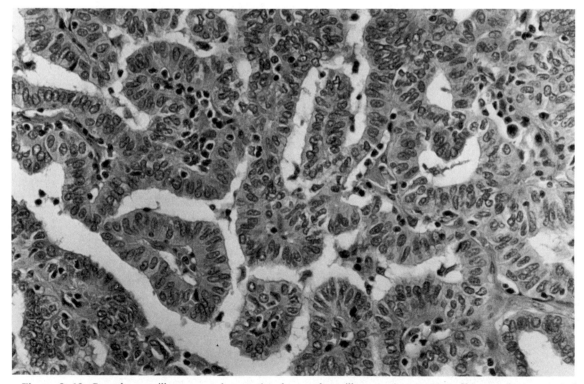

Figure 8–12. Complex papillary areas characterize the usual papillary carcinoma. Note fibrovascular cores, and elongated and overlapping nuclei. × 150, H & E.

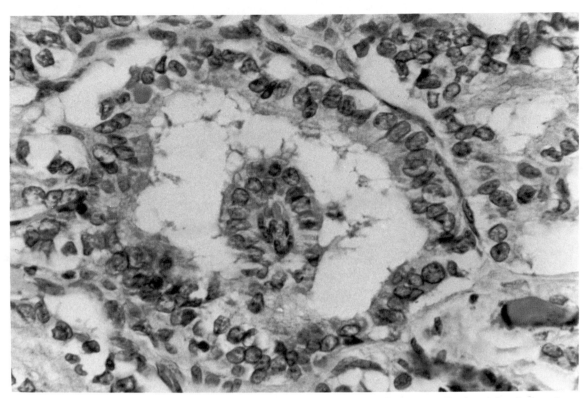

Figure 8–13. In some examples a follicular pattern predominates and only focal papilla formation is found. × 200, H & E.

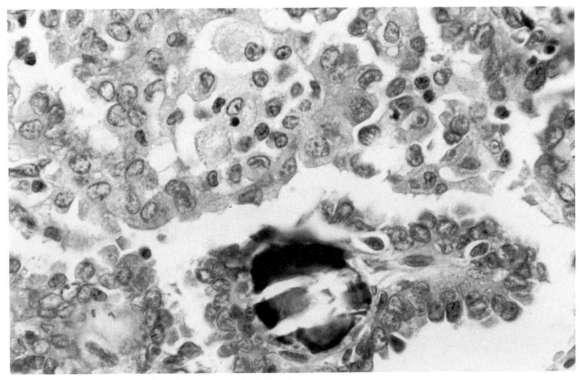

Figure 8–14. Psammoma body within fibrovascular core of papillae. × 200, H & E.

dead papillae, their presence in thyroid tissue, most likely in intrathyroidal lymphatic spaces (Figs. 8–15 and 8–16), indicates that a papillary carcinoma is very probably somewhere in the gland. Similarly, the finding of psammoma bodies in a lymph node should be seen as strong evidence of a papillary cancer in the thyroid.

About 10 to 12 percent of ordinary papillary carcinomas contain areas of solid growth,[21] which the current author believes represent areas of trabecular follicular pattern. Most of these foci are seen only focally; these areas contain cytologically bland cells and rare mitoses and must not be misinterpreted as dedifferentiation of the tumor. Very rarely these solid zones will constitute the greatest area of the tumor (see below).

Many papillary carcinomas contain foci of squamous differentiation.[21, 52, 130, 203, 212] Fransilla indicated that in his material these areas could be found in about 40 percent of cases.[52] Most other series indicate a range of percentage for this finding of about 15 to 45 percent.[130] These areas, often seen within neoplastic follicles or abutting papillae, resemble squamous morules in endometrial cancer. Rarely keratinization is found. At the ultrastructural level, Gould et al. identified features suggesting squamous differentiation in some of the papillary tumors they studied.[62] It is possible that these foci are responsible for some of the immuno-staining results, indicating the presence of epidermal type keratins in some papillary carcinomas. (See below and Chapter 18.)

Almost all usual papillary carcinomas show areas of desmoplasia either in the central portions of the tumor or more commonly at the peripheral zones of the lesions.[21, 52, 72, 129, 130, 203, 211–215] Such sclerotic foci are associated with invasive areas (Figs. 8–8 and 8–9). Even in partially encapsulated lesions, these zones of sclerosis may be identified at the areas of capsular penetration. Rarely, amyloid has been described in these tumors.[147] (Whether this lesion represents a true papillary tumor or a variant of medullary cancer is unclear; immunostains were not available when it was reported.)

It is common at these leading edges of invasion to find the presence of scattered lymphocytes.[52, 61, 72, 129, 130, 203, 211, 212] Rarely an intense lymphocytic infiltrate, even with the presence of germinal centers, will be seen. This infiltrate, however, is curiously localized to the invasive tumor foci and does not indicate a preexisting underlying chronic thyroiditis. It is likely, as postulated by Volpe,[205] that these immunocytes are reacting to altered cell surface antigens on the tumor cells or to abnormal tumor cell products (? altered thyroglobulin). Clark et al. identified the presence of thyrotropin receptor apparatus in tumorous thyroid tissue as well.[28] Pontius and Hawk noted the loss of microsomal antigen in papillary carcinoma.[148] Interesting in this regard is the finding of increased numbers of antigen-presenting dendritic cells in these lesions.[174] Kamma et al. noted HLA-DR expression in the tumor cells, and that the peritumor lymphocytes were predominantly of T cell type, all findings similar to those in chronic lymphocytic thyroiditis.[101] These studies suggest that a mechanism similar to that in autoimmune thyroid disease may be taking place in these tumors.

A few usual papillary cancers will be associated with histologic evidence of chronic thyroiditis (including not only lymphocytic infiltration, but also oncocytic change in nontumorous follicular epithelium and follicular atrophy) in areas of the gland, not only abutting the neoplasm but also in other noncancerous areas. Whether this represents an underlying autoimmune thyroiditis or an exaggerated diffuse response to the cancer cannot be answered in all cases; in some the former is true.[121, 141] However, as noted above, the coincidence of these two relatively common conditions does not prove an etiologic relationship. Abundant lymphoid

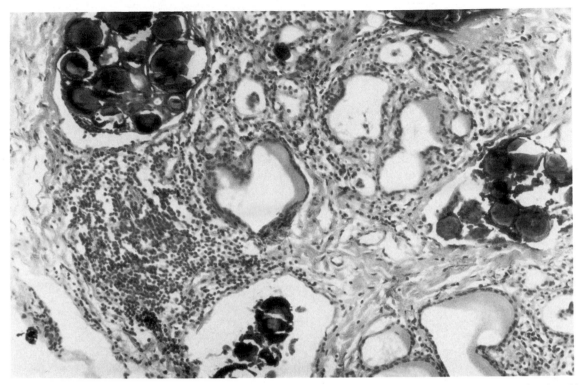

Figure 8–15. This example of psammoma bodies with minimal residual epithelium in lymphatics in thyroid removed from the main mass of tumor supports the contention that they represent the residua of dead tumor cells. Note lymphocytes nearby. × 100, H & E.

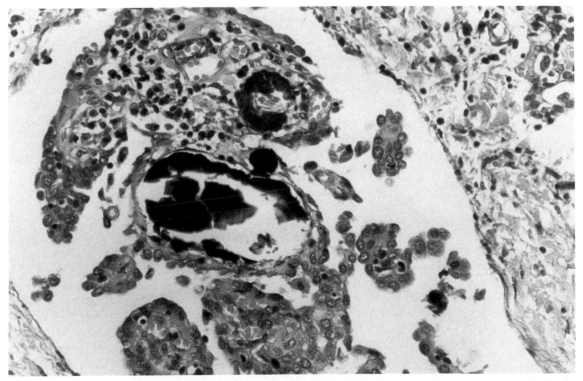

Figure 8–16. Another area of thyroid in same case as in Figure 8–15. Note tumor mass with psammoma bodies in lymphatic space. × 200, H & E.

infiltrate appears more commonly in children with thyroid cancer and may be a reflection of their better prognosis.[101, 203]

Distinctly different from true follicular carcinoma, which has a propensity to invade the venous system and bypass the thyroid lymphatics (see Chapter 9), papillary carcinoma has a propensity to invade the glandular lymphatics (Figs. 8–15 and 8–16).[49, 64, 88, 159] This feature leads to two commonly noted consequences of this tumor: so-called multifocality of the tumor and a high incidence of regional node metastases. Papillary carcinoma is not a lesion in which multiple clones of cells undergo neoplastic transformation at the same time; i.e., it is not a multicentric tumor. Studies by Fialkow using enzyme technology[51] and by Hicks et al. utilizing molecular biology techniques[77] have shown that, of those papillary cancers studied, all appear to be clonal proliferations. (These techniques are hampered by the fact that since they depend on the Lyon hypothesis [see Chapter 9], they can be performed on only a small sample of female patients; it is possible, but the present author feels it is unlikely, that some papillary tumors are multiclonal.)

The majority of papillary carcinomas, if not all of them, therefore, are clonal proliferations, and the multifocality must be due to intrathyroidal lymphatic spread. Whether this avidity for lymphatic spread and node metastasis predicts what therapy should be given to patients with this tumor has led to debate among surgeons and endocrinologists. Some argue that because of multifocal microscopic lesions in the gland, the entire gland should be excised;[27] others indicate that more conservative surgery followed by thyroid suppression is adequate since the tumor is often hormonally controllable.[33, 41, 160, 171, 204] In support of the latter school of thought is the low frequency of local recurrence in the opposite thyroid lobe[194] and the recent follow-up studies of conservatively treated patients showing excellent results.[30, 32, 33, 204] (Virtually all therapists agree that treatment of extrathyroidal or massive papillary cancer requires more radical procedures.[29, 60, 89, 197, 211, 212])

Venous invasion does occur in papillary cancer but in only about 7 percent of cases of the usual type.[52, 72, 130, 196] Whether this finding alone is predictive of a more aggressive behavior is unclear, since it is so uncommon.

Regional lymph node metastases are extremely common at initial presentation of usual papillary cancer; the literature indicates that about 50 percent or more of patients who present with intrathyroidal masses that are papillary carcinoma will have nodal metastases. However, in contrast to any other body site, this feature apparently does not adversely affect long-term prognosis.[52, 74, 122–126, 137] Hence, attempts at staging of papillary carcinoma may have minimal clinical significance.

As noted above, some patients will present with cervical node enlargement and will have no obvious clinical manifestation of a thyroid tumor. Not infrequently the nodal metastasis will involve one node, which may be cystic. Both the surgeon and the pathologist must be aware of papillary carcinoma presenting as a unilocular cystic node metastasis so that a misdiagnosis of branchial cleft cyst is not rendered.[120, 150] The histology of the nodal metastases in papillary cancer may appear papillary, mixed, or follicular; one cannot predict from examination of the primary lesion the histology of the metastatic disease. Similarly, the converse is true; i.e., one cannot predict the histologic appearance of the primary tumor by evaluating the metastases.

When discussing ordinary papillary carcinoma of the thyroid and not the subtypes, the question of tumor grading needs to be raised in order to indicate that it is of no use in this tumor, since over 95 percent of these lesions are grade

1.[203] In some tumors, either in the primary site or in recurrences, areas of poorly differentiated cancer characterized by solid growth of tumor, often with easily noted mitotic activity and with cytologic atypia, can be found. Such lesions, while falling short of anaplastic transformation of papillary cancer, portend a much more guarded prognosis. Anaplastic change in a papillary cancer can occur, although its frequency is fortunately uncommon.[135, 203, 216] Despite the fact that some classification schemes place such lesions in the papillary cancer category, the prognosis for the patient is equal to the extremely poor one associated with anaplastic carcinoma of the thyroid. (See Chapter 11.)

Distant metastases of papillary carcinoma occur in the lungs and bones most often.[122–126, 170, 203, 211, 212] The incidence of this ranges from 5 to 7 percent of cases; despite the presence of multiple metastases, however, the survival may still be prolonged, especially if the metastases can be treated with radioiodine.[41, 80, 156, 170] In ordinary papillary carcinoma death is uncommon; patients who do succumb usually will have pulmonary metastases that no longer respond to radioiodine therapy.[41, 161]

Ultrastructure. Several investigations of the electron microscopic appearance of papillary carcinoma have been published.[1, 5, 62, 93–97, 191] The nuclear features have been described above and include the dispersed chromatin and highly infolded nuclear membrane.[62, 95] The cytoplasm contains many mitochondria and numerous cytoplasmic filaments.[62] Reduplication of the basal lamina can be found; long and pleomorphic microvilli are noted in some tumors.[95] In tumors with squamous foci, cytoplasmic structures consistent with keratohyaline granules have been found.[62]

Special Stains. In ordinary papillary cancer special stains are of little use. Chan et al. found that 17.5 percent contained mucicarminophilic intracellular material.[93] This has been noted by others.

Immunostaining. Studies, utilizing either immunoperoxidase or immunofluorescent techniques, have shown that the great majority of papillary cancers (92 to 100 percent) contain thyroglobulin.[8, 209] Most also contain thyroxine and triiodothyronine. Staining to localize keratin has yielded confusing results.[15, 40, 76, 131, 145, 207, 209] Low-molecular-weight keratin is found in almost all examples of papillary carcinoma; the staining results show diffuse and intense positivity in these tumors. However, although some authors have found that epidermal (high-molecular-weight) keratins are also found in papillary carcinoma (possibly related to the squamous change in some of these lesions), others have not reproduced these findings. If the epidermal keratins were uniformly found in papillary carcinomas, this would be a relatively simple way of distinguishing between the follicular variant of papillary cancer (positive) and true follicular carcinoma or adenoma (negative) and between papillary hyperplastic nodule (negative) and papillary carcinoma (positive). The present author has found that keratin immunostaining is too unreliable to recommend for these important differential diagnoses.

Flow Cytometry. As discussed in Chapter 18, flow cytometry has been used as a prognostic indicator for papillary carcinoma.[90] Some tumors that are small lesions expected to have an excellent prognosis but that show aneuploid cell populations have behaved in a biologically aggressive fashion.[92, 98, 99]

Prognosis. Prognostic factors in usual papillary carcinoma include some that are clinical and some pathologic features.[67, 127, 136, 152, 158, 181, 182, 192, 193, 195, 198]

Age. Patients who are over age 50 at diagnosis of papillary carcinoma tend to have a more serious prognosis than younger individuals.[16–18, 34, 36, 108, 112, 116, 154–156, 169] Papillary carcinoma in children is associated with an excellent outlook, even in the presence of lung metastases;[14, 36] Kodama et al. identified only 10 fatal cases of thyroid cancer in children under the age of 15 in Japan in series through 1986.[108] Of these only seven were papillary in type, and these patients died of lung metastases.

Sex. Men tend to have more aggressive lesions than women in some series.[122]

Size. Larger lesions are more biologically aggressive as a rule. Some of these tumors are also grossly extending beyond the thyroid capsule, and it may be that these two factors combine to result in a more guarded prognosis. Grossly noted extrathyroidal extension is associated with a worse prognosis;[29, 30, 52, 57, 60, 71, 72, 89, 193, 196, 197] microscopic penetration of the gland capsule, however, does not appear to be associated with an unfavorable outlook.

Differentiation. The majority of papillary cancers are well differentiated and can contain and produce thyroglobulin.[41] Dedifferentiation, as defined above, is, of course, a poor indicator.[20, 21, 86, 87, 194] Aneuploidy, as indicated by flow cytometric measurements, is associated with a poor prognosis.[31]

It is not possible to define which of these features is an independent variable for prognosis. The best evidence seems to indicate that ploidy measurements may be. (Dedifferentiation is also, but here the tumor has changed its features morphologically and can be recognized as different.) It is curious that most large series have failed to segregate out the subtypes of papillary cancer that have been associated with poor outcomes—the tall cell variant and diffuse sclerosis variant. A notable exception to this is the paper by Hawk and Hazard,[72] which defined the tall cell variant as an aggressive lesion. In addition, in some papers there are insufficient numbers of cases to allow for multivariate analysis to define which if any variable is the most critical. Thus, in the paper that defined the tall cell variant, Hawk and Hazard noted that this lesion occurred in older patients, often was massive in size and extrathyroidal in extent, and showed vascular invasion;[72] which of these factors was the most important with regard to prognosis remains unknown.

Subtypes of Papillary Carcinoma

Certain histologic subtypes of papillary cancer occur that will be discussed below; some of these are associated with a more guarded prognosis.

Follicular Variant of Papillary Cancer. Initially defined by Lindsay[114, 116] in the 1950's, this variant was redescribed by Chen and Rosai in 1977.[25] Before the recognition of this tumor as papillary cancer, it was classified among the true follicular carcinomas. (The latter are clinically and biologically different.[168]) Grossly, the tumor may appear encapsulated, and this feature may be noted histologically as well.[25, 203] In the follicular variant, despite the almost total or complete follicular pattern in the primary site, there may be psammoma bodies (the ghosts of dead papillae), and even papillae in nodal metastases. Features that suggest that a follicular tumor is a follicular variant of papillary cancer include the clear nuclei, psammoma bodies, desmoplastic response at invasive areas, and lymphocytic infiltration. In this variant the follicles that compose the tumor often contain colloid with peripheral scalloping, mimicking the appearance of a hyperplastic gland. (However, such lesions are not hot on scan and are not associated with hyperfunction.) Also, clearing of the cytoplasm in addition to the nuclear clearing can be seen. The prognosis of the follicular variant is apparently similar to more usual papillary cancer, although some series indicate a greater propensity of this variant to metastasize outside the neck.[20, 21]

Tall Cell Variant (Table 8–7) (Figs. 8–17 and 8–18). Hawk and Hazard

Table 8–7. Tall Cell Variant of Papillary Thyroid Carcinoma

Incidence	9–10%
Age	older 57 vs. 36 (Hawk & Hazard[72])
Sex (F/M)	5:1
Size of lesion	large, often massive >6 cm.
Extrathyroidal	42%
Node metastasis	75%
Distant metastasis	17%
Deaths of tumor	25%

described the tall cell variant of papillary cancer and found that in their material this tumor made up about 10 percent of the papillary cancers.[72] At presentation, the tumor is often quite large (>6 cm.), extends extrathyroidally, and shows vascular invasion more often than usual papillary cancer. The tumor tends to occur in elderly patients.

The tumors are composed of cells that are twice as tall as they are wide, and the cytoplasm is often quite eosinophilic.[196] By electron microscopy, the cytoplasm of the tumor cells contains increased numbers of mitochondria, but they tend not to recapitulate true Hürthle cells.[196] Unlike usual papillary tumors, they can contain readily identifiable mitotic figures.[203] The tumors tend to be very papillary, and often a heavy lymphocytic infiltration is present in and/or around the tumor. In some examples, the lymphocytes are present within the cores of papillae (Fig. 8–17). Some tall cell tumors arise in glands with extensive histologic evidence of chronic thyroiditis.

The prognosis for this variant is more serious; these patients tend to suffer

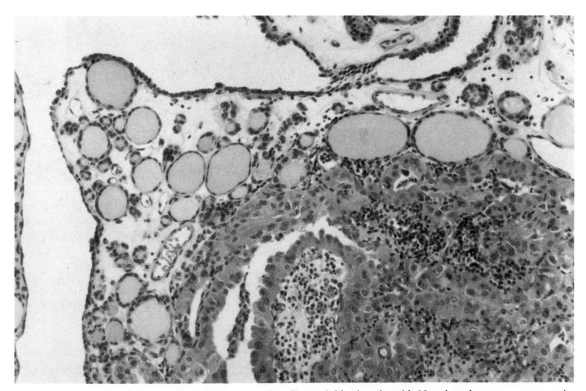

Figure 8–17. Tall cell variant of papillary cancer invading neighboring thyroid. Note lymphocytes accompanying the tumor. × 200, H & E.

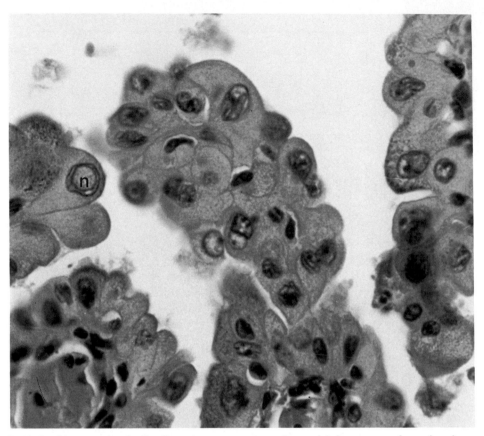

Figure 8–18. In this example of tall cell carcinoma, note irregular nuclei that are not clear, abundant cytoplasm, and intranuclear cytoplasmic invagination (*n*). × 400, H & E.

local recurrences in the neck, often with invasion of the trachea, and many will succumb to this complication. It is difficult to be sure that the histology alone is responsible for this prognosis or if the influence of older age, extrathyroidal growth and vascular invasion contribute; no studies using multivariate analysis have been published, probably because the number of available cases is too small.[72, 100]

Columnar Cell Variant of Papillary Cancer (Table 8–8). Only three published cases of this variant are available.[44, 185] In each, the affected patient was male, and in each case the patient died of metastatic tumor, usually in five years. The curious histologic features of this lesion are extreme papillarity, tall columnar cells, and nuclear stratification; I have noted in a case I studied, as well as in Evans' cases, that cytoplasmic clearing is present and the tumor cells resemble the cellular

Table 8–8. Columnar Cell Variant of Papillary Thyroid Carcinoma[44, 185]

Age	34, 47, 60
Sex (F/M)	all male
Size of lesion	10 cm., 8 cm., 6 cm.
Extrathyroidal	yes
Node metastasis	yes
Distant metastasis	yes—lungs, bone
Deaths of tumor	all (in less than 4 yrs.)

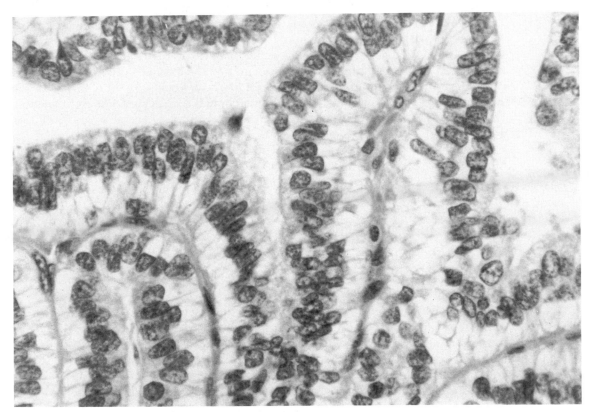

Figure 8–19. Columnar cell variant of papillary cancer. Note subnuclear vacuolization reminiscent of early secretory endometrium. × 400, H & E.

changes seen in secretory endometrium (Fig. 8–19). In the cases described by Evans zones of less well differentiated tumor were recognized.[44]

Diffuse Sclerosis Variant (Table 8–9). Vickery et al. described this tumor, which often affects children, as a more aggressive type of papillary cancer.[203] Such lesions often do not present with a dominant mass but rather with bilateral goiter. The tumor freely permeates the gland as though outlining the course of the lymphatic system of the thyroid. The tumor nests are composed of papillae with associated solid areas resembling endometrial morules (these have been referred to as squamous metaplasia); these solid zones may constitute over 50 percent of the lesion. Numerous psammoma bodies are found; the gross impression related to this is that of a gritty cut surface. A prominent lymphocytic infiltrate is found around the tumor foci. Chan et al. noted the presence of large numbers of S-100 stained dendritic cells in these lesions; in addition, two of their three patients had measurable titers of antithyroid antibodies in the serum.[24]

Table 8–9. Diffuse Sclerosis Variant of Papillary Thyroid Carcinoma

Number	11 cases*
Age	childhood to mid-thirties
Sex (F/M)	2:1
Size of lesion	diffuse
Extrathyroidal	yes
Node metastasis	100%
Distant metastasis	37%

*(Refs. 19, 24)

The lesions tend to recur in the neck and appear to have a somewhat more serious prognosis than usual childhood papillary cancer. Carcangiu et al., in comparing eight cases to their entire series of 241 cases of papillary cancer, noted that these tumors had a higher frequency of nodal metastases (100 percent versus 37.5 percent) and distant metastases (54 percent versus 14 percent) and less likelihood of disease-free survival (25 percent versus 77 percent) at eight years of follow-up.[19] The three patients reported by Chan et al. were alive and well, but the follow-up was under two years in these cases.[24]

A somewhat related lesion (some authors consider it a totally distinct tumor unrelated to papillary cancer and related to ultimobranchial body rests) is the mucoepidermoid carcinoma.[56] (See also Chapter 15.)

Solid Variant. Although solid areas resembling trabeculae or microfollicles devoid of colloid can be found focally in many papillary cancers, a tumor composed solely of a solid pattern is rare. Schroder et al. described a 1.4 centimeter thyroid tumor in a 24 year old woman who presented with nodal metastases.[173] The primary and metastatic lesions were associated with extensive band-like sclerosis. The follicular origin of this tumor was documented by immunostaining for thyroglobulin.

Clear Cell Variant. Papillary carcinoma composed of clear cells (in contradistinction to clear nuclei) has been described, usually in series on clear cell thyroid tumors. (See Chapter 15.) Variokjis et al. reported such a case in a 67 year old man.[200] These authors indicated that the cells were filled with glycogen and fat.

Oxyphil Variant. Papillary cancer composed of Hürthle cells (not just pink tall cells) can occur, but is unusual. These must be differentiated from papillary zones in otherwise classic follicular carcinomas of Hürthle cell type. Dickersin et al. described an apparently unique tumor that showed features of tall cell, oxyphil, and clear cells.[39] The cells had an oxyphilic basal zone, clear apex, and mid-placed nucleus. By electron microscopy, they showed characteristic large mitochondria of oxyphils at the base, but empty mitochondria at the apical zones.

Encapsulated Variant. This tumor, which presents the gross appearance of an adenoma, constitutes from 8 to 13 percent of papillary cancers.[11, 72, 172, 173] Microscopically, such lesions can also show total encapsulation; however, there are cytologic features of papillary cancer, including nuclear changes and psammoma bodies. Some of these lesions show focal invasion into the capsule.[45, 172]

The differential diagnosis is with papillary hyperplastic changes in a follicular nodule; for this distinction one must rely on the cytologic changes.

Although this subgroup of tumors is associated with an even better prognosis than papillary cancer in general, occasional lesions (25 percent in the series of Bocker et al.[11]) have shown lymph node metastases, and hence they are considered carcinomas.[45, 172] Distant spread or death due to tumor has not been documented.[11]

Do these lesions represent papillary cancer arising in an adenoma? Vickery indicates that some may.[203] Evans divided his series of 14 cases of papillary encapsulated tumors into three groups: five papillary cancers that showed focal invasion, one of which metastasized; two cases of papillary change in a benign adenoma; and a group he considered of uncertain malignant potential in which some features of papillary cancer but not all were present. Since in the material of Schroder et al.[172] an occasional tumor of this type apparently metastasized, Evans felt they should not simply be considered totally benign.[45]

Papillary Carcinoma with Lipomatous Stroma. An apparently unique papillary carcinoma was described by Vestfrid.[201] The 2.5 centimeter lesion occurred in a 53-year-old woman and appeared as an ordinary papillary cancer, except that many of the papillary cores contained mature fat. It apparently was a slowly

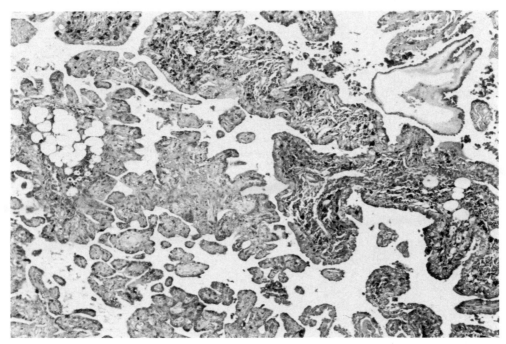

Figure 8–20. In this papillary cancer, abundant hemosiderin is seen in some stromal cores of papillae, and in one, mature fat is present. × 100, H & E.

growing tumor by history; no follow-up is presented. This lesion should be added to the thyroid tumors containing fat, the rest of which so far reported have been classified as benign: adenolipomas and hamartomas (Fig. 8–20). (See Chapter 15.)

It has been my experience that papillary cancers of the thyroid that arise in the setting of *immunoderegulation,* such as following chemotherapy for leukemia, tend to appear like ordinary papillary tumors but may behave clinically in a more serious manner.

PAPILLARY HYPERPLASIA

Papillary hyperplasia is best characterized as the lesion found in untreated autoimmune hyperthyroidism (Graves' disease). In this condition, the immunologic derangement leads to production of immunoglobulins, which attach to the thyrotropin (TSH) receptor on the follicular epithelial cell, simulating the actions of TSH; consequently, the follicular epithelium undergoes growth and also increases output of thyroid hormones. The cell growth involves hypertrophy and hyperplasia; the result is that there are too many enlarged cells to "fit" on the scaffolding of the follicle. Hence, infoldings, or "papillations," form (Figs. 8–21 and 8–22).

Papillary hyperplasia in Graves' disease is distinguished from papillary carcinoma by the preservation of the lobular architecture of the gland (both grossly and microscopically), the diffuse nature of the lesion, the round although enlarged nuclei present in the individual cells, and the presence of lymphoid cells, often with germinal centers scattered throughout the stroma of the gland.

In treated Graves' the papillary areas are scanty and focal. In toxic nodular goiter, the changes are similar to those in Graves' glands, but the lesion tends to be more focal. Here the nuclear characteristics need to be relied upon to differentiate the lesion from cancer.

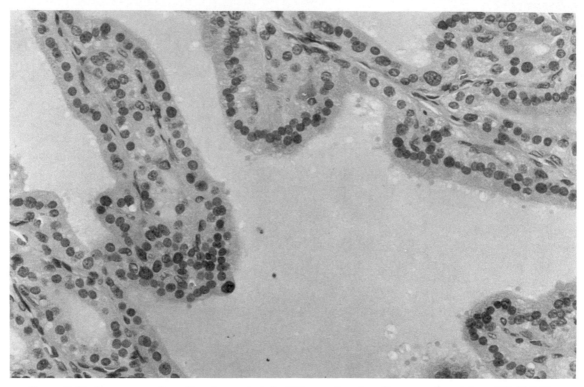

Figure 8–21. Low power of papillary hyperplasia in diffuse toxic goiter. Note round nuclei. × 100, H & E.

Papillary Hyperplasia in Follicular Nodule (Table 8–10). On occasion—and in my experience these lesions tend to occur more frequently in children and teenagers—a solitary thyroid nodule will be removed that will show a microscopic appearance of papillary growth. However, the nodule is always well circumscribed, often even encapsulated, unlike the usual papillary cancer. In addition, the papillae tend to contain extremely edematous stalks with follicles in them. The nuclei are round and not clear as in cancer (Fig. 8–22); there are no psammoma bodies. In contrast to papillary cancer wherein the papillae are often complex and arranged in different directions, the papillary foci in the benign follicular nodule are always directed toward the center of the nodule. Often the center is cystic. Such lesions may represent degenerative changes with edema and pseudopapillations; although the correlation between scan findings and histology is only fair, one might expect that some of these nodules would give a warm or hot appearance on scan; a number of them but not all have been hot nodules.[203] Such lesions need to be distinguished from microscopically encapsulated papillary carcinomas;[45, 82, 172] in most of the latter cases, nuclear characteristics and/or psammoma bodies can be relied upon to help in the differential diagnosis.

Table 8–10. Papillary Hyperplastic Nodule: Features

Clinically solitary; may be warm or hot on scan
Encapsulation
Often centrally cystic
Papillae with broad edematous cores
Subfollicle formation prominent
Papillae point to center of lesion
Nuclei round; not clear; not grooved

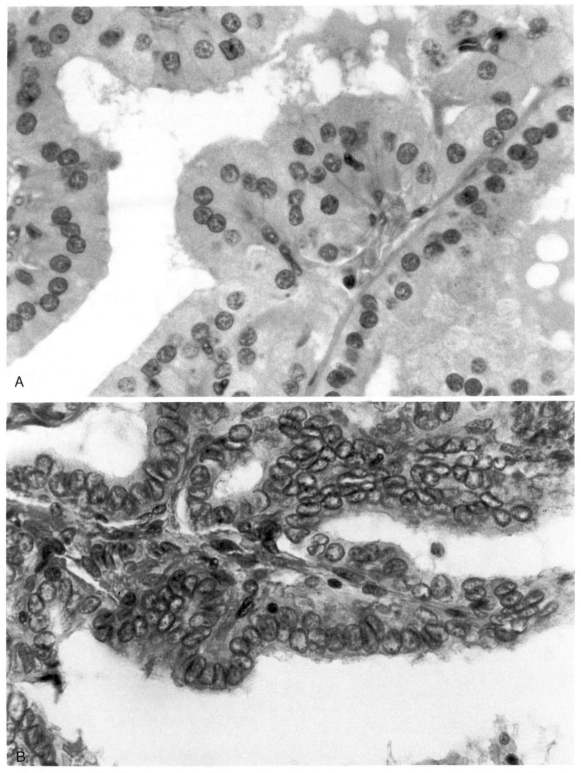

Figure 8–22. *A,* Papillary hyperplasia. Note round nuclei, abundant cytoplasm, and nuclei polarized to lower to mid part of cell. × 300, H & E.

B, Papillary cancer. Note fibrovascular core, large oval nuclei, clear and grooved nuclei, and their overlapping. × 300, H & E.

At times areas in nodular goiters will show a focally similar papillary appearance; these areas are often associated with hemorrhage and edema as well. Most of these areas cause less concern to the pathologist probably because of the associated background goiter.

Bennett et al. indicate that the use of immunostaining for monoclonal keratin may be useful in the distinction of papillary cancer from benign papillary change in follicular nodules.[7] In their study, keratin was identified in a diffuse staining pattern in the papillary cancers but was found only focally in the papillary hyperplastic nodules.

Are these lesions papillary adenomas? It is likely that such lesions have been diagnosed as adenomas by some. However, most pathologists prefer not to use this term since it has been applied to a host of lesions, from hyperplastic ones to encapsulated papillary carcinomas. Hence, it is preferable to avoid use of the term.

Papillary Variant of Medullary Carcinoma. This unusual tumor needs to be recognized as a medullary cancer. True papillae are formed; however, the nuclear characteristics are absent. This lesion is discussed in Chapter 10.

REFERENCES

1. Albores-Saavedra, J., Altamirano-Dimas, M., et al.: Fine structure of human papillary thyroid carcinoma. Cancer 28:763–774, 1971.
2. Arellano, L., and Ibaarra, A.: Occult carcinoma of the thyroid gland. Pathol. Res. Pract. 179:88–91, 1984.
3. Banik, S., Hasleton, P. S., and Lyon, R. L.: An unusual variant of multiple endocrine neoplasia syndrome. Histopathology 8:135–144, 1984.
4. Batsakis, J. G., Nishiyama, R. H., and Rich, C. R.: Microlithiasis (calcospherites) and carcinoma of the thyroid gland. Arch. Pathol. 69:493–498, 1960.
5. Beaumont, A., Othman, S. B., and Fragu, P.: The fine structure of papillary carcinoma of the thyroid. Histopathology 5:377–388, 1981.
6. Beaugie, J. M., Brown, C. L., et al.: Primary malignant tumours of the thyroid: the relationship between histological classification and clinical behaviour. Br. J. Surg. 63:173–181, 1976.
7. Bennett, W. P., Bhan, A. K., and Vickery, A. L.: Keratin expression as a diagnostic adjunct in thyroid tumors with papillary architecture. Lab. Invest. 58:9A, 1988 (abstract).
8. Berge-LeFranc, J. L., Cartouzou, G., et al.: Quantification of thyroglobulin messenger RNA by in situ hybridization in differentiated thyroid cancers. Cancer 56:345–350, 1985.
9. Block, M. A.: Well-differentiated carcinomas of the thyroid. Curr. Prob. Cancer 3:3–60, 1979.
10. Block, M. A., Miller, M. J., and Horn, R.: Carcinoma of the thyroid after external radiation to the neck in adults. Am. J. Surg. 118:764–768, 1969.
11. Bocker, W., Schroder, S., and Dralle, H.: Minimal thyroid neoplasia. Rec. Results Cancer Res. 106:131–138, 1988.
12. Bondeson, L. and Ljungberg, O.: Occult papillary thyroid carcinoma in the young and the aged. Cancer 53:1790–1792, 1984.
13. Brewer, D. B.: Papillary tumours of the thyroid gland. J. Pathol. Bacteriol. 77:149–162, 1959.
14. Buckwalter, J. A., Thomas, C. G., and Freeman, J. B.: Is childhood thyroid cancer a lethal disease? Ann. Surg. 181:632–635, 1975.
15. Buley, I. D., Gatter, K. C., et al.: Expression of intermediate filament proteins in normal and diseased thyroid glands. J. Clin. Pathol. 40:136–142, 1987.
16. Cady, B., Meissner, W. A., and Sala, L. E.: Thyroid cancer for forty-one years. N. Engl. J. Med. 299:901, 1978.
17. Cady, B., Sedgwick, C. E., et al.: Changing clinical, pathologic, therapeutic and survival patterns in differentiated thyroid carcinoma. Ann. Surg. 184:541–553, 1978.
18. Cady, B., Sedgwick, C. E., et al.: Risk factor analysis in differentiated thyroid cancer. Cancer 43:810–820, 1979.
19. Carcangiu, M. L., Bianchi, S., and Rosai, J.: Diffuse sclerosing papillary carcinoma: report of 8 cases of a distinctive variant of thyroid malignancy. Lab. Invest. 56:10A, 1987 (abstract).
20. Carcangiu, M. L., Zampi, G., et al.: Papillary carcinoma of the thyroid. A clinicopathologic study of 244 cases treated at the University of Florence, Italy. Cancer 55:805–828, 1985.

21. Carcangiu, M. L., Zampi, G., and Rosai, J.: Papillary thyroid carcinoma. A study of its many morphologic expressions and clinical correlates. Pathol. Annu. *20* (Pt. 1):1–44, 1985.
22. Chan, J. K. C., and Saw, D.: The grooved nucleus: A useful diagnostic criterion of papillary carcinoma of the thyroid. Am. J. Surg. Pathol. *10*:672–679, 1986.
23. Chan, J. K. C., and Tse, C. C. H.: Mucin production in metastatic papillary carcinoma of the thyroid. Hum. Pathol. *19*:195–200, 1988.
24. Chan, J. K. C., Tsui, M. S., and Tse, C. H.: Diffuse sclerosing variant of papillary carcinoma of the thyroid: a histological and immunohistochemical study of three cases. Histopathology *11*:191–202, 1987.
25. Chen, K. T. K., and Rosai, J.: Follicular variant of thyroid papillary carcinoma: A clinicopathologic study of six cases. Am. J. Surg. Pathol. *1*:123, 1977.
26. Christensen, S. B., Ljungberg, O., and Tibblin, S.: Thyroid carcinoma in Malmo, 1960–1977: Epidemiologic, clinical and prognostic findings in a defined urban population. Cancer *53*:1625–1633, 1984.
27. Clark, O. H.: Total thyroidectomy: the treatment of choice for patients with differentiated thyroid cancer. Ann. Surg. *196*:361–370, 1982.
28. Clark, O. H., Gerend, P. L., et al.: Characterization of the thyrotropin receptor adenylate cyclase system in neoplastic human thyroid tissue. J. Clin. Endocrinol. Metab. *57*:140–147, 1983.
29. Cody, H. S., and Shah, J. P.: Locally invasive, well differentiated thyroid cancer: 22 years' experience at Memorial Sloan-Kettering Cancer Center. Am. J. Surg. *142*:480–483, 1981.
30. Cohn, K. H., Backdahl, M., et al.: Biologic considerations and operative strategy in papillary thyroid carcinoma: Arguments against the routine performance of total thyroidectomy. Surgery *96*:957–970, 1984.
31. Cohn, K. H., Backdahl, M., et al.: Prognostic value of nuclear DNA content in papillary thyroid carcinoma. World J. Surg. *8*:474–480, 1984.
32. Crile, G.: Changing end results in patients with papillary carcinoma of the thyroid. Surg. Gynecol. Obstet. *132*:460–468, 1971.
33. Crile, G., Antunez, A. R., et al.: The advantages of subtotal thyroidectomy and suppression of TSH in the primary treatment of papillary carcinoma of the thyroid. Cancer *55*:2691–2697, 1985.
34. Crile, G., and Hazard, J. B.: Relationship of the age of the patient to the natural history and prognosis of carcinoma of the thyroid. Ann. Surg. *138*:33–38, 1953.
35. Cuello, C., Correa, P., and Eisenberg, H.: Geographic pathology of thyroid carcinoma. Cancer *23*:230–238, 1969.
36. DeKeyser, L. F. M., and van Herle, A. J.: Differentiated thyroid cancer in children. Head & Neck Surgery *8*:100–114, 1985.
37. Delides, G. S., Elemenglou, J., et al.: Occult thyroid carcinoma in a Greek population. Neoplasma *34*:119–125, 1987.
38. Deligeorgi-Politi, H.: Nuclear crease as a cytodiagnostic feature of papillary thyroid carcinoma in fine-needle aspiration biopsies. Diagn. Cytopathol. *3*:307–310, 1987.
39. Dickersin, G. R., Vickery, A. L., and Smith, S. B.: Papillary carcinoma of the thyroid, oxyphil cell type, "clear cell" variant. Am. J. Surg. Pathol. *4*:501–509, 1980.
40. Dockhorn-Dworniczak, B., Franke, W. W., et al.: Patterns of expression of cytoskeletal proteins in human thyroid gland and thyroid carcinomas. Differentiation *35*:53–71, 1987.
41. Dralle, H., Schwarzrock, R., et al.: Comparison of histology and immunohistochemistry with thyroglobulin serum levels and radioiodine uptake in recurrences and metastases of differentiated thyroid carcinomas. Acta Endocrinol. *108*:504–510, 1985.
42. Dugan, J. M., Atkinson, B. F., et al.: Psammoma bodies in fine needle aspirate of the thyroid in lymphocytic thyroiditis. Acta Cytol. *31*:330–334, 1987.
43. Dzwonkowski, P., O'Leary, J., and Farid, N. R.: Thyroid papillary carcinoma in HLA identical sibs. Lancet *2*:971, 1988.
44. Evans, H. L.: Columnar cell carcinoma of the thyroid: A report of two cases of an aggressive variant of thyroid carcinoma. Am. J. Clin. Pathol. *85*:77–80, 1986.
45. Evans, H. L.: Encapsulated papillary neoplasms of the thyroid: A study of 14 cases followed for a minimum of 10 years. Am. J. Surg. Pathol. *11*:592–597, 1987.
46. Exelby, P. E., and Frazell, E. L.: Carcinoma of the thyroid in children. Surg. Clin. N. Amer. *49*:249–259, 1969.
47. Farbota, L. M., Calandra, D. B., et al.: Thyroid carcinoma in Graves' disease. Surgery *98*:1148–1152, 1985.
48. Favus, M. J., Schneider, A. B., et al.: Thyroid cancer occurring as a late consequence of head and neck irradiation. N. Engl. J. Med. *294*:1019–1022, 1976.
49. Feind, C. R.: The head and neck. *In:* Haagensen, C. D., Feind, C. R., Herter, F. P., Slanetz, C. A., and Weinberg, J. A. (eds.): The Lymphatics in Cancer. Philadelphia, W. B. Saunders Co., 1972, pp. 59–230.
50. Ferenczy, A., Talens, M., Zoghby, M., and Hussain, S. S.: Ultrastructural studies on the morphogenesis of psammoma bodies in ovarian serous neoplasia. Cancer *39*:2451–2459, 1977.
51. Fialkow, P. J.: The origin and development of human tumor studies with cell markers. N. Engl. J. Med. *291*:26–33, 1974.
52. Franssila, K. O.: Value of histologic classification of thyroid cancer. Acta Pathol. Micro. Scand. Suppl. *225*:5–76, 1971.

53. Franssila, K. O.: Is the differentiation between papillary and follicular thyroid carcinoma valid? Cancer *32*:853–858, 1973.
54. Franssila, K. O.: Prognosis in thyroid carcinoma. Cancer *36*:1138–1146, 1975.
55. Franssila, K. O., and Harach, H. R.: Occult papillary carcinoma of the thyroid in children and young adults: A systemic autopsy study in Finland. Cancer *58*:715–719, 1986.
56. Franssila, K. O., Harach, H. R., and Wasenius, V. M.: Mucoepidermoid carcinoma of the thyroid. Histopathology *8*:847–860, 1984.
57. Frazell, E., and Duffy, B. J.: Invasive papillary cancer of the thyroid. J. Clin. Endocrinol. Metab. *14*:1362–1366, 1954.
58. Fukunaga, F. H., and Yatani, R.: Geographic pathology of occult thyroid carcinomas. Cancer *36*:1095–1099, 1975.
59. Gikas, P. W., Labow, S. S., et al.: Occult metastasis from occult papillary carcinoma of the thyroid. Cancer *20*:2100–2104, 1967.
60. Gionsberg, J., Pedersen, J. D., et al.: Cervical cord compression due to extension of a papillary thyroid carcinoma. Am. J. Med. *82*:156–158, 1987.
61. Goudie, R. B.: Thyroiditis and thyroid carcinoma. Int. Coll. Tum. Thyr. Gland. Marseilles, 1964. New York, Karger, Basel, pp. 292–298, 1966.
62. Gould, V. E., Gould, N. S., and Benditt, E. P.: Ultrastructural aspects of papillary and sclerosing carcinomas of the thyroid. Cancer *29*:1613–1625, 1972.
63. Gouygou, C.: Morphologic aspects of papillary tumors of the thyroid gland. Int. Coll. Tum. Thyr. Gland. Marseilles, 1964. New York, Karger, Basel, pp. 1–16, 1966.
64. Graham, A.: Malignant epithelial tumors of the thyroid; with special reference to invasion of blood vessels. Surg. Gynecol. Obstet. *39*:781–790, 1924.
65. Hammer, M., Wortsman, J., and Folse, R.: Cancer in cystic lesions of the thyroid. Arch. Surg. *117*:1020–1023, 1982.
66. Hanford, J. M., Quimby, E. H., and Frantz, V. K.: Cancer arising many years after radiation therapy. J.A.M.A. *181*:404–410, 1962.
67. Hannequin, P., Liehn, J. C., and Delisle, M. J.: Multifactorial analysis of survival in thyroid cancer: Pitfalls of applying the results of published studies to another population. Cancer *58*:1749–1755, 1986.
68. Hapke, M. R., and Dehner, L. P.: The optically clear nucleus: A reliable sign of papillary carcinoma of the thyroid? Am. J. Surg. Pathol. *3*:31–38, 1979.
69. Harach, H. R., Escalante, D. A., et al.: Thyroid carcinoma and thyroiditis in an endemic goitre region before and after iodine prophylaxis. Acta Endocrinol. *108*:55–60, 1985.
70. Harach, H. R., Franssila, K. O., and Wasenius, V.: Occult papillary carcinoma of the thyroid: A "normal" finding in Finland. A systematic autopsy study. Cancer *56*:531–538, 1985.
71. Har-El, G., Sidi, J., et al.: Thyroid cancer in patients 70 years of age or older. Ann. Otol. Rhinol. Laryngol. *96*:403–410, 1987.
72. Hawk, W. A., and Hazard, J. B.: The many appearances of papillary carcinoma of the thyroid. Cleveland Clin. Quart. *43*:207–216, 1976.
73. Hawkins, M. M., and Kingston, J. E.: Malignant thyroid tumours following childhood cancer. Lancet *2*:804, 1988.
74. Hay, I. D.: Nodal metastases from papillary thyroid carcinoma. Lancet *2*:1283, 1986.
75. Hazard, J. B.: Small papillary carcinoma of the thyroid. Lab. Invest. *9*:86–97, 1960.
76. Henzen-Logmans, S. C., Mullink, H., et al.: Expression of cytokeratins and vimentin in epithelial cells of normal and pathological thyroid tissue. Virch. Arch. Pathol. Anat. *410*:347–354, 1987.
77. Hicks, D. G., LiVolsi, V. A., et al.: Solitary follicular nodules of the thyroid are clonal proliferations. Lab. Invest. *60*:40A, 1989 (abstract).
78. Hirabayashi, R. N., and Lindsay, S.: Carcinoma of the thyroid gland: a statistical study of 390 patients. J. Clin. Endocrinol. Metab. *21*:1596–1610, 1961.
79. Hofstadter, F.: Frequency and morphology of malignant tumours of the thyroid before and after the introduction of iodine prophylaxis. Virch. Arch. Pathol. Anat. *385*:263–270, 1980.
80. Hoie, J., Stenwig, A. E., Kullman, G., and Lindegaard, M.: Distant metastases in papillary thyroid cancer. A review of 91 patients. Cancer *61*:1–6, 1988.
81. Holm, L. E., Wiklund, K. E., et al.: Thyroid cancer after diagnostic doses of iodine-131: A retrospective cohort study. J. Natl. Cancer Inst. *80*:1132–1138, 1988.
82. Horn, R. C.: Problems in the pathologic diagnosis of carcinoma of the thyroid. Arch. Pathol. *69*:481–492, 1960.
83. Howard, R. B., and Truels, W. P.: Thyroid cancer: 30 year review of 201 cases. Am. J. Surg. *138*:934–938, 1979.
84. Hubert, J. P., Kiernan, P. D., et al.: Occult papillary carcinoma of the thyroid. Arch. Surg. *115*:394–398, 1980.
85. Hull, O. H.: Critical analysis of two hundred twenty-one thyroid glands. Arch. Pathol. *59*:291–311, 1955.
86. Hutter, R. V. P., Tollefson, H. R., et al.: Spindle and giant cell metaplasia in papillary carcinoma of the thyroid. Am. J. Surg. *110*:660–668, 1965.
87. Ibanez, M. L., Russell, W. O., et al.: Thyroid carcinoma—biologic behavior and mortality: postmortem findings in 42 cases including 27 in which the disease was fatal. Cancer *19*:1039–1052, 1966.

88. Iida, F., Yonekura, M., and Miyakawa, M.: Study of intraglandular dissemination of thyroid cancer. Cancer 24:764–771, 1969.

89. Ishihara, T., Kikuchi, K., et al.: Resection of thyroid carcinoma infiltrating the trachea. Thorax 333:378–386, 1978.

90. Izuo, M., Okagaki, T., et al.: Nuclear DNA content of occult sclerosing and frank carcinoma of the thyroid. Cancer 27:902–909, 1971.

91. Jancic-Zguricas, M., and Jankovic, R.: Occult papillary carcinoma of the thyroid gland revisited by cancer pericarditis. Pathol. Res. Pract. 181:761–764, 1986.

92. Joensuu, H., Klemi, P., et al.: Influence of cellular DNA content on survival in differentiated thyroid cancer. Cancer 58:2462–2467, 1986.

93. Johannessen, J. V., Gould, V. E., and Jao, W.: The fine structure of human thyroid cancer. Hum. Pathol. 9:385–400, 1978.

94. Johannessen, J. V., and Sobrinho-Simoes, M.: The origin and significance of thyroid psammoma bodies. Lab. Invest. 43:287–296, 1980.

95. Johannessen, J. V., and Sobrinho-Simoes, M.: Papillary carcinoma of the human thyroid gland. Prog. Surg. Pathol. 1:111–128, 1980.

96. Johannessen, J. V., Sobrinho-Simoes, M., et al.: Papillary carcinomas of the thyroid have pore-deficient nuclei. Int. J. Cancer 30:409–411, 1982.

97. Johannessen, J. V., Sobrinho-Simoes, M., et al.: Ultrastructural morphometry of thyroid neoplasms. Am. J. Clin. Pathol. 79:162–167, 1983.

98. Johannessen, J. V., Sobrinho-Simoes, M., et al.: Anomalous papillary carcinoma of the thyroid. Cancer 51:1462–1467, 1983.

99. Johannessen, J. V., Sobrinho-Simoes, M., et al.: A flow cytometric DNA analysis of papillary thyroid carcinoma. Lab. Invest. 45:336, 1981.

100. Johnson, T. L., Lloyd, R. V., et al.: Prognostic implications of the tall cell variant of papillary thyroid carcinoma. Am. J. Surg. Pathol. 12:22–27, 1988.

101. Kamma, H., Fujii, K., and Ogata, T.: Lymphocytic infiltration in juvenile thyroid carcinoma. Cancer 62:1988–1993, 1988.

102. Kaplan, M. M., Garnick, M. B., et al.: Risk factors for thyroid abnormalities after neck irradiation for childhood cancer. Am. J. Med. 74:272–280, 1983.

103. Kasai, N., and Sakamoto, A.: New subgrouping of small thyroid carcinoma. Cancer 60:1767–1770, 1987.

104. Key, C. R.: Carcinoma of the thyroid. Hum. Pathol. 2:521–523, 1971.

105. Kini, S. R.: Guides to Clinical Aspiration Biopsy: Thyroid. New York, Igaku-Shoin, 1987.

106. Klinck, G. H., and Winship, T.: Occult sclerosing carcinoma of the thyroid. Cancer 8:701–706, 1955.

107. Klinck, G. H., and Winship, T.: Psammoma bodies and thyroid cancer. Cancer 12:656–662, 1959.

108. Kodama, T., Fujimoto, Y., et al.: Justification of conservative surgical treatment of childhood thyroid cancer: report of eleven cases and analysis of Japanese literature. Jpn. J. Cancer Res. (Gann) 77:799–807, 1986.

109. Komorowski, R. A., and Hanson, G. A.: Occult thyroid pathology in the young adult: An autopsy study of 138 patients without clinical thyroid disease. Hum. Pathol. 19:689–696, 1988.

110. Lang, W., Borrusch, H., and Bauer, L.: Occult carcinomas of the thyroid: Evaluation of 1020 sequential autopsies. Am. J. Clin. Pathol. 90:72–76, 1988.

111. Lee, T. K., Myers, R. T., et al.: The significance of mitotic rate: A retrospective study of 127 thyroid carcinomas. Hum. Pathol. 16:1042–1046, 1985.

112. Liechty, R. D., Safaie-Shirazi, S., and Soper, R. T.: Carcinoma of the thyroid in children. Surg. Gynecol. Obstet. 134:632–635, 1972.

113. Lindahl, F.: Papillary thyroid carcinoma in Denmark, 1943–1968. Cancer 36:540–552, 1975.

114. Lindsay, S.: Papillary thyroid carcinoma revisited. In: Hedinger, C. E. (ed.): Thyroid Cancer. Heidelberg, Springer-Verlag, 1969, p. 29.

115. Lindsay, S.: Microspectrophotometric measurements of deoxyribonucleic acid in human thyroid carcinoma. Surg. Gynecol. Obstet. 130:905–908, 1970.

116. Lindsay, S.: Carcinoma of the Thyroid Gland. Springfield, C. C. Thomas Publ., 1960.

117. Linos, D. A., van Heerden, J. A., and Edis, A. J.: Primary hyperparathyroidism and nonmedullary thyroid cancer. Am. J. Surg. 143:301–303, 1982.

118. LiVolsi, V. A., and Feind, C. R.: Parathyroid adenoma and nonmedullary thyroid carcinoma. Cancer 38:1391–1393, 1976.

119. Lloyd, R. V., and Beierwaltes, W. H.: Occult sclerosing carcinoma of the thyroid: Potential for aggressive biologic behavior. South. Med. J. 76:437–439, 1983.

120. Maceri, D. H., Babyak, J., and Ossakow, S. J.: Lateral neck mass: sole presenting sign of metastatic thyroid cancer. Arch. Otolaryngol. Head Neck Surg. 112:47–49, 1986.

121. Mauras, N., Zimmerman, D., and Goellner, J. R.: Hashimoto thyroiditis associated with thyroid cancer in adolescent patients. J. Pediatr. 106:895–898, 1985.

122. Mazzaferri, E. L.: Papillary thyroid carcinoma: Factors influencing prognosis and current therapy. Sem. Oncol. 14:315–332, 1987.

123. Mazzaferri, E. L., and Young, R. L.: Papillary thyroid carcinoma. A 10 year followup report of the impact of therapy in 576 patients. Am. J. Med. 70:511–518, 1980.

124. Mazzaferri, E. L., Young, R. L., et al.: Papillary thyroid carcinoma: the impact of therapy in 576 patients. Medicine *56*:171–196, 1977.
125. McConahey, W. M., Hay, I. D., et al.: Papillary thyroid cancer treated at the Mayo Clinic, 1946 through 1970: initial manifestations, pathologic findings, therapy and outcome. Mayo Clin. Proc. *61*:978–996, 1986.
126. McDermott, M. V., Morgan, W., et al.: Cancer of the thyroid. J. Clin. Endocrinol. Metab. *14*:1336–1360, 1954.
127. Mc Kenzie, A. D.: The natural history of thyroid cancer: A report of 102 cases analyzed 10 to 15 years after diagnosis. Arch. Surg. *102*:274–277, 1971.
128. Meissner, W. A.: Surgical pathology. *In:* Surgery of the Thyroid Gland. Philadelphia, W. B. Saunders, Co., 1974, p. 24.
129. Meissner, W. A., and Adler, A.: Papillary carcinoma of the thyroid: a study of the pathology of two hundred twenty-six cases. Arch. Pathol. *66*:518–525, 1958.
130. Meissner, W. A., and Warren, S.: Tumors of the Thyroid Gland, Fascicle 4, Second series. Armed Forces Institute of Pathology, Washington, D.C., 1969.
131. Miettenin, M., Franssila, K. O., et al.: Expression of intermediate filament proteins in thyroid gland and thyroid tumors. Lab. Invest. *50*:262–270, 1984.
132. Mills, S. E., and Allen, M. S.: Congenital occult papillary carcinoma of the thyroid gland. Hum. Pathol. *17*:1179–1181, 1986.
133. Naruse, T., Koike, A., et al.: Minimal thyroid carcinoma: A report of nine cases discovered by cervical lymph node metastases. Jpn. J. Surg. *14*:118–121, 1984.
134. Nielsen, B., and Zetterlund, B.: Malignant thyroid tumors at autopsy in a Swedish goitrous population. Cancer *55*:1041–1043, 1985.
135. Nishiyama, R. H., Dunn, E. L., and Thompson, N. W.: Anaplastic spindle cell and giant cell tumors of the thyroid gland. Cancer *30*:113–127, 1972.
136. Noguchi, S., Noguchi, A., and Murakami, N.: Papillary carcinoma of the thyroid. I. Developing pattern of metastasis. Cancer *26*:1053–1060, 1970.
137. Noguchi, S., Noguchi, A., and Murakami, N.: Papillary carcinoma of the thyroid. II. Value of prophylactic lymph node dissection. Cancer *26*:1061–1064, 1970.
138. Noguchi, M., Tanaka, S., et al.: Clinicopathological studies of minimal thyroid and ordinary thyroid cancers. Jpn. J. Surg. *13*:110–117, 1984.
139. Olen, E., and Klinck, G. H.: Thyroid carcinoma occurring in Graves' disease. Arch. Intern. Med. *117*:432–435, 1966.
140. Olson, J. L., Penney, D. P., and Averill, K. A.: Fine structural studies of a human thyroid adenoma with special reference to psammoma bodies. Hum. Pathol. *8*:103–111, 1977.
141. Ott, R. A., McCall, A. R., et al.: The incidence of thyroid carcinoma in Hashimoto's thyroiditis. Am. Surg. *53*:442–445, 1987.
142. Patchefsky, A. S., and Hoch, W. S.: Psammoma bodies in diffuse toxic goiter. Am. J. Clin. Pathol. *57*:551–556, 1972.
143. Patchefsky, A. S., Keller, I. B., and Mansfield, C. M.: Solitary vertebral column metastasis from occult sclerosing carcinoma of the thyroid gland. Am. J. Clin. Pathol. *53*:596–601, 1970.
144. Perkel, V. S., Gail, M. H., et al.: Radiation-induced thyroid neoplasms: Evidence for familial susceptibility factors. J. Clin. Endocrinol. Metab. *66*:1316–1322, 1988.
145. Permanetter, W., Nathrath, W. B. J., and Lohrs, U.: Immunohistochemical analysis of thyroglobulin and keratin in benign and malignant thyroid tumours. Virch. Arch. Pathol. Anat. *398*:221–228, 1982.
146. Petro, A. B., and Hardy, J. D.: The association of parathyroid adenoma and nonmedullary cancer of the thyroid. Ann. Surg. *181*:118–124, 1975.
147. Polliack, A., and Freund, U.: Mixed papillary and follicular carcinoma of the thyroid gland with stromal amyloid. Am. J. Clin. Pathol. *53*:592–595, 1970.
148. Pontius, K. I., and Hawk, W. A.: Loss of microsomal antigen in follicular and papillary carcinoma of the thyroid: An immunofluorescence and electron-microscopic study. Am. J. Clin. Pathol. *74*:620–629, 1980.
149. Prinz, R. A., Barbato, A. L., et al.: Prior irradiation and the development of coexistent differentiated thyroid cancer and hyperparathyroidism. Cancer *439*:874–877, 1982.
150. Reed, R. J., Russin, D. J., and Krementz, E. T.: Latent metastases from occult sclerosing carcinoma of the thyroid. J. A. M. A. *196*:233–237, 1966.
151. Reteloff, S., Harrison, J., and Karanfilski, B. T.: Continuing occurrence of thyroid carcinoma after irradiation to the neck in infancy and childhood. N. Engl. J. Med. *292*:171–175, 1975.
152. Ritzl, F., Siebers, G., et al.: Thyroid carcinoma: a followup study of 11 years. Radiat. Environ. Biophys. *26*:283–288, 1987.
153. Ron, E., Kleinerman, R. A., et al.: A population based case control study of thyroid cancer. J. Natl. Cancer Inst. *79*:1–12, 1987.
154. Rosai, J., Zampi, G., and Carcangiu, M.: Papillary carcinoma of the thyroid. Am. J. Surg. Pathol. *7*:809, 1983.
155. Rosen, I. B., Bowden, J., et al.: Aggressive thyroid cancer in low risk age population. Surgery *102*:1075–1080, 1987.
156. Ruegemer, J. J., Hay, I. D., et al.: Distant metastases in differentiated thyroid carcinoma: A multivariate analysis of prognostic variables. J. Clin. Endocrinol. Metab. *67*:501–508, 1988.

157. Ruiz-Velasco, R., Waisman, J., and van Herle, A.: Cystic papillary carcinoma of the thyroid gland. Acta Cytol. 22:38–42, 1978.
158. Russell, M. A., Gilbert, E. F., and Jaeschke, W. F.: Prognostic features of thyroid cancer: a longterm followup of 68 cases. Cancer 36:553–559, 1975.
159. Russell, W. O., Ibanez, M., et al.: Thyroid carcinoma. Classification, intraglandular dissemination and clinicopathological study based upon whole organ sections of 80 thyroid glands. Cancer 16:1425, 1963.
160. Samaan, N. A., Maheshwari, Y. K., et al.: Impact of therapy for differentiated carcinoma of the thyroid: an analysis of 706 cases. J. Clin. Endocrinol. Metab. 56:1131–1138, 1983.
161. Samaan, N. A., Schultz, P. N., et al.: A comparison of thyroid carcinoma in those who have and have not had head and neck irradiation in childhood. J. Clin. Endocrinol. Metab. 64:219–223, 1987.
162. Sampson, R. J., Oka, H., et al.: Metastases from occult thyroid carcinoma: an autopsy study from Hiroshima and Nagasaki, Japan. Cancer 25:803–811, 1970.
163. Sampson, R. J., Key, C. R., et al.: Thyroid carcinoma in Hiroshima and Nagasaki: I: Prevalence of thyroid carcinoma at autopsy. J. A. M. A. 209:65–70, 1969.
164. Sampson, R. J., Key, C. R., et al.: Smallest forms of papillary carcinoma of the thyroid. Arch. Pathol. 91:334–339, 1971.
165. Sampson, R. J., Key, C. R., et al.: Papillary carcinoma of the thyroid gland. Sizes of 525 tumors found at autopsy in Hiroshima and Nagasaki. Cancer 25:1391–1398, 1970.
166. Sampson, R. J., Woolner, L. B., et al.: Occult thyroid carcinoma in Olmsted County, Minnesota: Prevalence at autopsy compared with that in Hiroshima and Nagasaki, Japan. Cancer 34:2072–2076, 1974.
167. Satran, L., Sklar, C., et al.: Thyroid neoplasm after high dose radiotherapy. Am. J. Pediatr. Hematol. Oncol. 5:307–309, 1983.
168. Saxen, E., Franssila, K., et al.: Observer variation in histologic classification of thyroid cancer. Acta Pathol. Microbiol. Scand. Sect. A 86:483–486, 1978.
169. Schlumberger, M., DeVathaire, F., et al.: Differentiated thyroid carcinoma in childhood: Long term followup of 72 patients. J. Clin. Endocrinol. Metab. 65:1088–1094, 1987.
170. Schlumberger, M., Tubiana, M., et al.: Long term results of treatment of 283 patients with lung and bone metastases from differentiated thyroid carcinoma. J. Clin. Endocrinol. Metab. 63:980–987, 1986.
171. Schroder, D. M., Chambers, A., and France, C. J.: Operative strategy for thyroid cancer: is total thyroidectomy worth the price? Cancer 58:2320–2328, 1986.
172. Schroder, S., Bocker, W., et al.: The encapsulated papillary carcinoma of the thyroid. A morphologic subtype of the papillary thyroid carcinoma. Cancer 54:90–93, 1984.
173. Schroder, S., Pfannschmidt, N., et al.: Histopathologic types and clinical behaviour of occult papillary carcinoma of the thyroid. Pathol. Res. Pract. 179:81–87, 1984.
174. Schroder, S., Schwarz, W., et al.: Dendritic/Langerhans cells and prognosis in patients with papillary thyroid carcinomas. Immunocytochemical study of 106 thyroid neoplasms correlated to followup data. Am. J. Clin. Pathol. 89:295–300, 1988.
175. Segal, K., Sidi, J., et al.: Thyroid carcinoma in children and adolescents. Ann. Otol. Rhinol. Laryngol. 94:346–349, 1985.
176. Shapiro, S. J., Friedman, N. B., et al.: Incidence of thyroid carcinoma in Graves' disease. Cancer 26:1261–1270, 1970.
177. Shurbaji, M. S., Gupta, P. K., and Frost, J. K.: Nuclear grooves: a useful criterion in the cytopathologic diagnosis of papillary thyroid carcinoma. Diagn. Cytopathol. 4:91–94, 1988.
178. Siegal, A., and Modan, M.: Latent carcinoma of thyroid in Israel: A study of 260 autopsies. Isr. J. Med. Sci. 17:249–253, 1981.
179. Silverberg, E., and Lubera, J.: Cancer statistics. CA 36:9–25, 1986.
180. Silverberg, S. G., and Vidone, R. A.: Adenoma and carcinoma of the thyroid. Cancer 19:1053–1062, 1966.
181. Simpson, W. J., McKinney, S. E., et al.: Papillary and follicular thyroid cancer: Prognostic factors in 1578 patients. Am. J. Med. 83:479–488, 1987.
182. Simpson, W. J., Panzarella, T., et al.: Papillary and follicular thyroid cancer: impact of treatment in 1578 patients. Int. J. Radiat. Oncol. Biol. Phys. 14:1063–1075, 1988.
183. Sobel, R. J., Liel, Y., and Goldstein, J.: Papillary carcinoma and the solitary autonomously functioning nodule of the thyroid. Isr. J. Med. Sci. 21:878–882, 1985.
184. Sobrinho-Simoes, M. A., and Goncalves, V.: Nuclear bodies in papillary carcinomas of the human thyroid gland. Arch. Pathol. 98:94–99, 1974.
185. Sobrinho-Simoes, M., Nesland, J. M., and Johannessen, J. V.: Columnar cell carcinoma: another variant of poorly differentiated carcinoma of the thyroid. Am. J. Clin. Pathol. 89:264, 1988.
186. Soderstrom, N., and Biorklund, A.: Intranuclear cytoplasmic inclusions in some types of thyroid cancer. Acta Cytol. 17:191–197, 1973.
187. Sridama, V., Hara, Y., et al.: Association of differentiated thyroid carcinoma with HLA-DR7. Cancer 56:1086–1088, 1985.
188. Strate, S. M., Lee, E. L., and Childers, J. H.: Occult papillary carcinoma of the thyroid with distant metastases. Cancer 54:1093–1100, 1984.
189. Tallroth, E., Backdahl, M., et al.: Thyroid carcinoma in children and adolescents. Cancer 58:2329–2332, 1986.

190. Tang, T. T., Holcenberg, J. S., et al.: Thyroid carcinoma following treatment for acute lymphoblastic leukemia. Cancer 46:1572–1576, 1980.
191. Tasca, C., and Stefaneanu, L.: Ultrastructural pathology of the thyroid folliculopapillary and follicular carcinoma. Morphol. Embryol. (Bucur) 27:239–244, 1981.
192. Tennvall, J., Biorklund, A., et al.: Is the EORTC prognostic index of thyroid cancer valid in differentiated thyroid carcinoma? Cancer 57:1405–1414, 1986.
193. Tollefsen, H. R., DeCosse, J. J., and Hutter, R. V. P.: Papillary carcinoma of the thyroid: A clinical and pathological study of 70 fatal cases. Cancer 17:1035–1044, 1964.
194. Tollefsen, H. R., Shah, J. P., and Huvos, A. G.: Papillary carcinoma of the thyroid: Recurrence in the thyroid gland after initial surgical treatment. Am. J. Surg. 124:468–472, 1972.
195. Torres, J., Volpato, R. D., et al.: Thyroid cancer: survival in 148 cases followed for 10 years or more. Cancer 56:2298–2304, 1985.
196. Tscholl-Ducommun, J., and Hedinger, C.: Papillary thyroid carcinoma. Morphology and prognosis. Virch. Arch. Anat. Pathol. 396:19–39, 1982.
197. Tsumori, T., Nakao, K., et al.: Clinicopathologic study of thyroid carcinoma infiltrating the trachea. Cancer 56:2843–2848, 1985.
198. Tubiana, M., Schlumberger, M., et al.: Long term results and prognostic factors in patients with differentiated thyroid carcinoma. Cancer 55:794–804, 1985.
199. Vane, D., King, D. R., and Boles, E. T.: Secondary thyroid neoplasms in pediatric cancer patients: increased risk with improved survival. J. Pediatr. Surg. 19:855–860, 1984.
200. Variakojis, D., Getz, M. L., et al.: Papillary clear cell carcinoma of the thyroid. Hum. Pathol. 6:384–390, 1975.
201. Vestfrid, M. A.: Papillary carcinoma of the thyroid gland with lipomatous stroma: report of a peculiar histological type of thyroid tumour. Histopathology 10:91–100, 1986.
202. Vickery, A. L.: Thyroid papillary carcinoma. Pathological and philosophical controversies. Am. J. Surg. Pathol. 7:797–807, 1983.
203. Vickery, A. L., Carcangiu, M., et al.: Papillary carcinoma. Sem. Diagn. Pathol. 2:90–100, 1985.
204. Vickery, A. L., Wang, C. A., and Walker, A. M.: Treatment of intrathyroidal papillary carcinoma of the thyroid. Cancer 60:2587–2595, 1987.
205. Volpe, R.: The immunoregulatory disturbance in autoimmune thyroid disease. Autoimmunity 2:55–72, 1988.
206. Wahner, H. W., Cuello, C., et al.: Incidence of thyroid carcinoma in an endemic goiter area, Cali, Columbia. Am. J. Med. 40:58–72, 1966.
207. Wick, M. R., Mills, S. E., et al.: Follicular variant of papillary thyroid carcinoma: an immunohistochemical comparison with other thyroid tumors. Lab. Invest. 60:105A, 1989 (abstract).
208. Williams, E. D., Doniach, I., et al.: Thyroid cancer in an iodide rich area. Cancer 39:215–222, 1977.
209. Wilson, N. W., Pambakian, H., et al.: Epithelial markers in thyroid carcinoma. An immunoperoxidase study. Histopathology 10:815–829, 1986.
210. Wilson, S. M., Platz, C., and Block, G. M.: Thyroid carcinoma after irradiation. Arch. Surg. 100:330–334, 1970.
211. Woolner, L. B.: Thyroid carcinoma: pathologic classification with data on prognosis. Sem. Nucl. Med. 1:481–502, 1971.
212. Woolner, L. B., Beahrs, O. H., et al.: Classification and prognosis of thyroid carcinoma: a study of 885 cases observed in a thirty year period. Am. J. Surg. 102:354–387, 1961.
213. Yamashita, H., Nakayama, I., et al.: Thyroid carcinoma in benign thyroid diseases: An analysis from minute carcinoma. Acta Pathol. Jpn. 35:781–788, 1985.
214. Yamashita, H., Nakayama, I., et al.: Minute carcinoma of the thyroid and its development to advanced carcinoma. Acta Pathol. Jpn. 35:377–383, 1985.
215. Yamashita, H., Noguchi, S., et al.: Prognosis of minute carcinoma of the thyroid: Followup study of 49 patients. Acta Pathol. Jpn. 36:1469–1475, 1986.
216. Yaremchuk, K., and Goldman, M. E.: Transformation of papillary carcinoma. Ear, Nose and Throat J. 64:54–56, 1985.
217. Yasuda, G., Shionoiri, H., et al.: Bilateral pheochromocytoma associated with papillary adenocarcinoma of the thyroid gland: Report of an unusual case. Endocrinol. Jpn. 32:399–404, 1985.
218. Young, J. L., Percy, C. L., and Asire, A. J. (eds.): Surveillance epidemiology and end results: incidence and mortality data, 1973–1977. Natl. Cancer Inst. Monogr. 57:1–1082, 1981.
219. Young, S., and Inman, D. R.: Thyroid Neoplasia. London, Academic Press, 1968, p. 111.
220. Zimmerman, L. M., Shubik, P., et al.: Experimental production of thyroid tumors by alternating hyperplasia and involution. J. Clin. Endocrinol. Metab. 14:1367–1377, 1954.

9

FOLLICULAR LESIONS OF THE THYROID

This chapter will describe the various thyroid nodular lesions that are characterized by a totally or predominantly follicular pattern. The basic functional unit of the thyroid is the follicle. Although the majority of thyroid lesions (physiologic hyperplasias, benign nodular lesions, and neoplasms) display a macro- or micro-follicular pattern, some of these are totally or partly composed of trabeculae and/ or solid nests. These patterns recapitulate those seen in the development of the gland and are referred to as embryonal or fetal adenomas or adenomatous nodules. The importance of these various histologic appearances lies in their recognition as a family or spectrum of follicular lesions; criteria for their distinction into subgroups of nonneoplastic and neoplastic, benign and malignant nodules are similar. These will be discussed as a group in this chapter.

Most lesions of the thyroid are follicular. These range from changes in the follicles seen diffusely, as in hyperthyroidism associated with Graves' disease, to those lesions that present as multiple or single nodules.

The differential diagnosis of follicular lesions of the thyroid, therefore, includes those listed in Table 9–1.

HYPERPLASTIC GOITER

The thyroid lesions in this histologic category include those found in patients with congenital disorders of thyroid metabolism (inborn errors of thyroid metabolism; dyshormonogenetic goiter) and those in the thyroid in diffuse toxic goiter (autoimmune hyperthyroidism—Graves' disease; Basedow's disease). In some of these conditions, hypothyroidism is found; in others, hyperfunction; and in still others, euthyroidism is present.

When the thyroid cannot produce normal amounts of thyroid hormone to meet the body's needs, there is an *appropriate* physiologic response of the pituitary which secretes increased amounts of thyrotropin (TSH); TSH "drives" the thyroid follicular cells (apparent follicular cell receptor–TSH linkage remains intact in these situations) to produce more thyroid hormones, thyroxine and triiodothyronine (T_4 and T_3).[152, 216, 220] (Both hormones may be produced; occasionally T_3 predominates.[18]) The cells therefore undergo hyperplasia and hypertrophy. The thyroid gland enlarges; in some cases, nodules form.

Causes of this type of hyperplasia include congenital disorders of thyroid metabolism (dyshormonogenetic goiter), TSH-producing pituitary adenomas, trophoblastic disease, inadequate dietary iodine, and goitrogenic drugs.

Table 9–1. Follicular Lesions of the Thyroid

Hyperplastic goiter—associated with
dyshormonogenesis
Graves' disease
trophoblastic disease
pituitary disease
Nodular goiter—toxic, nontoxic
Adenomatous (adenomatoid) nodule
True follicular adenoma
Atypical adenoma
Follicular carcinoma
Follicular variant of papillary carcinoma
Follicular (glandular) variant of medullary carcinoma
Insular carcinoma
Mixed follicular and parafollicular carcinoma

In autoimmune hyperthyroidism (diffuse toxic goiter or Graves' disease), hyperplasia and hypertrophy result from TSH-mimicking immunoglobulins (thyrotropin receptor antibodies), which attach to the receptor on the follicular cell membrane and trigger the intracellular sequence of events that enables increased thyroid hormone production. Schroder et al. found decreased numbers of TSH binding sites in Graves' tissue.[232]

Inborn Errors of Thyroid Metabolism—Genetic Disorders

The interrelationships among the developing hypothalamus, pituitary, and thyroid glands are delicate and balanced in the normal state.[152] Defects in a variety of areas can interfere with these balances: antithyroid antibodies that pass through the placenta from mother to fetus;[8, 43, 87, 136] environmental and nutritional deficiencies; and genetic errors in thyroid metabolism. Each of these can be manifested as congenital hypothyroidism.[73]

Inborn errors of thyroid metabolism consist of a spectrum of biochemical abnormalities, which are inherited, and which can affect any step in the pathway of thyroid hormone synthesis, secretion, or action. Lever et al. discussed this topic in a scholarly review published in 1983.[158] The following discussion borrows heavily from their paper.

The pathways involved in thyroid metabolism constitute reactions controlled by specific proteins; mutations in the genes controlling these proteins result in the various syndromes of dyshormonogenesis.[158] The majority of these syndromes are inherited with a recessive pattern, although a few (including generalized resistance to thyroid hormone) appear to be inherited as autosomal dominant defects.

Differences in the clinical symptoms and presentations depend upon whether the defect is complete or incomplete, whether the change is qualitative or quantitative, which enzyme or protein is involved and the degree of compensation of the individual. If the defect is severe and poorly compensated, neonatal hypothyroidism with growth and mental retardation (cretinism) occurs.[10, 11, 73, 158, 310] In some families, the initial symptoms may present in adult life with goiter and minimal thyroid dysfunction.[158]

The following major defects have been described; some of these have subgroupings involving one or a few families, with clinical and laboratory distinctions that separate them from the main category. The main areas of dyshormonogenesis, then, include blocks or quantitative defects in the major steps in thyroid hormone synthesis and action (Table 9–2).

TSH Unresponsiveness. Lever et al. culled only three cases of this condition in their review.[158] Leger et al. added two more.[156] Each was a male, who had hypothyroidism and mental retardation, but none had goiter. Consanguinity was documented in two cases.[158, 253, 254]

Iodide Transport Defect. The transport of iodide ion into thyroid cells requires energy since the iodide enters against an electrochemical gradient. Iodide becomes concentrated within the thyroid follicular cells. Two forms of this defect have been described: complete and partial.[86, 177, 194, 224] In Lever's review, only 14 cases were accepted.[158, 272] Additional patients were accepted by Wolff,[297] bringing the total number of patients with this abnormality to 22. In each patient, large goiter and hypothyroidism were present. Only those patients with the partial form of this defect were mentally retarded; Lever et al. postulated that the latter could be caused by severe dietary iodine deficiency.[158] The patients were diagnosed at ages that varied from 15 months to 50 years. Family history of goiter was often noted; consanguinity was documented in some cases.

Organification Defect. The organification of iodide involves the oxidation of iodine and its covalent binding to tyrosyl residues on thyroglobulin. This process depends on several factors, an abnormality of one of which could result in the defect: intact activity of the membrane bound enzyme TPO; generation of an oxidizing agent, hydrogen peroxide; availability of iodide ion; and correct spatial relationships among these components.

Five subgroups of organification defect have been described.[158, 194, 210, 212, 274] These include quantitative defects in TPO enzyme (10 cases), qualitative defect in TPO (12 cases), deficiency of hydrogen peroxide generation (1 case), abnormal iodine receptor on thyroglobulin (4 cases), and Pendred's syndrome.

In addition to these which have been studied in detail and in which the biochemical abnormality is well documented, additional cases are recorded in which the exact defect is less well understood. Lever et al. accepted a total of 41 cases of organification defect.[158] These patients displayed variable clinical manifestations, ranging from hypo- to euthyroidism, presence or absence of physical and/or mental retardation, and variable sized goiters. Patients with partial defects fared better clinically.

Pendred's syndrome is defined as congenital sensorineural deafness and partial organification defect. The exact biochemical defect remains uncertain, and indeed this syndrome may include a number of heterogeneous subgroups.[38, 80] Most patients are euthyroid; the cause of the associated deafness is unknown. Several hundred cases of this syndrome have been reported;[158] two patients have apparently developed thyroid carcinoma.[60]

Rarely, defects in iodine organification can apparently be acquired: Horton et al. noted this in patients after therapy for hyperthyroidism with antithyroid medication.[114]

Table 9–2. Inherited Disorders of Thyroid Metabolism

Unresponsiveness to thyrotropin
Iodide transport defect
Organification defect (including Pendred's syndrome)
Coupling defect
Thyroglobulin defect
Deiodinase deficiency
Thyroid transport protein defect (abnormalities of thyroid binding globulins)
Resistance to thyroid hormone (pituitary, generalized)
Other
    Multinodular goiter
    Intrathyroidal calcification
    Iodide leak

Coupling Defect. Monoiodotyrosine and diiodotyrosine on thyroglobulin couple to form the hormones triiodotyrosine and thyroxine (T_3 and T_4). The reaction requires oxidation of the iodotyrosines, covalent binding, and fission of the completed product. Fifteen cases of this coupling defect have been reported; family history indicated thyroid disease and goiter in seven of these. All patients had goitrous hypothyroidism; a few were mentally retarded.

Abnormalities of Thyroglobulin Synthesis and Secretion. These may be quantitative or qualitative; there may be abnormal thyroglobulin transport or glycosylation.[31, 121, 156, 161] Thirty-nine cases of this general type of defect were accepted by Lever et al.[158] Three additional cases have been added.[31] Of these, 34 were hypothyroid; two were also deaf. A positive family history was documented in half the cases.

Deiodinase Defect. The recirculation of intrathyroidal iodine following release of monoiodotyrosine and diiodotyrosine from thyroglobulin requires deiodinase. About 80 percent of iodine is reused in this way; that is, the thyroid jealously conserves iodine. Seventeen cases of this defect were identified in the review of Lever et al.[158] They described three subgroups: isolated thyroid deiodinase deficiency, total body deiodinase deficiency, and a deiodinase defect involving diiodotyrosine but not monoiodotyrosine. Euthyroid goiter was noted in the patients with the isolated thyroid enzyme deficiency, whereas those with total body deficiency were also mentally retarded.

Abnormalities of Thyroid Hormone Transport. These usually involve absence or deficiency of thyroxine binding globulin, excess of this substance, or its abnormal chemical makeup.[158, 181, 196, 217, 218, 226, 227, 310] The mode of genetic transmission is X-linked dominant. Most affected patients are euthyroid, and without goiter. The patients are usually discovered to have the defect on routine thyroid function testing.

Other Defects. Patients with multinodular nontoxic goiter do not have a biochemically defined defect in hormonogenesis, but many do have a positive family history of goiter. In addition patients with dyshormonogenesis may have relatives with euthyroid multinodular goiters. So there may be families with subtle as yet undefined abnormalities of thyroid hormone synthesis or secretion. Whether environmental (dietary?) factors also play a role in some of these families remains to be determined.[10]

A curious group of patients with goiter but without identifiable dyshormonogenesis has been described. These four patients with positive family histories of goiter were all euthyroid but, on plain X-ray of the neck, a diffuse intraglandular calcification was noted. The defect, if any exists, remains undefined.[10, 158]

One family has been described in which dyshormonogenetic goiter was associated with iodide leak. These patients had an abnormal recirculation of intrathyroidal iodine, leading to relative iodine deficiency, goiter, and hypothyroidism. In two of these patients follicular carcinoma with metastases developed.[44]

Pathology

The morphology of the thyroid in patients with dyshormonogenesis who have goiter is strikingly similar despite the different biochemical abnormalities.[11, 140, 141, 187, 244]

The glands are usually enlarged. Virtually all glands show nodules grossly; some of the nodules show gross encapsulation, others do not. Secondary changes including hemorrhage, fibrosis, and, rarely, calcification can be found, especially in older patients.

Microscopically, the changes are also similar and consist of extreme follicular hyperplasia, with the internodular thyroid showing compression; lymphocytic infiltration is absent. The nodules can vary in appearance; most show microfollicular or trabecular patterns. The cells may be large but otherwise resemble follicular epithelium; clear cell change may be seen. Cytologic atypia is very common and may be so severe as to suggest a malignancy. However, true invasive growth is extremely rare, and documented clinically malignant behavior even more unusual.[44, 60, 284]

Endemic goiter regions of the world include those areas in which dietary iodine is deficient. It has been believed that the nutritional deficiency itself was sufficient to explain the goiters that occurred. However, differences among individuals in both goiter size and thyroid function, despite similar diets, have called this theory into question. It is possible that certain underlying dyshormonogenetic defects are present in certain families and population groups most affected in endemic goiter areas, partially explaining the different clinical manifestations noted.[46, 47, 72, 90, 92, 93, 95, 109, 116, 118, 119, 162, 219, 283]

HYPERTHYROIDISM

There are numerous causes of hyperthyroidism and these are listed in Table 9–3. In some of these the pathology of the gland is not characterized. The discussion below will emphasize those disorders in which the pathology is well documented.

Autoimmune Hyperthyroidism; Diffuse Toxic Goiter; Graves' Disease

This common cause of hyperthyroidism, which occurs predominantly in women (ratio about 9:1), is believed to be related to autoimmunity, as discussed in Chapter 5.[2, 3, 12, 13, 28, 51, 64–66, 74, 133, 145, 153, 168, 169, 197, 198, 201, 213, 229, 241–243, 249, 255, 258, 269, 281, 285, 286, 307] The autoimmunity theory is supported by (a) genetic predisposition to the disease (finding Graves' disease in several family members, or identifying in affected patients and their relatives an unusually high incidence of other "autoimmune disorders"—pernicious anemia, Addison's disease, rheumatoid arthritis, and chronic lymphocytic thyroiditis[26, 67, 159]); (b) an association with HLA-DR3;[66, 201, 241,

Table 9–3. Causes of Hyperthyroidism

Diffuse toxic goiter (Graves' disease)
Toxic nodular goiter
Solitary toxic nodule (adenoma or carcinoma)
Subacute thyroiditis
Painless thyroiditis (postpartum; other)
TSH-producing pituitary adenoma
Hypothalamic hyperthyroidism
Gestational trophoblastic disease
Struma ovarii
Iodine-induced hyperthyroidism
Rapidly growing thyroid tumors (primary or metastatic)
Exogenous thyroid hormone intake (factitious)
Ectopic production of TSH or TRH
Peripheral, pituitary, or generalized resistance to thyroid hormone

[255, 258] (c) finding circulating antibodies in the serum of affected individuals;[145, 213, 234, 235, 242, 276, 281, 285] and (d) infiltration of the thyroid by lymphocytes.[251] (For historical accuracy and modern diplomacy, the other name attached to this disorder is Basedow's disease.[159])

Similarities to Hashimoto's thyroiditis include an apparently genetically determined defect in suppressor T cells with consequent proliferation of thyroid directed B cells that produce antithyroid autoantibodies. These antibodies (thyroid receptor immunoglobulins), which are directed against the thyrotropin receptor complex of the follicular epithelial cell, apparently are stimulatory both to growth of the gland and to function. (Originally discovered about 30 years ago, the antibodies involved were called *long acting thyroid stimulators*—LATS.[24, 25, 175, 234, 303]) It is now known that these are a family of related immunoglobulins acting on the thyroid cell TSH receptor;[36, 52, 81, 243] they are collectively known as thyrotropin receptor antibodies (TRAbs). Hence the gland enlarges and secretes increased amounts of thyroid hormones, resulting in the clinical syndrome of hyperthyroidism.

What triggers the process of autoantibody production? Studies of the follicular epithelium in Graves' disease have shed some light on the issue.[292] Wick and Sawyer[292] identified expression of HLA-DR antigen on the epithelial cell surfaces.[101, 143] These authors expanded the work of Sobrinho-Simoes and Damjanov,[247] studying lectin binding to the normal and diseased thyroid epithelium. They found lectins bound to immunologically damaged follicular epithelium (i.e., follicles of Graves' disease thyroids) but not to normal control glands.

In addition, Wick and Sawyer identified differences in keratin and vimentin immunostaining patterns between immune-damaged tissue and normal tissue;[292] the former stained for both intermediate filaments, whereas normal follicular epithelium contained only vimentin. Buley et al.[23] and Henzen-Logmans et al.,[108] using different species of antibodies for immunostaining, did not confirm this result, however.

Hence, there are definite surface differences in follicular epithelium of Graves' glands. It is possible that the process begins with an inflammatory insult (?viral, ?Yersinia infection),[238, 291] which may lead to a T-cell response and production of gamma interferon. The latter substance induces the epithelial cells to ectopically express HLA-DR type II molecules on their surfaces.[94, 123, 124, 143, 173] These molecules, normally found only on immunocompetent cells, would allow T-helper cells to recognize the follicular epithelium as antigens with which to react.[188] These helper T cells then function as they should[168] and elaborate lymphokines, which attract B cells and induce these to differentiate into plasma cells and produce immunoglobulins—in this case thyrotropin receptor antibodies.

Pathology

The pathology of the thyroid in Graves' disease includes hyperplasia and hypertrophy. Grossly, the gland is diffusely and usually symmetrically enlarged, with weights of 50 to 150 grams (Figs. 9–1 and 9–2). The capsule is smooth; prominent vascular markings are noted.[298, 299, 308] Cut section discloses a deep red parenchyma.

Histologic examination shows retention of lobular architecture, prominent vascular congestion, and follicular hyperplasia. The follicular cells are columnar with pale cytoplasm and enlarged nuclei; some of the latter may show central clearing (Fig. 9–3). Colloid is virtually absent, so that in the untreated case recognition of the tissue as thyroid may be difficult. When colloid is present it is hardly ever in every follicular lumen; scalloping of the colloid where it abuts against the epithelium is seen. The latter is caused by fixation artifact since

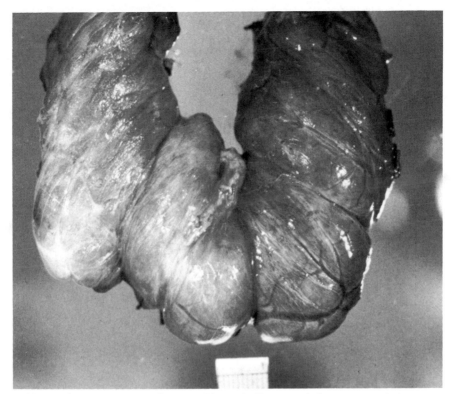

Figure 9–1. Diffuse toxic goiter (Graves' disease). This surgically resected 175 gram gland shows an intact capsule, lobular accentuation without nodularity, and very prominent vascular pattern.

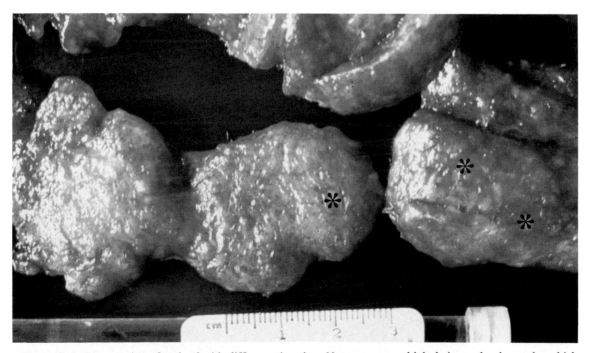

Figure 9–2. Cross section of a gland with diffuse toxic goiter. Note accentuated lobulation and pale specks, which microscopically represented lymphoid follicles (some denoted by asterisks).

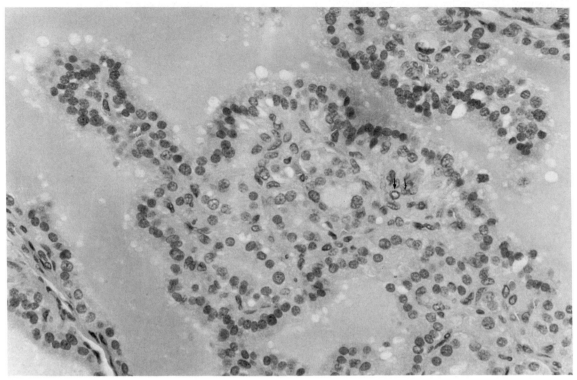

Figure 9–3. Diffuse toxic goiter. Individual cells are columnar; occasional nuclei show slight clearing (*arrow*), but this is rarely a widespread finding. × 150.

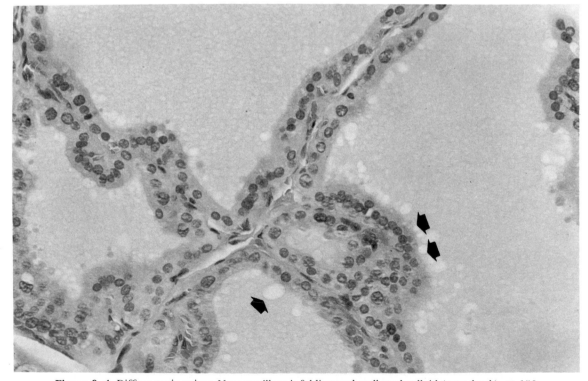

Figure 9–4. Diffuse toxic goiter. Note papillary infolding and scalloped colloid (*arrowheads*). × 150.

decreased amounts of colloid in the individual follicles cause greater shrinkage than in the normal gland. Papillary infoldings of the follicular epithelium are also seen in the untreated case (Fig. 9–4).[251] These are probably produced by the hypertrophied cells, which are present in increased numbers, and the basic "scaffolding" of the follicle cannot accommodate the cells; hence short nonbranching papillae form. These papillae and the occasional clear nucleus may suggest a diagnosis of papillary carcinoma. However, in Graves' disease the process is a diffuse one, sclerosis is rare, and the papillae are rarely complex and branching as they are in cancer. Rarely, psammoma bodies may be seen in Graves' thyroids without associated cancer.[202] (Although some studies have indicated a higher than expected incidence of thyroid cancer in Graves' disease[237]—as high as 9 percent—not all authors agree.)

Electron microscopic examination of the Graves' gland has shown the features of hyperplastic cells with increased cytoplasm, and increased endoplasmic reticulum and mitochondria.[263] Immune complexes have also been found on the basement membrane.[133]

In the perifollicular stroma, lymphocytes, often arranged in follicular or germinal centers, are seen. Kabel et al. have demonstrated increased numbers of antigen-presenting dendritic cells in Graves' disease tissue.[131] These cells were often seen in intimate contact with lymphocytes in the thyroid. A number of studies have defined the types of lymphocytes infiltrating the gland in autoimmune diseases.[120, 124, 168, 169] Within the follicular centers, B cells predominate; T lymphocytes are seen in a perifollicular location. Some studies have shown differences in the ratio of B/T cells in the thyroid as compared to peripheral blood in patients with Graves' disease.[169, 188, 198, 266] The numbers of helper subtype T lymphocytes are increased in Graves' thyroid tissue; this differs from Hashimoto's disease since in the latter the T cells infiltrating the gland are predominantly suppressor subtype.[198, 266]

Changes in the morphologic picture accompany treatment. If medical therapy is directed at the peripheral manifestations of thyroid hormone excess (beta blocker drugs, such as propanolol),[91, 154, 257] there is no effect on the thyroid pathology. If therapy involves interference with thyroid hormone synthesis (thiouracil drugs, etc.), the pathology of the gland is basically unchanged or more hyperplastic than in the untreated state. However, iodine therapy, usually in the form of potassium iodide, given for a short period, reduces the vascularity of the gland and causes involution; the follicular epithelium reverts toward cuboidal form and colloid storage is repleted.[40] Focally, small papillary projections persist; there may be considerable variability in response to treatment from area to area within the gland so that focally areas of marked hyperplasia may persist.[251, 305]

The morphologic changes that are seen after radioiodine treatment for Graves' disease are often dramatic. Although initially there may be little change, as time progresses continuing destruction of the gland and fibrosis occur. The thyroid follicles atrophy and random marked cytologic atypia of follicular epithelium is seen. (See Chapter 6.)

The extrathyroidal pathology in Graves' disease involves predominantly the eyes and the skin.[70, 195, 288] In the retroorbital tissues edema, fibrosis, lymphocytic infiltration, and the presence of mucopolysaccharides produce swelling leading to the exophthalmos so characteristic of the disease. In a small number of affected individuals, dermopathy (pretibial myxedema) occurs, especially on the legs. There is thickening of the skin owing to deposition of mucopolysaccharides.[195]

Nodular Thyroid Disease and Hyperthyroidism. The presence of clinical hyperthyroidism in patients with nodular glands, distinct from Graves' disease, has been described by both Plummer[293] and Goetsch.[98] The gland may be multinodular, or only a solitary clinical mass may be present. This type of hyperfunctioning gland is seen more often in endemic goiter areas of the world. Recent evidence has suggested that some patients with this disorder may share with Graves' disease an autoimmune etiology.[21, 50, 56, 148, 174, 178, 229, 246, 280] Other patients, probably the majority, harbor solitary or multiple nodules that autonomously hyperfunction; the nonnodular gland tends to be suppressed.[27, 98, 148, 157, 192, 209, 250]

Toxic Nodular Goiter. In this condition, the clinical symptom complex of hyperthyroidism is associated with a nodular gland.[130] This cause of hyperthyroidism is more commonly seen in older individuals.

The histology is similar to that of diffuse toxic goiter, with the changes occurring within nodules rather than throughout the gland. Secondary degenerative changes, including fibrosis and calcification, are more often seen in these glands than in diffuse goiter.

Toxic Nodule (Adenoma, Carcinoma). Rarely, a solitary nodule will function autonomously and produce clinical hyperfunction.[174, 192, 264, 267, 277] Most of these are benign nodules; only rare examples of documented follicular carcinomas producing hyperthyroidism are known.[39, 79, 96, 99, 245, 271] The histologic appearance of such hyperfunctioning nodules is similar to that of the nonfunctional ones described below; sometimes evidence of papillary hyperplasia may be found in these nodules. However, the success rate for predicting functional status of nodules from the histologic appearance is fair at best.[35] Hamburger noted that some hyperfunctioning adenomas may undergo spontaneous degeneration and hence spontaneous cure of the patient's thyrotoxicosis may result.[98]

Some patients with metastatic follicular carcinoma will develop hyperthyroidism, presumably due to activity of large amounts of functioning well-differentiated neoplastic thyroid tissue in the metastatic sites.[39, 172, 176, 271, 275]

Subacute Thyroiditis. As discussed in Chapter 4, during the course of subacute thyroiditis a phase of hyperthyroidism occurs. As the destructive process disrupts follicles, stored hormone is rapidly released into the circulation, producing chemical and sometimes clinical hyperthyroidism. In this condition, however, radioiodine uptake is depressed as the thyroid follicles are destroyed and not functional; this is one of the few causes of hyperthyroidism in which iodine uptake is low.

Central Hyperthyroidism. Pituitary and, more rarely, hypothalamic causes of hyperthyroidism have been documented in some patients.[15, 17, 37, 41, 61, 82, 84, 99, 100, 113, 134, 147, 211, 270]

Thyrotropin (TSH) producing pituitary adenomas can cause hyperthyroidism since excessive levels of circulating thyrotropin drive the thyroid follicular epithelium to produce increased levels of thyroid hormone. In a significant number of cases of thyrotropin secreting pituitary adenomas, prolactin or growth hormone is also produced, causing a multihormone–excess symptom complex.[37, 99, 113] Similarly, a lesion in the hypothalamus could cause excess levels of thyrotropin releasing hormone (TRH) in the portal circulation and stimulate the pituitary thyrotrophs to hypersecrete TSH.[211] TRH hypersecretion might be caused by excess production in the hypothalamus or inadequate regulation or inhibition of secretion; hence any lesion—neoplastic, granulomatous, or inflammatory—might cause such deregulation.

The thyroid in these cases would be enlarged, but is often only slightly bigger than normal. Histologically, the appearance mimics the hyperplasia seen in autoimmune hyperthyroidism, except that lymphocytic infiltration is absent or minimal.

Gestational Trophoblastic Disease. Human chorionic gonadotropin (HCG) shares certain biochemical similarities with TSH. The hormones are each composed of two subunits—alpha and beta; the latter confers biochemical identity to the specific hormone.[142, 184, 199, 203] Both HCG and TSH contain biochemically identical alpha subunits. Hence, in trophoblastic neoplasms in which large amounts of HCG are present, one side effect of this excess circulating hormone is that it mimics the effect of excess TSH.[7, 42, 111, 142, 184, 189, 199, 214, 282] Thus the thyroid responds as it would to TSH and undergoes hyperplasia; hyperthyroidism results. (Some studies have failed to show that HCG is the actual agent stimulating the thyroid; these reports postulate another substance produced by trophoblastic tissue which in fact is responsible for thyroid hyperplasia.[6]) Interestingly, therapy directed toward the trophoblastic neoplasm corrects the thyroid dysfunction. Both hydatidiform mole and choriocarcinoma have been associated with hyperthyroidism; the thyroid effects appear directly related to tumor burden and concentration of circulating HCG or, conversely, another TSH-like tumor product. In general, the larger the tumor mass, the more HCG, and the more likely hyperthyroidism will occur.

Iodine-induced Hyperthyroidism. In some normal and more often in abnormal thyroids, ingestion of excess iodine will produce hyperthyroidism.[75, 121, 155, 191, 228] It appears that iodine may induce vacuolization, necrosis, and desquamation of follicular epithelial cells with apparent release of hormone. Amiodarone therapy (amiodarone being an iodine-containing drug) has been associated with this phenomenon.[170] The mechanism for this hyperfunction is unknown: possible suggested causes are that iodine influences an underlying subclinical thyroiditis (autoimmune) or affects a relatively iodine-deficient gland by overloading it with iodine.

Painless Thyroiditis. This condition, originally classified among the subacute thyroiditis group, probably represents a type of autoimmune thyroid disease related to chronic lymphocytic thyroiditis. It is often seen in postpartum women and may regress and recur. This disorder is discussed in Chapter 5.

Struma Ovarii. The presence of thyroid tissue within ovarian teratomas has been estimated to occur in 5 to 20 percent of cases. Usually the thyroid appears normal or resembles nodular goiter with degenerative changes. Rarely, the ovarian thyroid will function and produce clinical hyperthyroidism.[138] (See Chapter 16.)

Rapidly Growing Tumors in the Thyroid. By a mechanism similar to that of subacute thyroiditis, hyperthyroidism may occur in patients who harbor rapidly growing malignancies in the thyroid. The tumors described that have been associated with this phenomenon include malignant lymphoma, anaplastic carcinoma of the thyroid, and metastatic tumors to the gland. As the tumor destroys preexisting normal thyroid, stored hormone is rapidly released into the circulation and hyperfunction occurs.

Exogenous Thyroid Hormone Intake. The ingestion of excess amounts of thyroid hormone will obviously cause clinical hyperthyroidism (factitious hyperthyroidism). The pathology in these patients is in their psyche and not in their thyroid gland.[309]

A recent intriguing detective story of a miniepidemic of hyperthyroidism traced to thyroid tissue admixed with commercially sold hamburger meat represents an extreme example of an exogenous cause for hyperthyroidism.[107]

Ectopic Production of TSH and TRH. Although theoretically possible as a cause of hyperthyroidism, documented cases of TSH or TRH production by nonpituitary neoplasms are not known. Some examples of cases suggesting this mechanism for hyperthyroidism are reported and include anaplastic carcinoma of the lung and hepatocellular carcinoma.

Resistance to Thyroid Hormone. This condition is found in three subtypes: pituitary resistance, generalized resistance, and both pituitary and generalized resistance to thyroid hormone.[55, 146] These individuals may present with chemical evidence of hyperthyroidism although their tissues are apparently functioning in a euthyroid state.

The usually familial syndromes of thyroid hormone resistance include three subgroups: generalized resistance; selective pituitary resistance; and peripheral but not pituitary resistance.[45, 122, 144, 217, 223, 302] (Among the patients with generalized resistance to thyroid hormone are included cases of Refetoff's syndrome; these individuals also have deafness and abnormal facial appearance.[158, 217, 236])

Patients with peripheral and/or generalized resistance to thyroid hormone have small goiters,[59, 85, 144, 304] and are really euthyroid or even hypothyroid but have elevated circulating thyroid hormone levels and inappropriately elevated thyrotropin (TSH) since their tissues do not respond to normal levels of circulating hormone.[182] In usual forms of hyperthyroidism, TSH levels are low to unmeasurable.

Patients in the subgroup with apparently isolated pituitary resistance to thyroid hormone show signs and symptoms of hyperthyroidism but inappropriately elevated thyrotropin.[100] These patients must be distinguished from individuals with thyrotropin secreting pituitary adenomas (see below). Radiologic examination of the sella turcica is essential.

In nonneoplastic TSH hypersecretion syndromes, therapy (surgery, radioiodine and thiouracil drugs) for diffuse toxic goiter is usually ineffective.[146] Recurrence of hyperthyroidism after surgery or radioablation is common because of continued TSH stimulation of the residual thyroid tissue. In addition, another theoretical fear is that constant hypersecretion of TSH by pituitary thyrotrophs may induce a pituitary neoplasm.[68, 146]

FOLLICULAR THYROID NODULES (NODULAR GOITER, ADENOMATOUS NODULES, AND TRUE FOLLICULAR ADENOMA)

Nodular Goiter

This very common condition can be defined in a variety of ways in order to get a handle on its frequency. If one limits the incidence of nodular goiter to those cases in which a patient presents with a clinically evident lump, then the incidence is somewhere around 2 to 4 percent of the population in developed countries.[278] (The incidence of goiter is much higher, of course, in endemic goiter [iodine-poor] regions of the world.) If one considers a diagnosis of nodular goiter from the gross pathology standpoint, about 10 percent of thyroids removed at autopsy will contain nodules, usually multiple. If one includes all cases of microscopically evident nodules also, then the incidence of nodular goiter is about 40 to 50 percent.[5, 14, 54, 115, 190, 278]

Multinodular goiter has been associated with hyperfunction[148] but is usually associated with a euthyroid state. In the clinically evident goiter, there may be one dominant nodule that draws attention to the thyroid, although pathologically many nodules of varying size may coexist.

Most nodules of the thyroid are benign; however, numerous studies have been performed to determine how best to discover malignancy in thyroid nodules—clinical parameters, radiologic tests, and most recently cytologic sampling have been used.[29, 30, 54, 88, 160, 183]

Pathology

Grossly nodular goiters range from slightly to massively enlarged glands (weights of 50 to over 800 grams can be found) with intact capsules and a bumpy external surface. Sectioning will show multiple nodules of varying consistency separated by variable amounts of normal-appearing thyroid (in huge goiters, no normal areas may be seen). The nodules are composed chiefly of brown thyroid tissue (Figs. 9–5 and 9–6). Variable amounts of fibrous tissue, often in bands, calcification, and even ossification will be noted. Areas of hemorrhage (recent or remote) and small or large cysts can also be found.

Microscopically, these features are recapitulated (Fig. 9–7). One finds colloid lakes alternating with normal- to hyperplastic-appearing foci of thyroid, hemorrhage,[248] siderosis, fibrosis, calcification, and bone. Sometimes fat is also present. In some longstanding goiters, especially in areas of dense scar, squamous metaplasia of follicular epithelium may be seen. Variable amounts of lymphocytic infiltrate will also be found; in some cases this may reflect an immunologic abnormality.[21, 178, 279] The appearance of the nodular thyroid is similar whether it

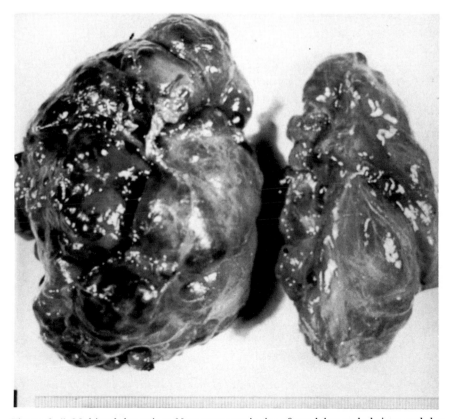

Figure 9–5. Multinodular goiter. Note asymmetric size of two lobes and obvious nodules.

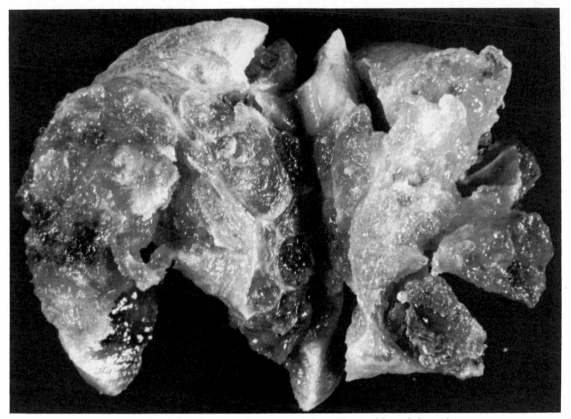

Figure 9–6. Colloid is abundant and appears shiny in this nodular goiter.

occurs in patients in nonendemic or endemic goiter regions; however, in the latter more numerous foci of hyperplasia are seen.[46, 287]

The pathogenesis of the initial events in the formation of nodules in the thyroid has elicited much interest; numerous studies utilizing a variety of techniques have been reported.[83, 205–208, 215, 265] Studer and his colleagues have worked on goitrous thyroid tissue from endemic goiter regions of Europe, and they indicate that their results may not be directly applicable to sporadic nodular goiter in other nonendemic goiter regions.[205–208, 215, 259–262] Investigators working in nonendemic goiter regions have postulated autoimmune mechanisms for the origin of nodules;[93, 148] others have found little evidence to support this hypothesis.[1] In the opinion of the present author, the underlying question that must be answered is: If all thyroid follicular epithelial cells are equal, why do some proliferate at the expense of their neighbors and produce nodules?

Are all follicular cells equal? Probably not; although biochemical, immunologic, and histochemical studies seem to indicate that they are. What then invokes inequality? The answer is unknown at present. The work of Studer suggests that certain follicular cells or groups thereof are *intrinsically* more rapidly growing than their neighbors. The initial proliferation is a polyclonal one involving one follicle or more likely a group of follicles. These proliferate, while adjacent follicles remain quiescent. Interfollicular stroma and the vessels contained therein participate in the process and vascular compression leads to focal ischemia, necrosis, and inflammatory and reparative changes. At later times, the same process may affect another group of follicles until large zones of the thyroid are affected. As the process continues the secondary phenomena so characteristic of longstanding nodular goiter take place: follicular destruction, hemorrhage, fibrosis, hemosiderosis, calcification, and even ossification. The associated follicular distortion by fibrous tissue may lead to diagnostic interpretative problems and be misinterpreted as invasion by follicular structures—hence a misdiagnosis of follicular carcinoma may be rendered.

While these changes occur, the hormonal stimuli to the gland continue. However, with distortion of vascular supply as well as the presence of dilated follicles filled with colloid (colloid lakes, as it were), the distribution of iodide and thyrotropin becomes uneven. Hence some portion of the gland will "see" excess thyrotropin and focal hyperplasia may occur; other areas will have relative iodide and/or thyrotropin deficiency, leading to zones of atrophy or inactivity. It seems that once the process begins, it is self-perpetuating. The question still of interest and still unanswered is: Why does it begin?

What can be said about solitary follicular nodules that histologically at least appear identical to the multiple nodules seen in nodular goiter? Are these then regenerative, proliferative nodules, but not neoplasms; or, alternatively, do these represent true benign follicular adenomas? Until recently this question could not be answered by the techniques available; hence many pathologists decided to use the term "adenomatous or adenomatoid follicular nodule" for such lesions, skirting the issue of histogenesis. From the clinical point of view, since these behave in a benign manner, it seemed an acceptable term to use.

Does it, however, have biological meaning if the solitary lesions are indeed neoplasms, i.e., adenomas? If they are true neoplasms, will they have a greater

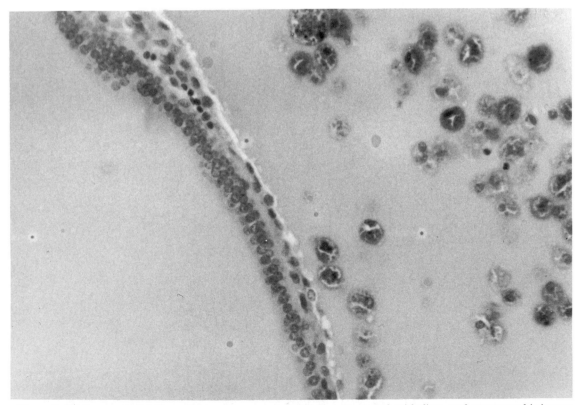

Figure 9–7. Microscopic field in nodular goiter—note colloid lakes, attenuated epithelium, and numerous histiocytes laden with hemosiderin (right). × 150.

tendency to transform into malignant tumors than nonneoplastic follicular proliferations? If so, should all clinically solitary follicular nodules be removed surgically? Obviously all of these questions cannot be easily answered. However, it
has been shown that at least some solitary follicular nodules are clonal and thus
neoplastic,[110, 193] whereas the nodules of multinodular glands are polyclonal and
hence not true neoplasms.

The methodology employed to answer the clonality question involves an understanding of the Lyon hypothesis.[166, 167, 268] This hypothesis assumes that in embryologic life in the female one of the two X chromosomes is inactivated. In some
cells, one X chromosome is activated; in other cells, the other is activated; this is
randomly distributed among all the cells of the body. If one could find a marker
(usually a gene for an enzyme or its product) that has different alleles on each of
the two X chromosomes, and one could distinguish between the two X chromosomes by Southern blot analysis, it would be possible to determine if a specific cell
or group of cells were the progeny of one cell (with a specific activated X) or of
several cells (random in their X activation). By Southern blot analysis, then, if a
lesion were clonal, all the cells in that lesion would carry the same activated X
which the gene for the marker enzyme can identify, and one band would result.
If one compares that single band to normal tissue or blood from the test patient
(which should contain two bands when reacted with the gene for the marker
enzyme, since the tissue present would contain randomly distributed numbers of
activated and inactivated X chromosomes), two bands would be seen. The differences between the test tissue and the normal (one band versus two) indicates
monoclonality in the test material.

Hicks et al.[110] and Namba and Fagin[193] utilized this technique, which had
previously been tested to prove the clonal origin of colonic adenomas[69] and
parathyroid adenomas[9, 171] to prove the clonal origin of solitary thyroid follicular
nodules. Incidentally, papillary and follicular carcinomas were also clonal, as
would be expected. (Namba and Fagin reported a case of nonclonal papillary
carcinoma, however; although these authors added the disclaimer that contami-
nation of their tumor sample with surrounding normal thyroid tissue may have
occurred.[193])

From the biologic and/or clinical standpoint, the behavior of these lesions is
benign. However, they have been removed entirely usually by unilateral thyroid
lobectomy. The biologic potential of these neoplasms if left undisturbed cannot
be known. In addition, since only women (and only 25 percent at most of women)
can have their nodules tested by this technique, it is unclear that one can
extrapolate the results obtained by Hicks et al.[110] to all solitary follicular thyroid
nodules. Hence it is premature to answer the question of whether surgical removal
of all clinically solitary follicular nodules seems appropriate.

Follicular Adenoma*

A follicular adenoma or solitary adenomatous or adenomatoid nodule is defined
as a benign encapsulated mass of follicles, usually showing a uniform pattern
throughout the confined nodule.[5, 179] Occasionally such a nodule will be associated
with clinical hyperthyroidism—so-called toxic adenoma.[27, 29, 35, 96–99, 160, 185, 200, 209, 221,
264, 267, 277, 280, 293] Virtually all solitary follicular nodules will contain thyroglobulin,

---

*Having established that at least some solitary follicular nodules are clonal and therefore neoplasms,
the clinically persistent term "follicular adenoma" may again be used for benign thyroid nodules.[71, 110]

T_3 and T_4 by immunostaining;[4, 19, 204] some will contain low molecular weight cytokeratin but not high molecular weight forms;[296] ultrastructural features will resemble those of normal thyroid although some nodules will have features suggesting significantly greater secretory activity than that of the normal gland.[19, 126, 137, 165, 186]

Adenomas are solitary (Figs. 9–8 to 9–10); indeed, if there are multiple nodules in a lobe or a thyroid gland, it is probably more appropriate to diagnose multinodular goiter with adenomatous change (adenomatous hyperplasia) and call attention to the discrete nodules in that way. The features that Meissner[179] used to distinguish histologically between adenoma and adenomatous nodules included: solitary versus multiple nodules; encapsulation versus merely circumscription; uniformity of pattern within the adenoma and divergence from surrounding thyroid; and compression of the surrounding gland by the adenoma and its capsule.

A variety of terms have been bestowed upon the patterns that may be seen in follicular adenomas: macrofollicular, simple, microfollicular, fetal, embryonal, and trabecular. Although these patterns can be recognized, they have no clinical significance and thus to subclassify thyroid adenomas is not recommended.

Follicular adenomas contain rare mitoses; the exception to this rule is in lesions that have recently been aspirated, since in areas of needle track, hemorrhage and reparative tissue changes may be associated with mitotic activity. The presence of mitoses in the absence of a history of attempted aspiration is a disturbing finding in a follicular adenoma; such lesions should be carefully evaluated for evidence of invasion, i.e., malignancy.

Other relatively common changes that may be found in adenomas include hemorrhage, edema, and fibrosis, especially in the central portions of the tumor

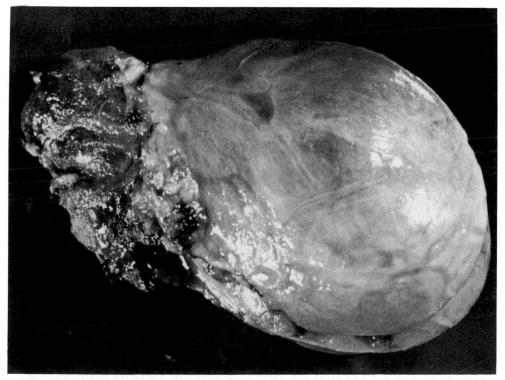

Figure 9–8. A solitary encapsulated nodule is shown.

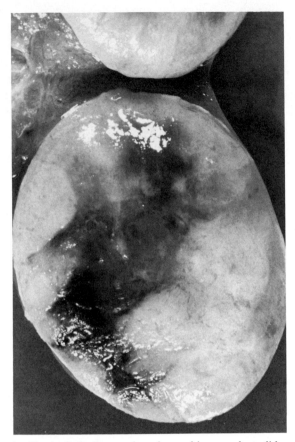

Figure 9–9. Same case as in Figure 9–8. Cut section shows thin capsule; solid center with track-like area of hemorrhage. Large bore needle biopsy had been performed preoperatively and diagnosis of follicular neoplasm was made. Final diagnosis in this case: follicular adenoma.

(Figs. 9–11 and 9–12). The extent of degenerative change can often be correlated with the length of time the lesion was present; older lesions may also contain areas of calcification and ossification. Some of these tumors may undergo spontaneous central cystic degeneration as well. Rarely, such lesions will contain dilated blood vessels engorged with blood (usually found in center of the lesions); this feature may be so pronounced as to suggest a vascular neoplasm.

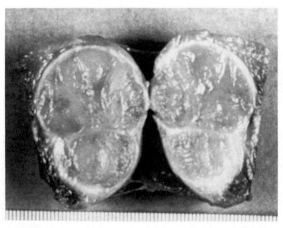

Figure 9–10. Well-demarcated follicular neoplasm; note relatively thick capsule. This lesion showed no invasion.

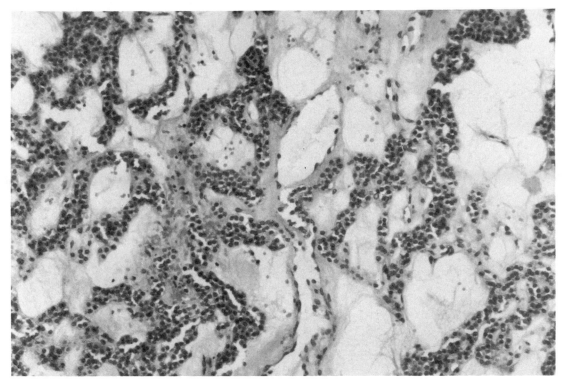

Figure 9–11. Central portion of follicular adenoma. Interspersed between small trabeculae of tumor cells is edematous and fibrous stroma. × 150.

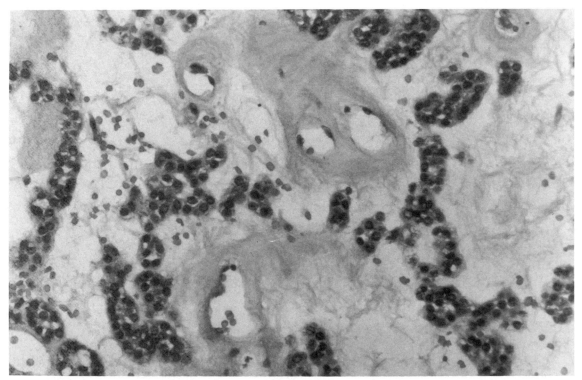

Figure 9–12. Higher power of Figure 9–11. × 300.

Some solitary adenomas, often those with cystic change, will contain areas of papillary growth pattern; these papillary areas tend to be oriented toward the center of the lesion, show edematous "cores" and follicles within the cores, and never contain clear nuclei, desmoplastic foci, or psammoma bodies. The term "papillary adenoma" may be suggested for such lesions, but the present author believes that term is too confusing to be meaningful. In an unpublished study involving a histopathologic review of 36 cases coded as "papillary adenoma" by the Connecticut Tumor Registry, 24 cases were classified as adenoma or goiter with areas of papillary hyperplasia; 10 represented papillary carcinoma; and the remainder were other benign lesions (Falcier and LiVolsi: unpublished observations). The term "follicular nodule" or "adenoma with papillary hyperplasia" is preferred.[16]

Whether some solitary follicular nodules have the biologic potential to become carcinoma or not cannot be known; the finding of aneuploid cell populations in 27 percent of such lesions suggests that some of these may represent carcinoma in situ.[125] However, since aneuploidy in endocrine lesions at various sites is quite common and the lesions behave in a biologically benign fashion, I think it is best not to overreact to such findings without much more data. The solitary follicular lesion which is removed by lobectomy, and which when adequately studied shows no evidence of invasion, will neither recur nor metastasize. (Enucleation of follicular adenomas should be mentioned here only to be condemned as a surgical procedure. The pathologic evaluation of these lesions requires analysis of the tumor-capsule-thyroid interface [Fig. 9–13]); if this interface is not present, an appropriate diagnosis cannot be rendered.)

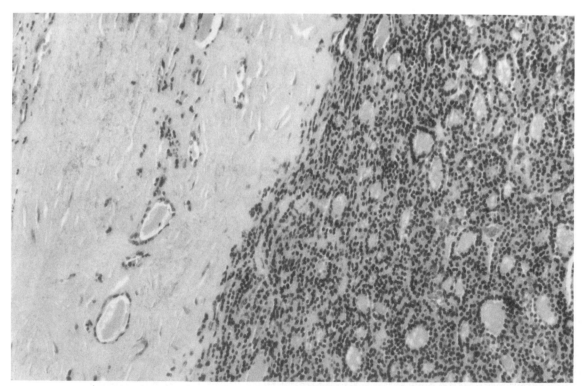

Figure 9–13. Follicular nodule with thin capsule; no invasion seen. A microfollicular tumor with thick capsule. The finding of follicles in the capsule without an edematous cellular "reactive stroma" is considered trapping and is not diagnostic of invasion. × 100.

Variants of follicular adenoma include Hürthle cell adenomas (discussed in Chapter 12), hyalinizing trabecular adenoma or paraganglioma-like adenoma (discussed in Chapter 15), signet ring cell adenoma and adenolipoma (discussed in Chapter 15), and adenoma with bizarre cells (considered analogous to the changes seen in parathyroid adenomas, i.e., a degenerative alteration). The follicular adenoma with bizarre cells shows random, often marked, cytologically atypical cells with huge hyperchromatic nuclei; sometimes multinucleated cells may be seen (Figs. 9–14 and 9–15).

Atypical Follicular Adenoma

This term proposed by Hazard[105] includes those follicular tumors that for one or more reasons are pathologically disturbing, *but that do not show invasive characteristics.* (See Fig. 9–13.) The features of these tumors that cause concern include the presence of spontaneous necrosis, infarction, numerous mitoses, or unusual cellularity (excluding bizarre cells noted above). Despite these findings, extensive evaluation of the capsule and edges of the tumor fails to disclose invasion. The overwhelming majority of the atypical adenomas (which truly fit in this category after adequate pathologic evaluation) behave in a benign fashion clinically.[78, 105, 132, 150, 151]

Follicular Carcinoma of the Thyroid

Follicular carcinoma represents about 5 percent of thyroid cancer in regions where sufficient iodide is present in the diet.[49, 294, 295] In endemic (iodide-deficient)

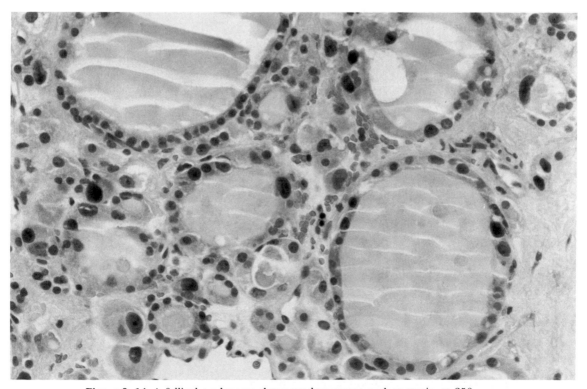

Figure 9–14. A follicular adenoma shows random severe nuclear atypia. × 250.

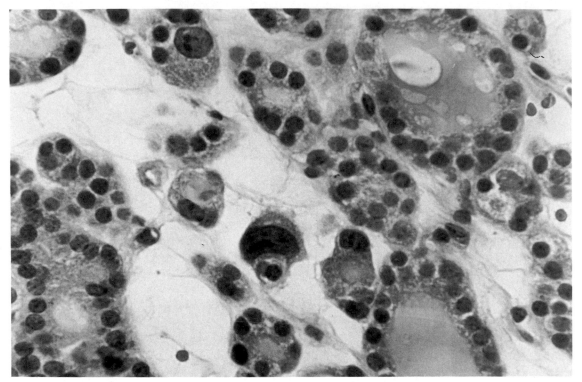

Figure 9–15. Similar nuclear atypia in adenomatous nodule in nontoxic nodular goiter. × 400.

areas, however, follicular carcinoma seems more prevalent, making up 25 to 40 percent of thyroid cancers.[49, 294, 295] When iodide is added to the diet, the change in incidence of cancer type is toward an increase in papillary cancer and corresponding decrease in follicular tumors.[102, 112, 294] (Interestingly, anaplastic cancer incidence decreases as well.) Of interest is that this follows closely the experience with induced thyroid tumors in animals—iodide-deprived animals with appropriately depressed thyroid hormone levels and elevated thyrotropin levels tend to develop follicular cancers.[240, 252, 294]

Other causative factors for follicular cancer are not easily identified. Does the presence of nodular goiter predispose to cancer? Do benign adenomas become cancer? Does external radiation play a role in the development of follicular cancer? The answers to these questions are not readily available: the first two cannot be answered since one cannot know whether the nodule was malignant from the outset and had an indolent biology. As for the role of radiation, most studies are flawed by the inclusion of follicular variants of papillary cancer as follicular carcinomas;[53, 57, 76] from the few data available it appears the radiation does not influence the development of follicular tumors.

Clinically, follicular carcinoma is usually a *solitary mass* in the thyroid, with the great majority of such tumors presenting as clinical "lumps." Although reported occasionally,[20] occult follicular carcinoma is very rare (in contradistinction to papillary cancer).*

The follicular carcinoma has a marked propensity for vascular invasion (not lymphatics). This phenomenon is not easily explained. Presumably derived from

---

*It must be pointed out that occult follicular cancer indicates a tumor not clinically evident or palpable—and does not refer to the unusual but not rare event of a patient presenting with metastatic follicular cancer in whom a thyroid mass is readily identified.

epithelium similar if not identical to that which gives rise to papillary carcinoma, the follicular tumor does not invade lymphatic channels. It is unknown if follicular cancers produce certain factors that alter the venous endothelium, allowing the tumor easy access; the study of Harach et al. that examined Factor VIII–related antigen staining in vessels invaded by follicular cancer[104] suggested such a possibility, since staining of endothelial cells in invaded vessels was often absent. In any event, follicular carcinoma *avoids* lymphatics—hence it is unifocal in the gland, and true embolic lymph node metastases are exceedingly rare.

Follicular carcinoma disseminates hematogenously and characteristically metastasizes to bone, lungs, brain, and liver.[62, 172, 222, 273] Depending upon the degree of differentiation of the tumor, these metastatic foci may take up radioiodine. (This can be used to scan patients for discovery of the metastases as well as to treat them.[79, 306])

The treatment of follicular carcinoma remains controversial. Follicular cancer metastases will usually be treatable by radioiodine if there is no normal thyroid tissue present in the neck.[79] For this reason, many surgeons consider total thyroidectomy appropriate therapy for encapsulated follicular cancers. Since it is very difficult if not impossible to render a definitive cancer diagnosis on a fine needle aspiration sample or frozen section of such a tumor, delayed completion thyroidectomy may be necessary.

Alternatively, since the disease-free interval after lobectomy and/or cure of these encapsulated lesions is so great, completion thyroidectomy may represent "overkill" in a large percentage of these patients.[22, 230, 231] Some endocrinologists and surgeons prefer radioablation of the residual thyroid, either when the definite diagnosis of cancer is made or if and when metastases first appear.[78, 245]

Total thyroidectomy appears warranted in those individuals who present with metastatic disease and in whom the primary is still present in the neck.

Certainly lymph node dissection is not warranted since these tumors do not spread to nodes; abnormal-appearing or enlarged nodes should, of course, be sampled.

Therapy for widely invasive follicular cancer that has spread beyond the gland is removal of as much tumor as possible (debulking) with total thyroidectomy and subsequent radioiodine treatment.

Patients who have follicular carcinoma that is widely invasive fare poorly.[77, 78, 149, 231] However, those individuals with encapsulated follicular tumors confined to the thyroid enjoy a prolonged survival (greater than 80 percent at 10 years).[78, 149, 231] However, if metastases are present at initial diagnosis—and some patients are referred for a complaint related to a metastasis (i.e., pathologic fracture)[62, 78, 132, 135, 149, 231]—or if the patient is elderly, the prognosis is less favorable.[62, 78, 149, 231]

Several studies have addressed those factors (clinical and pathologic) that are associated with a worse outcome.[32–34, 48, 77, 78, 106, 132, 149, 151, 222, 225, 230, 271, 300, 301] These include:

- old age at diagnosis
- male sex
- extrathyroidal growth at time of diagnosis
- degree of vascular invasion (many veins involved)
- solid or trabecular pattern of tumor (low histologic degree of "follicularity")
- aneuploid cell population (see Chapter 18)

Some follicular carcinomas may become less differentiated in recurrences or metastases; usually staining for thyroglobulin will be retained.[58] Harach and Franssila noted that immunostaining for thyroglobulin correlated with the degree of differentiation of the tumor. The less differentiated lesions showed little positive staining.[103] Franssila et al.[78] point out that in some cases, metastases, especially in bone, more closely resemble normal thyroid than does the primary tumor.*

An apparently rare but extremely significant complication that may occur in patients with follicular cancer is transformation into anaplastic cancer with its attendant dismal prognosis;[239] the incidence of this occurrence is not known but is considered quite unusual. As discussed in Chapter 11, this may occur *de novo* in an untreated follicular lesion, or even in metastatic sites. It is not clear whether therapy with radioiodine influences the development of transformation in treated low-grade lesions. (See Chapter 11.)

Pathology

For the pathologist, two main types of follicular carcinoma are recognized: so-called minimally invasive and widely invasive.

The widely invasive follicular carcinoma is a tumor that is clinically and surgically recognized as a cancer; the role of the pathologist in its diagnosis is to confirm that it is of thyroid origin and that it fits into a follicular neoplasm category. Such lesions grossly extend into cervical veins, or through the thyroid capsule. They often can only be subtotally resected. Such tumors often are fairly cellular, usually microfollicular and/or focally solid. (Some pathologists prefer to grade such lesions as "moderately" or "poorly" differentiated.[225]) The prognosis is guarded. In the series of Lang et al.,[149, 151] 80 percent of the patients with widely invasive cancers developed metastases and about 20 percent died of tumor. Woolner et al.[301] found a 50 percent fatality rate for widely invasive tumors[301] compared with only 3 percent for those with "minimal invasion."[300, 301]

The minimally invasive follicular carcinoma can be diagnosed only by the pathologist and, in the present author's opinion, only on the basis of well-fixed histologic sections. These lesions are not diagnosable by fine needle aspiration cytology since the diagnosis requires the demonstration of invasion at the edges of the lesion; therefore, sampling of the center, as is done in obtaining a cytologic sample, cannot be diagnostic. (See also Chapter 17.)

Similar problems exist in evaluating such lesions by frozen section. Some authors have recommended that intraoperative assessment of such lesions involves the examination of frozen sections from three or four separate areas of the nodule.[180] In the present author's view, this only wastes time and resources and rarely gives useful, i.e., diagnostic, information. The surgeon should have removed the lobe involved by the nodule and, if it is a follicular carcinoma that is only minimally invasive, the appropriate therapy has already been accomplished. Since only a small number of these lesions will show evidence of invasion at the time of permanent section (i.e., the majority of them are benign), and since overdiagnosis is more dangerous for the patient than is the delay in making a definitive diagnosis, we discourage frozen section evaluation for these nodules. When a surgeon insists a frozen section be performed, we do one and only one; if the lesion is follicular and cellular, we render a diagnosis of "follicular neoplasm: diagnosis deferred." In an ongoing study of our institution's experience with over 200 such cases, only in four was a final diagnosis of carcinoma made. (One of these was a follicular variant of papillary cancer.)

Grossly, the minimally invasive follicular carcinoma resembles a follicular adenoma; the lesion is well-defined, often encapsulated, and on cut section may bulge

---

*Historical footnote: Because of the degree of differentiation of the metastases, thyroid tumors of this type were diagnosed as "adenoma malignum" or "benign metastasizing goiter"—these terms are to be condemned since the tumors are indeed carcinomas.

from the confines of its capsule. (See Fig. 9–10.) The gross appearance may differ slightly in some cases from the benign nodule because of the thickness of the capsule. As Evans has pointed out in his paper, the follicular carcinoma tends to be surrounded by a wide thick capsule.[62] Calcification may be noted grossly in the capsule. The central portion of the lesion is usually homogeneous (except when hemorrhagic foci are present secondary to preoperative biopsy) tan to pink tissue. Although degenerative changes (such as cysts and calcification) may be seen, these are unusual; the central part of the tumor is usually solid.

Microscopically, the tumor again resembles the benign follicular adenoma; however, it is more likely to demonstrate a microfollicular or trabecular pattern throughout than does a benign adenoma. The follicles are usually regular, small and round; often they are arranged back to back. If the lesion shows trabecular areas, these are often irregular.[78, 149] On occasion papillary infoldings into follicles may be seen; these do not contain the classic nuclei of papillary cancer, however, and are only found focally. (See Chapter 8.) Centrally, edema may separate individual follicles. In some examples frank hemorrhage, necrosis, or even tumor infarction may be noted, although in very well differentiated lesions these features are uncommon. Significant mitotic activity is often found; this feature is very rare in benign adenomas.[78, 106, 132, 150] Whatever the central areas show, the tumor-capsule-thyroid interface is the arena in which the diagnostician must work, however (Figs. 9–16 and 9–17).

How is the diagnosis of minimally invasive follicular carcinoma made? In other words, what are the minimum criteria for making that diagnosis? I believe that invasion *of* the capsule, invasion *through* the capsule, and invasion *into* veins in or beyond the capsule represent the diagnostic criteria for carcinoma in a follicular thyroid neoplasm.

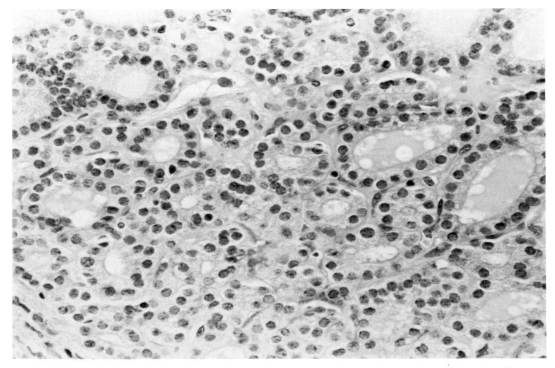

Figure 9–16. Center of follicular tumor. This area cannot predict biologic nature of the lesion. Invasion was not found. × 200.

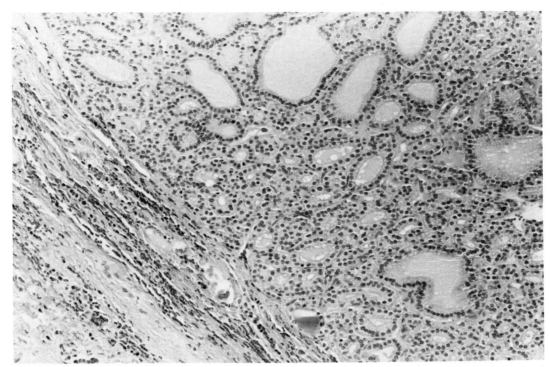

Figure 9–17. Edge of follicular nodule with thin to absent capsule. If this were one of several similar areas in a nodular goiter, it probably would represent focal hyperplasia. If this were a single lesion, it could be diagnosed as an "adenoma." × 150.

The criterion for *vascular* invasion applies solely and strictly to vessels in or beyond the capsule, since tumor plugs *within capillaries in the substance of the tumor have no apparent diagnostic and prognostic importance*—this finding alone is not associated with malignant behavior.[78] Kahn and Perzin[132] caution that because of edema in the center of these lesions what may appear to be tumor in vessels may represent follicles with surrounding separation artifact.[78, 132]

How is vascular invasion defined? (See Figs. 9–18 to 9–20.) The papers by Franssila et al.[78] and Kahn and Perzin[132] review the literature on this point[105, 106, 289, 290] and describe and illustrate the criteria necessary for the definition.

1. The invasive tumor should form a plug or polyp in a subendothelial location; a few cells or nests slightly impinging into a lumen are insufficient evidence for invasion.

2. The tumor thrombus is usually covered by endothelium. Although this is true in most cases, and tumor cells or small nests strewn freely in a vessel lumen probably represent artifacts,* Kahn and Perzin feel that some tumor thrombi are not covered by endothelium, probably because they have only recently invaded the vessel.[132] Franssila et al. prefer to see endothelialization of the tumor plug, but accept the noncovered tumor as invasion if other criteria are met: the plug has a smooth contour and/or it is attached to the vessel wall.[78]

3. The tumor thrombus does not have to be attached to the vessel wall to be acceptable as invasion.[132]

4. Kahn and Perzin as well as Franssila et al. agree that it is not necessary to detect the point of invasion into the vessel wall in order to diagnose invasion.[78, 132]

---

*The term "knife metastasis" was taught to me by my colleague Dr. Carolyn Meis—she was too kind to tell me if the knife was the one held by the surgeon or the pathologist.

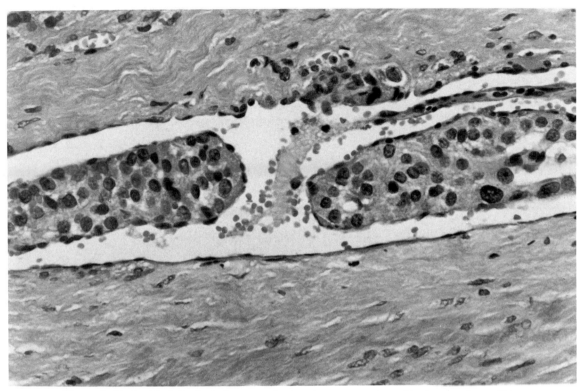

Figure 9–18. In this follicular lesion, vascular invasion was noted outside the capsule. × 100.

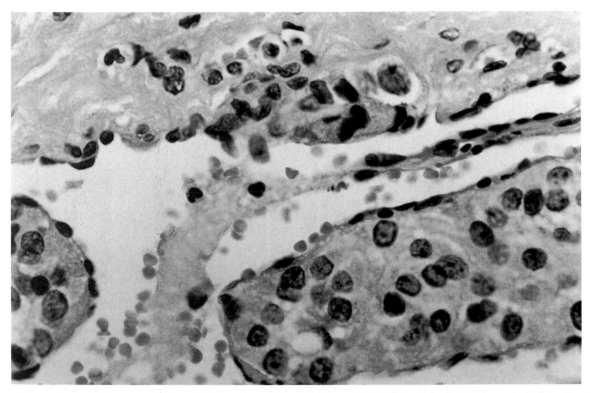

Figure 9–19. Higher power view of this area; note plug of tumor within vein lumen, covered by endothelial cells. × 200.

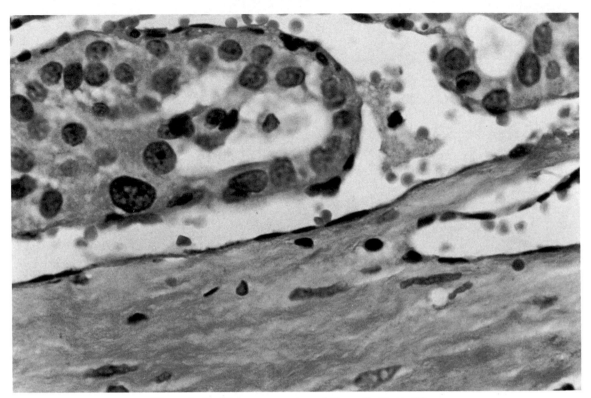

Figure 9–20. Higher power view of Figure 9–18. × 400.

Several studies have been published that attempted to define the vessel wall and endothelium in relationship to the follicular tumor nests near or in them.[78, 104] Staining for elastic tissue in the vein wall is usually futile since the size of the vessels involved is small enough that there is no significant amount of elastic lamina in its wall.[78] Immunostaining for Factor VIII–related antigen, a marker for vascular endothelium, is of limited use, since the endothelium of involved, i.e., invaded, veins rarely stains. (Vascular endothelium of uninvaded or partially invaded vessels does.) The reason for this result is unclear, but Harach et al. suggested the possibility that the tumor may elaborate some factor that alters the endothelium, allowing for invasion by tumor; this same factor(?s) may interfere with immunostaining and/or expression of Factor VIII–related antigen.[104] Other studies have claimed that immunostaining for *Ulex europaeus* lectin, laminin, or basement membrane collagen may prove more successful in defining the relationship of tumor to the endothelial lining of a questionably invaded vein.[89, 139, 256] The present author's experience recapitulates that of Harach et al.;[104] only a few veins in a few follicular carcinomas stain for Factor VIII–related antigen (Fig. 9–21). My experience with Ulex lectin is admittedly more limited, but it may prove to be successful in diagnostically problematic cases.

The diagnostic implications of "*capsular*" invasion have evoked great debate among pathologists—some require vascular invasion to render a diagnosis of follicular carcinoma; others need penetration *through* the capsule of the tumor and still others invasion *into* the capsule.[78, 132, 149–151, 233]

Kahn and Perzin found that in their series solely capsular invasion was associated with metastatic disease: "invasion only into the tumor capsule is a sufficient criterion to diagnose malignancy."[132] These authors define capsular invasion as

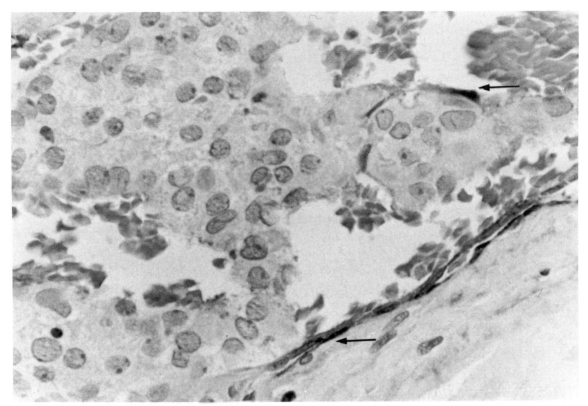

Figure 9–21. Immunoperoxidase stain for Factor VIII shows a few positive endothelial cells (*arrows*). Not all endothelial cells in the other invaded vessels stained. × 400.

irregular nests or fingers of tumor within the capsule outside the confines of the bulk of the lesion. Evans[62] and Schroder et al.[233] agreed that capsular invasion was an important diagnostic criterion. Hazard and Kenyon[106] noted that smooth, contoured islands of tumor in the capsule may represent vascular invasion; however, these authors felt that just the presence of these islands was insufficient to make the diagnosis and recommended further sectioning of the tumor to define malignancy.

Lang[149–151] and Franssila et al.[78] consider nests of tumor in the capsule to possibly represent trapping and distortion by fibrosis rather than invasion. (See Fig. 9–13.) These authors require *penetration* of the capsule to diagnose a follicular tumor as carcinoma, preferring not to overdiagnose such lesions. Iida noted that distinguishing capsular invasion from trapping may prove difficult; he required that the invasive tongues of tumor sever and deflect the collagen fibers in the capsule.[117] Thus, in Iida's opinion, a focal herniation into the capsule or the finding of a few follicles in the capsule without an apparent reactive fibrosis is insufficient to diagnose cancer.[117]

Is capsular invasion insufficient for the diagnosis of follicular cancer? What follow-up is available in series in which such lesions are diagnosed as cancer? Kahn and Perzin found one in seven patients with only capsular invasion demonstrated metastases (14 percent).[132] Evans noted that capsular invasion appeared as important if not more so than venous invasion since three of seven patients with this finding showed metastases.[62] However, in these three cases, *metastases were already present* at initial diagnosis.[62, 78]

On the other hand, those authors who diagnose tumors with capsular "invasion" only as atypical adenomas (if they are not cancer one can prefer the term capsular "impingement") indicate a benign clinical course after thyroid lobectomy. Periods of follow-up differ among various series. Data are not available in the literature on 20 to 30 year follow-up of large numbers of patients with a diagnosis of atypical adenoma of the thyroid. Will this diagnosis "backfire"? Twenty years from now? For the time being, it appears appropriate to be conservative, however.[132]

Although most recurrences or metastases will appear within five years after thyroidectomy,[78, 132, 149–151, 231] encapsulated follicular carcinomas notoriously can present as metastases many years after initial resection. (We recently analyzed a solitary vertebral metastasis in a 70-year-old woman who had undergone thyroid lobectomy for a follicular tumor 24 years before the bone lesion appeared! There had been no local recurrence in the neck or other evidence of disease during the entire follow-up period.)

It is of tremendous importance for the reader to recognize that the debate about the capsular invasion criterion must be limited to prospective pronouncements regarding the diagnosis and prognosis. Most pathologists have seen cases of follicular carcinoma presenting initially in metastatic sites; when the primary thyroid tumor is resected, extensive sampling may disclose only capsular invasion. To extrapolate from these cases to all follicular tumors confined to the thyroid at diagnosis may not be justified (although for every other tumor system we do exactly that).[78] It is possible that the small group of patients presenting with metastases and primary lesions showing only capsular invasion harbor tumors of different biologic nature or that unknown host factors are operational in these individuals.

Kahn and Perzin indicate that a few cellular follicular tumors that contain no or only a partial capsule can be diagnosed as carcinoma since they freely abut normal thyroid;[132] one of the cases in their series showed only this feature. Since hyperplastic follicular nodules in nodular goiter can show this feature, i.e., there is no capsule and they abut against the thyroid, one must be cautious—taking into consideration the size of the lesion and its intrinsic histology: mitoses, microfollicular or solid pattern, necrosis, etc. (See Figure 9–17.)

It is important to reiterate that the present author agrees with others[132] that diagnostic criteria for follicular carcinoma are identical for oxyphilic (Hürthle cell) tumors and primary clear cell neoplasms of the thyroid. (See also Chapters 12 and 15, respectively.) It has been my experience that for oxyphilic tumors the criteria for malignancy are met much more frequently than for nonoxyphilic encapsulated follicular neoplasms.

Considering the debate in the published literature, the practicing pathologist needs to ask the following:

1. How many sections (blocks) are needed of an encapsulated follicular lesion in order to prove there is no definite invasion. Although earlier published reports suggested three or five or eight blocks,[106, 290] Lang et al.[149] and Franssila et al.[78] recommend 10 blocks be examined. (As noted above, however, these sections should represent the tumor-capsule-thyroid interface in order to be considered adequate and representative.)

Ten blocks from a 3 centimeter mass may sample 50 to 60 percent of the tumor, whereas the same number of blocks from a 6 centimeter mass samples only 30 percent. Kahn and Perzin consider as adequate blocks of the entire capsule.[132] In our laboratory sampling of the whole capsule is undertaken in all cellular follicular lesions, regardless of size. For practical purposes, however, the larger the lesion, if it is malignant, the more easily invasion will be found, and I believe the recommended 10 blocks of the capsule will probably not miss a significant cancer.

Of course, if any of the 10 blocks show irregular tongues of tumor in the capsule or a suspicious area for invasion, further blocks should be examined from the lesion.

2. Do any of the modern ancillary techniques assist one in defining benign from malignant follicular tumors? Currently—no! Ultrastructural, morphometric, and flow cytometric analyses have not helped in separating these lesions.[125, 127–129, 137, 163, 164] It may be possible that studies of oncogene expression[63] or more refined image analysis techniques and/or flow cytometric analysis of multiple parameters may guide us diagnostically in the future.

Follicular Variant of Papillary Carcinoma. This entity is discussed in detail in Chapter 8. This tumor, although follicular in pattern, shares histologic and biologic characteristics with papillary cancer (nuclear features, infiltrative growth pattern, lymphatic invasion) and thus should be classified as a variant of papillary thyroid cancer.

Follicular (Glandular) Variant of Medullary Carcinoma. This unusual lesion is discussed in Chapter 10. To distinguish this tumor from follicular carcinoma requires immunostaining for calcitonin.

Insular Carcinoma. This lesion is discussed in Chapter 15. It has been categorized by some pathologists as a variant of follicular carcinoma; however, some of these tumors have shown papillary differentiation either in the primary site, in previous tumor foci, or in recurrences. Until more data are available on this lesion, it probably is best to consider it a separate entity derived from follicular epithelium and with an aggressive clinical behavior.

Mixed Follicular and Medullary Carcinoma. This tumor is discussed in Chapters 10 and 15. The existence of this lesion has been questioned but it probably does occur. Some early reports, however, which indicated its incidence was significant among thyroid tumors, were flawed by immunostaining results using antisera with inappropriate cross-reactivity with thyroglobulin.

REFERENCES

1. Aguayo, J., Sakatsuma, Y., et al.: Nontoxic nodular goiter and papillary thyroid carcinoma are not associated with peripheral blood lymphocyte sensitization to thyroid cells. J. Clin. Endocrinol. Metab. *68:*145–149, 1989.
2. Ahmann, A. J., and Burman, K. D.: The role of T lymphocytes in autoimmune thyroid disease. Endocrinol. Metab. Clin. N. Amer. *16:*287–326, 1987.
3. Akamizu, T., Ishii, H., et al.: Abnormal thyrotropin-binding immunoglobulins in two patients with Graves' disease. J. Clin. Endocrinol. Metab. *59:*240–245, 1984.
4. Albores-Saavedra, J., Nadji, M., et al.: Thyroglobulin in carcinoma of the thyroid. Hum. Pathol. *14:*62–66, 1983.
5. Al-Moussa, M., and Beck, J. S.: Histometry of thyroids containing few and multiple nodules. J. Clin. Pathol. *39:*483–488, 1986.
6. Amir, S. M., Osathanondh, R., et al.: Human chorionic gonadotropin and thyroid function in patients with hydatidiform mole. Am. J. Obstet. Gynecol. *150:*723–728, 1984.
7. Anderson, N. R., Lokich, J. J., et al.: Gestational choriocarcinoma and thyrotoxicosis. Cancer *44:*304–306, 1979.
8. Arisaka, O., Arisaka, M., et al.: Thyrotropin binding inhibitor immunoglobulin. Am. J. Dis. Child. *140:*998–1000, 1986.
9. Arnold, A., Staunton, C. E., et al.: Monoclonality and abnormal parathyroid hormone genes in parathyroid adenomas. N. Engl. J. Med. *318:*658–662, 1988.
10. Barsano, C. P., and DeGroot, L. G.: Dyshormonogenetic goiter. Clin. Endocrinol. Metab. *8:*145–165, 1979.
11. Batsakis, J. G., Nishiyama, R. H., and Schmidt, R. W.: "Sporadic goiter syndrome": a clinicopathologic analysis. Am. J. Clin. Pathol. *30:*241–251, 1963.
12. Bech, K.: Immunological aspects of Graves' disease and importance of thyroid stimulating immunoglobulins. Acta Endocrinol. *103:* Suppl.254, 1–40, 1983.
13. Bech, K., and Madsen, S. N.: Thyroid adenylate cyclase stimulating immunoglobulins in thyroid diseases. Clin. Endocrinol. *11:*47–58, 1979.

14. Beckers, C.: Thyroid nodules. Clin. Endocrinol. Metab. *8:*181–192, 1979.
15. Beck-Peccoz, P., Mariotti, S., et al.: Treatment of hyperthyroidism due to inappropriate secretion of thyrotropin with the somatostatin analog, SM S201–995. J. Clin. Endocrinol. Metab. *68:*208–214, 1989.
16. Bennett, W. P., Bhan, A. K., and Vickery, A. L.: Keratin expression as a diagnostic adjunct in thyroid tumors with papillary architecture. Lab. Invest. *58.*9A, 1988 (abstract).
17. Bigos, S. T., Ridgway, E. C., et al.: Spectrum of pituitary alterations with mild and severe thyroid impairment. J. Clin. Endocrinol. Metab. *46:*317–325, 1978.
18. Blank, M. S., and Tucci, J. R.: A case of thyroxine thyrotoxicosis. Arch. Intern. Med. *147:*863–864, 1987.
19. Bocker, W., Dralle, H., et al.: Immunohistochemical and electron microscopic analysis of adenomas of the thyroid. Virch. Arch. Pathol. Anat. *380:*205–220, 1978.
20. Boehm, T., Rothouse, L., and Wartofsky, L.: Metastatic occult follicular thyroid carcinoma. J.A.M.A. *235:*2420–2421, 1976.
21. Brown, R. S., Jackson, I. M. D., et al.: Do thyroid stimulating immunoglobulins cause nontoxic and toxic multinodular goiter? Lancet *1:*904–906, 1978.
22. Buckwalter, J. A., and Thomas, C. G.: Selection of surgical treatment for well differentiated thyroid carcinomas. Ann. Surg. *176:*565–578, 1972.
23. Buley, I. D., Gatter, K. C., et al.: Expression of intermediate filament proteins in normal and diseased thyroid glands. J. Clin. Pathol. *40:*136–142, 1987.
24. Burke, G.: The long acting thyroid stimulator of Graves' disease. Am. J. Med. *45:*435–450, 1968.
25. Burke, G.: The cell membrane: a common site of action of thyrotropin (TSH) and long acting thyroid stimulator (LATS). Metabolism *18:*720–729, 1969.
26. Burke, G., and Feldman, J. M.: Addison's disease and hyperthyroidism. Am. J. Med. *38:*470–474, 1965.
27. Burke, G., and Szabo, M.: Dissociation of in vivo and in vitro "autonomy" in hyperfunctioning thyroid nodules. J. Clin. Endocrinol. Metab. *35:*199–202, 1972.
28. Burman, K. D., and Baker, J. R.: Immune mechanisms in Graves' disease. Endocrinol. Rev. *6:*183–232, 1985.
29. Burman, K. D., Earll, J. M., et al.: Clinical observations on the solitary autonomous thyroid nodule. Arch. Intern. Med. *134:*915–919, 1974.
30. Burrow, G. N., Mujtaba, Q., et al.: The incidence of carcinoma in solitary "cold" thyroid nodules. Yale J. Biol. Med. *51:*13–17, 1978.
31. Cabrer, B., Brocas, H., et al.: Normal level of thyroglobulin messenger ribonucleic acid in a human congenital goiter with thyroglobulin deficiency. J. Clin. Endocrinol. Metab. *63:*931–940, 1986.
32. Cady, B., Rossi, R., et al.: Further evidence of the validity of risk group definition in differentiated thyroid carcinoma. Surgery *98:*1171–1178, 1985.
33. Cady, B., Sedgwick, C. E., et al.: Changing clinical, pathologic, therapeutic and survival patterns in differentiated thyroid carcinoma. Ann. Surg. *184:*541–553, 1976.
34. Cady, B., Sedgwick, C. E., et al.: Risk factor analysis in differentiated thyroid cancer. Cancer *43:*810–820, 1979.
35. Campbell, W. L., Santiago, H. E., et al.: The autonomous thyroid nodule. Radiology *107:*133–138, 1973.
36. Carayon, P., Adler, G., et al.: Heterogeneity of the Graves' immunoglobulins directed toward the thyrotropin receptor adenylate cyclase system. J. Clin. Endocrinol. Metab. *56:*1202–1208, 1983.
37. Carlson, H. E., Linfoot, J. A., et al.: Hyperthyroidism and acromegaly due to a thyrotropin and growth hormone secreting pituitary tumor. Am. J. Med. *74:*915–923, 1983.
38. Cave, W. T., and Dunn, J. T.: Studies on the thyroidal defect in an atypical form of Pendred's syndrome. J. Clin. Endocrinol. Metab. *41:*590–599, 1975.
39. Cerietty, J. M., and Listwasn, W. J.: Hyperthyroidism due to functioning metastatic thyroid carcinoma. J.A.M.A. *242:*269–270, 1979.
40. Chang, D. C. S., Wheeler, M. H., et al.: The effect of preoperative Lugol's iodine on thyroid blood flow in patients with Graves' hyperthyroidism. Surgery *102:*1055–1061, 1987.
41. Chanson, P., Li, J. Y., et al.: Absence of receptors for thyrotropin (TSH) releasing hormone in human TSH secreting pituitary adenomas associated with hyperthyroidism. J. Clin. Endocrinol. Metab. *66:*447–450, 1988.
42. Clore, J. N., Sharpe, A. R., et al.: Thyrotropin induced hyperthyroidism. Am. J. Med. Sci. *298:*3–5, 1988.
43. Connors, M. H., and Styne, D. M.: Transient neonatal athyreosis resulting from thyrotropin binding inhibitory immunoglobulins. Pediatrics *78:*287–290, 1986.
44. Cooper, D. S., Axelrod, L., et al.: Congenital goiter and the development of metastatic follicular carcinoma with evidence for a leak of nonhormonal iodide: clinical, pathological, kinetic and biochemical studies and a review of the literature. J. Clin. Endocrinol. Metab. *52:*294–303, 1981.
45. Cooper, D. S., Ladenson, P. W., et al.: Familial thyroid hormone resistance. Metabolism *31:*504–513, 1982.
46. Correa, P., and Castro, S.: Survey of the pathology of thyroid glands from Cali, Colombia—a goiter area. Lab. Invest. *10:*39–50, 1961.

47. Costa, A., Benedetto, V., et al.: Immunological features of endemic goiter. Clin. Immunol. Immunopathol. *41:*265–272, 1986.
48. Crile, G., Pontius, K. I., and Hawk, W. A.: Factors influencing the survival of patients with follicular carcinoma of the thyroid gland. Surg. Gynecol. Obstet. *160:*409–412, 1985.
49. Cuello, C., Correa, P., and Eisenberg, H.: Geographic pathology of thyroid carcinoma. Cancer *23:*230–239, 1969.
50. Dali, S. M., Chopra, P., and Nayak, N. C.: Thyroiditis in adcnomatous goitre and adenoma of the thyroid. Indian J. Med. Res. *80:*670–676, 1984.
51. Davies, T. F., and Piccinini, L. A.: Intrathyroidal MHC class II antigen expression and thyroid autoimmunity. Endocrinol. Metab. Clin. N. Amer. *16:*247–268, 1987.
52. DeBruin, T. W. A.: Differences in species specificity of TSH receptor antibodies in Graves' disease and Hashimoto's thyroiditis. J. Endocrinol. Invest. *11:*403–408, 1988.
53. DeGroot, L. J., and Paloyan, E.: Thyroid carcinoma and radiation: a Chicago epidemic. J.A.M.A. *225:*487–491, 1973.
54. DeHaven, J. W., and Sherwin, R. S.: The thyroid nodule: Approach to diagnosis and therapy. Conn. Med. *43:*761–767, 1979.
55. DeNayer, P., Lambot, M. P., et al.: Sex hormone binding protein in hyperthyroxinemic patients: A discriminator for thyroid status in thyroid hormone resistance and familial dysalbuminemic hyperthyroxincmia. J. Clin. Endocrinol. Metab. *62:*1309–1312, 1986.
56. DeRubertis, F. R., and Geyer, S. J.: Unilateral multinodular toxic goiter. Am. J. Med. Sci. *291:*183–186, 1986.
57. Donohue, J. H., Goldfien, S. D., et al.: Do the prognoses of papillary and follicular thyroid carcinomas differ? Am. J. Surg. *148:*168–173, 1984.
58. Dralle, H., Schwarzrock, R., et al.: Comparison of histology and immunohistochemistry with thyroglobulin serum levels and radioiodine uptake in recurrences and metastases of differentiated thyroid carcinomas. Acta Endocrinol. *108:*504–510, 1985.
59. Elewaut, A., Mussche, M., and Vermeulen, A.: Familial partial target organ resistance to thyroid hormones. J. Clin. Endocrinol. Metab. *43:*575–581, 1976.
60. Elman, D. S.: Familial association of nerve deafness with nodular goiter and thyroid carcinoma. N. Engl. J. Med. *259:*219–223, 1958.
61. Emerson, C. H., and Utiger, R. D.: Hyperthyroidism and excessive thyrotropin secretion. N. Engl. J. Med. *287:*328–333, 1972.
62. Evans, H. L.: Follicular neoplasms of the thyroid. Cancer *54:*535–540, 1984.
63. Fagin, J. A., Namba, H., et al.: Protooncogene mutations in human thyroid neoplasms: H-ras amplification and gene rearrangements. Clin. Res. *37:*107A, 1989.
64. Farid, N. R.: Immunogenetics of autoimmune thyroid disorders. Endocrinol. Metab. Clin. N. Amer. *16:*229–245, 1987.
65. Farid, N. R., Munro, R. E., et al.: Rosette inhibition test for the demonstration of thymus dependent lymphocyte sensitization in Graves' disease and Hashimoto's thyroiditis. N. Engl. J. Med. *289:*1111–1117, 1973.
66. Farid, N. R., Sampson, L., et al.: A study of human leukocyte-D locus related antigens in Graves' disease. J. Clin. Invest. *63:*108–113, 1979.
67. Fatourechi, V., and Gharib, H.: Hyperthyroidism following hypothyroidism. Arch. Intern. Med. *148:*976–978, 1988.
68. Fatourechi, V., Gharib, H., et al.: Pituitary thyrotropic adenoma associated with congenital hypothyroidism. Am. J. Med. *76:*725–728, 1984.
69. Fearon, E. R., Hamilton, S. R., and Vogelstein, B.: Clonal analysis of human colorectal tumors. Science *123:*193–197, 1987.
70. Felberg, N. T., Sergott, R. C., et al.: Lymphocyte subpopulations in Graves' ophthalmopathy. Arch. Ophthalmol. *103:*656–659, 1985.
71. Ferriman, D., Hennebry, T. M., and Tassopoulos, C. N.: True thyroid adenoma. Quart. J. Med. *162:*127–139, 1972.
72. FierrBenitez, R., Penafiel, W., et al.: Endemic goiter and endemic cretinism in the Andean region. N. Engl. J. Med. *280:*296–302, 1969.
73. Fisher, D. A., and Klein, A. H.: Thyroid development and disorders of thyroid function in the newborn. N. Engl. J. Med. *304:*702–712, 1981.
74. Foley, T. P., White, C., and New, A.: Juvenile Graves' disease. J. Pediatr. *110:*378–386, 1987.
75. Fradkin, J. E., and Wolff, J.: Iodide-induced thyrotoxicosis. Medicine *62:*1–20, 1983.
76. Franssila, K. O.: Value of histologic classification of thyroid cancer. Acta Pathol. Microbiol. Immunol. Scand. *225* (Suppl. A):1–76, 1971.
77. Franssilla, K. O.: Prognosis in thyroid carcinoma. Cancer *36:*1138–1146, 1975.
78. Franssila, K. O., Ackerman, L. V., et al.: Follicular carcinoma. Sem. Diagn. Pathol. *2:*101–122, 1985.
79. Frantz, V. K., Quimby, E. H., and Evans, T. C.: Radioactive iodine studies of functional thyroid carcinoma. Radiology *51:*532–552, 1948.
80. Fraser, G. R., Morgans, M. E., and Trotter, W. R.: The syndrome of sporadic goitre and congenital deafness. Quart. J. Med. *29:*279–295, 1960.
81. Furmaniak, J., Nakajima, Y., et al.: The TSH receptor: structure and interaction with autoantibodies in thyroid disease. Acta Endocrinol. Suppl. *281:*157–165, 1987.

82. Furth, J., Moy, P., et al.: Thyrotropic tumor syndrome. Arch. Pathol. *96:*217–226, 1973.
83. Gerber, H., Peter, H. J., et al.: Apparently clonal thyroid adenomas may contain heterogeneously growing and functioning cell subpopulations. In: Frontiers in Thyroidology, Vol 2, ed by Medeiros-Neto, G., and Gaitan, E. New York: Plenum Medical Book Co., 1987. Pp. 901–905.
84. Gharib, H., and Abboud, C. F.: Primary idiopathic hypothalamic hypothyroidism. Am. J. Med. *83:*171–174, 1987.
85. Gheri, R. G., Bianchi, R., et al.: A new case of familial partial generalized resistance to thyroid hormones. J. Clin. Endocrinol. Metab. *58:*563–569, 1984.
86. Gilboa, Y., Ber, A., et al.: Goitrous myxedema with defect in iodide trapping and hormonogenesis. Isr. J. Med. Sci. *2:*145–151, 1966.
87. Ginsberg, J. M., Walfish, P. G., et al.: Thyrotrophin blocking antibodies in the sera of mothers with congenitally hypothyroid infants. Clin. Endocrinol. *25:*189–194, 1986.
88. Goldstein, R., and Hart, I. R.: Followup of solitary autonomous thyroid nodules treated with 131–I. N. Engl. J. Med. *309:*1473–1476, 1983.
89. Gonzalez-Campora, R., Montero, C., et al.: Demonstration of vascular endothelium in thyroid carcinomas using Ulex europaeus I agglutinin. Histopathology *10:*261–266, 1986.
90. Goslings, B. M., Djokomoeljanto, R., et al.: Hypothyroidism in an area of endemic goiter and cretinism in central Java, Indonesia. J. Clin. Endocrinol. Metab. *44:*481–490, 1977.
91. Grossman, W., Robin, N. I., et al.: Effects of beta blockade on the peripheral manifestations of thyrotoxicosis. Ann. Intern. Med. *74:*875–879, 1971.
92. Grubeck-Loebenstein, B., Derfler, K., et al.: Immunological features of nonimmunogenic hyperthyroidism. J. Clin. Endocrinol. Metab. *60:*150–155, 1985.
93. Grubeck-Loebenstein, B., Kassal, H., et al.: The prevalence of immunological abnormalities in endemic simple goitre. Acta Endocrinol. *113:*508–513, 1986.
94. Grubeck-Loebenstein, B., Londei, M., et al.: Pathogenetic relevance of HLA class II expressing thyroid follicular cells in nontoxic goiter and in Graves' disease. J. Clin. Invest. *81:*1608–1614, 1988.
95. Gutekunst, R., Smolarek, H., et al.: Goitre epidemiology: thyroid volume, iodine excretion, thyroglobulin and thyrotropin in Germany and Switzerland. Acta Endocrinol. *112:*494–501, 1986.
96. Hamburger, J. I.: Solitary autonomously functioning thyroid lesions. Am. J. Med. *58:*740–748, 1975.
97. Hamburger, J. I.: The autonomously functioning thyroid adenoma. N. Engl. J. Med. *309:*1312–1313, 1983.
98. Hamburger, J. I.: The autonomously functioning thyroid nodule: Goetsch's disease. Endocrinol. Rev. *8:*439–447, 1987.
99. Hamilton, C. R., and Maloof, F.: Unusual types of hyperthyroidism. Medicine *52:*195–214, 1973.
100. Hamon, P., Bovier-LaPierre, M., et al.: Hyperthyroidism due to selective pituitary resistance to thyroid hormones in a 15-month-old boy. J. Clin. Endocrinol. Metab. *67:*1089–1093, 1988.
101. Hanafusa, T., Pujol-Borrell, R., et al.: Aberrant expression of HLA-DR antigen on thyrocytes in Graves' disease: relevance for autoimmunity. Lancet *2:*1111–1115, 1983.
102. Harach, H. R., Escalante, D. A., et al.: Thyroid carcinoma and thyroiditis in an endemic goitre region before and after iodine prophylaxis. Acta Endocrinol. *108:*55–60, 1985.
103. Harach, H. R., and Franssila, K. O.: Thyroglobulin immunostaining in follicular thyroid carcinoma. Histopathology *13:*43–54, 1988.
104. Harach, H. R., Jasani, B., and Williams, E. D.: Factor VIII as a marker of endothelial cells in follicular carcinoma of the thyroid. J. Clin. Pathol. *36:*1050–1054, 1977.
105. Hazard, J. B., and Kenyon, R.: Atypical adenoma of the thyroid. Arch. Pathol. *58:*554–563, 1954.
106. Hazard, J. B., and Kenyon, R.: Encapsulated angioinvasive carcinoma (angioinvasive adenoma) of the thyroid gland. Am. J. Clin. Pathol. *24:*755–766, 1954.
107. Hedberg, C. W., Fishbein, D. B., et al.: An outbreak of thyrotoxicosis caused by the consumption of bovine thyroid gland in ground beef. N. Engl. J. Med. *316:*993–998, 1987.
108. Henzel-Logmans, S. C., Millink, H., et al.: Expression of keratin and vimentin in epithelial cells of normal and pathological thyroid tissue. Virch. Arch. Pathol. Anat. *410:*347–354, 1987.
109. Hetzel, B. S.: Iodine deficiency disorders and their eradication. Lancet *2:*1126–1129, 1983.
110. Hicks, D. G., LiVolsi, V. A., et al.: Solitary follicular nodules of the thyroid are monoclonal proliferations. Lab. Invest. *60:*40A, 1989.
111. Himelman, R. B., and Chappell, D. A.: Hyperthyroidism in a healthy pregnant woman. Hosp. Pract. *21:*38–45, 1986.
112. Hofstadter, F.: Frequency and morphology of malignant tumours of the thyroid before and after the introduction of iodine prophylaxis. Virch. Arch. Pathol. Anat. *385:*263–270, 1980.
113. Horn, K., Erhardt, F., et al.: Recurrent goiter, hyperthyroidism, galactorrhea and amenorrhea due to a thyrotropin and prolactin producing pituitary tumor. J. Clin. Endocrinol. *43:*137–143, 1976.
114. Horton, P. W., Millar, W. T., et al.: Iodine organification defect following treatment of thyrotoxicosis with antithyroid drugs. Clin. Endocrinol. *4:*357–362, 1975.
115. Hull, O. H.: Critical analysis of two hundred and twenty-one thyroid glands: study of thyroid glands obtained at necropsy in Colorado. Arch. Pathol. *59:*291–311, 1955.

116. Ibbertson, H. K.: Endemic goitre and cretinism. Clin. Endocrinol. Metab. 8:97–128, 1979.
117. Iida, F.: The fate and surgical significance of adenoma of the thyroid gland. Surg. Gynecol. Obstet. *136:*536–540, 1973.
118. Ingenbleek, Y., Luypaert, B., and DeNayer, P.: Nutritional status and endemic goitre. Lancet *1:*388–392, 1980.
119. Ingenbleek, Y., and DeVisscher, M.: Hormonal and nutritional status: critical conditions for endemic goiter epidemiology? Metabolism *28:*9–19, 1979.
120. Ishikawa, N., Eguchi, K., et al.: Reduction in the suppressor-inducer T cell subset and increase in the helper T cell subset in thyroid tissue from patients with Graves' disease. J. Clin. Endocrinol. Metab. *65:*17–23, 1987.
121. Itikawa, A., and Kawada, J.: Role of thyroidal lysosomes in the hydrolysis of thyroglobulin and its relation to the development of iodide goiter. J. Clin. Endocrinol. Metab. *95:*1574–1581, 1974.
122. Jackson, J. A., Verdonk, C. A., and Spiekerman, A. M.: Euthyroid hyperthyroxinemia and inappropriate secretion of thyrotropin. Arch. Intern. Med. *147:*1311–1313, 1987.
123. Jackson, R. A., Haynes, B. F., et al.: Ia+ T cells in new onset Graves' disease. J. Clin. Endocrinol. Metab. *59:*187–190, 1984.
124. Jansson, R., Karlsson, A., and Forsum, U.: Intrathyroidal HLA-DR expression and T lymphocyte phenotypes in Graves' thyrotoxicosis, Hashimoto's thyroiditis and nodular colloid goitre. Clin. Exp. Immunol. *58:*264–272, 1984.
125. Joensuu, H., Klemi, P., and Eerola, E.: DNA aneuploidy in follicular adenomas of the thyroid gland. Am. J. Pathol. *124:*373–376, 1987.
126. Johannessen, J. V., and Sobrinho-Simoes, M.: The fine structure of follicular thyroid adenomas. Am. J. Clin. Pathol. *78:*299–310, 1982.
127. Johannessen, J. V., and Sobrinho-Simoes, M.: Follicular carcinoma of the human thyroid gland. An ultrastructural study with emphasis on scanning electron microscopy. Diagn. Histopathol. *5:*113–127, 1982.
128. Johannessen, J. V., and Sobrinho-Simoes, M.: Well-differentiated thyroid tumors: Problems in diagnosis and understanding. Pathol. Annu. *18:*(part 1):255–285, 1983.
129. Johannessen, J. V., Sobrinho-Simoes, M., et al.: The diagnostic value of flow cytometric DNA measurements in selected disorders of the human thyroid. Am. J. Clin. Pathol. *77:*20–25, 1982.
130. Johnson, J. R.: Adenomatous goiters with and without hyperthyroidism. Arch. Surg. *59:*1088–1099, 1949.
131. Kabel, P. J., Voorbij, H. A. M., et al.: Intrathyroidal dendritic cells. J. Clin. Endocrinol. Metab. *65:*199–207, 1988.
132. Kahn, N., and Perzin, K. H.: Follicular carcinoma of the thyroid: An evaluation of the histologic criteria used for diagnosis. Pathol. Annu. *18*(Part 1):221–253, 1983.
133. Kalderon, A. E., and Bogaars, H. A.: Immune complex deposits in Graves' disease and Hashimoto's thyroiditis. Am. J. Med. *63:*729–734, 1977.
134. Kamoi, K., Mitsuma, T., et al.: Hyperthyroidism caused by a pituitary thyrotropin secreting tumour with excessive secretion of thyrotropin releasing hormone and subsequently followed by Graves' disease in a middle aged woman. Acta Endocrinol. *110:*373–382, 1985.
135. Kaplan, A. S., vanHeerden, J. A., et al.: Follicular carcinoma of the thyroid presenting with hematuria. Surgery *100:*572–575, 1986.
136. Karlsson, F. A., Wibell, L., and Wide, L.: Hypothyroidism due to thyroid-hormone binding antibodies. N. Engl. J. Med. *296:*1146–1148, 1977.
137. Kay, S., and Terz, J. J.: Ultrastructural observations on a follicular carcinoma of the thyroid gland. Am. J. Clin. Pathol. *65:*328–336, 1976.
138. Kempers, R. D., Dockerty, M. B., et al.: Struma ovarii—ascitic, hyperthyroid and asymptomatic syndromes. Ann. Intern. Med. *72:*883–892, 1970.
139. Kendall, C. H., Sanderson, P. R., et al.: Follicular thyroid tumours: a study of laminin and type IV collagen in basement membrane and endothelium. J. Clin. Pathol. *38:*1100–1105, 1985.
140. Kennedy, J. S.: The pathology of dyshormonogenetic goitre. J. Pathol. *99:*251–264, 1969.
141. Ketelbant-Balasse, P., Glinoer, D., and Neve, P.: Ultrastructural aspects of the thyroid in a case of human congenital goitre with cretinism. Pathol. Europ. *10:*155–165, 1975.
142. Ketalslegers, J. M., Nisula, B. C., and Kohler, P. O.: Investigation of choriocarcinoma clonal cell lines in vitro and choriocarcinoma transplants in the hamster for the secretion of a thyroid stimulating factor. Endocrinology *96:*808–810, 1975.
143. Khoury, E. L., Greenspan, J. S., and Greenspan, F. S.: Ectopic expression of HLA class II antigens on thyroid follicular cells: induction and transfer in vitro by autologous mononuclear leukocytes. J. Clin. Endocrinol. Metab. *67:*992–1004, 1988.
144. Kleinhaus, N., Faber, J., et al.: Euthyroid hyperthyroxinemia due to a generalized 5'-deiodinase defect. J. Clin. Endocrinol. Metab. *66:*684–688, 1988.
145. Knight, J., Laing, P., et al.: Thyroid stimulating autoantibodies usually contain only lambda chains: evidence for the "forbidden clone" theory. J. Clin. Endocrinol. Metab. *62:*342–347, 1986.
146. Kourides, I. A.: A patient with thyroid stimulating hormone (TSH) hypersecretion. Med. Grand Rounds 2:222–228, 1983.
147. Kourides, I. A., Ridgway, E. C., et al.: Thyrotropin-induced hyperthyroidism: use of alpha and

beta subunit levels to identify patients with pituitary tumors. J. Clin. Endocrinol. Metab. *45:*534–543, 1977.

148. Kraiem, Z., Glaser, B., et al.: Toxic multinodular goiter: a variant of autoimmune hyperthyroidism J. Clin. Endocrinol. Metab. *65:*659–664, 1987.

149. Lang, W., Choritz, H., and Hundeshagen, H.: Risk factors in follicular thyroid carcinomas. A retrospective followup study covering a 14 year period with emphasis on morphological findings. Am. J. Surg. Pathol. *10:*246–255, 1986.

150. Lang, W., Georgii, G., et al.: The differentiation of atypical adenomas and encapsulated follicular carcinomas in the thyroid gland. Virch. Arch. Pathol. Anat. *385:*125–141, 1980.

151. Lang, W., and Georgii, G.: Minimal invasive cancer in the thyroid. Clin. Oncol. *1:*527–537, 1982.

152. Larsen, P. R.: Thyroid-pituitary interaction. N. Engl. J. Med. *306:*23–32, 1982.

153. Leclere, J., Bene, M. C., et al.: Behaviour of thyroid tissue from patients with Graves' disease in nude mice. J. Clin. Endocrinol. Metab. *59:*175–177, 1984.

154. Lee, K. S., Kim, K., et al.: The role of propanolol in the preoperative preparation of patients with Graves' disease. Surg. Gynecol. Obstet. *162:*365–369, 1986.

155. Leger, F. A., Massin, J. P., et al.: Iodine-induced thyrotoxicosis. Eur. J. Clin. Invest. *14:*449–455, 1984.

156. Leger, F. A., Thomas, G., et al.: Hypothyroidie congenitale avec probable anomalie de la receptivite thyroidienne a l'hormone thyrotrope. Presse Med. *13:*491–494, 1984.

157. Lerro, S., Losa, M., et al.: Free thyroid hormone levels and TSH response to TRH in patients with autonomous thyroid adenomata and normal T3 and T4. Clin. Endocrinol. *23:*373–378, 1985.

158. Lever, E. G., Medeiros-Neto, G. A., and De Groot, L. J.: Inherited disorders of thyroid metabolism. Endocrinol. Rev. *4:*213–239, 1983.

159. Leovey, A., Bako, G., et al.: The common incidence of Basedow's-Graves' disease and chronic lymphocytic thyroiditis. Radiobiol. Radiother. (Berl) *25:*769–774, 1984.

160. Liechty, R. D., Stoffel, P. T., et al.: Solitary thyroid nodules. Arch. Surg. *112:*59–61, 1977.

161. Lissitzky, S., Torresani, J., et al.: Defective thyroglobulin export as a cause of congenital goitre. Clin. Endocrinol. *4:*363–392, 1975.

162. London, W. T., Koutras, D. A., et al.: Epidemiologic and metabolic studies of a goiter endemic in eastern Kentucky. J. Clin. Endocrinol. *25:*1001–1010, 1965.

163. Luck, J. B., Mumaw, V. C., and Frable, W. J.: Video-plan image analysis on fine needle aspiration biopsies of the thyroid gland. Acta Cytol. *25:*718–722, 1981.

164. Lukacs, G. L., Balazs, G., Zs-Nagy, I.: Cytofluorimetric measurements on the DNA contents of tumor cells in human thyroid gland. J. Cancer Res. Clin. Oncol. *95:*265–271, 1979.

165. Lupulescu, A. P., and Boyd, C. B.: Follicular adenomas. Arch. Pathol. *93:*492–502, 1972.

166. Lyon, M. F.: Clones and X-chromosomes. J. Pathol. *155:*97–99, 1988.

167. Lyon, M. F.: X-chromosome inactivation and the location and expression of X-linked genes. Am. J. Hum. Genet. *42:*8–16, 1988.

168. MacKenzie, W. A., Schwartz, A. E., et al.: Intrathyroidal T cell clones from patients with autoimmune thyroid disease. J. Clin. Endocrinol. Metab. *64:*818–824, 1987.

169. Madec, A. M., Allannic, H., et al.: T-lymphocyte subsets at various stages of hyperthyroid Graves' disease. J. Clin. Endocrinol. Metab. *62:*117–121, 1986.

170. Mahmoud, I., Colin, I., et al.: Direct toxic effect of iodide excess on iodine-deficient thyroid glands: epithelial necrosis and inflammation associated with lipofuscin accumulation. Exper. Molec. Pathol. *44:*259–271, 1986.

171. Marx, S. J.: Genetic defects in primary hyperparathyroidism. N. Engl. J. Med. *318:*609–611, 1988.

172. Massin, J. P., Savoie, J. C., et al.: Pulmonary metastases in differentiated thyroid carcinoma. Cancer *53:*982–992, 1984.

173. Matsunaga, M., Eguchi, K., et al.: Class II major histocompatibility complex antigen expression and cellular interactions in thyroid glands of Graves' disease. J. Clin. Endocrinol. Metab. *62:*723–728, 1986.

174. McKenzie, J. M.: Hyperthyroidism caused by thyroid adenomata. J. Clin. Endocrinol. Metab. *26:*779–781, 1966.

175. McKenzie, J. M.: Does LATS cause hyperthyroidism in Graves' disease? Metabolism *21:*883–894, 1972.

176. McLaughlin, R. P., Scholz, D. A., et al.: Metastatic thyroid carcinoma with hyperthyroidism. Mayo Clin. Proc. *45:*328–335, 1970.

177. Medeiros-Neto, G. A., Bloise, W., and Ulhoa-cintra, A. B.: Partial defect of iodide trapping mechanism in two siblings with congenital goiter and hypothyroidism. J. Clin. Endocrinol. Metab. *35:*370–377, 1972.

178. Medeiros-Neto, G. A., Halpern, A., et al.: Thyroid growth immunoglobulins in large multinodular endemic goiters. J. Clin. Endocrinol. Metab. *63:*644–650, 1986.

179. Meissner, W. A.: Surgical pathology. *In:* Sedgwick, C. E. (ed.): Surgery of the Thyroid Gland. Philadelphia, W. B. Saunders Company, 1974, pp. 24–40.

180. Meissner, W. A.: Follicular carcinoma of the thyroid; frozen section diagnosis. Am. J. Surg. Pathol. *1:*171–175, 1977.

181. Mendel, C. M., and Cavalieri, R. R.: Thyroxine distribution and metabolism in familial dysalbuminemic hyperthyroxinemia. J. Clin. Endocrinol. Metab. *59:*499–504, 1984.

182. Menezes-Ferreira, M. M., Eil, C., et al.: Decreased nuclear uptake of I-125 triiodo-L-thyronine in fibroblasts from patients with peripheral thyroid hormone resistance. J. Clin. Endocrinol. Metab. *59:*1081–1087, 1984.

183. Miller, J. M., Kini, S. R., and Hamburger, J. I.: The diagnosis of malignant follicular neoplasms of the thyroid by needle biopsy. Cancer *55:*2812–2817, 1985.

184. Miyai, K., Tanizawa, O., et al.: Pituitary-thyroid function in trophoblastic disease. J. Clin. Endocrinol. Metab. *42:*254–259, 1976.

185. Monaco, F., Monaco, G., and Andreoli, M.: Thyroglobulin biosynthesis in "cold" and "hot" nodules in the human thyroid gland. J. Clin. Endocrinol. Metab. *41:*253–259, 1975.

186. Monaco, P. B., Martin, J. H., and Lieberman, Z. H.: Convoluted secretory material in thyroid follicular epithelial tumors. Am. J. Surg. Pathol. *3:*279–281, 1979.

187. Moore, G. H.: The thyroid in sporadic goitrous cretinism. Arch. Pathol. *74:*35–58, 1962.

188. Mori, H., Amino, N., et al.: Decrease of immunoglobulins G-Fc receptor-bearing T lymphocytes in Graves' disease. J. Clin. Endocrinol. Metab. *55:*399–402, 1982.

189. Morley, J. E., Jacobson, R. J., et al.: Choriocarcinoma as a cause of thyrotoxicosis. Am. J. Med. *60:*1036–1040, 1976.

190. Mortensen, J. D., Woolner, L. B., and Bennett, W. A.: Gross and microscopic findings in clinically normal thyroid glands. J. Clin. Endocrinol. Metab. *15:*1270–1280, 1955.

191. Mu, L., Chengyi, Q., et al.: Endemic goitre in central China caused by excessive iodine intake. Lancet *2:*257–259, 1987.

192. Muller-Gartner, H. W., Baisch, H., et al.: Increased deoxyribonucleic acid synthesis of autonomously functioning thyroid adenomas: Independent of but further stimulable by thyrotropin. J. Clin. Endocrinol. Metab. *68:*39–45, 1989.

193. Namba, H., and Fagin, J. A.: Clonal origin of human thyroid tumors; Determination by X-chromosome inactivation analysis. Clin. Res. *37:*108A, 1989.

194. Niepomniszcze, H., Rosenbloom, A. L., et al.: Differentiation of two abnormalities in thyroid peroxidase causing organification defect and goitrous hypothyroidism. Metabolism *24:*57–67, 1975.

195. Noppakun, N., Bancheun, K., and Chandraprasert, S.: Unusual locations of localized myxedema in Graves' disease. Arch. Dermatol. *122:*85–88, 1986.

196. Nusynowitz, M. L., Clark, R. F., et al.: Thyroxine-binding globulin deficiency in three families and total deficiency in a normal woman. Am. J. Med. *50:*458–464, 1971.

197. Ochi, Y., and DeGroot, L. J.: Long acting stimulator of Graves' disease. N. Engl. J. Med. *278:*718–721, 1968.

198. Okita, N., How, J., et al.: Suppressor T lymphocytes dysfunction in Graves' disease: role of the H-2 histamine receptor-bearing suppressor T lymphocytes. J. Clin. Endocrinol. Metab. *53:*1002–1007, 1981.

199. Orgiazzi, J., Rousset, B., et al.: Plasma thyrotropic activity in a man with choriocarcinoma. J. Clin. Endocrinol. Metab. *39:*653–657, 1974.

200. Pamke, T. W., Croxson, M. S., et al.: Triiodothyronine secreting (toxic) adenoma of the thyroid gland. Cancer *41:*528–537, 1978.

201. Papasteriades, C., Alevizaki-Harhalaki, M. N., et al.: HLA antigens in Greek patients with thyrotoxicosis (Graves' disease and toxic nodular goiter). J. Endocrinol. Invest. *7:*283–286, 1984.

202. Patchefsky, A. S., and Hoch, W. S.: Psammoma bodies in diffuse toxic goiter. Am. J. Clin. Pathol. *57:*551–556, 1972.

203. Pekonen, F., Alfthan, H., et al.: Human chorionic gonadotropin (hCG) and thyroid function in early human pregnancy: circadian variation and evidence for intrinsic thyrotropic activity of hCG. J. Clin. Endocrinol. Metab. *66:*853–856, 1988.

204. Permanetter, W., Nathrathm, W. B. J., and Lohrs, U.: Immunohistochemical analysis of thyroglobulin and keratin in benign and malignant thyroid tumours. Virch. Arch. Pathol. Anat. *398:*221–228, 1982.

205. Peter, H. J., Gerber, H., et al.: Autonomy of growth and of iodine metabolism in hyperthyroid feline goiters transplanted onto nude mice. J. Clin. Invest. *80:*491–498, 1987.

206. Peter, H. J., Gerber, H., et al.: Pathogenesis of heterogeneity in human multinodular goiter. J. Clin. Invest. *76:*1992–2002, 1985.

207. Peter, H. J., Studer, H., et al.: The pathogenesis of "hot" and "cold" follicles in multinodular goiters. J. Clin. Endocrinol. Metab. *55:*941–946, 1982.

208. Peter, H. J., Studer, H., and Groscurth, P.: Autonomous growth, but not autonomous function in embryonic human thyroids: A clue to understanding autonomous goiter growth? J. Clin. Endocrinol. Metab. *66:*968–973, 1988.

209. Pickardt, C. R., Erhardt, F., et al.: Stimulation of TSH secretion by TRH in autonomous thyroid adenoma. Deutsche Med. Wochenschr. *98:*152–157, 1973.

210. Pittman, C. S., and Pittman, J. A.: A study of the thyroglobulin, thyroidal protease and iodoproteins in two congenital cretins. Am. J. Med. *40:*49–56, 1966.

211. Pittman, J. A.: Hypothalamic hyperthyroidism (?). N. Engl. J. Med. *287:*356–357, 1972.

212. Pommier, J. Tourniaire, J., et al.: A defective thyroid peroxidase solubilized from a familial goiter with iodine organification defect. J. Clin. Endocrinol. Metab. *39:*69–80, 1974.

213. Raines, K. B., Baker, J. R., et al.: Antithyrotropin antibodies in the sera of Graves' disease patients. J. Clin. Endocrinol. Metab. *61:*217–222, 1985.

214. Rajatanavin, R., Chailurkit, L., et al.: Trophoblastic hyperthyroidism: Clinical and biochemical features of five cases. Am. J. Med. *85*:237–241, 1988.

215. Ramelli, F., Studer, H., and Bruggisser, D.: Pathogenesis of thyroid nodules in multinodular goiter. Am. J. Pathol. *109*:215–223, 1982.

216. Rapoport, B., and Ingbar, S. H.: Production of triiodothyronine in normal human subjects and in patients with hyperthyroidism. Am. J. Med. *56*:586–590, 1974.

217. Refetoff, S., DeGroot, L. G., and Barsano, C. P.: Defective thyroid hormone feedback regulation in the syndrome of peripheral resistance to thyroid hormone. J. Clin. Endocrinol. Metab. *51*:41–45, 1980.

218. Refetoff, S., and Murata, Y.: X-chromosome linked inheritance of the variant thyroxine binding globulin in Australian aborigines. J. Clin. Endocrinol. Metab. *60*:356–360, 1985.

219. Report of the subcommittee for the study of endemic goitre and iodine deficiency of the European Thyroid Association. Goitre and iodine deficiency in Europe. Lancet *1*:1289–1293, 1985.

220. Roger, P. P., and Dumont, J. E.: Thyrotropin is a potent growth factor for normal human thyroid cells in primary culture. Biochem. Biophys. Res. Comm. *149*:707–711, 1987.

221. Rosenthal, D.: Kinetic analysis of iodine and thyroxine metabolism in "hot" thyroid nodules. Metabolism *30*:384–392, 1981.

222. Ruegemer, J. J., Hay, I. D., et al.: Distant metastases in differentiated thyroid carcinoma: a multivariate analysis of prognostic variables. J. Clin. Endocrinol. Metab. *67*:501–508, 1988.

223. Ruiz, M., Rajatanavin, R., et al.: Familial dysalbuminemic hyperthyroxinemia. N. Engl. J. Med. *306*:635–639, 1982.

224. Saito, H., Yamamoto, K., et al.: Goitrous hypothyroidism due to iodide trapping defect. J. Clin. Endocrinol. Metab. *53*:1267–1272, 1981.

225. Sakamoto, A., Kasai, N., and Sugano, H.: Poorly differentiated carcinoma of the thyroid. Cancer *52*:1849–1855, 1983.

226. Sarne, D., Barokas, K., et al.: Elevated serum thyroglobulin in congenital thyroxine binding globulin deficiency. J. Clin. Endocrinol. Metab. *57*:665–667, 1983.

227. Sarne, D. H., Refetoff, S., et al.: A new inherited abnormality of thyroxine-binding globulin (TBG-San Diego) and decreased affinity for thyroxine and triiodothyronine. J. Clin. Endocrinol. Metab. *68*:114–119, 1989.

228. Savoie, J. C., Massin, J. P., et al.: Iodine induced thyrotoxicosis in apparently normal thyroid glands. J. Clin. Endocrinol. Metab. *41*:685–691, 1975.

229. Schicha, H., Emrich, D., and Schreivogel, I.: Hyperthyroidism due to Graves' disease and due to autonomous goiter. J. Endocrinol. Invest. *8*:399–497, 1085.

230. Schmidt, R. J., and Wang, C. A.: Encapsulated follicular carcinoma of the thyroid: Diagnosis, treatment and results. Surgery *100*:1068–1076, 1986.

231. Schroder, S., Baisch, H., et al.: Morphologie und Prognose des folliculären Schilddrusencarcinoms–Eine klinisch-pathologische und DNS-cytometrische Untersuchung an 95 Tumoren. Langenbecks Arch. Chir. *370*:3–24, 1987.

232. Schroder, S., MullerGartner, H. W., et al.: Morphological demonstration and quantification of TSH binding sites in neoplastic and non-neoplastic thyroid tissue. Virch. Arch. Pathol. Anat. *409*:555–570, 1986.

233. Schroder, S., Pfannschmidt, N., et al.: The encapsulated follicular carcinoma of the thyroid. Virch. Arch. Pathol. Anat. *402*:259–273, 1984.

234. Sellers, E. A., Awad, A. G., and Schonbaum, E.: Long acting stimulator in Graves' disease. Lancet *2*:335–338, 1970.

235. Sellschopp, C., Derwahl, M., et al.: Direct immunostaining of TSH receptor related autoantibodies in Graves' disease. Acta Endocrinol. *114*:132–137, 1987.

236. Shane, S. R., Jones, J. E., and Flink, E. B.: Familial goiter and congenital nerve deafness. J. Clin. Endocrinol. *25*:1085–1090, 1965.

237. Shapiro, S. J., Friedman, N. B., et al.: Incidence of thyroid carcinoma in Graves' disease. Cancer *26*:1261–1270, 1970.

238. Shenkman, L., and Bottone, E. J.: Antibodies to Yersinia enterocolitica in thyroid disease. Ann. Intern. Med. *85*:735–739, 1976.

239. Silverberg, S. G., Hutter, R. V. P., and Foote, F. W.: Fatal carcinoma of the thyroid: histology, metastases and causes of death. Cancer *25*:792–802, 1970.

240. Sinha, D., Pascal, R., and Furth, J.: Transplantable thyroid carcinoma induced by thyrotropin. Arch. Pathol. *79*:192–198, 1965.

241. Skillern, P. G.: Genetics of Graves' disease. Mayo Clin. Proc. *47*:848–849, 1972.

242. Smith, B. R., and Hall, R.: Thyroid stimulating immunoglobulins in Graves' disease. Lancet *2*:427–431, 1974.

243. Smith, B. R., McLachlan, S. M., and Furmaniak, J.: Autoantibodies to the thyrotropin receptor. Endocrinol. Rev. *9*:106–121, 1988.

244. Smith, J. F.: The pathology of the thyroid in the syndrome of sporadic goitre and congenital deafness. Quart. J. Med. *29*:297–303, 1960.

245. Smith, R., Blum, C., et al.: Radioactive iodine treatment of metastatic thyroid carcinoma with clinical thyrotoxicosis. Clin. Nucl. Med. *10*:874–875, 1985.

246. Smyth, P. P. A., Neylan, D., and O'Donovan, D. K.: The prevalence of thyroid stimulating antibodies in goitrous disease assessed by cytochemical section bioassay. J. Clin. Endocrinol. Metab. *54*:357–361, 1982.

247. Sobrinho-Simoes, M., and Damjanov, I.: Lectin histochemistry of papillary and follicular carcinoma of the thyroid gland. Arch. Pathol. Lab. Med. *110:*722–729, 1986.
248. Soderstrom, N., Lindgren, J., and Tibblin, S.: Hemorrhagic thyroid cysts in nodular goitre. Lancet *2:*531–532, 1974.
249. Solomon, D. H., and Kleeman, K. E.: Concepts of pathogenesis of Graves' disease. Adv. Intern. Med. *22:*273–299, 1976.
250. Soltec, M., Tislaric, D., et al.: Increased thyroidal T4/T3 ratio in nodular and paranodular tissues of nontoxic goiter following suppressive treatment with thyroid hormones. Hormone Res. *25:*147–151, 1987.
251. Spjut, H. J., Warren, W. D., and Ackerman, L. V.: Clinical-pathologic study of 76 cases of recurrent Graves' disease, toxic (nonexophthalmic) goiter, and nontoxic goiter. Am. J. Clin. Pathol. *27:*367–392, 1957.
252. Stanbury, J. B.: Thyroid specific metabolic incompetence and tumour development. *In:* Thyroid Cancer. Hedinger, C. (ed.) Berlin, Springer-Verlag, 1969, pp. 183–190.
253. Stanbury, J. B., and Chapman, E. M.: Congenital hypothyroidism with goitre. Lancet *1:*1162–1165, 1960.
254. Stanbury, J. B., Rocmans, P., et al.: Congenital hypothyroidism with impaired thyroid response to thyrotropin. N. Engl. J. Med. *279:*1132–1136, 1968.
255. Stenszky, V., Kozma, L., et al.: The genetics of Graves' disease: HLA and disease susceptibility. J. Clin. Endocrinol. Metab. *61:*735–740, 1985.
256. Stephenson, T. J., Griffiths, D. W. R., and Mills, P. M.: Comparison of Ulex europaeus I lectin binding and factor VIII-related antigen as markers for vascular endothelium in follicular carcinoma of the thyroid. Histopathology *10:*251–260, 1986.
257. Stout, B. D., Wiener, L., and Cox, J. W.: Combined alpha and beta sympathetic blockade in hyperthyroidism. Ann. Intern. Med. *70:*963–970, 1969.
258. Strakosch, C. R., Wenzel, B. E., et al.: Immunology of autoimmune thyroid disease. N. Engl. J. Med. *307:*1499–1507, 1982.
259. Studer, H.: Growth control and follicular cell neoplasia. *In:* Frontiers in Thyroidology, Vol. 1, Medeiros-Neto, G., and Gaitan, E. (eds.). New York, Plenum Medical Book Company, pp. 131–137, 1986.
260. Studer, H., Hunziker, H. R., and Ruchti, C.: Morphologic and functional substrate of thyrotoxicosis caused by nodular goiters. Am. J. Med. *65:*227–234, 1978.
261. Studer, H., Peter, H. J., and Gerber, H.: Morphologic and functional changes in developing goiters. *In:* Thyroid Disorders Associated with Iodine Deficiency and Excess, Hall, R., and Kobberling, J. (eds.). New York, Raven Press, pp. 229–241, 1985.
262. Studer, H. and Ramelli, F.: Simple goiter and its variants: euthyroid and hyperthyroid. Endocrinol. Rev. *3:*40–61, 1982.
263. Tachiwaki, O., and Wollman, S. H.: Shedding of dense cell fragments into follicular lumen early in involution of the hyperplastic thyroid gland. Lab. Invest. *47:*91–98, 1982.
264. Taylor, H. C.: Solitary hyperfunctioning thyroid adenoma in a child. J.A.M.A. *234:*1253–1255, 1975.
265. Teuscher, J., Peter, H. J., et al.: Pathogenesis of nodular goiter and its implications for surgical management. Surgery *103:*87–93, 1988.
266. Tezuka, H., Eguchi, K., et al.: Natural killer and natural killer-like cell activity of peripheral blood and intrathyroidal mononuclear cells from patients with Graves' disease. J. Clin. Endocrinol. Metab. *66:*702–707, 1988.
267. Thomas, C. G., Combesi, W., et al.: Biological characteristics of adenomatous nodules, adenomas and hyperfunctioning nodules as defined by adenylate cyclase activity and TSH receptors. World J. Surg. *8:*445–451, 1984.
268. Thomas, G. A., Williams, D., and Williams, E. D.: The demonstration of tissue clonality by X-linked enzyme histochemistry. J. Pathol. *155:*101–108, 1988.
269. Tibaldi, J. M., Barzel, U. S., et al.: Thyrotoxicosis in the very old. Am. J. Med. *81:*619–622, 1986.
270. Tolis, G., Bird, C., et al.: Pituitary hyperthyroidism. Am. J. Med. *64:*177–181, 1978.
271. Tollefson, H. R., Shah, J. P., and Huvos, A. G.: Follicular carcinoma of the thyroid. Am. J. Surg. *126:*523–528, 1973.
272. Toyoshima, K., Matsumoto, Y. et al.: Five cases of absence of iodine concentrating mechanism. Acta Endocrinol. *84:*527–537, 1977.
273. Tubiana, M., Schlumberger, M., et al.: Long-term results and prognostic factors in patients with well differentiated thyroid carcinoma. Cancer *55:*794–804, 1985.
274. Valenta, L. J., Bode, H., et al.: Lack of thyroid peroxidase activity as the cause of congenital goitrous hypothyroidism. J. Clin. Endocrinol. Metab. *36:*830–844, 1973.
275. Valenta, L., Lemarchand-Beraud, T., et al.: Metastatic thyroid carcinoma provoking hyperthyroidism, with elevated circulating thyrostimulators. Am. J. Med. *48:*72–76, 1970.
276. Valente, W. A., Vitti, P., et al.: Antibodies that promote thyroid growth: distinct population of thyroid stimulating antibodies. N. Engl. J. Med. *309:*1028–1034, 1983.
277. Van den Hove-Vandenbroucke, M. F., DeVisscher, M., and Couvreur-Eppe, M.: Secretory activity of isolated thyroid adenomas. J. Clin. Endocrinol. Metab. *43:*178–181, 1976.
278. Vander, J. B., Gaston, E. A., and Dawber, T. R.: The significance of nontoxic thyroid nodules. Ann. Intern. Med. *69:*537–540, 1968.

279. Van der Gaag, R. D., von Blomberg-van der Flier, M., et al.: T-suppressor cell defects in euthyroid nonendemic goiters. Acta Endocrinol. *112:*83–86, 1986.
280. Van Sande, J., Lamy, F., et al.: Pathogenesis of autonomous thyroid nodules: in vitro study of iodine and adenosine 3'5'-monophosphate metabolism. J. Clin. Endocrinol. Metab. *66:*570–579, 1988.
281. van Ouwerkerk, B. M., Krenning, E. P., et al.: Cellular and humoral immunity in patients with hyperthyroid Graves' disease before, during and after antithyroid drug treatment. Clin. Endocrinol. *26:*385–394, 1987.
282. Vergadoro, F., Tabacchi, L., et al.: Thyroid function in gestational trophoblastic tumors. Tumori *72:*205–209, 1986.
283. Vermiglio, F., Benvenga, S., et al.: Increased serum thyroglobulin concentrations and impaired thyrotropin response to thyrotropin-releasing hormone in euthyroid subjects with endemic goiter in Sicily: their relation to goiter size and nodularity. J. Endocrinol. Invest. *9:*389–396, 1986.
284. Vickery, A. L.: The diagnosis of malignancy in dyshormonogenetic goitre. Clin. Endocrinol. Metab. *10:*317–335, 1981.
285. Vitti, P., Chiovato, L., et al.: Thyroid stimulating antibody mimics thyrotropin in its ability to desensitize the adenosine 3'5' monophosphate response to acute stimulation in continuously cultured rat thyroid cells (FRT-L5). J. Clin. Endocrinol. Metab. *63:*454–458, 1986.
286. Volpe, R., Edmonds, M., et al.: The pathogenesis of Graves' disease. Mayo Clin. Proc. *47:*824–834, 1972.
287. Wahner, E. W., Cuello, C., et al.: Thyroid carcinoma in an endemic goiter area, Cali, Colombia. Am. J. Med. *40:*566, 1966.
288. Wang, P. W., Hiromatsu, Y., et al.: Immunologically mediated cytotoxicity against human eye muscle cells in Graves' ophthalmopathy. J. Clin. Endocrinol. Metab. *63:*316–322, 1986.
289. Warren, S.: Significance of invasion of blood vessels of the thyroid gland. Arch. Pathol. *11:*255–257, 1931.
290. Warren, S.: Invasion of blood vessels in thyroid cancer. Am. J. Clin. Pathol. *26:*64–65, 1956.
291. Weiss, M., Ingbar, S. H., et al.: Demonstration of a saturable binding site for thyrotropin in Yersinia enterocolitica. Science *219:*1331–1333, 1983.
292. Wick, M. R., and Sawyer, M. D.: Antigenic alterations in autoimmune thyroid diseases. Arch. Pathol. Lab. Med. *113:*77–81, 1989.
293. Wiener, J. D.: Plummer's disease: localized thyroid autoimmunity. J. Endocrinol. Invest. *10:*207–224, 1987.
294. Williams, E. D.: Pathology and natural history. *In:* Thyroid Cancer, Duncan, W. (ed.). Berlin, Springer-Verlag, 1980, pp. 47–55.
295. Williams, E. D., Doniach, I., et al.: Thyroid cancer in an iodide rich area. Cancer *39:*215–222, 1977.
296. Wilson, N. W., Pameakian, H., et al.: Epithelial markers in thyroid carcinoma. An immunoperoxidase study. Histopathology *10:*815–829, 1986.
297. Wolff, J.: Congenital goiter with defective iodide transport. Endocrinol. Rev. *4:*240–254, 1983.
298. Wollman, S. H., and Herveg, J. P.: Thyroid capsule changes during the development of thyroid hyperplasia in the rat. Am. J. Pathol. *93:*639–654, 1978.
299. Wollman, S. H., Herveg, J. P., et al.: Blood capillary enlargement during the development of thyroid hyperplasia in the rat. Endocrinology *103:*2306–2314, 1978.
300. Woolner, L. B.: Thyroid carcinoma: Pathologic consideration with data on prognosis. Sem. Nucl. Med. *1:*481–502, 1971.
301. Woolner, L. B., Beahrs, O. H., et al.: Classification and diagnosis of thyroid carcinoma. Am. J. Surg. *102:*354–387, 1961.
302. Wortsman, J., Premachandra, B. N., et al.: Familial resistance of thyroid hormone associated with decreased transport across the plasma membrane. Ann. Intern. Med. *98:*904–908, 1983.
303. Wu, S. Y., Reggio, R., et al.: Stimulation of thyroidal iodothyronine 5' monodeiodinase by long acting thyroid stimulator (LATS). Acta Endocrinol. *114:*193–200, 1987.
304. Yabu, Y., Amir, S. M., et al.: Heterogeneity of thyroxine binding by serum albumins in normal subjects and patients with familial dysalbuminemic hyperthyroxinemia. J. Clin. Endocrinol. Metab. *60:*451–459, 1985.
305. Young, R. J., Beck, J. S., and Michie, W.: The predictive value of histometry of thyroid tissue in anticipating hypothyroidism after subtotal thyroidectomy for primary thyrotoxicosis. J. Clin. Pathol. *28:*94–98, 1975.
306. Young, R. L., Mazzaferri, E. L., et al.: Pure follicular thyroid carcinoma. Impact of therapy in 214 patients. J. Nucl. Med. *21:*733–737, 1980.
307. Zakarija, M., Garcia, A., and McKenzie, J. M.: Studies on multiple thyroid cell membrane directed antibodies in Graves' disease. J. Clin. Invest. *76:*1885–1891, 1985.
308. Zeliga, J. D., and Wollman, S. H.: Microhemorrhage in the hyperplastic thyroid gland of the rat. Am. J. Pathol. *85:*317–332, 1976.
309. Zellmann, H. E.: Iatrogenic and factitious thyroidal disease. Med. Clin. N. Amer. *63:*329–335, 1979.
310. Zonana, J., and Rimoin, D. L.: Genetic disorders of the thyroid. Med. Clin. N. Amer. *59:*1263–1274, 1975.

MEDULLARY CARCINOMA

10

Although some recent articles have cast doubt on the dual histogenesis of thyroid neoplasms (follicular derived and C cell derived) by implicating a common precursor stem cell for these lesions,[68, 166, 205, 206, 284, 287, 325, 355, 414, 450] the evidence is not yet totally conclusive.[192, 279] From the practical standpoint, therefore, this chapter devoted predominantly to medullary carcinoma and its relatives considers the status of these investigations as preliminary; the discussions therefore reflect the theory of origin of medullary carcinoma from C cells.

Topics discussed in this chapter are outlined in Table 10–1.

INTRODUCTION AND BACKGROUND

For decades, physiologists recognized that serum calcium is carefully maintained within narrow limits. The major factor known to be involved in calcium homeostasis was parathyroid hormone, which raised serum calcium levels. Analogy to other endocrine systems suggested that another factor (? factors) should exist which would antagonize and balance the effects of parathyroid hormone. Hence, a calcium-lowering hormone was sought. In the early 1960's, several groups of investigators, including biochemists, physiologists, and endocrinologists, discovered the calcium-lowering hormone and named it calcitonin.[19, 73, 90, 132, 142, 156, 200, 385] At first it was unclear whether the source of this substance was actually the parathyroid, the thyroid, the thymus or any combination of these;[93] hence some articles refer to thyrocalcitonin to indicate that hormone produced in the thyroid.[23, 143, 144, 156, 201, 362] Numerous experiments disclosed that the major source of calcitonin is the thyroid; hence the term calcitonin was substituted for thyrocalcitonin. (As discussed below, calcitonin-containing cells and measurable hormone levels can be found normally and in small amounts in other tissues.)

Some of the physiologic actions of calcitonin are known; this hormone acts at the levels of the bone, the kidney, and the gastrointestinal tract, and at each site

Table 10–1. C Cell Lesions and Medullary Carcinoma

C cells
Medullary thyroid carcinoma and variants
C cell adenoma
C cell hyperplasia
Mixed medullary and follicular carcinoma

the effect is to lower serum calcium.[17, 177, 200, 201] Thus in the bone calcitonin inhibits bone resorption, although it apparently acts independently of parathyroid hormone. In the kidney, which contains receptors specific for calcitonin, the hormone increases excretion of calcium and phosphate. At the level of the gastrointestinal tract, calcitonin inhibits calcium absorption. Experiments indicate that the most important of these three effects is on the skeleton.[278, 362, 432] Despite the data that have accumulated on the effects of this hormone, it plays a minor role in the maintenance of calcium homeostasis in the adult human (when compared to the effects of parathyroid hormone and vitamin D metabolites).[155, 347]

The question of what factors control the secretion of calcitonin has been at least partially answered. In animal studies, hypercalcemia, especially if acute, causes increased release of the hormone.[71, 133, 241] Whether chronic hypercalcemia affects secretion is still poorly understood. (See C cell hyperplasia—below.) In rats, thyroid stimulating hormone (TSH) can produce increases in calcitonin levels; the mechanism of action of TSH is not clear. (Calcitonin can conversely inhibit TSH secretion.[504])

The relationship between the newly identified hormone and its cell of origin in the thyroid was subsequently recognized.

At about the same time, pathologists were defining the morphologic parameters of the tumor now known as medullary carcinoma.[150, 189, 190, 207, 264] Certainly the tumor existed before 1959,[150, 207, 264] when the classic description of the lesion was published by Hazard et al.[190] Horn had reported the tumor eight years earlier but the name medullary carcinoma was not used by him.[207] This neoplasm had been previously included among spindle cell anaplastic cancers, or small cell carcinomas of the thyroid.[150] In 1967, Williams proposed that medullary carcinoma might be derived from the C cell and predicted that if the C cell was the source of calcitonin, the tumors might also produce this hormone.[476]

As we now understand, he was correct. Over the next decade, medullary carcinoma was recognized as C cell derived,[189, 307, 335, 348, 477, 487] diagnosed by calcitonin assay clinically[5, 6, 23, 43, 88, 100, 104, 120, 130, 134, 147, 223, 302, 357–359, 408, 409, 416, 421, 436, 437, 440, 456, 462–465, 467] and immunostaining pathologically.[14, 63, 102, 130, 145, 181, 261, 399] Sporadic and familial cases were defined.[21, 56, 57, 75, 76, 78–80, 82, 96, 97, 124, 127, 128, 188, 199, 215, 216, 247, 252, 253, 293, 295, 305, 329, 331, 386, 388–390, 398, 406, 420, 453, 466, 473] In addition, the tumor was found to produce other hormones and proteins which gave rise to a variety of clinical effects and symptom complexes.[131, 141, 304, 374, 419, 431, 447, 480] In familial cases, precursor and preinvasive lesions were recognized and provocative tests for identifying these were developed.[21, 57, 74–76, 78–80, 82, 96, 110, 146, 148, 154, 172, 175, 181, 188, 199, 223, 226, 232, 249, 253, 273, 283, 285, 302, 305, 346, 382, 384, 386, 388, 392, 416, 420, 437] Genetic analyses identified defects in familial cases and allowed for a better understanding of the epidemiology and etiology of the tumors and associated lesions.[15, 222, 453, 464, 466, 467, 478, 487]

Finally, pathologic studies defined a myriad of histologic patterns in these tumors; immunostaining and *in vitro* experiments showed the numerous substances which these lesions may produce, molecular probes defined the genetic makeup of the tumor cells, and clinicopathologic studies of large groups of affected patients outlined clinical and pathologic prognostic parameters.[13, 24, 56, 62, 85, 94, 101, 111, 122, 127, 130, 140, 169, 171, 197, 203, 232, 247, 272, 328, 376–382, 384, 392, 407, 438, 449, 479, 490, 491]

The problems still to be addressed included (a) the definition of C cell hyperplasia, (b) the question as to whether it is always a precursor to medullary cancer, (c) the problem of identification of tumors of mixed histogenesis, and defining an embryologic and/or anatomic background for such lesions, and (d) from the clinical viewpoint the necessity and frequency of screening and determining the best and most cost-effective screening techniques.

In this chapter, emphasis is placed on the pathologic manifestations of this group of thyroid lesions, and clinical and prognostic information is provided, especially as it pertains to their morphologic expressions.

C CELLS (SO-CALLED PARAFOLLICULAR CELLS) OF THE THYROID

The C cell was perhaps recognized in animal thyroids in the last century, but was confused with follicular derived elements such as oncocytes.[370, 371] Its function was not known.

Synonyms included parenchymatous cell, interfollicular cell, argyrophil cell, light cell, and mitochondrion rich cell[18, 326, 370, 371, 423, 442, 498]; it was Nonidez who coined it the parafollicular cell from his studies in the dog thyroid.[326] Since many of these cells lie within the follicular basement membrane, the preferred term is C cell (for calcitonin-producing cell).[113, 260]

The C cells are apparently derived embryologically from the remnants of the ultimobranchial body and ultimately from the neural crest.[44, 67, 92, 165, 196, 220, 231, 269, 320, 344, 349, 351, 424, 451, 461, 471] In avian and piscine species, most of these cells are found in the ultimobranchial body, which persists as a separate organ and is located outside of the thyroid gland.[91, 210, 211, 242] Numerous biochemical assays and immunohistochemical studies in many different species, including many mammals, have confirmed the close association of these C cells with the ultimobranchial body or its remnants.[67, 227, 322, 323, 348, 351, 445, 446]

In humans, evidence to support the ultimobranchial origin of the C cells is derived from studies of patients with DiGeorge syndrome.[44, 60, 86, 118, 321, 368] The DiGeorge anomaly consists of complete or partial absence of derivatives of the third, fourth, and fifth (fourth-fifth complex) pharyngeal pouches[60, 368, 424]; hence, there are hypoplastic or absent thymus and parathyroid glands. In addition, cardiac anomalies can also be found. Robinson postulated that if C cells were derived from the fifth (or fourth-fifth complex) pouch, these cells would be absent in infants affected with DiGeorge syndrome.[368] The study of Burke et al. supports this hypotheses: only 3 of 11 (27 percent) infants with the DiGeorge anomaly showed immunoreactive C cells in the thyroid, whereas 82 percent of control infants did.[60] Patients with partial defects can have some C cells in their thyroid. Of interest, however, is the finding by Burke et al. that both normals and infants affected with DiGeorge syndrome had normal numbers of calcitonin immunoreactive cells in their bronchi.[60]

The C cells represented one of the hallmarks of the APUD theory of Pearse.[173, 349, 351] The theory considered a variety of cells which were widely dispersed throughout the body as related because of certain morphologic, biochemical, and presumed embryologic similarities. Thus the cells contain membrane-bound secretory granules as seen by electron microscopy, have the capacity for amine precursor uptake and decarboxylation (hence, the eponym, APUD), and produce polypeptide hormones. Although embryologic and anatomic studies have now definitely proved that all the cells included as part of this dispersed system were not neural crest derived,[266, 422] similarities exist among the members and between them and cells of the nervous system.[113] The currently preferred terminology, therefore, for these widely and diffusely dispersed cells is "neuroendocrine" cells.[113, 208, 411]

In mammals, the distribution of C cells varies among species.[89, 243, 335] In some animals, they are distributed throughout the thyroid; in others, including humans, they are found chiefly along the lateral aspects of the thyroid lobes in the upper two-thirds of the gland—the area believed to represent the area of contribution to the thyroid of the ultimobranchial body.[424] Kalisnik et al. have noted by stereologic analysis studies that in mammals, C cells are found in the mid portion of the thyroid lobes where the most active follicles are present.[239] These authors suggest that the C cells may play a role in the regulation of follicular cell function. Wolfe et al. showed excellent correlation between immunohistochemical localization of these cells and calcitonin content of the area of the thyroid in which they were found.[486, 488] The cells are rarely if ever normally found in the poles of the thyroid or in the isthmus. The C cells constitute less than 0.1 percent of the thyroid mass in humans.[190, 371, 486, 488]

By light microscopy, these cells are difficult to identify by routine hematoxylin and eosin stains. They may be confused with tangentially cut follicular cells or even histiocytes. Silver stains or immunostaining discloses these cells in tissue sections.[240, 474] DeLellis and Wolfe indicate that in glutaraldehyde fixed material the C cells are more readily seen since their cytoplasm tends to appear basophilic as compared to the follicular epithelium, which is eosinophilic.[113] The C cells are pale, round to oval elements found singly or in groups of 3 to 5 in an intrafollicular location. Wolfe et al. had suggested from light microscopic evidence that 75 percent of C cells in adults and about 4 to 8 percent in children were interfollicular.[486] Ultrastructural studies have revealed that virtually all of them are situated within the follicular basement membrane. However, their cytoplasm does not abut against the colloid; rather the cytoplasm of the follicular cells intervenes.[113, 486]

Most C cells are round or polygonal and measure up to 40 micra in size. A second type of C cell originally noted by Ljungberg consists of a more spindled shaped element with tapered ends.[282] This second type is apparently more common in adults than in children.[113]

The number of C cells in the thyroid differs according to age.[69, 300, 486, 488] Wolfe et al. have performed careful analyses of this question and identified larger numbers of these cells in infants and children under the age of six than in adults[486, 488]; it has been postulated that the increased calcitonin levels and C cells in the neonatal thyroid may reflect a physiologic role of calcitonin in the developing fetal and neonatal skeleton.[106, 113, 250, 332, 341, 486] Groups of up to six cells can be seen, with as many as 100 cells noted in a low power microscopic field.[162, 486, 488] Most adult glands contain no more than 10 cells in a low power field.[113]

Clusters of C cells in adults have been described in apparently endocrinologically normal adults without evidence of familial tumors. Gibson identified nodular aggregates of these C cells in some normal thyroids[162]; the significance of this finding is unclear but may produce problems in evaluating the upper limit of normal C cell distribution, as discussed below. O'Toole et al. examined thyroid glands from forensic autopsies and attempted to correlate numbers of C cells with age and sex.[343] Although they recognized a trend toward increased numbers of these cells in older individuals (over age 60), they noted that the large standard deviations (caused by wide variations in numbers of cells among the individuals studied) precluded statistical significance. Of note, however, was that this study also identified aggregates or clusters of C cells in older persons; this finding may be related to osteoporosis in older adults, although this is merely a hypothesis at present.

Calcitonin-containing cells have been described in extrathyroidal sites in normal tissues in several species, including humans. Thus, they have been found in thymus, parathyroid, prostate, adrenal medulla, pituitary, and bronchus.[60, 103, 112, 139, 269]

Special stains show that the C cells are argyrophilic, staining with Grimelius and Sevier-Munger techniques.[107, 179, 348] Histochemical studies have shown that they contain cholinesterases, decarboxylases, and dehydrogenases, as do many neuroendocrine cells.[348, 354] They exhibit masked metachromasia with toluidine blue after acid hydrolysis (reflecting content of polypeptides with high content of carboxyl side chains). In addition they exhibit formalin-induced fluorescence following incubation with L-dopa and exposure to formalin vapor.[65, 81, 107, 183]

Ultrastructural studies of C cells have shown that they are intrafollicular in location, and contain the hallmarks of polypeptide-producing cells—membrane-bound neurosecretory granules.[12, 427, 443, 468] Their cytoplasm is filled with many mitochondria and abundant endoplasmic reticulin with lamellar stacking.[51, 110, 113, 129, 442] Both large (250–280 nanometers) and smaller (130 nanometers) granules can be found; both contain calcitonin.[110, 113] These features are identical to the ultrastructural characteristics of medullary carcinoma and hyperplastic C cells.[108, 110] In normal C cells, the larger granules are more numerous than in the cells of medullary carcinoma.[110, 113] Experiments in several animal species have shown degranulation of the C cells in response to acute hypercalcemia.[71, 72, 133, 333, 429]

Immunocytochemical studies of normal C cells have shown that, as expected, they contain calcitonin;[110, 113, 428] indeed, as DeLellis and Wolfe point out,[113] normal C cells tend to stain more intensely than medullary carcinoma cells. In addition, C cells can contain a variety of other factors including somatostatin, calcitonin gene–related peptide, and carcinoembryonic antigen.[111, 113, 257, 274] All these substances and others as well have been identified in medullary carcinomas (see below).

MEDULLARY THYROID CARCINOMA

Epidemiology. Medullary thyroid carcinoma is an unusual type of thyroid neoplasm. Its incidence ranges from 3 to 10 percent of all thyroid malignancies, although in the general population the lower figure is probably more accurate.[149, 197] In institutions wherein kindreds with the familial forms of the disease are followed and treated, the percentage of thyroid cancers that are medullary lesions will be higher (closer to 10 percent).

Medullary carcinoma has been reported in animals (bulls, horses, cows, and rats).[39, 45–47, 59, 265, 288, 334] In some species a multiple endocrine neoplasia syndrome analogous to Sipple's syndrome has been documented.[271, 452]

Etiology. There is no known or suspected etiology for medullary carcinoma. Exogenous factors such as radiation have not been implicated in this disease. However, in a small but significant minority of cases, a genetic basis for the tumor can be identified. It is estimated that 10 to 20 percent of patients with medullary carcinoma have one of the multiple endocrine neoplasia syndromes and a positive family history of thyroid tumors, or evidence of hypercalcemia or pheochromocytoma. There are two syndromes in which medullary carcinoma is a major component: these have been termed multiple endocrine neoplasia, type 2a and type 2b or 3. (See Table 10–2.)

These syndromes are distinguished from the type 1 described by Wermer, in which neoplasms of parathyroid, pituitary, pancreatic islets, and adrenal cortex are present.[50, 188] Originally termed multiple endocrine adenomatosis, or MEA, it

Table 10–2. Multiple Endocrine Neoplasia Syndromes*

MEN 2a (Sipple's Syndrome)
Medullary thyroid carcinoma
Adrenal pheochromocytoma
Parathyroid hyperplasia
Associated precursor lesions:
C cell hyperplasia
Adrenal medullary hyperplasia
MEN 2b (MEN 3)
Medullary thyroid carcinoma
Adrenal pheochromocytoma
Mucosal neuromas
Gastrointestinal ganglioneuromas
Musculoskeletal abnormalities
Melanosis
Associated precursor lesions:
C cell hyperplasia
Adrenal medullary hyperplasia
MEN 1 (Wermer's Syndrome)
Parathyroid hyperplasia
Pituitary adenoma
Pancreatic islet cell tumors (benign; malignant)
Adrenal cortical adenomas

*Variants of these syndromes exist and include, among others, families with medullary carcinoma and parathyroid disease but without pheochromocytoma; MEN 2b with adenomatous polyposis of the colon; patients with parts of MEN 1 and MEN 2a but with paragangliomas; medullary carcinoma with nesidioblastosis of the pancreas; C cell hyperplasia and pheochromocytoma without medullary carcinoma; and patients with MEN plus carcinoid tumors.[121, 135, 228, 292, 295, 363]

was recognized that many of the neoplasms which occur in these syndromes are indeed malignant; hence, as Wermer noted,[469] the preferred designation is multiple endocrine neoplasia (MEN).

Clinical Features.[4, 85, 94, 101, 122, 140, 152, 169, 171, 197, 199, 203, 216, 252, 253, 283, 407, 420, 438, 441, 475, 490, 491] The clinical features in both sporadic and familial cases which are symptomatic are similar. Medullary carcinoma can affect patients of any age; most affected individuals are adults, with an average age of about 50 years. However, in familial cases, children can be affected; also in these instances, the age at diagnosis tends to be younger than in the sporadic cases (mean age: about 20 years versus 50 years).

Although in the sporadic variety, there is a slight female predominance as in most thyroid cancers, in medullary carcinoma the ratio of female to male is lower, about 1.5:1. In familial cases, since an autosomal dominant mode of inheritance is present, the sex ratio is equal.

Most patients will present with a thyroid nodule which is painless but firm. In up to 50 percent of cases, obvious nodal metastases will be present at the time of diagnosis. Distant metastases, such as to lung, bone, or liver, may also be noted initially in about 15 to 25 percent of cases. When the tumor produces excess hormone other than calcitonin, the presenting symptoms may be related to that hormone hypersecretion; as an example, the patient with an adrenocorticotropin (ACTH) producing medullary carcinoma may present as Cushing's syndrome.[167, 234, 304, 431, 481] Williams et al.[480] and others[245, 246] have noted the frequent (up to 30 percent) symptom of diarrhea. Although excess calcitonin can apparently produce this symptom,[100] some studies suggest that medullary carcinoma can also secrete prostaglandins, which may be responsible for the diarrhea.[480]

In familial cases, the presenting symptom complex may be related to other associated lesions, such as renal stones in hyperparathyroidism, or severe hypertension caused by a pheochromocytoma.

In those patients in whom the presenting problem is merely a thyroid mass, the history may indicate that the mass had been present for a long time—even many years before the patient came for treatment. In other instances, the mass may be of relatively recent onset and may have grown rapidly.

Genetics. Numerous studies have shown that MEN 2a is inherited as an autosomal dominant disorder with a high degree of penetrance.[25, 30, 124, 127, 157, 274] Jackson et al. have postulated that the underlying endocrine hyperplasia (of C cells and/or adrenal medulla) results from genetic mutation;[222] a second somatic mutation is needed to further transform the initially mutated cell into a cancer.[25, 222, 353, 478]

Recent studies have shown that the gene responsible for familial medullary carcinoma is located on chromosome 10.[298, 403, 404]

Chromosomal abnormalities are common in medullary carcinoma cells; specific marker chromosome anomalies remain to be defined.[383, 434, 492]

Associations. As noted above, in the familial forms there are associated endocrine and/or neuroendocrine lesions.

Sipple in 1961 described a patient with pheochromocytoma and thyroid adenocarcinoma which he considered undifferentiated.[406] Since that time many series have defined this syndrome as familial (transmitted as an autosomal dominant with an almost complete penetrance), and consisting of the following lesions: medullary thyroid cancer and C cell hyperplasia, adrenal pheochromocytoma and adrenal medullary hyperplasia, and parathyroid hyperplasia (Sipple's syndrome, MEN 2 or 2a).[37, 82, 97, 213, 225, 273, 285, 293, 295, 305, 363, 386, 388–390] Although most affected patients will have the complete syndrome, not every affected patient need manifest each of these lesions, and certain individuals in certain families may show clinical evidence of only one affected organ or system. The medullary carcinoma is the most clinically virulent of the tumors that these patients can have; however, if the patients with pheochromocytomas are not treated for them, they may die of consequences of hypertension from these histologically "benign" tumors.[420, 482]

Multiple endocrine neoplasia type 2b consists of medullary thyroid carcinoma and C cell hyperplasia, pheochromocytoma and adrenal medullary hyperplasia and mucosal neuromas, gastrointestinal ganglioneuromas, and musculoskeletal abnormalities.[21, 22, 41, 42, 56, 57, 74–76, 78–80, 96, 137, 141, 148, 172, 262, 329, 352, 388, 398, 453, 466, 473] These patients may or may not have familial disease (over 50 percent do)[115]; some arise apparently as spontaneous mutations. These patients, however, have biologically aggressive medullary carcinoma and may succumb to metastases at an early age; not all affected individuals have such prognostically unfavorable tumors.[262]

This syndrome shows some overlap with von Recklinghausen's disease, since in neurofibromatosis similar lesions to those in MEN 2b are found in the gastrointestinal tract and pheochromocytomas are common.[482] Nerve growth factor has been identified in some medullary carcinomas of these patients; it has been postulated that this product of the tumor may be responsible for the neural lesions seen in the MEN 2b patients.[36, 95, 115] However, the neural lesions often precede by many years the development of medullary cancer.[78] Some of the nonfamilial cases of MEN 2b may present with manifestations of gastrointestinal disease, with alternating diarrhea and constipation; misdiagnosis of Hirschsprung's disease, Crohn's colitis, or other intrinsic bowel disease may be rendered unless the clinician recognizes the characteristic facies of these patients due to the mucosal neuromas.

As noted in Table 10–2, variants and permutations of these two major syndromes have been described.

The pathologist may contribute to the determination of familial rather than sporadic disease if, upon examining a medullary carcinoma of the thyroid, he or she notes multifocal and/or bilateral tumors and the presence of C cell hyperplasia.[128, 131, 145, 305] Some studies but not all have claimed that the pathologic appearance of the thyroid in a patient with medullary cancer can distinguish familial from sporadic disease, since C cell hyperplasia should be found only in the former situation.[128, 131, 145] Unfortunately, because the histologic definition of C cell hyperplasia is still problematical except in florid cases (see below), other studies have found that the prediction of familial or sporadic medullary carcinoma from pathologic examination of the thyroid cannot always be accurate.[128, 131]

Although it is beyond the scope of this monograph, a brief mention will be made of the adrenal and parathyroid lesions seen in these syndromes. Adrenal medullary hyperplasia may occur as a sporadic lesion at any age or in either sex. However, the lesion is characteristic in the multiple endocrine neoplasia syndromes type 2 where it represents the precursor lesion to pheochromocytoma.[79, 80, 226] The lesion may be asymptomatic or may present with signs and symptoms of pheochromocytoma, including episodic hypertension. In the syndrome, this lesion and the pheochromocytomas are multiple and bilateral.[79, 80, 114, 459, 483]

Grossly and histologically, in adrenal medullary hyperplasia the medulla is expanded and nodules may be found.[79, 80, 114] The individual medullary cells are large and may show pleomorphism similar to that in the cells in a well-developed pheochromocytoma. For early cases, morphometric measurements estimating medullary weight and medullary:cortical ratios are required.[114]

The parathyroid hyperplasia seen in these syndromes is believed to represent a genetically defined event and not a response to hypercalcitoninemia,[281, 439] since in some patients the hyperparathyroidism precedes the development of calcitonin elevations.

All four parathyroid glands are affected in a process similar to nodular or diffuse chief cell hyperplasia; however, the lesions may manifest involvement of only one parathyroid gland at any one time, leading to the erroneous diagnosis of an isolated parathyroid adenoma. Carney et al. indicate that in their series of multiple endocrine neoplasia type 2b patients, the parathyroid abnormalities were minimal.[76] In classic Sipple's syndrome, the hyperparathyroidism is clinically and pathologically more significant.[76, 278]

Pathology of Medullary Carcinoma[2, 37, 85, 145, 149, 152, 169, 171, 189, 190, 197, 215, 216, 232, 282, 301, 328, 382, 384, 392, 420, 449, 475–477, 479, 490, 491]

Since the morphologic expressions of the sporadic and familial are similar, they will be discussed as a group. The major differences in the pathologic manifestations between sporadic and familial cases include the multifocal and bilateral tumors present and the C cell hyperplasia commonly seen in the latter. Some studies suggest that glandular and follicular variants of medullary carcinoma are more common in the familial setting.[145–147]

Gross Pathology (Fig. 10–1, *A* and *B*). The tumor is usually located in the area of highest C cell concentration, i.e., the lateral upper two-thirds of the gland. In familial cases, multiple small nodules may be detected grossly and, rarely, lesions in the isthmus may be found.[223] The tumors range in size from barely visible to several centimeters. The former variety is found in familial cases, in which the tumor is identified only through biochemical screening.[223, 273, 487]

Many medullary carcinomas are grossly circumscribed although not encapsu-

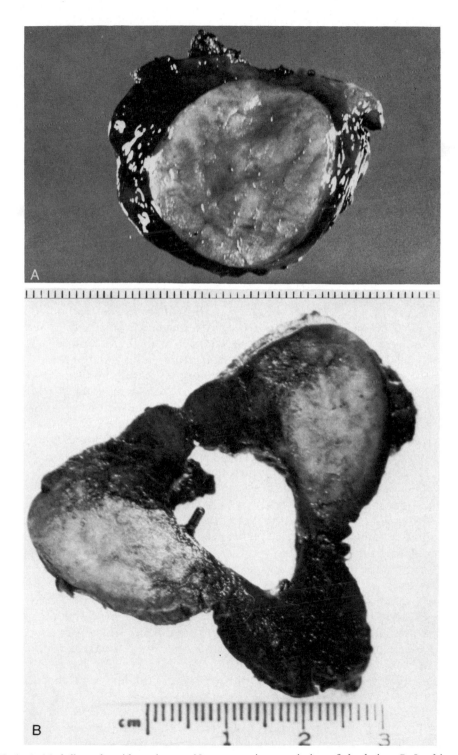

Figure 10–1. *A,* Medullary thyroid carcinoma. Note gross circumscription of the lesion. *B,* In this example the tumor is infiltrative.

lated; some show infiltrative borders. They have a white or white-gray color, but some are yellow or tan. The tumors are firm but rarely are hard. Granular calcification can occur; rarely, bone formation is found.[189, 282] Some tumors show necrosis and hemorrhage, but this is rare unless the lesion is large, poorly differentiated and often infiltrative in macroscopic appearance.

Histology (Figs. 10–2 to 10–4). The only consistent statement that can be made about the histologic appearance of medullary thyroid carcinoma is that the appearance is extremely variable. Table 10–3 lists the descriptive terms applied to describe these tumors. I have divided them into "variations in pattern" and "variations in product"; the reader should recognize that the two lists are not mutually exclusive, however—hence, one can have a giant cell medullary carcinoma that contains mucin.

Variations in Pattern

The typical medullary carcinoma may be microscopically circumscribed or, more likely, is freely infiltrating into the surrounding thyroid. The pattern of growth is of tumor cells arranged in nests separated by varying amounts of stroma. A prominent small capillary vasculature may be found permeating through the stroma (Fig. 10–2).

The tumor nests are composed of round, oval, or angulated cells or of spindle cells with tapered ends; in some tumors both round and spindled cell foci are found. Plasmacytoid cells with eccentric nuclei are also seen; this is especially prominent in fine needle aspirate samples from these tumors.[256] Although the cytology of the tumor cells is often uniform and quite bland in the classical variant, there often is isolated cellular pleomorphism, with the finding of enlarged nuclei or even multinucleated cells. The nuclei are uniform, round-to-oval in most of the tumor except for these atypical elements; the nuclear/cytoplasmic ratio is low. Intranuclear cytoplasmic inclusions are commonly noted.[256] Mitoses can be seen, but this is a variable feature. The cytoplasm has ill-defined margins and may appear granular; it may be amphophilic or eosinophilic.

Necrosis is rare in the usual medullary carcinoma.

The tumor stroma, which is composed of collagen, may contain masses of homogeneous eosinophilic material with the staining properties of amyloid. Calcification, often in the amyloid, can be found; some calcium deposits may be found in tumor nests and resemble psammoma bodies, although lamellations are not always present.

The tumors commonly invade lymphatics and veins in the thyroid and beyond the gland as well.

Variations in the histologic patterns of medullary carcinoma have been briefly discussed in a number of reports on series of cases, or individual patterns have been detailed by some authors. One of the most complete but concise histologic descriptions of common medullary carcinoma variants can be found in a clinicopathologic review of medullary cancer by Saad et al.[382] These authors divided their tumors into the following categories: classical, insular, trabecular, epithelial, and amyloid rich.

The *classical* pattern consists of uniform round-to-oval cells with eosinophilic or amphophilic granular cytoplasm admixed with spindle-shaped cells; these epithelial cells are arranged in nests separated by fibrous stroma containing amyloid (Figs. 10–2 and 10–3).

The *insular* variety resembles classical carcinoid and shows nodules of tumors separated by strands of a vascular fibrous stroma.

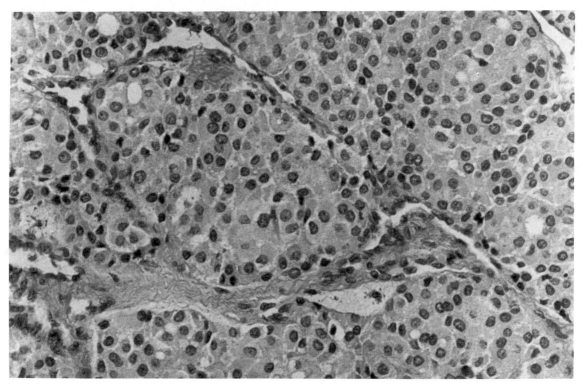

Figure 10–2. Classic medullary thyroid carcinoma with nests of uniform round to oval cells. × 200. H & E.

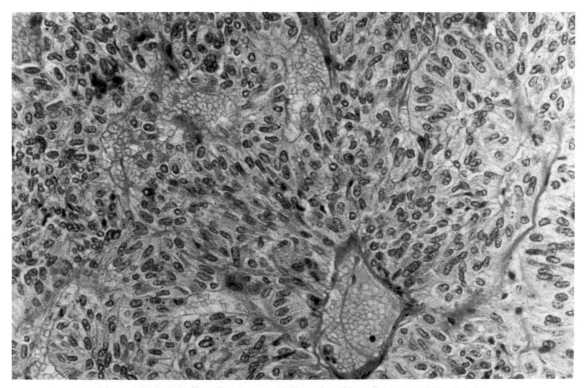

Figure 10–3. Spindle cell pattern medullary thyroid carcinoma. × 200. H & E.

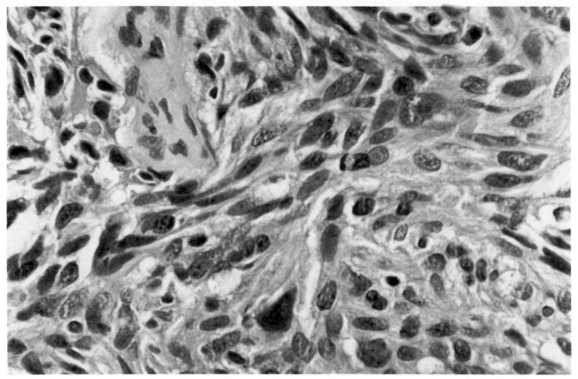

Figure 10–4. Medullary thyroid carcinoma—spindle cell pattern with pleomorphism. × 350. H & E.

The *trabecular* pattern shows ribbons of tumor cells, often large and polygonal but occasionally spindled, forming cords of two to three cells thick.

An *epithelial* pattern was defined by Saad et al. as sheets and masses of tumor cells with scant stroma, mimicking a poorly differentiated carcinoma.[382]

The amyloid rich type is discussed below.

Encapsulated medullary carcinomas can occur; in these, the gross encapsulation is recapitulated microscopically. Some of these tumors have fibrous stroma and contain amyloid; however, others do not. These lesions may show a zellballen pattern and have been mistaken for intrathyroidal paragangliomas.[248, 316] In addition, the recently described follicular derived hyalinizing trabecular adenoma or paraganglioma-like adenoma of the thyroid[54, 77] can be mistaken for encapsulated medullary cancer. The latter have been included under the term "atypical adenoma" of the thyroid in the older literature. The report of Mendelsohn and

Table 10–3. Variations of Medullary Thyroid Carcinoma

Variations in Pattern	Variations in Product
Classical	Mucin-producing
Carcinoid-like	Melanin-producing
Trabecular	Amyloid-rich
Carcinoma-like	Amyloid-free
Encapsulated type	Multihormone-producing
Papillary	Calcitonin-free
Glandular or follicular	
Giant cell	
Small cell	
Clear cell	
Oncocytic	
(Other)	

Oertel on a series of encapsulated thyroid lesions classified as atypical adenomas showed that many of these were medullary cancers containing immunoreactive calcitonin.[308] The follow-up in these encapsulated medullary carcinomas indicates that they have a more benign prognosis than usual medullary tumors. The question of whether such lesions should be designated C cell adenoma is discussed below.

Other patterns of medullary carcinoma have often formed the basis of specific reports.

The *papillary* variant can occur in two forms: the more common pseudopapillary type and a tumor forming true papillae.[236] Since many medullary cancers are extremely cellular and the tumor nests contain little stroma, incomplete fixation of the tissue can produce artifactual splitting of the tissue and the formation of pseudopapillary structures.[189, 441] However, Kakudo et al. described two cases in which the epithelial cells were arranged on fibrovascular stalks:[236] hence true papillae were formed (Fig. 10–5). These were associated with solid areas in the lesions which were characteristic of the classical medullary tumor. Electron microscopic examination showed characteristic findings for medullary differentiation; plasma calcitonin was elevated in both patients, and in one instance the calcitonin content of the tumor was increased (27 microgram/gram tissue).

The differential diagnosis of this lesion is with classic papillary (follicular derived) carcinoma; the clear nuclei of the latter are extremely useful in this distinction. Certainly immunostaining is important also.

Harach and Williams defined the *glandular* (*tubular, follicular*) subtype of medullary carcinoma in 1983.[187] These tumors showed large areas of "tubular" or follicular differentiation within the neoplasm, not solely at the periphery of the tumor (the latter could be interpreted as trapped normal thyroid gland). Immu-

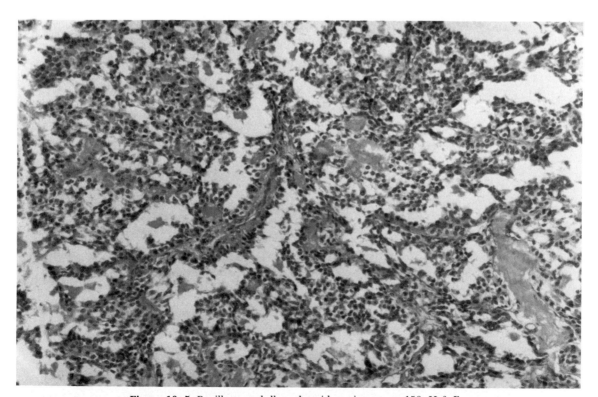

Figure 10–5. Papillary medullary thyroid carcinoma. × 150. H & E.

nostaining showed the presence of calcitonin in all three of their cases, and electron microscopy was confirmatory. Thyroglobulin immunoreactivity was found only at the edges of the lesion in trapped residual normal thyroid follicles.

Giant cell medullary carcinoma has been described by Kakudo et al.[235] Although random nuclear and/or cellular pleomorphism can be found in classic medullary cancer (Fig. 10–4), these giant cell lesions have a predominant pattern of large cell cancer, with some cells resembling choriocarcinoma.[235] (These giant cells are obviously neoplastic and should not be confused with foreign body giant cells often seen in the stromal amyloid.) However, as Kakudo et al. noted,[235] these tumors should not be classified as anaplastic carcinoma of giant cell type,[296, 306, 324, 503] since the former show characteristics of medullary cancer—including intermingling with classic medullary cancer pattern of tumor, infrequent mitoses, nuclear invaginations of cytoplasm, and amyloid stroma.[235] As discussed in Chapter 11, it is very rare for anaplastic thyroid cancers to show evidence of medullary differentiation by either electron microscopy or immunostaining. The prognosis of the giant cell medullary carcinoma is better than that of anaplastic carcinoma; although many of the patients have died of metastases, the survival is measured in years, not months.

The *small cell* variant of medullary carcinoma is composed of relatively small cells with little cytoplasm. The size of the cells is similar to the intermediate cell type of small cell lung cancer. Amyloid is rarely seen in these tumors; necrosis is more common than in most other variants. Some authors believe that the prognosis is less favorable in small cell type than in other variants.[2]

Landon and Ordonez[263] described a *clear* cell tumor in a middle-aged woman, which they documented by immunostaining to represent a medullary carcinoma.

Harach and Bergholm recently described a small series of medullary carcinomas which had cytologic features of *oncocytic* follicular tumors.[186] Granular cytoplasm in large eosinophilic almost plate-like cells had been noted in some medullary tumors, and these could be misdiagnosed as Hürthle cell lesions.[278] Harach and Bergholm illustrated that the characteristics of these tumors placing them in the medullary group included prominent nuclear cytoplasmic invagination, amyloid, argyrophilia, and, of course, immunostaining results.[186]

Albores-Saavedra et al. described one case of medullary carcinoma with oncocytic cells and considered this as an expansion of the myriad patterns medullary thyroid carcinoma can present.[1] In addition, these authors reported a medullary cancer with *squamous* differentiation and another case in which clear nuclei reminiscent of classical papillary thyroid carcinoma were identified.[1, 116a]

Variations in Product

Mucin production documented by mucicarmine stain can be found in up to 40 percent of medullary cancers.[138, 166, 499] In most cases, the mucin is found extracellularly; however, in 8 to 10 percent intracytoplasmic mucin can be found.[499] It is thus important to recall that the old dictum that thyroid cancers do not contain mucicarminophilic material is incorrect; a pathologist faced with a cervical lymph node containing mucin positive cancer must consider the thyroid and specifically (although not exclusively) medullary carcinoma.

Melanin production by medullary carcinoma was documented by Marcus et al.,[294] and other cases have been described.[254, 297, 360] These lesions are very rare, but serve to strengthen the theory of overlap between endocrine cells and neural crest derivatives. (Pigmented thymic carcinoids, pulmonary carcinoids, and others are lesions supporting this relationship.[20, 119, 176, 202]) In these cases, black areas can be seen grossly; the pigment stains as melanin; premelanosomes can be found in the tumor cells by electron microscopic examination.[294] The case reported by Kimura et al.[254] is unique in that the tumor contained, in addition to pigmented zones, two separate areas—one classic medullary and another glandular, each staining for calcitonin and carcinoembryonic antigen, and not for thyroglobulin.

Amyloid rich medullary carcinoma may be confused with amyloid goiter—a mass of amyloid found in the thyroid in patients with systemic amyloidosis.[224, 251] In the former, careful search will disclose tumor cells focally admixed with the masses of amyloid. Conversely, about 25 percent of medullary cancers do not contain demonstrable amyloid (at least at the light microscopic but also in some at the ultrastructural level). These *amyloid free* variants, documented as medullary lesions by immunostaining and electron microscopic studies,[328] may be biologically more aggressive tumors than classic medullary cancer.

Numerous studies have proved the production of *many polypeptides,* and other factors by medullary carcinoma. These studies have either disclosed the production of these products by medullary cancer cells grown in vitro, by immunostaining, or by in-situ hybridization.[14, 204, 221, 261, 289, 399, 449] The list of factors secreted or found in medullary carcinoma includes but is not limited to*: calcitonin,[13, 26, 27, 35, 62, 63, 66, 70, 83, 98, 100, 102, 123, 125, 168, 181, 191, 365, 393, 409] carcinoembryonic antigen,[13, 14, 35, 61, 62, 102, 181, 217, 218, 365, 394, 396, 433] ACTH,[38, 66, 70, 83, 102, 117, 167, 234, 304, 374] prostaglandins,[180] beta endorphin,[15, 337, 375] bradykinin, synaptophysin,[84, 174] chromogranins,[11, 255, 291, 336, 391, 402, 458] katacalan,[7] calcitonin gene related peptide,[123, 126, 163, 182, 214, 230, 275, 276, 318, 361, 418, 502] bombesin or gastrin releasing peptide,[161, 209, 299, 425, 494] somatostatin,[35, 70, 83, 243, 426] prolactin-like activity,[38] vasoactive intestinal peptide, substance P,[238, 410] human chorionic gonadotropin,[493] serotonin,[70] mucin,[499] histaminase,[24, 26, 28, 136, 272, 307] dopa decarboxylase,[16, 28, 272] proopiomelanocortin,[417] enolases,[290, 342, 500, 501] C-thyroglobulin,[244] and thyroglobulin itself.[109, 204, 449] (See also below—mixed tumors.) In some tumors many of the substances are made; production of more than one factor by the same neoplastic cells is also well documented.[70, 327]

It seems impossible that one could define a tumor as medullary carcinoma if it did not produce calcitonin (*calcitonin-free* medullary carcinoma). However, occasional lesions (and often these are small cell type) do not contain immunoreactive calcitonin. In order to accept a calcitonin-free tumor of the thyroid as a medullary carcinoma, it should arise in a familial setting or occur in a thyroid with unequivocal C cell hyperplasia. Immunoreactivity for calcitonin gene related peptide would add proof of the medullary nature of such a lesion.[2, 261, 399]

(It should be noted that there exist occasional small cell cancers of thyroid origin which can neither be pigeonholed into C cell or follicular origin; these very rare lesions if truly primary in the thyroid, may be categorized as small cell carcinoma, although they may represent small cell medullary cancers without calcitonin arising in a nonfamilial setting.)

The frequency of the various patterns is difficult to estimate from the literature. Some varieties, such as the clear cell medullary cancer, consist of one well-documented case. However, the extreme variability in proven medullary tumors accentuates the need for appropriate immunostaining for both thyroglobulin and calcitonin in any thyroid tumor which is not easily classifiable.

Special Studies

Special stains in medullary carcinoma show small amounts of glycogen in the tumor cells; alcian blue and even mucicarmine-positive material can show intra-

---

*Since new ones are reported virtually daily.

and extracellular mucin in some tumors.[499] Formalin-induced fluorescence can be demonstrated.[183, 319]

The stromal amyloid can be stained with Congo red, metachromatic stains such as crystal violet, and thioflavin T.[107]

Histochemical stains indicate masked metachromasia when stained with toluidine blue after acid hydrolysis. Argyrophilia can be demonstrated by Grimelius or Sevier-Munger methods.[107, 189, 278, 319]

Immunostaining. As discussed above, many peptides and other substances can be demonstrated in medullary cancer cells. Most reports indicate that medullary carcinoma stains for low molecular weight keratins.[261]

Ultrastructural studies of medullary cancer[48, 52, 212, 229, 233, 237, 310–312, 395] have shown a resemblance of the tumor cells to C cells. The tumor cells contain nuclei with clumped chromatin, lamellar arrangement of the rough endoplasmic reticulum, conspicuous Golgi with associated granules, a complement of mitochondria, and the characteristic neurosecretory granules. These are composed of a central electron-dense core, surrounded by a clear space and a single delimiting membrane. Immunoelectron microscopic studies have proved that these granules contain calcitonin.[311, 312] In the extracellular stroma, amyloid fibrils may be present.

Flow cytometric analyses of small series of medullary thyroid carcinoma are available[435]; as expected, some tumors show diploid cell populations and about 40 to 50 percent contain aneuploid cells. Some of the reported series indicate that the latter are associated with a more guarded prognosis.[392, 435]

Other studies. Lloyd has reviewed the technique of in-situ hybridization and specifically the data on its use in the medullary carcinoma.[289] Such studies confirm that in the tumor cells and in normal human C cells the gene for calcitonin and calcitonin gene related peptide are found within the same cell.[418, 502] Recently Noel et al. reported that the genes for both calcitonin and thyroglobulin have been localized to the same cells in mixed tumors of the thyroid[325]; this exciting work awaits confirmation.

Cytology of Medullary Carcinoma. Reports of the appearance of medullary carcinoma in fine needle aspiration samples are few but disclose several common features of the tumor which should lead to a definitive or "highly suspicious" diagnosis of medullary cancer.[159, 256] The pattern of medullary cancer in smears is very variable, reflecting the tumor's variable histology. The aspirate is usually a cellular sample and the cells are often obviously malignant. The cells occur as isolated elements or as loosely cohesive groups. Neither a papillary nor a follicular pattern is seen. The cells can be oval, round, spindled, or plasmacytoid. In some cells the cytoplasm is granular; immunostaining will demonstrate calcitonin.

The nuclei of medullary carcinoma are eccentrically located in the cell; occasional binucleation is seen. Intranuclear invaginations of cytoplasm are characteristic (Fig. 10–6).

In the background of a smear of medullary cancer, finely granular acellular material can be found which represents amyloid. Although this cannot be definitively differentiated from colloid in routine preparations, if medullary tumor is suspected, stains for amyloid can be performed.[159, 256, 387]

Amyloid

About 50 to 80 percent of medullary carcinomas contain stromal amyloid. This feature was stressed as important to the diagnosis in the initial descriptions of the lesion.[189, 190] Amyloid was considered necessary for the diagnosis until Norman et al. and others[328, 454] identified immunoreactive calcitonin and classic electron

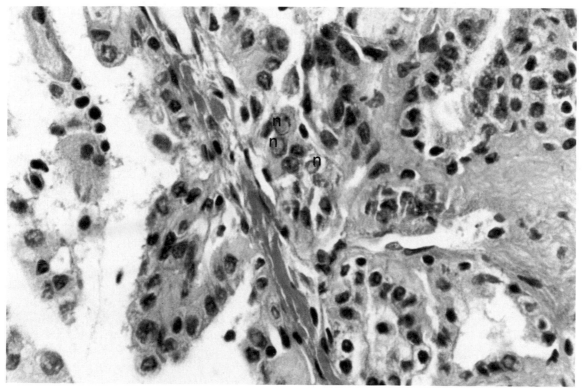

Figure 10–6. Medullary thyroid carcinoma—note intranuclear cytoplasmic invaginations (*n*), × 300. H & E.

microscopic features in amyloid-free tumors, confirming the existence of medullary cancer without amyloid.

Numerous studies of the amyloid in endocrine tumors indicate that it differs from plasma cell dyscrasia associated amyloid, which is a product of immunoglobulin light chains.[164, 350] Endocrine amyloid is found in tumors which produce certain hormones, including calcitonin; the common feature of these hormones seems to be that they are initially secreted or manufactured as prohormones or preprohormones. The protein in medullary cancer and other amyloids shares a conformation of rigid fibrils arranged in a beta-pleated sheet structure; the latter bestows on the amyloid its characteristic staining properties (apple green birefringence when stained with Congo red and examined with polarized light[470]).

Biochemical and physiochemical data indicate that the medullary carcinoma amyloid is a fibril protein of about 6000 dalton molecular weight[219, 339, 372, 412, 470]; this is twice the molecular mass of calcitonin. The amyloid protein in medullary cancer is believed to be related to or represent procalcitonin, following cleavage of the preprohormone.[10, 470] Immunogold staining has shown immunoreactive calcitonin in the amyloid fibrils of medullary carcinoma.[58]

Differential Diagnosis

From the preceding discussion of variants of medullary carcinoma, it should be obvious to the reader that the differential diagnosis of medullary thyroid cancer includes almost all primary thyroid neoplasms. Hence, it can resemble papillary, follicular, and Hürthle cell neoplasms, hyalinizing trabecular adenoma, and even nonneoplastic amyloid goiter. Since medullary cancer can mimic metastatic carcinoma, this must also be ruled out.

It is essential that whenever a pathologist is faced with a thyroid lesion which is atypical in appearance or when all the criteria for a particular diagnosis are not present, immunostaining for both thyroglobulin and calcitonin be performed to help in arriving at a definitive diagnosis. It is important to diagnose a thyroid cancer as medullary because of prognostic implications not only for the patient but also the patient's family. The survival rate for medullary carcinoma is in general worse than that for papillary and follicular carcinoma, but much better than that for anaplastic cancer (about 50 percent at five years if all variants and sporadic and familial cases are included).

Follicular Tumors. As noted above, some medullary cancers contain follicles not only at the periphery but within the center of the neoplasm. Some of these lesions have been classified as follicular or mixed medullary and follicular tumors (see mixed tumors—below). The centrally located follicles do not contain thyroglobulin in the follicular variants of medullary cancer, but Kameda et al. demonstrated immunoreactivity for C-thyroglobulin,[244] a product apparently related to calcitonin.

Papillary Carcinoma. Most papillary variants of medullary carcinoma represent artifacts due to poor fixation of the tumor, and, therefore, pseudopapillae. Usually at the better fixed areas or at the edges of the tumor, a diagnosable medullary pattern can be found. Some true papillary medullary cancers do occur. In these, the nuclear changes of true (follicular derived) papillary cancer need to be sought.

Large Cell Tumors. Oncocytic neoplasms of follicular derivation are much more common than the medullary lesions resembling them. In cases that are unusual, immunostaining will have to be relied upon. Anaplastic giant and spindle cell tumors are most often related to follicular neoplasms, not C cells, despite some reports to the contrary.[306, 324, 503] As noted by Kakudo et al., certain features such as amyloid and nuclear invaginations are found in the giant cell medullary carcinomas[235]; these features and appropriate immunostaining results will aid in the diagnosis. Large cell malignant lymphomas rarely cause diagnostic confusion.

Small Cell Tumors. Small cell lymphomas are usually diffusely growing neoplasms that should not easily be mistaken for medullary carcinoma. In such a case, staining for lymphocytic markers should assist in the diagnosis. The insular carcinoma discussed in Chapter 15 has been diagnosed as medullary since in areas it can assume an organoid pattern, follicular since it can produce follicles, and mixed because both patterns may coexist. It has been shown unequivocally to represent a follicular derived tumor; calcitonin immunoreactivity is not found in these lesions.

Hyalinizing Trabecular Adenoma. This curious benign neoplasm demonstrates a zellballen and trabecular pattern in an encapsulated thyroid tumor. Misdiagnosed in the past as atypical adenoma, paraganglioma, and encapsulated medullary carcinoma, it needs to be recognized as a peculiar histologic variant of follicular adenoma.* Immunostaining may be critical to define the lesion.

Prognostic Factors[13, 24, 62, 101, 128, 197, 272, 376–378, 380–382, 392, 407, 449, 479, 490, 491]

A number of studies have examined both clinical and pathologic factors which appear related to prognosis in medullary thyroid carcinoma. Although not all the studies agree on all points, certain factors emerge as important prognostic indicators.

From the clinical standpoint, stage is the most important variable: a tumor confined to the thyroid without nodal or distant metastases is associated with a

*It is possible malignant variants of this tumor will be described in the future.

long survival; most tumors which are intrathyroidal are relatively small, a few centimeters in greatest diameter. Several workers have found that younger patients (under age 40), especially women, fare somewhat better than the whole group of medullary cancer patients.

Patients who are discovered by screening because they are members of affected families often have very small tumors and can be cured by thyroidectomy.[88, 175, 223, 232, 302, 303, 330, 357–359, 384, 397, 408, 416, 436, 437, 440, 456, 462–465, 467, 472] However, even some families whose tumors are not discovered by screening will have lesions which are either extremely indolent or very virulent; this may reflect genetically determined events or poorly defined immunologic factors.[160, 369]

When comparing familial and sporadic cases, a number of investigators have found that patients with Sipple's syndrome tend to have less aggressive tumors than the sporadic group[305]; the patients with multiple endocrine neoplasia type 2b have extremely aggressive lesions and a very low five-year survival rate, less than 5 percent at five years,[247, 331] although not all studies confirm the latter point.[262]

Therapy may also affect outlook.[314] The recommended treatment for medullary carcinoma is total thyroidectomy.[9, 379, 405] Since multifocal disease and multiple foci of the precursor C cell hyperplasia cannot be predicted preoperatively (except in known familial cases in which these findings are expected and total thyroidectomy is undertaken anyway[41–43, 101]), it must be assumed that any patient with such a tumor is at risk for multiple areas of disease in the gland, and therefore complete removal of the gland is necessary.* If thyroidectomy and lymph node sampling remove all gross tumor and if postoperative calcitonin and carcinoembryonic antigen levels remain low, it is possible the patient is cured.[317, 365, 376, 380, 421]

Those patients who have subtotal removal of the tumor or who have known distant metastases, or in whom postoperative calcitonin or carcinoembryonic antigen levels remain elevated, have a guarded prognosis.[62, 378] Some of these patients may live for long periods of time with their tumor—this is especially true in some kindreds with familial medullary cancer in which the affected members seem to have extremely indolent tumors.

Pathologic features which have been related to prognosis include tumor type, amyloid content, pleomorphism, necrosis, and mitotic activity.[215, 267, 479] Small cell medullary carcinomas, those tumors with extensive areas of necrosis and marked cellular pleomorphism, are associated with poor prognosis. Lesions which have uniform cytology, much amyloid, and especially those in which the amyloid shows calcification tend to be indolent tumors.[215] Mendelsohn and Oertel have suggested that patients with encapsulated medullary cancers enjoy prolonged disease free survivals.[308]

Recent studies have shown that immunostaining results have significant predictive value in medullary carcinoma. Thus those tumors which show diffuse and intense calcitonin staining (Fig. 10–7) tend to be indolent and those with little staining behave as rapidly metastasizing lesions.[13, 24, 62, 111, 272, 380–382, 384, 392, 444] Mendelsohn et al. found that calcitonin and carcinoembryonic antigen (CEA) have an even distribution in C cell hyperplasia and medullary carcinoma confined to the thyroid (early medullary carcinoma).[309] In both primary and metastatic sites

---

*Postoperative radioiodine therapy can be administered if it is assumed that small foci of thyroid were not removed and C cell hyperplasia may recur in the residual thyroid tissue. Even though it is doubtful that the C cells take up radioiodine, the nearby thyroid does; it has been calculated that sufficient radioactivity is delivered to the C cells from the normal thyroid nearby to destroy them.[105, 194] Some case reports indicate that hormonal therapy can cause tumor regression in medullary carcinoma.[116, 457, 496]

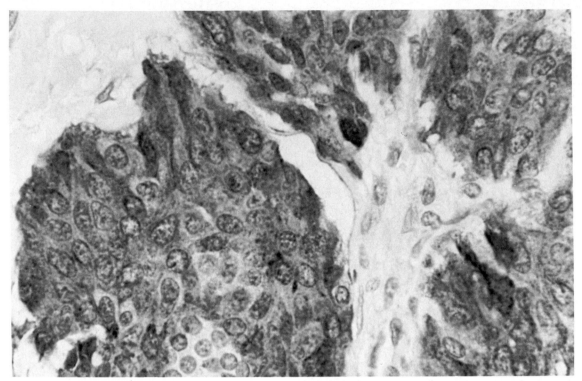

Figure 10–7. Sporadic medullary thyroid carcinoma, immunostained for calcitonin. Note less concentrated immunoreactivity than in Figures 10–9 and 10–10. × 250. Calcitonin immunoperoxidase.

there is an inverse relationship between calcitonin and CEA, with the latter being retained and calcitonin immunoreactivity decreasing as tumor becomes more widely metastatic.[111, 272, 309, 381, 382] The tissue results can be correlated directly with the plasma levels of calcitonin and CEA.[13, 24, 309, 381, 382]

The markers histaminase and dopa decarboxylase that are found in medullary carcinoma were considered to be good indicators of virulence; however, many studies now indicate that the two best predictive markers are calcitonin and CEA.

The study of Schroder et al. found that another important predictive factor is the finding of an aneuploid cell population in the tumor by flow cytometric analysis.[392] This feature was associated with poor outcome.

Hence, it appears that pathologic prognostic indicators in medullary carcinoma include pathologic stage, tumor necrosis, cellular pleomorphism, mitotic activity, immunostaining results (for calcitonin and CEA), and flow cytometric data.

C Cell Adenoma

Rare cases diagnosed and reported as C cell adenoma are found in the literature.[32, 33, 258, 259] All these are grossly encapsulated lesions which, by immunostaining or electron microscopy or both, are C cell lesions. However, as Carney has pointed out,[258] it is probably best to classify such lesions as encapsulated medullary cancers since on occasion such tumors may metastasize, although often after many years of disease-free follow-up.

Mixed Follicular and Medullary Carcinoma

There exists continuing controversy in the literature as to the nature of some unusual thyroid tumors which demonstrate features of both follicular and C cell differentiation. (Follicles are present in the center of the tumor, not only at the invasive edge, but there are areas of the tumor which have a carcinoid-like or spindle cell appearance, suggesting medullary carcinoma.) These tumors, originally reported as isolated cases, show thyroglobulin and calcitonin immunoreactivity and ultrastructural evidence of differentiation along two cell lines.[64, 166, 184, 356, 450] Some of the series of these tumors may have involved confusing trapping of follicles at the invading edge of the medullary carcinoma and diffusion of thyroglobulin into the medullary carcinoma; this may result in diagnoses of mixed tumors showing immunostaining with both hormones. In some series the antibodies used may have given spurious results.[284, 287]

Most of these mixed tumors have been diagnosed in the thyroid.[205, 206, 449] However, a few cases of dual differentiation have been noted in metastatic sites[355, 449]; DeLellis et al. suggest thyroglobulin may get into cervical lymph nodes via lymphatic pathways from a gland that because of tumor may have destroyed follicles and release of thyroglobulin.[109] However, in a few reported cases, dual differentiation has been found in metastatic sites away from the neck;[449] hence, this cannot be explained away. Harach and Bergholm,[186] LiVolsi,[279] and Hedinger et al.[192] still suggest caution in making a diagnosis of mixed thyroid carcinoma. Indeed, the second edition of the WHO classification of thyroid tumors indicates "the identification of a single unexpected peptide in an otherwise typical tumor is not used in other sites to define a separate subtype of tumor. The identification of immunoreactive thyroglobulin in a tumor which is otherwise a typical calcitonin positive medullary carcinoma is therefore not considered adequate to establish the diagnosis of mixed medullary-follicular carcinoma."[192]

The debate will, of course, continue. Evidence on both sides will be accrued. For instance, the recent report by Noel et al. showing coexpression of thyroglobulin and calcitonin gene in a mixed carcinoma[325] is extremely intriguing. Further developments are anticipated.

C Cell Hyperplasia

The term C cell hyperplasia has been challenged by Carney et al. who state correctly that the lesion is really preinvasive cancer;[78] hence, a preferred term would be C cell disease rather than C cell hyperplasia. However, the term C cell hyperplasia is so ingrained in the literature that it will continue to be used despite its semantic inaccuracy.

What is C cell hyperplasia?[273, 478] The definition of this lesions suffers at both ends of the spectrum:

a. the definition of the lower limit of C cell hyperplasia and the upper limit of normal C cell mass is not clear. Various studies show C cell clusters in adults which, taken by themselves, could fit into the category of C cell hyperplasia. Yet O'Toole et al.[343] and Gibson et al.[162] noted these clusters of C cells in apparently endocrinologically normal individuals at autopsy.

b. the lower limit of medullary carcinoma and upper limit of C cell hyperplasia is difficult to define. Although DeLellis and Wolfe state that C cell hyperplasia ranges from diffuse increase in the cells to nodules of C cells replacing follicles and that once the basement membrance of the follicle is breached medullary carcinoma should be diagnosed,[113] Carney et al. correctly point out it is not always obvious that the basement membrane has been crossed.[78] It is known that C cell hyperplasia shows intense and diffuse immunoreactivity for calcitonin of a degree much greater than usual medullary cancer; however, this is a matter of degree and very early medullary carcinoma may stain intensely also.[309]

In the classic case, and this is usually found in patients with multiple endocrine neoplasia, i.e., the C cell hyperplasia has been discovered by screening and provocative testing,[8, 195] the lesion appears as multifocal areas of increased numbers of amphophilic large cells replacing follicular epithelium and also replacing follicles completely, forming nodules (Figs. 10–8 to 10–11).

Outside of the spectrum of endocrine neoplasia syndromes, C cell hyperplasia has been described in hyperparathyroidism, in chronic hypercalcemia from other causes, and in residual thyroid tissue following removal of a medullary cancer (sporadic type).[29, 34, 55, 134, 280, 281, 286, 439, 448, 485] In some of these situations, plasma hypercalcitoninemia has been documented, but many of the studies have been based solely upon histologic examination. Provocative testing for exaggerated calcitonin response, as is done for family screening, has not been systematically carried out in the chronic hypercalcemic patients who have "morphologic evidence" of C cell hyperplasia.

Recent articles have reported C cell hyperplasia in Hashimoto's thyroiditis[270] and in thyroid near nonmedullary carcinoma.[3] In addition, one report of medullary carcinoma arising in a thyroiditis gland has been published.[460] In the context of the work of Janzer et al.,[227] Nadiz et al.,[322, 323] Harach,[185, 495] and others, indicating the close relationship between ultimobranchial body rests (solid cell nests) and C cells, it is interesting to speculate that the hyperplasia of solid cell nests in thyroiditis may in some individuals be accompanied by a corresponding hyperplasia of neighboring C cells (perhaps a common response to growth and/ or proliferation factors, which may be produced in the inflammatory process affecting the gland; it is important not to diagnose solid cell nests as small medullary carcinoma[153]). The present author has seen a case of C cell hyperplasia and early medullary carcinoma arising in a woman with a long history of chronic

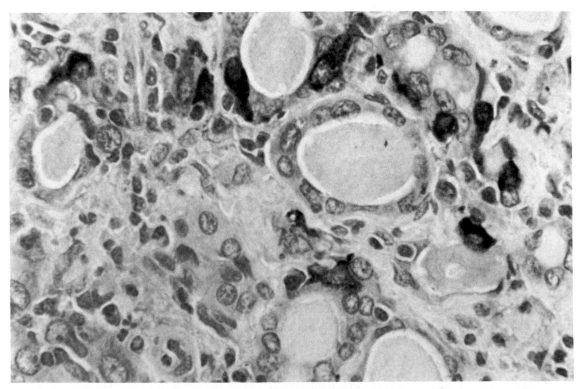

Figure 10–8. C cells are prominent; note intrafollicular location. × 300. Calcitonin immunoperoxidase.

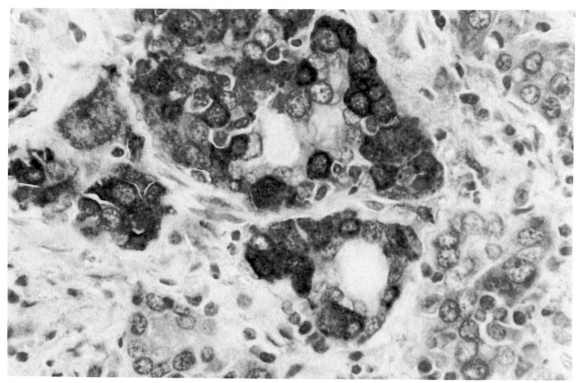

Figure 10–9. C-cell hyperplasia. Thyroid near medullary thyroid carcinoma—familial case. × 300. Calcitonin immunoperoxidase.

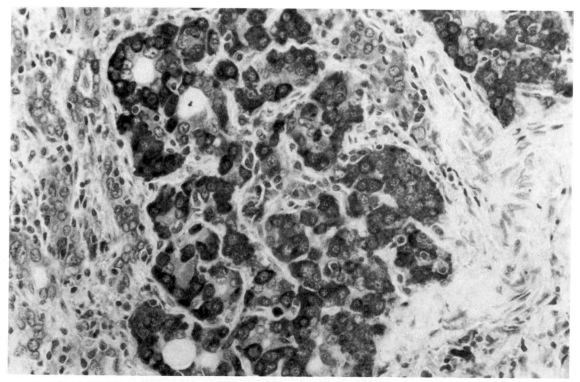

Figure 10–10. Small medullary thyroid carcinoma. One of multiple foci in gland with several 1 to 2 mm lesions and C-cell hyperplasia. Patient from Sipple family. × 200. Calcitonin immunoperoxidase

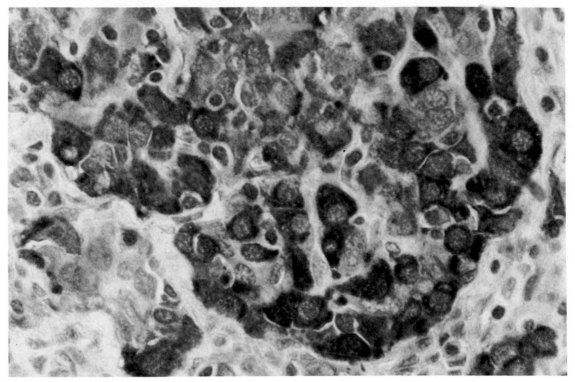

Figure 10–11. Higher power of Figure 10–9. Note dense immunostaining. × 350. Calcitonin immunoperoxidase.

thyroiditis and hypothyroidism; her family history included several members who had had medullary carcinoma.

Albores-Saavedra et al. have described C cell hyperplasia and in some instances hypercalcitoninemia in patients with nonmedullary carcinoma.[3] In their evaluation, about one-third of their cases of nonmedullary carcinoma showed increased numbers of immunoreactive C cells in the gland near the tumor. The pathophysiology of this phenomenon is difficult to explain; perhaps the tumor produces certain factors which stimulate the C cells; perhaps the carcinogenic influences associated with the development of the original tumor were operating on the C cells also.

Thyrotropin probably influences the development or maintenance of nonmedullary carcinoma of the thyroid. The effect of thyrotropin on C cells is difficult to understand but it is known that this pituitary hormone does stimulate the C cells as well as the follicular epithelium. Although not thyrotropin, the stimulus (immunoglobulin) to hyperplasia in patients with hyperthyroidism also seems able to affect C cells; such patients can have plasma calcitonin elevations (two to three times normal).[151] A recent paper reported the first case of medullary thyroid cancer arising in a patient with Graves' disease.[396a]

Calcitonin

Calcitonin itself has been identified both by immunoassay and by immunostaining in a variety of normal tissues (bronchial epithelium, prostate, pituitary[103, 139, 484]) and in a number of endocrine and nonendocrine tumors (pancreatic islet cell tumors, small cell lung cancer and others[31, 49, 87, 158, 170, 198, 313, 340, 373, 400, 401, 497]). In the latter cases it is believed that the hormone is produced by the neoplastic cells ectopically.[193] Elevations of plasma calcitonin in patients with breast or lung cancer may be related to production of the hormone by the tumor, to the presence of bone metastases and reaction to them, or to stimulation of thyroid C cells to hypersecrete.[400, 401]

Some authors have considered tumors analogous to medullary carcinoma to arise in the lung,[170, 176] thymus,[112, 202, 268] larynx,[53, 315, 345, 415, 430, 489] and the ovary-strumal carcinoid.[40, 99, 178, 179, 277, 364, 366, 367, 413]

The spectrum of calcitonin physiology and pathophysiology and its use as a pharmacologic agent, as in the therapy of hypercalcemia[455] and Paget's disease of bone, is beyond the scope of this monograph and can be found in textbooks of general medicine and endocrinology.

SUMMARY

This chapter has described those thyroid lesions currently classified as C cell lesions and has included the normal, hyperplastic, and neoplastic counterparts. The author has attempted to introduce the concept of mixed tumors and their histogenesis while indicating that current evidence does not warrant a separate category of mixed tumor as yet.

REFERENCES

1. Albores-Saavedra, J., Gould, E., and Dominguez-Malagon, H.: Three new cell types in medullary thyroid carcinoma. Lab. Invest. *60*:2A, 1989 (abstract).
2. Albores-Saavedra, J., LiVolsi, V. A., and Williams, E. D.: Medullary carcinoma. Sem. Diag. Pathol. *2*:137–150, 1985.
3. Albores-Saavedra, J., Monforte, H., et al.: C-Cell hyperplasia in thyroid tissue adjacent to follicular cell tumors. Hum. Pathol. *19*:795–799, 1988.
4. Aldabagh, S. M., Trujillo, Y. P., and Taxy, J. B.: Occult medullary thyroid carcinoma: Unusual histologic variants presenting with metastatic disease. Am. J. Clin. Pathol. *85*:247–250, 1986.
5. Aliapoulios, M. A., and Kacoyanis, G. P.: Primary and metastatic medullary thyroid carcinoma: Determination of thyrocalcitonin content by bioassay. Arch. Surg. *106*:105–108, 1973.
6. Aliapoulios, M. A., Voelkel, E. F., and Munson, P. L.: Assay of human thyroid glands for thyrocalcitonin activity. J. Clin. Endocrinol. Metab. *26*:897–901, 1966.
7. Ali-Rachedi, A., Varndell, I. M., et al.: Immunocytochemical localization of katacalcin, a calcium-lowering hormone cleaved from the human calcitonin precursor. J. Clin. Endocrinol. Metab. *57*:680–682, 1983.
8. AlSaadi, A. A.: Ultrastructure in C Cell hyperplasia in asymptomatic patients with hypercalciton-inemia and a family history of medullary thyroid carcinoma. Hum. Pathol. *12*:617–622, 1981.
9. AlSaadi, A.: Management and prevention of familial medullary carcinoma of the thyroid. Prog. Clin. Biol. Res. *34*:343–350, 1979.
10. Amara, S. G., Jonas, V., et al.: Alternative RNA processing in calcitonin gene expression generates mRNAs encoding different polypeptide products. Nature *298*:240–244, 1982.
11. Angeletti, R. H.: Chromogranins and neuroendocrine secretion. Lab. Invest. *55*:387–390, 1986.
12. Aoi, T.: Electron microscopic studies of the follicle cells and parafollicular cells of the thyroid gland of the primates. Folia Anat. Jpn. *42*:63–89, 1966.
13. Argemi, B., Vagneur, J. P., et al.: Les marquers tumoraux plasmatiques (calcitonin et antigene carcino-embryonnaire) au cours des cancers medullaires thyroidiens. Bull. Cancer (Paris) *71*:133–139, 1984.
14. ArnaMonreal, F. M., Goltzman, D., et al.: Immunohistologic study of thyroidal medullary carcinoma and pancreatic insulinoma. Cancer *40*:1060–1070, 1977.
15. Aron, D. C., Mendelsohn, G., and Roos, B. A.: Elaboration of nonsomatostatin peptides containing the amino-terminal portion of prosomatostatin in a somatostatin-secreting human medullary thyroid carcinoma cell line. J. Clin. Endocrinol. Metab. *62*:1237–1242, 1986.
16. Atkins, F. L., Beaven, M. A., and Keiser, H. R.: DOPA decarboxylase in medullary carcinoma of the thyroid. N. Engl. J. Med. *289*:545–548, 1973.
17. Austin, L. A., and Heath, H.: Calcitonin: Physiology and pathophysiology. N. Engl. J. Med. *304*:269–278, 1981.
18. Baber, E. C.: Contributions to the minute anatomy of the thyroid gland of the dog. Proc. Soc. Lond. (Biol.) *24*:240–241, 1876.

19. Baghdiantz, A., Foster, G. V., et al.: Extraction and purification of calcitonin. Nature *203*:1027–1028, 1964.

20. Bagnara, J. T., Matsumoto, J., et al.: Common origin of pigment cells. Science *203*:410–415, 1979.

21. Bartlett, R. D., Myall, R. W. T., et al.: A neuroendocrine syndrome: Mucosal neuromas, pheochromocytoma and medullary thyroid carcinoma. Oral Surg. *31*:206–220, 1971.

22. Baum, J. L.: Abnormal intradermal histamine reaction in the syndrome of pheochromocytoma, medullary carcinoma of the thyroid gland and multiple mucosal neuromas. N. Engl. J. Med. *284*:963–964, 1971.

23. Bauer, W. C., and Teitelbaum, S. L.: Thyrocalcitonin activity of particulate fraction of the thyroid gland. Lab. Invest. *15*:323–329, 1966.

24. Baylin, S. B., Beaven, M. A., et al.: Elevated histaminase activity in medullary carcinoma of the thyroid gland. N. Engl. J. Med. *283*:1239–1244, 1972.

25. Baylin, S. B., Hsu, S. H., et al.: Inherited medullary thyroid carcinoma: a final monoclonal mutation in one of multiple clones of susceptible cells. Science *199*:429–431, 1978.

26. Baylin, S. B., Beaven, M. A., et al.: Serum histaminase and calcitonin levels in medullary carcinoma of the thyroid. Lancet *1*:455–458, 1972.

27. Baylin, S. B., Hsu, T. H., et al.: The effect of L-DOPA on in vitro and in vivo calcitonin release from medullary thyroid carcinoma. J. Clin. Endocrinol. Metab. *48*:408–414, 1979.

28. Baylin, S. B., Mendelsohn, G., et al.: Levels of histaminase and L-DOPA decarboxylase activity in the transition from C Cell hyperplasia to familial medullary thyroid carcinoma. Cancer *44*:1315–1321, 1979.

29. Becker, K. L., Silva, O. L., et al.: The surgical implications of hypercalcitoninemia. Surg. Gynecol. Obstet. *154*:897–908, 1982.

30. Berger, C. L., deBustros, A., et al.: Human medullary thyroid carcinoma in culture provides a model relating growth dynamics, endocrine cell differentiation and tumor progression. J. Clin. Endocrinol. Metab. *59*:338–343, 1984.

31. Bertagna, X. Y., Nicholson, W. E., et al.: Ectopic production of high molecular weight calcitonin and corticotrophin by human small cell carcinoma cells in tissue culture: Evidence for separate precursors. J. Clin. Endocrinol. Metab. *47*:1290–1293, 1978.

32. Beshid, M.: C cell adenoma of the human thyroid gland. Oncology *36*:19–22, 1979.

33. Beshid, M., Lorenc, R., and Rosciszewska, A.: A thyroid C cell adenoma in man. J. Pathol. *103*:343–346, 1971.

34. Beshid, M., Hartwig, W., and Sadowski, J.: Electron microscopic and ultracytochemical investigations of thyroid C cells in primary hyperparathyroidism. Endokrinologie *74*:369–375, 1979.

35. Bethge, N., Ahuja, S., and Diel, F.: Occurrence of calcitonin, somatostatin-like immunoreactivity and carcinoembryonic antigen in two sisters suffering from familial thyroid medullary carcinoma. Exp. Clin. Endocrinol. *88*:365–372, 1986.

36. Bigazzi, M., Revoltella, R., et al.: High level of a nerve growth factor in the serum of a patient with medullary carcinoma of the thyroid gland. Clin. Endocrinol. *6*:105–111, 1977.

37. Bigner, S. H., Cox, E. B., et al.: Medullary carcinoma of the thyroid in the multiple endocrine neoplasia II A syndrome. Am. J. Surg. Pathol. *5*:459–472, 1981.

38. Birkenhager, J. C., Upton, G. V., et al.: Medullary thyroid carcinoma: Ectopic production of peptides with ACTH-like, corticotropin-releasing factor-like and prolactin production-stimulating activities. Acta Endocrinol. *83*:280–292, 1976.

39. Black, H. E., Capen, C. C., and Young, D. M.: Ultimobranchial thyroid neoplasms in bulls. Cancer *32*:865–878, 1973.

40. Blaustein, A.: Calcitonin secreting strumal carcinoid tumor of the ovary. Hum. Pathol. *10*:222–228, 1979.

41. Block, M. A., Horn, R. C., et al.: Familial medullary carcinoma of the thyroid. Ann. Surg. *166*:403–412, 1967.

42. Block, M. A., Jackson, C. E., et al.: Clinical characteristics distinguishing hereditary from sporadic medullary thyroid carcinoma: treatment implications. Arch. Surg. *115*:142–148, 1980.

43. Block, M. A., Jackson, C. E., and Tashjian, A. H.: Medullary thyroid carcinoma detected by calcitonin assay. Arch. Surg. *104*:957–958, 1972.

44. Bolande, R. P.: The neurocristopathies: a unifying concept of disease arising in neural crest maldevelopment. Hum. Pathol. *5*:409–429, 1974.

45. Boorman, G. A., Heersche, J. N. M., and Hollander, C. F.: Transplantable calcitonin secreting medullary carcinomas of the thyroid in the WAG-Rij rat. J. Natl. Cancer Inst. *53*:1011–1015, 1974.

46. Boorman, G. A., and Hollander, C. F.: Medullary carcinoma of the thyroid in the rat. Am. J. Pathol. *83*:237–240, 1976.

47. Boorman, G. A., and Hollander, C. F.: Naturally occurring medullary thyroid carcinoma in the rat. Arch. Pathol. *94*:35–41, 1972.

48. Bordi, C., Anversa, P., and Vitali-Mazza, L.: Ultrastructural study of a calcitonin secreting tumor. Virch. Arch. Pathol. Anat. *357*:145–161, 1972.

49. Bower, B. F., and Gordan, G. S.: Hormonal effects of non-endocrine tumors. Ann. Rev. Med. *16*:83–118, 1965.

50. Brandi, M. L., Marx, S. J., et al.: Familial multiple endocrine neoplasia type I: A new look at pathophysiology. Endocr. Rev. *8*:391–405, 1987.

51. Braunstein, H., and Stephens, C. L.: Parafollicular cells of the human thyroid. Arch. Pathol. *86*:659–666, 1968.
52. Braunstein, H., Stephens, C. L., and Gibson, R. L.: Secretory granules in medullary carcinoma of the thyroid: Electron microscopic demonstration. Arch. Pathol. *85*:306–313, 1968.
53. Brisigotti, M., Fabbretti, G., et al.: Atypical carcinoid of the larynx. Tumori *73*:417–421, 1987.
54. Bronner M., LiVolsi, V. A., and Jennings, T.: Paraganglioma-like adenomas of the thyroid. Surg. Pathol *1*:383–389, 1988.
55. Broulik, P. D., Hradec, E., and Pacovsky, V.: Calcitonin activity of the thyroid gland in primary hyperparathyroidism. Acta Endocrinol. *89*:122–125, 1978.
56. Brown, J. S., and Steiner, A. L.: Medullary thyroid carcinoma and the syndromes of multiple endocrine adenomas. Disease-A-Month *28*:8–35, 1982 (August).
57. Brown, R. S., Colle, E., and Tashjian, A. H.: The syndrome of multiple mucosal neuromas and medullary thyroid carcinoma in childhood. J. Pediatr. *86*:77–83, 1975.
58. Butler, M., and Khan, S.: Immunoreactive calcitonin in amyloid fibrils of medullary carcinoma of the thyroid gland. An immunogold staining technique. Arch. Pathol. Lab. Med. *110*:647–649, 1986.
59. Bundza, A., and Stead, R. H.: Medullary thyroid carcinoma in two cows. Vet. Pathol. *23*:90–92, 1986.
60. Burke, B. A., Johnson, D., et al.: Thyrocalcitonin containing cells in the DiGeorge anomaly. Hum. Pathol. *18*:355–360, 1987.
61. Burtin, P., Calmettes, C., and Fondaneche, M. C.: CEA and nonspecific cross reacting antigen (NCA) in medullary carcinomas of the thyroid. Int. J. Cancer *23*:741–745, 1979.
62. Busnardo, B., Girelli, M. E., et al.: Nonparallel patterns of calcitonin and carcinoembryonic antigen in the follow up of medullary thyroid carcinoma. Cancer *53*:278–285, 1984.
63. Bussolati, G., Foster, G. V., et al.: Immunofluorescent localization of calcitonin in medullary (C cell) thyroid carcinoma using antibody to the pure porcine hormone. Virch. Arch. Abt. B Zellpathol. *2*:234–238, 1969.
64. Bussolati, G., and Monga, G.: Medullary carcinoma of the thyroid with atypical patterns. Cancer *44*:1769–1777, 1979.
65. Bussolati, G., Monga, G., et al.: Histochemical and electron microscopical study of C cells in organ culture. *In:* Taylor, S., and Foster, G. (eds.): Calcitonin 1969: Proceedings of the Second International Symposium. London, Heinemann Publishing, 1970, pp. 240–251.
66. Bussolati, G., Van Noorden, S., and Bordi, C.: Calcitonin and ACTH producing cells in a case of medullary carcinoma of the thyroid. Virch. Arch. Pathol. Anat. *360*:123–127, 1973.
67. Caillou, B., Calmettes, C., et al.: Mise en evidence dans un cancer de la thyroide de formations vesiculaires comparable de type ultimobranchial decrites chez la Souris. C. R. Acad. Sci. Paris *292*:999–1004, 1981.
68. Calmettes, C., Caillou, B., et al.: Calcitonin and carcinoembryonic antigen in poorly differentiated follicular carcinoma. Cancer *49*:2342–2348, 1982.
69. Cannarozzi, D. B., Canale, D. D., and Donabedian, R. K.: Hypercalcitoninemia in infancy. Clin. Chim. Acta *66*:387–392, 1976.
70. Capella, C., Bordi, C., et al.: Multiple endocrine cell types in thyroid medullary carcinoma. Evidence for calcitonin, somatostatin, ACTH, 5HT, and small granule cells. Virch. Arch. Pathol. Anat. *377*:111–128, 1978.
71. Capen, C. C., and Young, D. M.: The ultrastructure of the parathyroid glands and thyroid parafollicular cells of cows with parturient paresis and hypocalcemia. Lab. Invest. *17*:717–737, 1967.
72. Capen, C. C., and Young, D. M.: Fine structural alterations in thyroid parafollicular cells in cows in response to experimental hypercalcemia induced by Vitamin D. Am. J. Pathol. *57*:365–382, 1969.
73. Care, A. D.: Secretion of thyrocalcitonin. Nature *205*:1289–1291, 1965.
74. Carney, J. A., and Hales, A. B.: Alimentary tract manifestations of multiple endocrine neoplasia, type 2b. Mayo Clin. Proc. *52*:543–548, 1977.
75. Carney, J. A., Hales, A. B., et al.: Abnormal cutaneous innervation in multiple endocrine neoplasia, type 2b. Ann. Intern. Med. *94*:262–263, 1981.
76. Carney, J. A., Roth, S. I., et al.: The parathyroid glands in multiple endocrine neoplasia, type 2b. Am. J. Pathol. *99*:387–398, 1980.
77. Carney, J. A., Ryan, J., and Goellner, J. R.: Hyalinizing trabecular adenoma of the thyroid gland. Am. J. Surg. Pathol. *10*:672–679, 1986.
78. Carney, J. A., Sizemore, G. W., and Hales, A. B.: Multiple endocrine neoplasia, type 2b. Pathobiol. Annu. *8*:105–153, 1978.
79. Carney, J. A., Sizemore, G. W., and Sheps, S. G.: Adrenal medullary disease in multiple endocrine neoplasia, type 2. Am. J. Clin. Pathol. *66*:279–290, 1976.
80. Carney, J. A., Sizemore, G. W., and Tyce, G. M.: Bilateral adrenal medullary hyperplasia in multiple endocrine neoplasia, type 2; The precursor of bilateral pheochromocytoma. Mayo Clin. Proc. *50*:3–10, 1975.
81. Carvalheira, A. F., and Pearse, A. G. E.: Comparative cytochemistry of C cell esterases in the mammalian thyroid-parathyroid complex. Histochemie *8*:175–182, 1967.
82. Catalona, W. J., Engelman, K., et al.: Familial medullary thyroid carcinoma, pheochromocytoma and parathyroid adenoma (Sipple's syndrome). Cancer *28*:1245–1254, 1971.

83. Charpin, C., Andrac, L., et al.: Calcitonin, somatostatin, and ACTH immunoreactive cells in a case of familial bilateral thyroid medullary carcinoma. Cancer 50:1806–1814, 1982.
84. Chejfec, G., Falkmer, S., et al.: Synaptophysin. Am. J. Surg. Pathol. 11:241–247, 1987.
85. Chong, C. C., Beahrs, O. H., et al.: Medullary carcinoma of the thyroid gland. Cancer 35:695–703, 1975.
86. Conley, M. E., Beckwith, M. D., et al.: The spectrum of the DiGeorge syndrome. J. Pediatr. 94:833–890, 1979.
87. Coombs, R. C., Hillyard, C., et al.: Plasma immunoreactive calcitonin in patients with nonthyroid tumours. Lancet 1:1080–1083, 1974.
88. Cooper, C. W., Schwesinger, W. H., et al.: Thyrocalcitonin: stimulation of secretion by pentagastrin. Science 172:1238–1240, 1971.
89. Copp, H. D.: Calcitonin: Comparative Endocrinology. In: DeGroot, L. J., Cahill, G. F., et al. (eds.): Endocrinology. New York, Grune and Stratton, 1979, Vol. 2, pp. 637–640.
90. Copp, D. H., Cameron, E. C., et al.: Evidence for calcitonin—a new hormone from the parathyroid that lowers serum calcium. Endocrinology 70:638–649, 1962.
91. Copp, D. H., Cockcroft, D. W., and Kuch, Y.: Calcitonin from ultimobranchial glands of dogfish and chickens. Science 158:924–925, 1967.
92. Copp, D. H., Cockcroft, D. W., et al.: Calcitonin-ultimobranchial hormone. In: Taylor, S. (ed.): Calcitonin: Proceedings of the Symposium on Thyrocalcitonin and the C Cells. London, Heinmann Publishing, 1968, pp. 306–321.
93. Copp, D. H., and Henze, K. G.: Parathyroid origin of calcitonin—evidence from perfusion of sheep glands. Endocrinology 75:49–55, 1964.
94. Corwin, T. R.: Medullary carcinoma of the thyroid. Surg. Gynecol. Obstet. 138:453–458, 1974.
95. Cramer, S. F., Bradshaw, R. A., et al.: Nerve growth factor in medullary carcinoma of the thyroid. Hum. Pathol. 10:731–736, 1979.
96. Cunliffe, W. J., Hudgson, P., et al.: A calcitonin secreting medullary thyroid carcinoma associated with mucosal neuromas, Marfanoid features, myopathy, and pigmentation. Am. J. Med. 48:120–126, 1970.
97. Cushman, P.: Familial endocrine tumors. Report of two unrelated kindreds affected with pheochromocytomas, and also with multiple thyroid carcinomas. Am. J. Med. 32:352–360, 1962.
98. Dammrich, J., Ormanns, W., and Schaffer, R.: Electron microscopic demonstration of calcitonin in human medullary carcinoma of thyroid by the immunogold staining method. Histochemistry 81:369–372, 1984.
99. Dayal, Y., Tashjian, A. H., and Wolfe, H. J.: Immunocytochemical localization of calcitonin producing cells in a strumal carcinoid with amyloid stroma. Cancer 43:1331–1338, 1979.
100. Deftos, L. J.: Radioimmunoassay for calcitonin in medullary thyroid carcinoma. J. A. M. A. 227:403–406, 1974.
101. Deftos, L. J.: Medullary thyroid carcinoma. Basel, Karger, Inc., 1983.
102. Deftos, L. J., Bone, H. G., et al.: Immunohistological studies of medullary thyroid carcinoma and C cell hyperplasia. J. Clin. Endocrinol. Metab. 51:857–862, 1980.
103. Deftos, L. J., Burton, D., et al.: Demonstration by immunoperoxidase immunocytochemistry of calcitonin in the anterior lobe of the rat pituitary. J. Clin. Endocrinol. Metab. 47:457–460, 1978.
104. Deftos, L. J., Bury, A. F., et al.: Immunoassay for calcitonin. II. Clinical studies. Metabolism 20:1129–1137, 1971.
105. Deftos, L. J., and Stein, M. F.: Radioiodine as an adjunct to the surgical treatment of medullary thyroid carcinoma. J. Clin. Endocrinol. Metab. 50:967–968, 1980.
106. Deftos, L. J., Weisman, M. H., et al.: Influence of age and sex on plasma calcitonin in human beings. N. Engl. J. Med. 302:1351–1353, 1980.
107. DeLellis, R. A., and Balogh, K.: Histochemical characteristics of parafollicular cells and medullary thyroid carcinoma. Am. J. Pathol. 72:119–128, 1973.
108. DeLellis, R. A., May, L., et al.: C cell granule heterogeneity in man. Lab. Invest. 38:263–269, 1978.
109. DeLellis, R. A., Moore, F. M., and Wolfe, H. J.: Thyroglobulin immunoreactivity in human medullary thyroid carcinoma. Lab. Invest. 48:20A, 1983 (abstract).
110. DeLellis, R. A., Nunnemacher, G., and Wolfe, H. J.: C cell hyperplasia: an ultrastructural analysis. Lab. Invest. 36:237–248, 1977.
111. DeLellis, R. A., Rule, A. H., et al.: Calcitonin and carcinoembryonic antigen as tumor markers in medullary thyroid carcinoma. Am. J. Clin. Pathol. 70:587–594, 1978.
112. DeLellis, R. A., and Wolfe, H. J.: Calcitonin in spindle cell thymic carcinoid tumors. Arch. Pathol. Lab. Med. 100:340, 1976 (letter).
113. DeLellis, R. A., and Wolfe, H. J.: Pathobiology of the human calcitonin (C) cell: A review. Pathol. Annu. 16: Pt 2:25–52, 1981.
114. DeLellis, R. A., Wolfe, H. J., et al.: Adrenal medullary hyperplasia. Am. J. Pathol. 83:177–190, 1976.
115. Deschryver-Keckemeti, K., Clouse, R. E., et al.: Intestinal ganglioneuromatosis. A manifestation of overproduction of nerve growth factor? N. Engl. J. Med. 308:635–639, 1983.
116. Didolkar, M. S., and Moore, G. E.: Hormone dependent medullary carcinoma of the thyroid. Am. J. Surg. 128:100–102, 1974.

116a. Dominquez-Malagon, H., Delgado-Chavez, R., et al.: Oxyphil and squamous variants of medullary thyroid carcinoma. Cancer *63*:1183–1188, 1989.
117. Donahower, G. F., Schumacher, O. P., and Hazard, J. B.: Medullary carcinoma of the thyroid—a cause of Cushing's syndrome: Report of two cases. J. Clin. Endocrinol. Metab. *28*:119–124, 1968.
118. Donnell, R. M., Kasselberg, A. G., and Rogers, L. W.: DiGeorge syndrome: variable presence of thyroid C cells related to pharyngeal pouch dysembryogenesis. Lab. Invest. *40*:16A, 1979 (abstract).
119. Dooling, E. C., Chi, J. G., and Gilles, F. H.: Melanotic neuroectodermal tumor of infancy. Cancer *39*:1535–1541, 1977.
120. Dube, W. J., Bell, G. O., and Aliapoulios, M. A.: Thyrocalcitonin activity in metastatic medullary thyroid carcinoma. Arch. Intern. Med. *123*:423–427, 1969.
121. Duh, Q. Y., Hybarger, C. P., et al.: Carcinoids associated with multiple endocrine neoplasia syndromes. Am. J. Surg. *154*:142–148, 1987.
122. Dunn, E. L., Nishiyama, R. H., and Thompson, N. W.: Medullary carcinoma of the thyroid gland. Surgery *73*:848–858, 1973.
123. Edbrooke, M. R., Parker, D., et al.: Expression of the human calcitonin/CGRP gene in lung and thyroid carcinoma. EMBO J. *4*:715–724, 1985.
124. Editorial: Sipple families. Lancet *1*:939–940, 1977.
125. Editorial: Plasma calcitonin in medullary thyroid carcinoma. Lancet *1*:338–339, 1983.
126. Editorial: Calcitonin gene related peptide. Lancet *2*:25–26, 1985.
127. Editorial: Genetic markers in multiple endocrine neoplasia type 2. Lancet *1*:396, 1988.
128. Ekblom, M., Valimaki, M., et al.: Familial and sporadic medullary thyroid carcinoma: Clinical and immunohistological findings. Quart. J. Med. *247*:899–910, 1987.
129. Ekblom, R., and Ericson, L. E.: The ultrastructure of the parafollicular cells of the thyroid gland in the rat. J. Ultrastruct. Res. *23*:378–402, 1968.
130. Emmertsen, K.: Medullary thyroid carcinoma and calcitonin. Dan. Med. Bull. *32*:1–28, 1985.
131. Emmertsen, K., Erno, H., et al.: C Cells for differentiation between familial and sporadic medullary thyroid carcinoma. Dan. Med. Bull. *30*:353–356, 1983.
132. Englund, N. E., Nilsson, G., et al.: Human thyroid C cells: Occurrence and amine formation studies by perfusion of surgically removed goitrous glands. J. Clin. Endocrinol. Metab. *35*:90–96, 1972.
133. Ericson, L. E.: Degranulation of the parafollicular cells of the rat thyroid by Vitamin D-2 induced hypercalcemia. J. Ultrastruct. Res. *24*:145–149, 1968.
134. Ericsson, M., Berg, M., et al.: Basal and pentagastrin stimulated levels of calcitonin in thyroid and peripheral veins during normocalcemia and chronic hypercalcemia in humans. Ann. Surg. *194*:129–133, 1981.
135. Farhi, F., Dikman, S. H., et al.: Paragangliomatosis associated with multiple endocrine adenomas. Arch. Pathol. Lab. Med. *100*:495–498, 1976.
136. Farndon, J. R., Lewis, K. R., et al.: Histamine and calcitonin release from medullary thyroid carcinoma. Cancer *51*:1221–1225, 1983.
137. Fassina, A. S., Scapinello, A., et al.: Medullary thyroid carcinoma in multiple endocrine neoplasia type II syndromes. Tumori *71*:397–401, 1985.
138. Fernandes, B. F., Bedard, Y. C., and Rosen, I.: Mucus producing medullary cell carcinoma of the thyroid gland. Am. J. Clin. Pathol. *78*:536–540, 1982.
139. Fetissof, F., Bertrand, G., et al.: Calcitonin immunoreactive cells in prostate gland and cloacal derived tissues. Virch. Arch. Pathol. Anat. *409*:523–533, 1986.
140. Fletcher, J. R.: Medullary (solid) carcinoma of the thyroid gland. Arch. Surg. *100*:257–262, 1970.
141. Forsman, P. J., and Jenkins, M. E.: Medullary carcinoma of the thyroid with Marfan-like habitus. Pediatrics *52*:188–191, 1973.
142. Foster, G. V.: Calcitonin (thyrocalcitonin). N. Engl. J. Med. *279*:349–360, 1968.
143. Foster, G. V., Baghdiantz, A., et al.: Thyroid origin of calcitonin. Nature *202*:1303–1305, 1964.
144. Foster, G. V., MacIntyre, I., and Pearse, A. G. E.: Calcitonin production and the mitochondrion rich cell of the dog. Nature *203*:1029–1030, 1964.
145. Franc, B., and Caillou, B.: Le cancer medullaire de la thyroide: definitions morphologiques et immunohistochimiques. Le role du pathologiste en 1987. Ann. Endocrinol. *49*:22–33, 1988.
146. Franc, B., Caillou, B., et al.: Immunohistochemistry in medullary thyroid carcinoma: Prognosis and distinction between hereditary and sporadic tumors. Henry Ford Hosp. Med. J. *35*:139–142, 1987.
147. Franc, B., Houcke, M., and Caillou, B.: Conditions diagnostiques des cancers medullaires et apparentes du corps thyroide. Ann. Pathol. *4*:393–398, 1984.
148. Frank, K., Raue, F., et al.: Importance of early diagnosis and followup in multiple endocrine neoplasia (MEN IIB). Eur. J. Pediatr. *143*:112–116, 1984.
149. Franssila, K.: Value of histologic classification of thyroid cancer. Acta Pathol. Microbiol. Scand. Suppl. *225*:5–76, 1971.
150. Frantz, V. K., and Yannopoulos, K.: Carcinoma of the thyroid: A clinicopathologic study of 216 cases with a ten year followup. Advances Thyroid Research. New York, Pergamon Press, 1961, 377–384.
151. Fraser, S. A., and Wilson, G. M.: Plasma calcitonin in disorders of thyroid function. Lancet *1*:725–726, 1971.

152. Freeman, D.: Medullary carcinoma of the thyroid gland. A clinicopathological study of 33 patients. Arch. Pathol. *80*:575–582, 1965.
153. Fukunaga, F. H., and Lockett, L. J.: Thyroid carcinoma in the Japanese in Hawaii. Arch. Pathol. *92*:6–13, 1971.
154. Gagel, R. F., Tashjian, A. H., et al.: The clinical outcome of prospective screening for multiple endocrine neoplasia type 2a. N. Engl. J. Med. *318*:478–484, 1988.
155. Galante, L., Gudmundsson, T. V., et al.: Effect of calcitonin on vitamin D metabolism. Nature *238*:271–273, 1972.
156. Galante, L., Gudmundsson, T. V., et al.: Thymic and parathyroid origin of calcitonin in man. Lancet *2*:537–538, 1968.
157. Galera, H., Gonzalez-Campora, R., et al.: Multiple endocrine neoplasia type 2b in twins. Histopathology *6*:111–119, 1982.
158. Galmichi, J. P., Chayvialle, J. A., et al.: Calcitonin producing pancreatic somatostatinoma. Gastroenterology *78*:1577–1583, 1980.
159. Geddie, W. R., Bedard, Y. C., and Strawbridge, H. T. G.: Medullary carcinoma of the thyroid in fine needle aspiration biopsies. Am. J. Clin. Pathol. *82*:552–558, 1984.
160. George, J. M., Williams, M. A., et al.: Medullary carcinoma of the thyroid: Cellular immune response to tumor antigen in a heritable human cancer. Cancer *36*:1658–1661, 1975.
161. Ghatei, M. A., Springall, D. R., et al.: Gastrin releasing peptide like immunoreactivity in medullary thyroid carcinoma. Am. J. Clin. Pathol. *84*:581–586, 1985.
162. Gibson, W. C. H., Peng, T. C., and Croker, B. P.: C cell nodules in adult human thyroid: a common autopsy finding. Am. J. Clin. Pathol. *73*:347–351, 1980.
163. Girgis, S. I., Macdonald, D. W. R., et al.: Calcitonin gene related peptide: potent vasodilator and major product of calcitonin gene. Lancet *2*:14–16, 1985.
164. Glenner, G. G.: Amyloid deposits and amyloidosis. N. Engl. J. Med. *302*:1283–1292, 1333–1342, 1980.
165. Godwin, M. C.: Complex IV in the dog with special emphasis on the relation of the ultimobranchial body to the interfollicular cells in the postnatal thyroid glands. Am. J. Anat. *60*:299–339, 1937.
166. Golouh, R., Us-Krasovec, M., et al.: Amphicrine-composite calcitonin and mucin producing carcinoma of the thyroid. Ultrastruct. Pathol. *8*:197–206, 1985.
167. Goltzman, D., Huang, S. N., et al.: Adrenocorticotropin and calcitonin in medullary thyroid carcinoma: frequency of occurrence and localization in the same cell type by immunocytochemistry. J. Clin. Endocrinol. Metab. *49*:364–370, 1979.
168. Goltzman, D., Potts, J. T., et al.: Calcitonin as a tumor marker. N. Engl. J. Med. *290*:1035–1039, 1974.
169. Gonzalez-Licea, A., Hartman, W. H., and Yardley, J. H.: Medullary carcinoma of the thyroid gland. Am. J. Clin. Pathol. *49*:512–520, 1968.
170. Gordon, H. W., Miller, R., and Mittman, C.: Medullary carcinoma of the lung with amyloid stroma: A counterpart of medullary carcinoma of the thyroid. Hum. Pathol. *4*:431–436, 1973.
171. Gordon, P. R., Huvos, A. G., and Strong, E. W.: Medullary carcinoma of the thyroid gland. Cancer *31*:915–924, 1973.
172. Gorlin, R. J., Sedano, H. O., et al.: Multiple mucosal neuromas, pheochromocytoma and medullary carcinoma of the thyroid. A syndrome. Cancer *22*:293–299, 1968.
173. Gould, R. P.: The APUD cell system. Rec. Adv. Histopathol. *10*:1–22, 1978.
174. Gould, V. E., Wiedenmann, B., et al.: Synaptophysin expression in neuroendocrine neoplasms as determined by immunocytochemistry. Am. J. Pathol. *126*:243–257, 1987.
175. Graze, K., Spiler, I. J., et al.: Natural history of familial medullary thyroid carcinoma. N. Engl J. Med. *299*:980–985, 1978.
176. Grazer, R., Cohen, S. M., et al.: Melanin containing peripheral carcinoid of the lung. Am. J. Surg. Pathol. *6*:73–78, 1982.
177. Gray, T. K., and Munson, P. L.: Thyrocalcitonin: evidence for physiological function. Science *166*:512–514, 1969.
178. Greco, M. A., LiVolsi, V. A., et al.: Strumal carcinoid of the ovary. An analysis of its components. Cancer *43*:1380–1388, 1979.
179. Grimelius, L.: The argyrophil reaction in islet cells of adult human pancreas studied with a new silver nitrate procedure. Acta Soc. Med. Upsalien. *73*:271–294, 1968.
180. Grimley, P. M., Deftos, L. J., et al.: Growth in vitro and ultrastructure of cells from a medullary carcinoma of the human thyroid gland. Transformation by simian virus 40 and evidence of thyrocalcitonin and prostaglandins. J. Natl. Cancer Inst. *42*:663–680, 1969.
181. Guliana, J. M., and Modigliani, E.: Les marqueurs tumoraux du cancer medullaire du corps thyroide. Ann. Endocrinol. *49*:34–50, 1988.
182. Guliana, J. M., Taboulet, J., et al., for the French Medullary Study Group: Secretion of calcitonin gene-related peptide in medullary thyroid carcinoma: its value as tumoral marker. Ann. Endocrinol. *49*:196, 1988 (abstract).
183. Halanson, R., Owman, C., and Sundler, F.: Fluorescence histochemical and microspectrofluorometric evidence of tryptophyl peptides in thyroid C cells of cat and pig. J. Histochem. Cytochem. *20*:205–210, 1972.
184. Hales, M., Rosenau, W., et al.: Carcinoma of the thyroid with a mixed medullary and follicular pattern. Cancer *50*:1352–1359, 1982.

185. Harach, H. R.: Solid cell nests in the thyroid. J. Pathol. *155*:191–200, 1988.
186. Harach, H. R., and Bergholm, U.: Medullary (C cell) carcinoma of the thyroid with features of follicular oxyphilic tumours. Histopathology *13*:645–656, 1988.
187. Harach, H. R., and Williams, E. D.: Glandular (tubular and follicular) variants of medullary carcinoma of the thyroid. Histopathology *7*:83–97, 1983.
188. Harrison, T. S., and Thompson, N. W.: Multiple endocrine adenomatosis I and II. Curr. Prob. Surg. 5–51, August 1975.
189. Hazard, J. B.: The C cells (parafollicular cells) of the thyroid gland and medullary thyroid carcinoma. Am. J. Pathol. *88*:214–249, 1977.
190. Hazard, J. B., Hawk, W. A., and Crile, G.: Medullary (solid) carcinoma of the thyroid: A clinicopathologic entity. J. Clin. Endocrinol. Metab. *19*:152–161, 1959.
191. Heath, H., Sizemore, G. W., et al.: Immunochemical heterogeneity of calcitonin in tumor, tumor effluent and peripheral blood of patients with medullary thyroid carcinoma. J. Lab. Clin. Med. *93*:390–401, 1979.
192. Hedinger, C., Williams, E. D., and Sobin, L. H.: The WHO histological classification of thyroid tumors: A commentary on the second edition. Cancer *63*:908–911, 1989.
193. Heitz, P. U., Kloppel, G., et al.: Ectopic hormone production by endocrine tumors. Cancer *48*:2029–2037, 1981.
194. Hellman, D. E., Kartchner, M., et al.: Radioiodine in the treatment of medullary carcinoma of the thyroid. J. Clin. Endocrinol. Metab. *48*:451–455, 1979.
195. Hellman, J. F., Gray, T. K., et al.: Stimulation of thyrocalcitonin secretion by pentagastrin and calcium in two patients with medullary carcinoma of the thyroid. J. Clin. Endocrinol. Metab. *36*:200–203, 1973.
196. Heuser, C. H.: A human embryo with 14 pairs of somites. Contrib. Embryol. *131*:135–154, 1930.
197. Hill, C. S., Ibanez, M. L., et al.: Medullary (solid) carcinoma of the thyroid gland: an analysis of the M. D. Anderson Hospital experience with patients with the tumor, its special features and its histogenesis. Medicine *52*:141–171, 1973.
198. Hillyard, C. J., Coombes, R. C., et al.: Calcitonin in breast and lung cancer. Clin. Endocrinol. *5*:1–8, 1978.
199. Hillyard, C. J., Evans, I. M. A., et al.: Familial medullary thyroid carcinoma. Lancet *1*:1009–1011, 1978.
200. Hirsch, P. F., and Munson, P. L.: Thyrocalcitonin. Physiol. Rev. *49*:548–622, 1969.
201. Hirsch, P. F., Voelkel, E. F., and Munson, P. L.: Thyrocalcitonin: hypocalcemic hypophosphatemic principle in the thyroid gland. Science *146*:412–413, 1964.
202. Ho, F. C. S., and Ho, J. C. I.: Pigmented carcinoid tumour of the thymus. Histopathology *1*:363–369, 1977.
203. Hollenberg, C. H.: Medullary carcinoma of the thyroid. Arch. Otolaryngol. *109*:103–105, 1983.
204. Holm, R., Sobrinho-Simoes, M., et al.: Medullary thyroid carcinoma of the thyroid gland. An immunocytochemical study. Ultrastruct. Pathol. *8*:25–41, 1985.
205. Holm, R., Sobrinho-Simoes, M., et al.: Medullary carcinoma of the thyroid gland with thyroglobulin immunoreactivity. A special entity? Lab. Invest. *57*:258–268, 1987.
206. Holm, R., Sobrinho-Simoes, M., et al.: Concurrent production of calcitonin and thyroglobulin by the same neoplastic cells. Ultrastruct. Pathol. *10*:241–251, 1986.
207. Horn, R. C.: Carcinoma of the thyroid. Description of a distinctive morphological variant and report of seven cases. Cancer *4*:697–707, 1951.
208. Horvath, E., Kovacs, K., and Ross, R. C.: Medullary cancer of the thyroid and its possible relations to carcinoids. Virch. Arch. Pathol. Anat. *356*:281–292, 1972.
209. Howlett, T. A., Price, J., et al.: Pituitary ACTH dependent Cushing's syndrome due to ectopic production of a bombesin-like peptide by a medullary carcinoma of the thyroid. Clin. Endocrinol. *22*:91–101, 1985.
210. Hoyt, R. F., Hamilton, D. W., and Tashjian, A. H.: Distribution of thyroid, parathyroid and ultimobranchial hypocalcemic factors in birds. II. Morphology, histochemistry and hypocalcemic activity of pigeon thyroid glands. Anat. Rec. *176*:1–34, 1973.
211. Hoyt, R. F., Tashjian, A. H., and Hamilton, D. W.: Distribution of thyroid, parathyroid and ultimobranchial hypocalcemic factors in birds. I. Thyroid, and ultimobranchial calcitonins in pigeons and pullets. Endocrinology *91*:770–783, 1972.
212. Huang, S. N., and Goltzman, D.: Electron and immunoelectron microscopic study of thyroidal medullary carcinoma. Cancer *41*:2226–2235, 1978.
213. Huang, S. N., and McLeish, W. A.: Pheochromocytoma and medullary carcinoma of the thyroid. Cancer *21*:302–311, 1968.
214. Hurley, D. L., Katz, H. H., et al.: Cosecretion of calcitonin gene products. J. Clin. Endocrinol. Metab. *66*:640–644, 1988.
215. Ibanez, M. L.: Medullary carcinoma of the thyroid gland. Pathol. Annu. *9*:263–290, 1974.
216. Ibanez, M. L., Cole, V. W., et al.: Solid carcinoma of the thyroid gland: Analysis of 53 cases. Cancer *20*:706–723, 1967.
217. Isaacson, P., and Judd, M. A.: Carcinoembryonic antigen in medullary carcinoma of thyroid. Lancet *2*:1016–1017, 1976.
218. Ishikawa, N., and Hamada, S.: Association of medullary carcinoma of the thyroid with carcinoembryonic antigen. Br. J. Cancer *34*:111–115, 1976.

219. Isobe, T., Fukasa, M., and Fujita, T.: Amyloid fibril protein from medullary carcinoma of the thyroid. Jpn. J. Med. *24*:8–12, 1985.
220. Ito, M., Kameda, Y., and Tagawa, T.: An ultrastructural study of the cysts in chicken ultimobranchial glands, with special reference to C cells. Cell Tissue Res. *246*:39–44, 1986.
221. Iwanaga, T., Koyama, H., et al.: Production of several substances by medullary carcinoma of the thyroid. Cancer *41*:1106–1112, 1978.
222. Jackson, C. E., Block, M. A., et al.: The two mutational event theory in medullary thyroid cancer. Am. J. Hum. Genet. *31*:704–710, 1979.
223. Jackson, C. E., Tashjian, A. H., and Block, M. A.: Detection of medullary thyroid carcinoma by calcitonin assay in families. Ann. Intern. Med. *78*:845–852, 1973.
224. James, P. D.: Amyloid goitre. J. Clin. Pathol. *25*:683–688, 1972.
225. Jansson, S., Hansson, G., et al.: Prevalence of C cell hyperplasia and medullary thyroid carcinoma in a consecutive series of pheochromocytoma patients. World J. Surg. *8*:493–500, 1984.
226. Jansson, S., Tissell, L. E., et al.: Early diagnosis of and surgical strategy for adrenal medullary disease in MEN II gene carriers. Surgery *103*:11–18, 1988.
227. Janzer, R. C., Weber, E., and Hedinger, C.: The relation between solid cell nests and C cells of the thyroid gland. Cell Tissue Res. *197*:295–312, 1979.
228. Jerkins, T. W., Sacks, H. S., et al.: Medullary carcinoma of the thyroid, pancreatic nesidioblastosis and microadenosis and pancreatic polypeptide hypersecretion. J. Clin. Endocrinol. Metab. *64*:1313–1319, 1989.
229. Johannessen, J. V., Gould, V. E., and Jao, W.: The fine structure of human thyroid cancer. Hum. Pathol. *9*:385–400, 1978.
230. Johannsen, I., Schroder, H. D., and Schifter, S.: Calcitonin gene related peptide and calcitonin in MEN 2 and sporadic pheochromocytomas: An immunohistochemical study. Henry Ford Hosp. Med. J. *35*:115–117, 1987.
231. Johnson, F. P.: A human embryo of 24 pairs of somites. Contrib. Embryol. *19*:125–166, 1917.
232. Kakudo, K., Carney, J. A., and Sizemore, G. W.: Medullary carcinoma of the thyroid. Biologic behavior of the sporadic and familial neoplasm. Cancer *55*:2818–2821, 1985.
233. Kakudo, K., Miyauchi, A., et al.: Ultrastructural study of poorly differentiated medullary carcinoma of the thyroid. Virch. Arch. Pathol. Anat. *410*:455–460, 1987.
234. Kakudo, K., Miyauchi, A., et al.: Medullary carcinoma of the thyroid with ectopic ACTH syndrome. Acta Pathol. Jpn. *32*:793–800, 1982.
235. Kakudo, K., Miyauchi, A., et al.: Medullary carcinoma of the thyroid: Giant cell type. Arch. Pathol. Lab. Med. *102*:445–447, 1978.
236. Kakudo, K., Miyauchi, A., et al.: C cell carcinoma of the thyroid: papillary type. Acta Pathol. Jpn. *29*:653–659, 1979.
237. Kakudo, K., Spurlock, B. O., et al.: Unusual cytoplasmic inclusion bodies in medullary carcinoma of the thyroid gland. Acta Pathol. Jpn. *32*:319–326, 1982.
238. Kakuda, K., and Vacca, L.: Immunohistochemical study of substance P-like immunoreactivity in human thyroid and medullary carcinoma of the thyroid. J. Submicrosc. Cytol. *15*:563–568, 1983.
239. Kalisnik, M., Vraspir-Porenta, O., et al.: The interdependence of the follicular, parafollicular and mast cells in the mammalian thyroid gland: A review and a synthesis. Am. J. Anat. *183*:148–157, 1988.
240. Kameda, Y.: Parafollicular cells of the thyroid as studied with Davenport's silver impregnation. Nippon Soshikigaku Kiroku. *30*:83–94, 1968.
241. Kameda, Y.: Increased mitotic activity of the parafollicular cells of the dog thyroid in experimentally induced hypercalcemia. Nippon Soshikigaku Kiroku. *32*:179–192, 1970.
242. Kameda, Y.: Immunohistochemical study of cyst structures in chick ultimobranchial glands. Arch. Histol. Jpn. *47*:411–419, 1984.
243. Kameda, Y.: Development of immunoreactive somatostatin in C cell complexes in the thyroid gland of the dog. Cell Tissue Res. *238*:263–269, 1984.
244. Kameda, Y., Harada, T., et al.: Immunohistochemical study of the medullary thyroid carcinoma with reference to C-thyroglobulin reaction of tumor cells. Cancer *44*:2071–2082, 1979.
245. Kaplan, E. L., and Peskin, G. W.: Physiologic implications of medullary carcinoma of the thyroid gland. Surg. Clin. N. Amer. *51*:125–137, 1971.
246. Kaplan, E. L., Sizemore, G. W., et al.: Humoral similarities of carcinoid tumors and medullary carcinomas of the thyroid. Surgery *74*:21–29, 1973.
247. Kaufman, F. R., Roe, T. F., et al.: Metastatic medullary carcinoma in young children with mucosal neuroma syndrome. Pediatr. *70*:263–267, 1982.
248. Kay, S., Montague, J. W., and Dodd, R. W.: Nonchromaffin paraganglioma (chemodectoma) of the thyroid region. Cancer *36*:582–585, 1975.
249. Keiser, H. R., Beaven, M. A., et al.: Sipple's syndrome: Medullary thyroid carcinoma, pheochromocytoma and parathyroid disease. Ann. Intern. Med. *78*:561–579, 1973.
250. Kendall, C. H., Homer, C. E., et al.: Age related peptide production by human thyroid C cells: An immunohistochemical study. Virch. Arch. Pathol. Anat. *410*:97–101, 1986.
251. Kennedy, J. S., Thomson, J. A., and Buchanan, W. M.: Amyloid in the thyroid. Quart. J. Med. *43*:127–143, 1974.
252. Keynes, W. M., and Till, A. S.: Medullary carcinoma of the thyroid. Quart. J. Med. *159*:443–456, 1971.

253. Khairi, M. R. S., Dexter, R. N., et al.: Mucosal neuroma, pheochromocytoma and medullary thyroid carcinoma: Multiple endocrine neoplasia type 3. Medicine *54*:89–112, 1975.
254. Kimura, N., Ishioka, K., et al.: Melanin producing medullary thyroid carcinoma with glandular differentiation. Acta Cytol. *33*:61–66, 1989.
255. Kimura, N., Sosano, N., et al.: Immunohistochemical study of chromogranin in 100 cases of pheochromocytoma, carotid body tumour, medullary thyroid carcinoma and carcinoid tumour. Virch. Arch. Pathol. Anat. *413*:33–38, 1988.
256. Kini, S. R., Miller, J. M., et al.: Cytopathologic features of medullary carcinoma of the thyroid. Arch. Pathol. Lab. Med. *108*:156–159, 1984.
257. Kodama, T., Fujino, M., et al.: Identification of carcinoembryonic antigen in the C cell of the normal thyroid. Cancer *45*:98–101, 1980.
258. Kodama, T., Okamoto, T., et al.: C cell adenoma of the thyroid: A rare but distinct clinical entity. Surgery *104*:997–1003, 1988.
259. Kodama, T., Tamura, M., et al.: A case of calcitonin producing adenoma of the thyroid. Endocrinol. Jpn. *31*:63–70, 1984.
260. Kracht, J., Hachmeiser, U., and Christ, U.: C cells in the human thyroid. In: Taylor, S., and Foster, G. (eds.): Calcitonin 1969: Proceedings of the Second International Symposium. London, Heinemann, 1970, pp. 274–280.
261. Krisch, K., Krisch, I., et al.: The value of immunohistochemistry in medullary thyroid carcinoma: a systematic study of 30 cases. Histopathology *9*:1077–1090, 1985.
262. Kullberg, B. J., and Nieuwenhuijzen-Kruseman, A. C.: Multiple endocrine neoplasia type 2b with a good prognosis. Arch. Intern. Med. *147*:1125–1127, 1987.
263. Landon, G., and Ordonez, N. G.: Clear cell variant of medullary carcinoma of the thyroid. Hum. Pathol. *16*:844–847, 1985.
264. Laskowski, J.: Carcinoma hyalinicum thyroideae. Nowotwory *7*:23–28, 1957.
265. Leav, I., Schiller, A. L., et al.: Adenomas and carcinoma of the canine and feline thyroid. Am. J. Pathol. *83*:61–122, 1976.
266. LeDourain, N. M., and Teillet, M. A.: The migration of neural crest cells to the wall of the digestive tract in the avian embryo. J. Embryol. Exp. Morphol. *30*:31–48, 1973.
267. Lee, T. K., Myers, R. T., et al.: The significance of mitotic rate: a retrospective study of 127 thyroid carcinomas. Hum. Pathol. *16*:1042–1046, 1985.
268. Levine, G. D., and Rosai, J.: A spindle cell variant of thymic carcinoid tumor. Arch. Pathol. Lab. Med. *100*:293–300, 1976.
269. Leitz, H.: C cells: Source of calcitonin. Curr. Topics Pathol. *55*:109–146, 1971.
270. Libbey, N. P., Nowakowski, K. J., and Tucci, J. R.: C cell hyperplasia of the thyroid in a patient with goitrous hypothyroidism and Hashimoto's thyroiditis. Am. J. Surg. Pathol. *13*:71–77, 1989.
271. Lindsay, S., and Nichols, C. W.: Medullary thyroid carcinoma and parathyroid hyperplasia in rats. Arch. Pathol. *88*:402–406, 1969.
272. Lippman, S. M., Mendelsohn, G., et al.: The prognostic and biological significance of cellular heterogeneity in medullary thyroid carcinoma. A study of calcitonin, L-DOPA decarboxylase and histaminase. J. Clin. Endocrinol. Metab. *54*:233–240, 1982.
273. Lips, C. J. M., Leo, J. R., et al.: Thyroid C cell hyperplasia and micronodules in close relatives of MEN-2A patients: Pitfalls in early diagnosis and reevaluation of criteria for surgery. Henry Ford Hosp. Med. J. *35*:133–138, 1987.
274. Lips, C. J. M., Steenbergh, P. H., et al.: Evolutionary pathway of the calcitonin genes. Molec. Cell. Endocrinol. *57*:1–6, 1988.
275. Lips, C. J. M., Steenbergh, P. H., et al.: The molecular basis of polypeptide hormone production by medullary thyroid cancer. Henry Ford Hosp. Med. J. *32*:269–272, 1984.
276. Lips, C. J. M., vander Sluys-Veer, J., et al.: Common precursor molecule as origin for the ectopic hormone producing tumour syndrome. Lancet *1*:16–18, 1978.
277. Livnat, E. J., Scommegna, A., et al.: Ultrastructural observations of the so-called strumal carcinoid of the ovary. Arch. Pathol. Lab. Med. *101*:585–589, 1977.
278. LiVolsi, V. A.: Calcitonin: the hormone and its significance. Prog. Surg. Pathol. *1*:71–103, 1980.
279. LiVolsi, V. A.: Mixed thyroid tumors: a real entity? Lab. Invest. *57*:237–239, 1987.
280. LiVolsi, V. A., and Feind, C. R.: Incidental medullary thyroid carcinoma in sporadic hyperparathyroidism. Am. J. Clin. Pathol. *71*:595–599, 1979.
281. LiVolsi, V. A., Feind, C. R., et al.: Demonstration by immunoperoxidase staining of hyperplasia of parafollicular cells in the thyroid gland in hyperparathyroidism. J. Clin. Endocrinol. Metab. *37*:550–559, 1973.
282. Ljungberg, O.: On medullary carcinoma of the thyroid. Acta Pathol. Microbiol. Scand. (A) Suppl. *231*:1–57, 1972.
283. Ljungberg, O.: Two cell types in familial medullary thyroid carcinoma: a histochemical study. Virch. Arch. Pathol. Anat. *349*:312–322, 1970.
284. Ljungberg, O., Bondeson, L., and Bondeson, A. G.: Differentiated thyroid carcinoma, intermediate type: a new tumor entity with features of follicular and parafollicular cell carcinoma. Hum. Pathol. *15*:218–228, 1984.
285. Ljungberg, O., Cederquist, E., and VonStudnitz, E.: Medullary thyroid carcinoma and pheochromocytomas: A familial chromaffinosis. Br. Med. J. *1*:279–281, 1967.

286. Ljungberg, O., and Dymling, J. F.: Pathogenesis of C cell neoplasia in thyroid gland: C cell proliferation in a case of chronic hypercalcemia. Acta Pathol. Microbiol. Scand. *80*:577–588, 1972.

287. Ljungberg, O., Ericsson, U. B., et al.: A compound follicular-parafollicular cell carcinoma of the thyroid: a new tumor entity? Cancer *52*:1053–1061, 1983.

288. Ljungberg, O., and Nilsson, P. O.: Hyperplastic and neoplastic changes in ultimobranchial remnants and in parafollicular (C) cells in bulls: a histologic and immunohistochemical study. Vet. Pathol. *22*:95–103, 1985.

289. Lloyd, R. V.: Use of molecular probes in the study of endocrine disease. Hum. Pathol. *18*:1199–1211, 1987.

290. Lloyd, R. V., Sisson, J. C., and Marangos, P. J.: Calcitonin, carcinoembryonic antigen and neuron specific enolase in medullary thyroid carcinoma. Cancer *51*:2234–2239, 1983.

291. Lloyd, R. V., and Wilson, B. S.: Specific endocrine tissue marker defined by a monoclonal antibody. Science *222*:628–630, 1983.

292. Macgillwray, J. B., and Anderson, C. J. B.: Medullary carcinoma of the thyroid with parathyroid adenoma and hypercalcemia. J. Clin. Pathol. *24*:851–855, 1971.

293. Manning, P. C., Molnar, G. D., et al.: Pheochromocytoma, hyperparathyroidism and thyroid carcinoma occurring coincidentally. N. Engl. J. Med. *268*:68–72, 1963.

294. Marcus, J., Dise, C. A., and LiVolsi, V. A.: Melanin production in a medullary thyroid carcinoma. Cancer *49*:2518–2526, 1982.

295. Markey, W. S., Ryan, W. G., et al.: Familial medullary carcinoma and parathyroid adenoma without pheochromocytoma. Ann. Intern. Med. *78*:898–901, 1973.

296. Martinelli, G., Bazzocchi, F., et al.: Anaplastic type of medullary thyroid carcinoma: an ultrastructural and immunohistochemical study. Virch. Arch. Pathol. Anat. *400*:61–67, 1983.

297. Martins, M. I. B., Goncalves, V., and Trincao, R.: Un marcador histologico do carcinoma medular da tireoide. Arq. Patal. Geral Anat. Patal Univ. de Coimbra. *17*:61–72, 1979–80.

298. Mathew, C. G. P., Chin, K. S., et al.: A linked genetic marker for multiple endocrine neoplasia type 2A on chromosome 10. Nature *328*:527–528, 1987.

299. Matsubayashi, S., Yanaihara, C., et al.: Gastrin-releasing peptide reactivity in medullary thyroid carcinoma. Cancer *53*:2472–2477, 1984.

300. McMillan, P. J., Hooker, W. M. and Deftos, L. J.: Distribution of calcitonin containing cells in the human thyroid. Am. J. Anat. *140*:73–80, 1974.

301. Meissner, W. A., and Warren, S.: Tumors of the thyroid gland. *In:* Armed Forces Institute of Pathology, series 2, fasc. 4, Washington, D.C., 1969.

302. Melvin, K. E. W., Miller, H. H., and Tashjian, A. H.: Early diagnosis of medullary carcinoma of the thyroid by means of calcitonin assay. N. Engl. J. Med. *285*:1115–1120, 1971.

303. Melvin, K. E. W., and Tashjian, A. H.: The syndrome of excessive calcitonin produced by medullary carcinoma of the thyroid. Proc. Natl. Acad. Sci. *59*:1261–1262, 1968.

304. Melvin, K. E. W., Tashjian, A. H., et al.: Cushing's syndrome caused by ACTH and calcitonin secreting medullary carcinoma of the thyroid. Metabolism *19*:831–838, 1972.

305. Melvin, K. E. W., Tashjian, A. H., and Miller, H. H.: Studies in familial medullary thyroid carcinoma. Rec. Progr. Horm. Res. *28*:399–470, 1972.

306. Mendelsohn, G., Bigner, S. H., et al.: Anaplastic variants of medullary thyroid carcinoma. Am. J. Surg. Pathol. *4*:333–341, 1980.

307. Mendelsohn, G., Eggleston, J. C., et al.: Calcitonin and histaminase in C-cell hyperplasia and medullary thyroid carcinoma. A light microscopic and immunohistochemical study. Am. J. Pathol. *92*:35–52, 1978.

308. Mendelsohn, G., and Oertel, J. E.: Encapsulated medullary thyroid carcinoma. Lab. Invest *44*:43A, 1981 (abstract).

309. Mendelsohn, G., Wells, S. A., and Baylin, S. B.: Relationship of tissue carcinoembryonic antigen and calcitonin to tumor virulence in medullary thyroid carcinoma. An immunohistochemical study in early, localized and virulent disseminated stages of disease. Cancer *54*:657–662, 1984.

310. Meyer, J. S.: Fine structure of two amyloid forming medullary carcinomas of the thyroid gland. Cancer *21*:406–425, 1968.

311. Meyer, J. S., and Abdel-Bari, W.: Granules and thyrocalcitonin like activity in medullary carcinoma of the thyroid gland. N. Engl. J. Med. *278*:523–529, 1968.

312. Meyer, J. S., Hutton, W. E., and Kenny, A. D.: Medullary carcinoma of the thyroid gland. Subcellular distribution of calcitonin and relationship between granules and amyloid. Cancer *31*:433–441, 1973.

313. Milhaud, G., Calmette, C., et al.: Hypersecretion of calcitonin in neoplastic conditions. Lancet *1*:462–463, 1974.

314. Miller, H. H., Melvin, K. E. W., et al.: Surgical approach to early familial medullary carcinoma of the thyroid gland. Am. J. Surg. *123*:438–443, 1972.

315. Mills, S. E., and Johns, M. E.: Atypical carcinoid of the larynx. Arch. Pathol. Lab. Med. *110*:58–62, 1984.

316. Mitsudo, S. M., Grajower, M. M., et al.: Malignant paraganglioma of the thyroid gland. Arch. Pathol. Lab. Med. *111*:378–380, 1987.

317. Miyauchi, A., Onishi, T., et al.: Relation of doubling time of plasma calcitonin levels to prognosis and recurrence of medullary thyroid carcinoma. Ann. Surg. *199*:461–466, 1984.

318. Morris, H. R., Panico, M., et al.: Isolation and characterization of human calcitonin gene related peptide. Nature *308*:746–748, 1984.

319. Mosca, L., Capella, C., et al.: Histological detection of thyroid medullary carcinoma by selective stainings. Acta Med. Cost. *15*:215–219, 1972.

320. Moseley, J. M., Matthews, E. W., et al.: The ultimobranchial origin of calcitonin. Lancet *1*:108–110, 1968.

321. Muller, W., Peter, H. H., et al.: The DiGeorge syndrome. Eur. J. Pediatr. *147*:496–502, 1988.

322. Nadiz, J., Weber, E., and Hedinger, C.: C cells in vestiges of the ultimobranchial body in human thyroid glands. Virch. Arch. Cell Pathol. *27*:189–191, 1978.

323. Nadiz, J., Weber, E., and Hedinger, C.: Morphologic and morphometric studies on human C cells in disorders of calcium metabolism. Virch. Arch. Cell Pathol. *29*:151–165, 1978.

324. Nieuwenhuijzen-Kruseman, A. C., Bosman, F. T., et al.: Medullary differentiation of anaplastic thyroid carcinoma. Am. J. Clin. Pathol. 77:541–547, 1982.

325. Noel, M., Delehaye, M. C., et al.: Demonstration of the coexpression of calcitonin and thyroglobulin gene in mixed follicular and medullary thyroid carcinoma. Ann. Endocrinol. *49*:195, 1988 (abstract).

326. Nonidez, J. F.: The origin of the "parafollicular" cell: a second epithelial component of the thyroid gland of the dog. Am. J. Anat. *49*:479–505, 1932.

327. Norman, T., and Johannessen, J. V.: Cell types in medullary thyroid carcinoma. Acta Pathol. Microbiol. Scand. *85*:561–571, 1977.

328. Norman, T., Johannessen, J. V., et al.: Medullary carcinoma of the thyroid. Diagnostic problems. Cancer *38*:366–377, 1976.

329. Norman, T., and Ontnes, B.: Intestinal ganglioneuromatosis, diarrhea and medullary thyroid carcinoma. Scand. J. Gastroenterol. *4*:553–559, 1969.

330. Norton, J. A., Doppmann, J. L., and Brennan, M. F.: Localization and resection of clinically inapparent medullary carcinoma of the thyroid. Surgery *87*:616–622, 1980.

331. Norton, J. A., Froome, B. A., et al.: Multiple endocrine neoplasia type IIb; the most aggressive form of medullary thyroid carcinoma. Surg. Clin. N. Amer. *59*:109–118, 1979.

332. Nunez, E. A., and Gershon, M. D.: Secretion of parafollicular cells beginning at birth: ultrastructural evidence from developing canine thyroid. Am. J. Anat. *147*:372–392, 1976.

333. Nunez, E. A., Hedhammer, A., et al.: Ultrastructure of the parafollicular (C) cells and the parathyroid cell in growing dogs on a high calcium diet. Lab. Invest. *31*:96–108, 1974.

334. Nunez, E. A., Payette, R., and Quimby, F.: Thyroid medullary carcinoma of the Djungarian hamster, Phodopus sungorus: ultrastructural evidence for the production of normal and atypical intracellular granules. Virch. Arch. Cell Pathol. *54*:284–294, 1988.

335. Nunez, E. A., Payette, R., et al.: Ultrastructural immunocytochemical studies of the localization and distribution of somatostatin, calcitonin, calcitonin gene related peptide and substance P in the bat thyroid follicle. Anat. Rec. *221*:707–713, 1988.

336. O'Connor, D. T., and Deftos, L. J.: Secretion of chromogranin by peptide producing endocrine neoplasms. N. Engl. J. Med. *314*:1145–1151, 1986.

337. Ohashi, M., Yanase, T., et al.: Alpha endorphin-like immunoreactivity in medullary carcinoma of the thyroid. Cancer *59*:277–280, 1987.

338. Oishi, S., Shimada, T., et al.: Elevated serum calcitonin levels in patients with thyroid disorders. Acta Endocrinol. *107*:476–481, 1984.

339. O'Leary, T. J., and Levin, I. W.: Secondary structure of endocrine amyloid: infrared spectroscopy of medullary carcinoma of the thyroid. Lab. Invest. *53*:240–242, 1985.

340. Ooi, A., Nakanishi, I., et al.: Calcitonin producing insulinoma. Acta Pathol. Jpn. *36*:1897–1903, 1986.

341. Orimo, H., and Hirsch, P. F.: Thyrocalcitonin and age. J. Clin. Endocrinol. Metab. *93*:1206–1211, 1973.

342. Oskam, R., Rijksen, G., et al.: Enolase isoenzymes in differentiated and undifferentiated medullary thyroid carcinomas. Cancer *55*:394–399, 1985.

343. O'Toole, K., Fenoglio-Preiser, C., and Pushpraj, N.: Endocrine changes associated with the human aging process. III. Effect of age on the number of calcitonin immunoreactive cells in the thyroid gland. Hum. Pathol. *16*:991–1000, 1985.

344. Pages, A.: Pathologie de la crete neurale. Ann. Pathol. *1*:109–119, 1981.

345. Paladugu, R. O., Nathwani, B. N., et al.: Carcinoma of the larynx with mucosubstance production and neuroendocrine differentiation. Cancer *49*:343–349, 1982.

346. Palmer, B. V., Harmer, C. L., and Shaw, H. J.: Calcitonin and carcinoembryonic antigen in the followup of patients with medullary carcinoma of the thyroid. Br. J. Surg. *71*:101–104, 1984.

347. Parthemore, J. G., and Deftos, L. J.: Calcitonin secretion in normal human subjects. J. Clin. Endocrinol. Metab. *47*:184–188, 1978.

348. Pearse, A. G. E.: The cytochemistry of the thyroid C cells and their relationship to calcitonin. Proc. Soc. Lond. *164*:478–487, 1966.

349. Pearse, A. G. E.: Common cytochemical and ultrastructural characteristics of cells producing polypeptide hormones (the APUD series) and their relevance to thyroid and ultimobranchial C cells and calcitonin. Proc. Roy. Soc. Lond. *170*:71–80, 1968.

350. Pearse, A. G. E., Ewen, S. W. B., and Polak, J. M.: The genesis of apudamyloid in endocrine polypeptide tumors: histochemical distinction from immunoamyloid. Virch. Arch. Cell Pathol. *10*:93–107, 1972.

351. Pearse, A. G. E., and Polak, J. M.: Cytochemical evidence for the neural crest origin of mammalian ultimobranchial C cells. Histochemie 27:96–102, 1976.
352. Perkins, J. T., Blackstone, M. O., and Riddell, R. H.: Adenomatous polyposis coli and multiple endocrine neoplasia type 2B. Cancer 55:375–381, 1985.
353. Perrier, P., Thomas, J. L., et al.: Lack of linkage between HLA and multiple endocrine neoplasia type 2 in a French family. Tissue Antigens 29:13–17, 1987.
354. Petko, J. T.: The use of 1:9 dimethyl methylene blue for the demonstration of thyroid C cells. Stain Tech. 49:65–67, 1974.
355. Pfaltz, M., Hedinger, C. E., and Muhlethaler, J. P.: Mixed medullary and follicular carcinoma of the thyroid. Virch. Arch. Pathol. Anat. 400:53–59, 1983.
356. Polliack, A., and Freund, U.: Mixed papillary and follicular carcinoma of the thyroid gland with stromal amyloid. Am. J. Clin. Pathol. 53:592–597, 1970.
357. Ponder, B. A. J.: Screening for familial medullary thyroid carcinoma: a review. J. Roy. Soc. Med. 77:585–594, 1984.
358. Ponder, B. A. J., Finer, N., et al.: Family screening in medullary thyroid carcinoma presenting without a family history. Quart. J. Med. 252:299–308, 1988.
359. Ponder, B. A. J., Ponder, M. A., et al.: Risk estimation and screening in families of patients with medullary thyroid carcinoma. Lancet 1:397–400, 1988.
360. Posen, J. A., Adamthwaite, D. N., and Greeff, H.: Melanin-producing medullary carcinoma of the thyroid gland. S. Afr. Med. J. 65:57–59, 1984.
361. Poston, G. J., Seitz, P. K., et al.: Calcitonin gene related peptide: Possible tumor marker for medullary thyroid cancer. Surgery 102:1049–1054, 1987.
362. Queener, S. F., and Bell, N. H.: Calcitonin: a general survey. Metabolism 24:555–567, 1975.
363. Ram, M. D., Rao, K. N., and Brown, L.: Hypercalcitoninemia, pheochromocytoma and C cell hyperplasia. A new variant of Sipple's syndrome. J. A. M. A. 239:2155–2156, 1978.
364. Ranchod, M., Kempson, R. L., and Dorgeloh, J. R.: Strumal carcinoid of the ovary. Cancer 37:1912–1922, 1976.
365. Raue, F., Boller, G., et al.: Secretion of calcitonin and carcinoembryonic antigen in longterm organ culture of human medullary thyroid carcinoma. Klin. Wochenstr. 63:205–210, 1985.
366. Robboy, S. J., Norris, H. J., and Scully, R. E.: Insular carcinoid in the ovary. A clinicopathologic analysis of 48 cases. Cancer 36:404–418, 1975.
367. Robboy, S. J., Scully, R. E., and Norris, H. J.: Primary trabecular carcinoid of the ovary. Obstet. Gynecol. 49:202–207, 1977.
368. Robinson, H. B.: DiGeorge's or the III–IV pharyngeal pouch syndrome. Persp. Pediatr. Pathol. 2:173–203, 1975.
369. Rocklin, R. E., Gagel, R., et al.: Cellular immune response in familial medullary thyroid carcinoma. N. Engl. J. Med. 296:835–838, 1977.
370. Roediger, W. E. W.: A comparative study of the normal human neonatal and the canine C cell. J. Anat. 115:255–276, 1973.
371. Roediger, W. E. W.: The oxyphil and C cells of the human thyroid gland: a cytochemical and histopathologic review. Cancer 36:1758–1770, 1975.
372. Roos, B. A., Huber, M. B., et al.: Medullary thyroid carcinomas secrete a noncalcitonin peptide corresponding to the carboxyl-terminal region of preprocalcitonin. J. Clin. Endocrinol. Metab. 56:802–807, 1983.
373. Roos, B. A., Lindall, A. W., et al.: Plasma immunoreactive calcitonin in lung cancer. J. Clin. Endocrinol. Metab. 50:659–666, 1980.
374. Rosenberg, E. M., Hahn, T. J., et al.: ACTH secreting medullary carcinoma of the thyroid presenting as severe idiopathic osteoporosis and senile purpura. J. Clin. Endocrinol. Metab. 47:255–262, 1978.
375. Roth, K. A., Bensch, K. G., and Hoffman, A. R.: Characterization of opioid peptides in human thyroid medullary carcinoma. Cancer 59:1594–1598, 1987.
376. Rougier, P., Calmettes, C., et al.: The value of calcitonin and carcinoembryonic antigen in the treatment and management of nonfamilial medullary thyroid carcinoma. Cancer 51:855–862, 1983.
377. Rougier, P., Parmentier, C., et al.: Medullary thyroid carcinoma: Prognostic factors and treatment. Int. J. Rad. Oncol. Biol. Phys. 9:161–169, 1983.
378. Ruppert, J. M., Eggleston, J. C., et al.: Disseminated calcitonin poor medullary thyroid carcinoma in a patient with calcitonin rich primary tumor. Am. J. Surg. Pathol. 10:513–518, 1986.
379. Russell, C. F., Van Heerden, J. A., et al.: The surgical management of medullary thyroid carcinoma. Ann. Surg. 197:42–48, 1983.
380. Saad, M. F., Fritsche, H. A., and Samaan, N. A.: Diagnostic and prognostic values of carcinoembryonic antigen in medullary carcinoma of the thyroid. J. Clin. Endocrinol. Metab. 58:889–894, 1984.
381. Saad, M. F., Ordonez, N. G., et al.: The prognostic value of calcitonin immunostaining in medullary carcinoma of the thyroid. J. Clin. Endocrinol. Metab. 59:850–856, 1984.
382. Saad, M. F., Ordonez, N. G., et al.: Medullary carcinoma of the thyroid. A study of the clinical features and prognostic factors in 161 patients. Medicine 63:319–342, 1984.
383. Samaan, N. A., Hsu, T. C., et al.: Chromosomal instability in medullary carcinoma of the thyroid. World J. Surg. 8:487–492, 1984.

384. Samaan, N. A., Schultz, P. N., and Hickey, R. C.: Medullary thyroid carcinoma: Prognosis of familial versus sporadic disease and the role of radiotherapy. J. Clin. Endocrinol. Metab. 67:801–805, 1988.

385. Sanderson, P. H., Marshall, F., and Wilson, R. E.: Calcium and phosphorus homeostasis in the parathyroidectomized dog: evaluation by means of ethylene diamine tetraacetate and calcium tolerance test. J. Clin. Invest. 39:662–670, 1960.

386. Sarosi, G., and Doe, R. P.: Familial occurrence of parathyroid adenomas, pheochromocytoma, and medullary carcinoma of the thyroid with amyloid stroma (Sipple's syndrome). Ann. Intern. Med. 68:1305–1308, 1968.

387. Schaffer, R., Muller, H. A., et al.: Cytological findings in medullary carcinoma of the thyroid. Pathol. Res. Pract. 178:461–466, 1984.

388. Schimke, R. N.: Multiple endocrine adenomatosis syndromes. Adv. Intern. Med. 21:249–265, 1976.

389. Schimke, R. N., and Hartman, W. H.: Familial amyloid producing medullary thyroid carcinoma and pheochromocytoma: a distinct genetic entity. Ann. Intern. Med. 63:1027–1039, 1965.

390. Schimke, R. N., Hartman, W. H., et al.: Syndrome of bilateral pheochromocytoma, medullary thyroid carcinoma and multiple neuromas. N. Engl. J. Med. 279:1–17, 1968.

391. Schmid, K. W., Fischer-Colbie, R., et al.: Chromogranin A and B and Secretogranin II in medullary carcinomas of the thyroid. Am. J. Surg. Pathol. 11:551–556, 1987.

392. Schroder, S., Bocker, W., et al.: Prognostic factors in medullary thyroid carcinomas: Survival in relation to age, sex, stage, histology, immunocytochemistry and DNA content. Cancer 61:806–816, 1988.

393. Schroder, S., and Delling, O.: Bone metastases of differentiated and medullary thyroid gland carcinomas: usefulness and limitation of immunohistology performed on undecalcified plastic embedded tissue specimens. Virch. Arch. Pathol. Anat. 409:767–776, 1986.

394. Schroder, S., and Kloppel, G.: Carcinoembryonic antigen and nonspecific cross reacting antigen in thyroid cancer. Am. J. Surg. Pathol. 11:100–108, 1987.

395. Schurch, W., Babei, F., et al.: Light, electron microscopic and cytochemical studies on the morphogenesis of familial medullary thyroid carcinoma. Virch. Arch. Pathol. Anat. 376:29–46, 1977.

396. Schurr, W., Rix, E., et al.: Metastatic C cell carcinoma: Calcitonin and CEA production in monolayer culture. J. Cancer Res. Clin. Oncol. 111:284–288, 1986.

396a. Schwartz, R. W., Kenady, D. E., et al.: Medullary thyroid cancer and Graves' disease. Surgery 105:804–807, 1989.

397. Schwerk, W. B., Grun, R., and Wahl, R.: Ultrasound diagnosis of C cell carcinoma of the thyroid. Cancer 55:614–630, 1985.

398. Sciubba, J. J., D'Amico, E., and Attie, J. N.: The occurrence of multiple endocrine neoplasia type IIb in two children of an affected mother. J. Oral Pathol. 16:310–316, 1987.

399. Sikri, K. L., Varndell, I. M., et al.: Medullary carcinoma of the thyroid. An immunocytochemical and histochemical study of 25 cases using eight separate markers. Cancer 56:2481–2491, 1985.

400. Silva, O. L., Becker, K. L., et al.: Increased serum calcitonin levels in bronchogenic cancer. Chest 69:495–499, 1976.

401. Silva, O. L., Becker, K. L., et al.: Hypercalcitoninemia in bronchogenic cancer: evidence for thyroid origin of the hormone. J.A.M.A. 234:183–185, 1975.

402. Silver, M. M., Hearn, S. A., et al.: Calcitonin and chromogranin A localization in medullary carcinoma of the thyroid by immunoelectron microscopy. J. Histochem. Cytochem. 36:1031–1036.

403. Simpson, N. E.: Genetic studies of multiple endocrine neoplasia type 2 syndromes. Henry Ford Hosp. Med. J. 32:273–276, 1984.

404. Simpson, N. E., Kidd, K. K., et al.: Assignment of multiple endocrine neoplasia type 2A to chromosome 10 by linkage. Nature 328:528–529, 1987.

405. Simpson, W. J., Palmer, J. A., et al.: Management of medullary carcinoma of the thyroid. Am. J. Surg. 144:420–422, 1982.

406. Sipple, J. H.: The association of pheochromocytoma with carcinoma of the thyroid gland. Am. J. Med. 31:163–166, 1961.

407. Sizemore, G. W.: Medullary carcinoma of the thyroid gland. Sem. Oncol. 14:306–314, 1987.

408. Sizemore, G. W., and Go, V. L. W.: Stimulation tests for the diagnosis of medullary thyroid carcinoma. Mayo Clin. Proc. 50:53–56, 1975.

409. Sizemore, G. W., and Heath, H.: Immunochemical heterogeneity of calcitonin in plasma of patients with medullary thyroid carcinoma. J. Clin. Invest. 55:1111–1118, 1975.

410. Skrabanek, P., Cannon, D., et al.: Substance P in medullary carcinoma of the thyroid. Experientia 35:1259–1260, 1979.

411. Skrabanek, P., Nat, D. R., and Powell, D.: Unifying concept of nonpituitary ACTH secreting tumors: evidence of common origin of neural crest tumors, carcinoids and oat cell carcinomas. Cancer 42:1263–1269, 1978.

412. Sletten, K., Westermark, P., and Natvig, J. B.: Characterization of amyloid fibril proteins from medullary carcinoma of the thyroid. J. Exp. Med. 143:993–1000, 1976.

413. Snyder, R. R., and Tavassoli, F. A.: Ovarian strumal carcinoid: immunohistochemical, ultrastructural and clinicopathologic observations. Int. J. Gynecol. Pathol. 5:187–199, 1986.

414. Sobrinho-Simoes, M., Nesland, J., and Johannessen, J. V.: Farewell to the dual histogenesis of thyroid tumors. Ultrastruct. Pathol. 8:iii–v, 1985.
415. Stanley, R. J., Scheithauer, B. W., et al.: Neural and neuroendocrine tumors of the larynx. Ann. Otol. Rhinol. Laryngol. 96:630–638, 1987.
416. Starling, J. R., Harris, C., and Granner, D. K.: Diagnosis of occult familial medullary carcinoma of the thyroid using pentagastrin. Arch. Surg. 113:241–143, 1978.
417. Steenbergh, P. H., Hoppener, J. W. M., et al.: Expression of the proopiomelanocortin gene in human medullary thyroid carcinoma. J. Clin. Endocrinol. Metab. 58:904–908, 1984.
418. Steenbergh, P. H., Hoppener, J. W. M., et al.: Calcitonin gene related peptide coding sequence is conserved in the human genome and is expressed in medullary thyroid carcinoma. J. Clin. Endocrinol. Metab. 59:358–360, 1984.
419. Steinfeld, C. M., Moertel, C. G., and Woolner, L. B.: Diarrhea and medullary carcinoma of the thyroid. Cancer 31:1237–1239, 1973.
420. Steiner, A. L., Goodman, A. D., and Powers, S. R.: Study of a kindred with pheochromocytoma, medullary thyroid carcinoma, hyperparathyroidism and Cushing's disease: Multiple endocrine neoplasia type 2. Medicine 47:371–409, 1968.
421. Stepanas, A. V., Samaan, N. A., et al.: Medullary thyroid carcinoma: importance of serial calcitonin measurement. Cancer 43:825–837, 1979.
422. Stevens, R. E., and Moore, G. E.: Inadequacy of APUD concept in explaining production of peptide hormones by tumours. Lancet 1:118–119, 1983.
423. Stux, M., Thompson, B., et al.: The "light cell" of the thyroid gland in the rat. Endocrinology 68:292–308, 1961.
424. Sugiyama, S.: The embryology of the human thyroid gland including ultimobranchial body and others related. Erg. Anat. Entwick. 44:6–111, 1971.
425. Sunday, M. E., Wolfe, H. J., et al.: Gastrin-releasing peptide gene expression in developing, hyperplastic and neoplastic thyroid C cells. Endocrinology 122:1551–1558, 1988.
426. Sundler, F., Alumets, J., et al.: Somatostatin immunoreactive cells in medullary carcinoma of the thyroid. Am. J. Pathol. 88:381–386, 1977.
427. Sussman, K. E., Draznin, B., et al.: The endocrine secretion granule revisited—postulating new functions. Metabolism 31:959–967, 1982.
428. Suzuki, T., Ito, S., et al.: Ultrastructural demonstration of calcitonin in osmium fixed human medullary carcinoma of thyroid by the protein A colloidal gold technique. Virch. Arch. Pathol. Anat. 407:497–417, 1985.
429. Swarup, K., Tewari, N. P., and Srivastav, A. K.: Ultimobranchial body and parathyroid gland of the parrot Psittacula psittacula in response to experimental hypercalcemia. Archiv. Anat. Micr. Morphol. Exper. 75:271–277, 1986–87.
430. Sweeney, E. C., McDonnell, L., and O'Brien, C.: Medullary carcinoma of the thyroid presenting as tumours of the pharynx and larynx. Histopathology 5:263–275, 1981.
431. Szijj, I., Csapo, Z., et al.: Medullary cancer of the thyroid gland associated with hypercorticism. Cancer 24:167–173, 1969.
432. Taggart, H. M., Chesnut, C. H., et al.: Deficient calcitonin response to calcium stimulation in postmenopausal osteoporosis? Lancet 1:475–477, 1982.
433. Talerman, A., Lindeman, J., et al.: Demonstration of calcitonin and carcinoembryonic antigen (CEA) in medullary carcinoma of the thyroid (MCT) by immunoperoxidase technique. Histopathology 3:503–510, 1979.
434. Tanaka, K., Baylin, S. B., et al.: Cytogenetic studies of a human medullary thyroid carcinoma cell line. Cancer Genet. Cytogenet. 25:27–35, 1987.
435. Tangen, K. O., Lindmo, T., et al.: A flow cytometric DNA analysis of medullary thyroid carcinoma. Am. J. Clin. Pathol. 79:172–177, 1983.
436. Tashjian, A. H.: Immunoassay of thyrocalcitonin I. The method and its serological specificity. Endocrinology 84:140–148, 1969.
437. Tashjian, A. H., Howland, B. G., et al.: Immunoassay of human calcitonin. Clinical measurement, relation to serum calcium and studies in patients with medullary carcinoma. N. Engl. J. Med. 283:890–895, 1970.
438. Tashjian, A. H., and Melvin, K. E. W.: Medullary carcinoma of the thyroid gland. N. Engl. J. Med. 279:279–283, 1968.
439. Tashjian, A. H., and Voelkel, E. F.: Decreased thyrocalcitonin in thyroid glands from patients with hyperparathyroidism. J. Clin. Endocrinol. Metab. 27:1353–1357, 1967.
440. Tashjian, A. H., Wolfe, H. J., and Voelkel, E. F.: Human calcitonin: immunologic assay, cytologic localization and studies on medullary carcinoma. Am. J. Med. 56:840–849, 1974.
441. Tateishi, R., Takashi, Y., and Noguchi, A.: Histologic and ultracytochemical studies on thyroid medullary carcinoma. Cancer 30:755–763, 1972.
442. Teitelbaum, S. L., Moore, K. E., and Shieber, W.: Parafollicular cells in the normal human thyroid. Nature 230:334–345, 1971.
443. Treilhou-Lahille, F., Pidoux, E., et al.: Granular and extragranular forms of immunoreactive calcitonin in normal rat "C" cells. Biology of the Cell 57:221–230, 1986.
444. Trump, D. L., Mendelsohn, G., and Baylin, S. B.: Discordance between plasma calcitonin and tumor cell mass in medullary thyroid carcinoma. N. Engl. J. Med. 301:253–254, 1979.
445. Tsuchiya, T., Shiomura, Y., et al.: Immunocytochemical study on the C cells in pig thyroid glands. Acta Anat. 120:138–141, 1984.

446. Tsuchiya, T., Takahashi, Y., et al.: Enzyme histochemical studies on the parathyroid gland and thyroid C cells in the common dolphin (Delphinus delphis). Tohoku J. Agricult. Res. *33*:146–151, 1983.

447. Tucker, L. E., O'Neal, L. W., and Martin, S. A.: Pseudocarcinoid syndrome due to medullary carcinoma of the thyroid. Mo. Med. *81*:607–608, 620, 1984.

448. Ulbright, T. M., Kraus, F. T., and O'Neal, L. W.: C cell hyperplasia developing in residual thyroid following resection for sporadic medullary carcinoma. Cancer *48*:2076–2079, 1981.

449. Uribe, M., Grimes, M., et al.: Medullary carcinoma of the thyroid gland: Clinical, pathological and immunohistochemical features with review of the literature. Am. J. Surg. Pathol. *9*:577–594, 1985.

450. Valenta, L. J., Michel-Bechet, M., et al.: Microfollicular thyroid carcinoma with amyloid rich stroma resembling the medullary carcinoma of the thyroid (MCT). Cancer *39*:1573–1586, 1977.

451. Van Dyke, J. H.: Behavior of ultimobranchial tissue in the postnatal thyroid gland: the origin of thyroid cystadenomata in the rat. Anat. Rec. *88*:369–391, 1944.

452. Van Zweiten, M. J., Frith, C. H., et al.: Medullary thyroid carcinoma in female BALB/c mice. Am. J. Pathol. *110*:219–229, 1983.

453. Vasen, H. F. A., Nieuwenhuijzen-Kruseman, A. C., et al.: Multiple endocrine neoplasia syndrome type 2: The value of screening and central registration. Am. J. Med. *83*:847–852, 1987.

454. Vassar, P. S., and Culling, C. F.: The significance of amyloid in carcinoma of the thyroid gland. Am. J. Clin. Pathol. *36*:244–247, 1961.

455. Vaughn, C. B., and Vaitkevicius, V. K.: The effects of calcitonin in hypercalcemia in patients with malignancy. Cancer *34*:1268–1271, 1974.

456. Verdy, M., Cholette, J. P., et al.: Calcium infusion and pentagastrin injection in diagnosis of medullary thyroid carcinoma. Canad. Med. Assoc. J. *119*:29–35, 1978.

457. Wahner, H. W., Cuello, C., and Aljure, F.: Hormone induced regression of medullary (solid) thyroid carcinoma. Am. J. Med. *45*:789–794, 1968.

458. Walts, A. E., Said, J. W., et al.: Chromogranin as a marker of neuroendocrine cells in cytologic material—an immunocytochemical study. Am. J. Clin. Pathol. *84*:273–277, 1985.

459. Webb, T. A., Sheps, S. G., and Carney, J. A.: Differences between sporadic pheochromocytoma and pheochromocytoma in multiple endocrine neoplasia, type 2. Am. J. Surg. Pathol. *4*:121–126, 1980.

460. Weiss, L. M., Weinberg, D. S., and Warhol, M. J.: Medullary carcinoma arising in a thyroid with Hashimoto's disease. Am. J. Clin. Pathol. *80*:534–538, 1983.

461. Weller, G. L.: Development of the thyroid, parathyroid and thymus gland in man. Contrib. Embryol. *24*:93–118, 1933.

462. Wells, S. A., Baylin, S. B., et al.: Medullary thyroid carcinoma: relationship of method of diagnosis to pathologic staging. Ann. Surg. *188*:377–383, 1978.

463. Wells, S. A., Baylin, S. B., et al.: Thyroid venous catheterization in the early diagnosis of familial medullary thyroid carcinoma. Ann. Surg. *196*:505–510, 1982.

464. Wells, S. A., Baylin, S. B., et al.: The importance of early diagnosis in patients with hereditary medullary thyroid carcinoma. Ann. Surg. *195*:595–599, 1982.

465. Wells, S. A., Haagensen, D. E., et al.: The detection of elevated plasma levels of carcinoembryonic antigen in patients with suspected or established medullary thyroid carcinoma. Cancer *42*:1498–1503, 1978.

466. Wells, S. A., and Ontjes, D. A.: Multiple endocrine neoplasia type II. Annu. Rev. Med. *27*:263–268, 1976.

467. Wells, S. A., Ontjes, D. A., et al.: The early diagnosis of medullary carcinoma of the thyroid gland in patients with multiple endocrine neoplasia type II. Ann. Surg. *182*:362–370, 1975.

468. Welsch, U., and Pearse, A. G. E.: Comparative studies on the ultrastructure of the thyroid parafollicular cells. J. Microsc. *89*:83–94, 1969.

469. Wermer, P.: Multiple endocrine adenomatosis: multiple hormone producing tumors, a familial syndrome. Clin. Gastroenterol. *3*:671–684, 1974.

470. Westermark, P., and Johnson, K. H.: The polypeptide hormone derived amyloid forms. Acta Pathol. Microbiol. Scand. *96*:475–483, 1988.

471. Weston, J. A.: The regulation of normal and abnormal neural crest cell development. Adv. Neurol. *29*:77–95, 1981.

472. White, I. L., Vimadalal, S. D., et al.: Occult medullary carcinoma of thyroid: an unusual clinical and pathologic presentation. Cancer *47*:1364–1368, 1981.

473. Whittle, T. S., and Goodwin, M. N.: Intestinal ganglioneuromatosis with the mucosal neuroma–medullary thyroid carcinoma–pheochromocytoma syndrome. Am. J. Gastroenterol. *65*:249–257, 1976.

474. Wilander, E., Juntti-Berggren, L., et al.: Staining of rat thyroid parafollicular (C) cells with the Sevier Munger silver technique. Acta Pathol. Microbiol. Scand. *88*:339–340, 1980.

475. Williams, E. D.: A review of 17 cases of carcinoma of the thyroid and pheochromocytoma. J. Clin. Pathol. *18*:288–292, 1965.

476. Williams, E. D.: Histogenesis of medullary carcinoma of the thyroid. J. Clin. Pathol. *19*:114–118, 1966.

477. Williams, E. D.: The origin and associations of medullary carcinoma of the thyroid. *In:* Smithers, D. (ed.): Tumours of the Thyroid Gland. London, E. & S. Livingstone, 1970, pp. 130–140.

478. Williams, E. D.: C cell hyperplasia. Bull. Cancer (Paris) 71:122–124, 1984.
479. Williams, E. D., Brown, C. L., and Doniach, I.: Pathological and clinical findings in a series of 67 cases of medullary carcinoma of the thyroid. J. Clin. Pathol. 19:103–113, 1966.
480. Williams, E. D., Karim, S. M. M., and Sandler, M.: Prostaglandin secretion by medullary carcinoma of the thyroid: a possible cause of the associated diarrhea. Lancet 1:22–23, 1968.
481. Williams, E. D., Morales, A. M., and Horn, R. C.: Thyroid carcinoma and Cushing's syndrome. J. Clin. Pathol. 21:129–135, 1968.
482. Williams, E. D., and Pollock, D. J.: Multiple mucosal neuromata with endocrine tumors: A syndrome allied to von Recklinghausen's disease. J. Pathol. Bacteriol. 91:71–80, 1966.
483. Wilson, R. A., and Ibanez, M. L.: A comparative study of 14 cases of familial and nonfamilial pheochromocytomas. Hum. Pathol. 9:181–188, 1978.
484. Wolfe, H. J., DeLellis, R. A., et al.: Immunocytochemical localization of calcitonin-like material in the pituitary gland. Lab. Invest. 41:56A, 1979 (abstract).
485. Wolfe, H. J., DeLellis, R. A., et al.: C cell hyperplasia in chronic hypercalcemia in man. Am. J. Pathol. 78:20A, 1975 (abstract).
486. Wolfe, H. J., DeLellis, R. A., et al.: Distribution of calcitonin containing cells in the normal neonatal human thyroid gland: A correlation of morphology with peptide content. J. Clin. Endocrinol. Metab. 41:1076–1081, 1975.
487. Wolfe, H. J., Melvin, K. E. W., et al.: C cell hyperplasia preceding medullary thyroid carcinoma. N. Engl. J. Med. 289:437–441, 1973.
488. Wolfe, H. J., Voelkel, E. F., and Tashjian, A. H.: Distribution of calcitonin containing cells in the normal adult human thyroid gland: a correlation of morphology and peptide content. J. Clin. Endocrinol. Metab. 38:688–694, 1974.
489. Woodruff, J. M., Shah, J. P., et al.: Neuroendocrine carcinomas of the larynx. A study of two types one of which mimics thyroid medullary carcinoma. Am. J. Surg. Pathol. 9:771–790, 1985.
490. Woolner, L. B.: Thyroid carcinoma: pathologic classification with data on prognosis. Sem. Nucl. Med. 1:481–502, 1971.
491. Woolner, L. B., Beahrs, O. H., et al.: Classification and prognosis of thyroid carcinoma. Am. J. Surg. 102:354–387, 1961.
492. Wurster-Hill, D. H., Noll, W. W., et al.: Cytogenetics of medullary carcinoma of the thyroid. Cancer Genet. Cytogenet. 20:247–253, 1986.
493. Wurzel, H. M., Kourides, I. A., and Brooks, J. S. J.: Medullary carcinomas of the thyroid contain immunoreactive human chorionic gonadotropin alpha subunit. Horm. Metab. Res. 16:677, 1984.
494. Yamaguchi, K., Abe, K., et al.: Concomitant production of immunoreactive gastrin releasing peptide and calcitonin in medullary carcinoma of the thyroid. Metabolism 33:724–727, 1984.
495. Yamaoka, Y.: Solid cell nest (SCN) of the human thyroid gland. Acta Pathol. Jpn. 23:493–506, 1973.
496. Yang, K. P., Pearson, C. E., and Samaan, N. A.: Estrogen receptor and hormone responsiveness of medullary thyroid carcinoma cells in continuous culture. Cancer Res. 48:2760–2763, 1988.
497. Yiakoumakis, E., Proukakis, C., et al.: Calcitonin concentrations in lung cancer and nonmalignant pulmonary diseases. Oncology 44:145–149, 1987.
498. Young, B. A., and LeBlond, C. P.: The light cell as compared to the follicular cell of the thyroid gland of the rat. Endocrinology 73:669–686, 1963.
499. Zaatari, G. S., Saigo, P. E., and Huvos, A. G.: Mucin production in medullary carcinoma of the thyroid. Arch. Pathol. Lab. Med. 107:70–74, 1983.
500. Zabel, M., and Dietal, M.: S-100 protein and neuron specific enolase in parathyroid glands and C cells of the thyroid. Histochemistry 86:389–392, 1987.
501. Zabel, M., and Schafer, H.: Ultrastructural immunocytochemical localization of neuron specific enolase in parafollicular cells of the rat thyroid. Histochemistry 83:77–80, 1985.
502. Zajac, J. D., Penschow, J., et al.: Identification of calcitonin and calcitonin gene related peptide messenger ribonucleic acid in medullary thyroid carcinomas by hybridization histochemistry. J. Clin. Endocrinol. Metab. 62:1037–1043, 1986.
503. Zeman, V., Nemec, J., et al.: Anaplastic transformation of medullary thyroid cancer. Neoplasma 25:249–255, 1978.
504. Zofkova, I., and Bednar, J.: Calcitonin inhibits TRH-induced TSH secretion. Exp. Clin. Endocrinol. 83:263–268, 1984.

11

UNDIFFERENTIATED OR ANAPLASTIC CARCINOMA OF THE THYROID

Anaplastic or undifferentiated carcinoma of the thyroid has traditionally been divided into two distinct categories: spindle and giant cell carcinoma and small cell carcinoma.[3, 11, 26, 34, 35, 42, 51, 54, 61, 68, 71, 76, 90, 105, 108]

In the spindle and giant cell tumor category, there exists a wide variety of histologic patterns which can be appropriately considered in the spectrum of anaplastic thyroid carcinoma, and the present author refers to these as epithelial predominant and sarcoma-like. Table 11–1 lists these patterns, some of which are illustrated in this chapter. The clinicopathologic similarities among these various tumors support their continued placement as a category of thyroid neoplasms.

Small cell carcinoma of the thyroid has become an entity whose major fame in recent years is that its existence is to be denied![8, 10, 55, 60, 84, 105] Indeed, numerous electron microscopic and immunohistochemical studies have shown conclusively that many tumors that would have been classified as small cell carcinoma 30 years ago do represent either medullary carcinoma, malignant lymphoma, or poorly differentiated carcinoma, insular variant.[9, 10, 12, 81, 86] In a few cases, especially in series including autopsy results, the small cell carcinoma represents a metastasis to the thyroid from a lung primary.[86] Hence, does small cell carcinoma of the thyroid exist? The answer to this question is in my opinion a qualified "yes"—it is, however, an extremely rare primary thyroid neoplasm.

ANAPLASTIC THYROID CARCINOMA—LARGE CELL TYPE; SPINDLE AND GIANT CELL CARCINOMA

Etiologic Considerations

Some indications exist in the literature on anaplastic thyroid cancer that external irradiation may play a role in its development.[5, 6, 28, 32, 46, 50, 88, 96, 103] Large series on this tumor show that a small but significant number of affected individuals have a history of irradiation to the neck.[3, 51, 71, 76] More significantly, several reports indicate that radiotherapy administered as treatment for low grade thyroid cancer may induce the development of the high grade lesion.[46, 66] This latter event is apparently quite rare and Vickery cautions that the fear of anaplastic carcinoma

Table 11–1. Patterns Seen in Large Cell Anaplastic Carcinoma of Thyroid

A. Epithelial
B. "Sarcomatous"
    1. Fibrosarcoma-like
    2. Hemangiopericytoma-like
    3. Malignant fibrous histiocytoma-like
    4. Rhabdomyosarcoma-like
    5. Angiosarcoma-like
    6. Osteoclastoma-like

should not deter physicians from treating low grade thyroid cancer with radiation if the latter is indicated for other reasons.[15]

Geographic differences also exist; anaplastic carcinoma is more frequent in regions of iodine deficiency.[35]

Clinical Features

This tumor constitutes about 3 to 5 percent of all thyroid tumors and about 10 percent of malignant ones.[3, 11, 35, 42, 51, 61, 68, 71, 76, 81, 90, 108] Epidemiologic studies have disclosed geographic differences in the incidence of this tumor. Thus, this lesion is relatively more frequent in endemic goiter regions of the world.[35, 46] Most studies indicate an origin in abnormal thyroid glands. A history of "goiter," usually of long standing, is found in about 80 percent of affected patients.[3, 11, 35, 42, 46, 61, 68, 71, 76, 81, 90, 100, 108]

Aldinger et al. described five possible clinical presentations for anaplastic carcinomas in their series of 84 cases.[3] These include:

1. The most common (31 of 84 cases) was a recent rapid growth in a longstanding goiter.
2. In 25 patients, a rapidly growing mass appeared in a patient with no prior thyroid disease.
3. In 18 cases, the patient had a history of a low grade thyroid cancer and suddenly developed a "superimposed" highly malignant tumor.
4. Five patients were found to have an unsuspected focus of anaplastic cancer within a thyroid removed for other reasons.
5. Finally, five patients were diagnosed as having metastatic anaplastic carcinoma without obvious primary site. The thyroid primary was discovered at autopsy.

Individuals with this tumor are usually elderly (over 50 years of age); it is an unusual lesion in young patients. Indeed, the diagnosis of anaplastic carcinoma of the thyroid in a patient whose age is under 40 should be questioned.[3, 11, 14, 35, 42, 46, 61, 68, 71, 76, 81, 90, 100, 108] A female proponderance is noted (ratio about 4:1 female:male).

The clinical scenario commonly encountered in these patients is exemplified as follows: An elderly woman who has had a goiter for many years presents with the recent (weeks to months) onset of dyspnea and/or dysphagia associated with enlargement of the neck mass. Physical examination usually discloses a huge mass obviously extrathyroidal; reddening or actual ulceration of the overlying skin may be present. Biopsy discloses the nature of the tumor, and, despite valiant attempts at therapy including radiation and chemotherapy, the patient succumbs in weeks or months to uncontrollable local disease and/or metastases.[3, 52, 81] Modern therapeutic approaches with radical surgery, radiation, and chemotherapy in relatively young patients may offer palliation.[16, 29, 44, 48, 80, 92, 93]

The striking association both by history and by histology of a preexisting low grade lesion and high grade cancer has led many authors to the conclusion that the pathogenesis of many anaplastic thyroid tumors results from the *transformation* of a benign or low grade lesion into a highly anaplastic one.[13, 15, 42, 66, 71, 73, 102, 108] Such transformation may be enhanced by external radiation.[3, 32, 46, 66, 71, 109]

A small number of case reports describe the occurrence of hyperthyroidism in patients with anaplastic carcinoma.[47, 72] In these cases, the pathogenesis of the hyperthyroidism is attributed to rapid destruction of the thyroid and release of stored thyroid hormone; this resembles the production of hyperthyroidism seen in subacute thyroiditis. (See Chapter 4.)

Pathology

Gross Pathology. These tumors present as large masses which freely infiltrate extrathyroidal tissues; thus, involvement of the trachea, soft tissues and lymph nodes is seen often.[3, 11, 35, 42, 46, 61, 68, 71, 76, 81, 90, 100, 108] The tumors appear white-tan and fleshy; hemorrhage and necrosis are often encountered (Fig. 11–1). An encapsulated nodule, representing the preexisting lesion may be found in intimate association with the aggressive tumor. (It should be remembered that most of these tumors are not amenable to attempts at surgical removal, so that often a biopsy only is performed; in fact, in the modern era fine needle aspiration biopsy may suffice; hence the opportunity to see the gross spectrum of these lesions is now quite rare.)

Occasionally, however, anaplastic carcinoma will be recognized as a microscopic focus in a thyroid removed for a low grade cancer or a benign nodule.[3, 11, 81] Such a case is seen in Figures 11–2, *A* and *B.*

Histology. A wide spectrum of patterns is seen (Figs. 11–3 to 11–11). About 20 to 30 percent show obvious epithelial features, whereas 50 to 60 percent show spindle cell or giant cell features or both.[11, 42, 54] In all cases, numerous mitoses

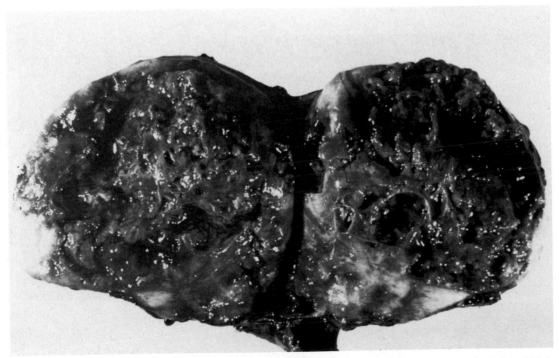

Figure 11–1. Gross appearance of anaplastic carcinoma. Fleshy tumor occupies almost all of bisected thyroid lobe; tumor extended into neighboring soft tissues. Residual recognizable thyroid is at left.

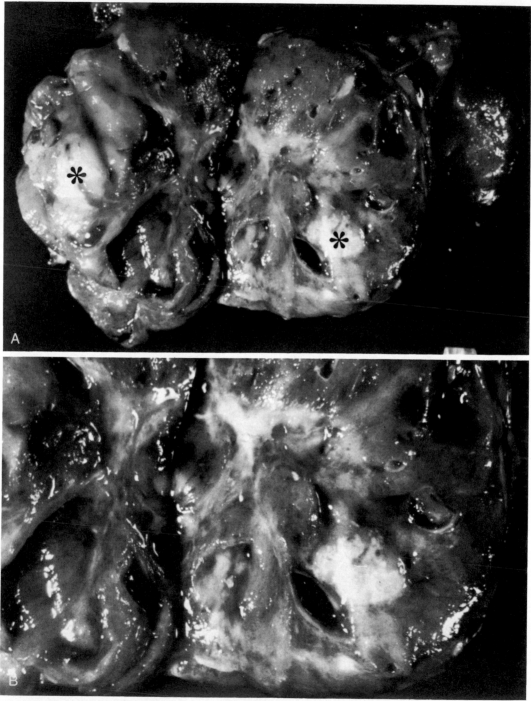

Figure 11–2. *A,* Low grade follicular carcinoma comprises most of this thyroid mass. White areas (asterisks) histologically were anaplastic carcinoma.
B, Close-up of Figure 11–2, *A.*

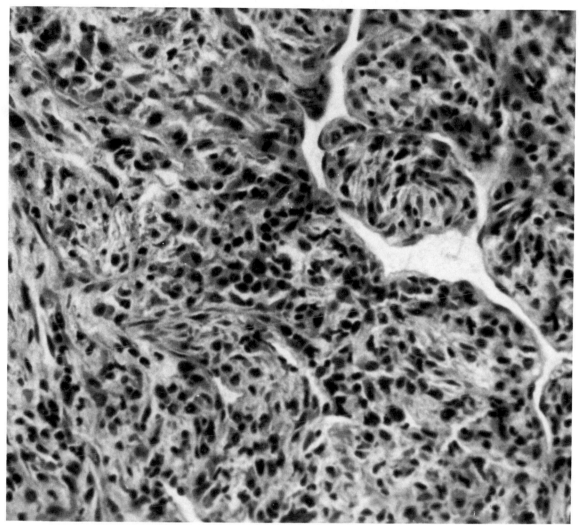

Figure 11–3. A common pattern in anaplastic carcinomas is that of pericytoma, seen here. Note irregularly shaped blood vessel at right. ×250, H & E.

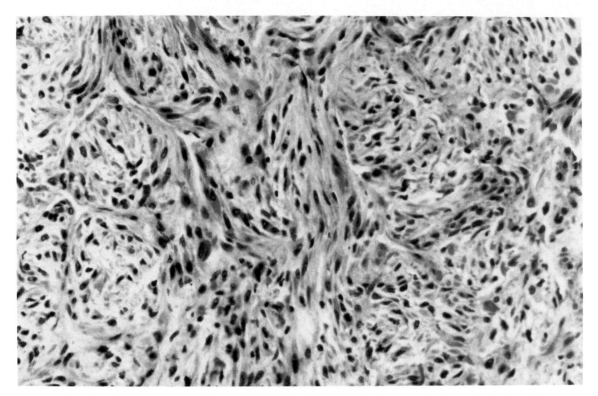

Figure 11–4. Storiform pattern reminiscent of fibrohistiocytic tumors is also common in anaplastic thyroid cancers. ×300, H & E.

(Fig. 11–5, *C*), often abnormal, are seen.[81] Cytologic anaplasia is common; bizarre tumor cells are often noted (Fig. 11–8). Necrosis is usual and may be so extensive that the only viable recognizable tumor is seen around blood vessels. The tumors show a marked propensity for invasion: thus thyroid, fat, muscle, and vascular invasion are encountered regularly. The tumor cells have a peculiar propensity to invade veins and arteries and replace endothelial cells.[11, 81] Rosai et al. indicate that this histologic feature may be helpful in distinguishing anaplastic cancer from sarcomas.[81] Of course, this type of vascular penetration can produce occlusion and subsequent infarction-like necrosis in the tumor.

The epithelial types resemble large cell undifferentiated carcinoma of other organs such as lung. Nests and clusters of cohesive tumor cells are seen; by ordinary stains and especially by reticulin staining, the grouping of the neoplastic cells is prominent. These tumors are easily recognized as epithelial; differentiation into glands is not identified, although occasionally trabeculae form or "squamoid" differentiation is noted[11, 40, 69, 81] (18 percent in the Carcangiu et al. series[11]). (Some authors include squamous cell carcinoma in this group. I do not since, although clinical similarities exist, the recognition of the squamous elements in most or all of the tumor enables one to render a more precise diagnosis.[40]) In some examples, the epithelial areas blend imperceptibly with spindle cell zones, resembling the sarcoma-like subgroup.

The sarcoma-like group may exhibit patterns suggesting a variety of sarcomas (Table 11–1); the most frequently seen are hemangiopericytoma (Fig. 11–3) or fibrous histiocytoma patterns (Fig. 11–4). When tumor giant cells are present the lesion may resemble pleomorphic rhabdomyosarcoma or malignant fibrous histiocytoma, giant cell type (Fig. 11–8). Angiosarcomatous areas may be seen.[11, 54, 68, 81, 108] (True angiosarcoma of the thyroid, however, exists and for epidemiologic

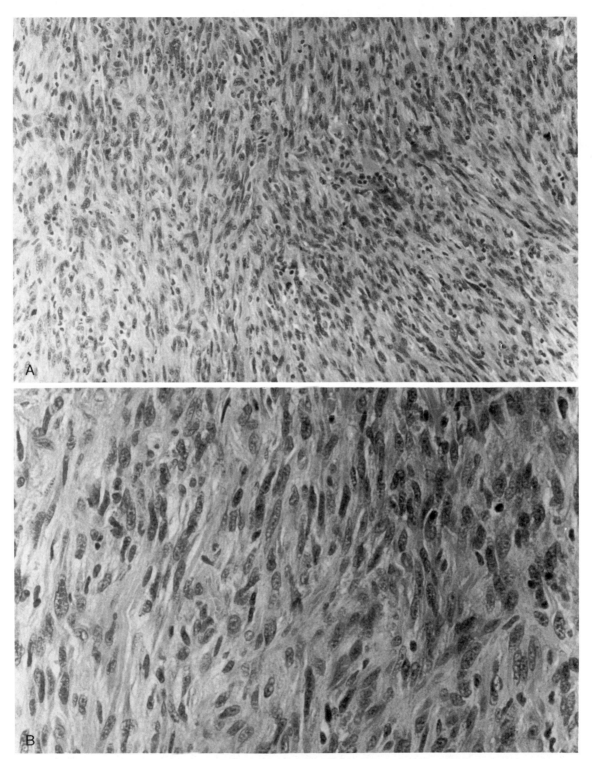

Figure 11–5. *A,* Another common pattern is spindle cell sarcoma without specific features. ×200, H & E. *B,* Higher power view of Figure 11–5, *A.* ×300, H & E.

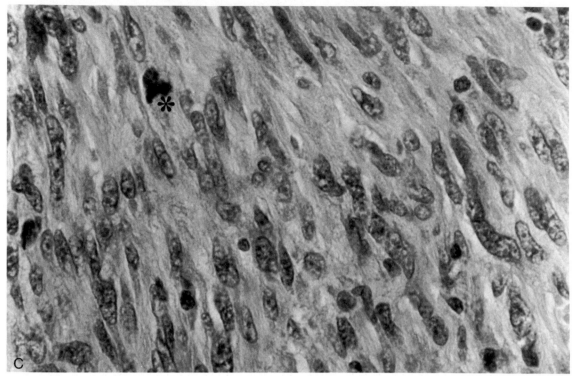

Figure 11–5 *Continued C,* Numerous and atypical mitoses are common (asterisk). ×400, H & E. Same case as in Figures 11–5, *A* and 11–5, *B.*

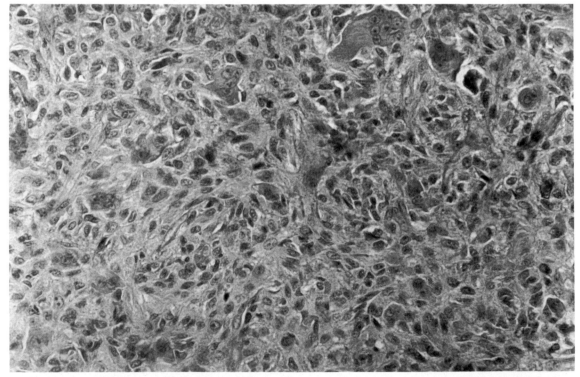

Figure 11–6. Anaplastic carcinoma with osteoclastic giant cells. The nature of the giant cells remains disputed. ×200, H & E.

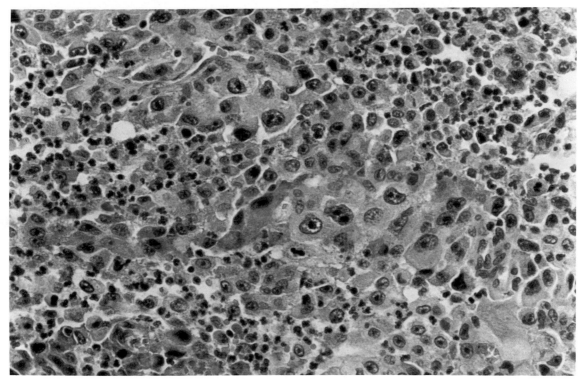

Figure 11–7. Epithelial nests of this anaplastic carcinoma may be seen throughout the tumor or merging with spindle cell areas. ×250, H & E.

reasons should be separated from this group [see below]). Mitoses, often abnormal, are commonly found. Hemorrhage and necrosis are usually seen.

Another unusual variant of the giant cell carcinoma is the so-called osteoclastic type (Fig. 11–6)[20, 24, 31, 33, 49, 61, 91]; this lesion, which resembles similar tumors that occur in the pancreas and breast,[2, 7, 39, 100, 104, 106] is believed by most authors to represent a variant of carcinoma.

The nature of the osteoclastic giant cell in these thyroid tumors remains debated.[12, 49, 81] Several authors consider them benign reactive cells of histiocytic origin[33, 61, 81]; some electron microscopic and immunohistologic evidence supports this view. Hashimoto et al. described high levels of acid phosphatase activity, and phagocytic capacity in these cells.[33] Ultrastructural features of histiocytes include many small mitochondria, lysosomes, and vacuoles and absence of intercellular junctions.[20, 33]

However, others, notably Albores-Saavedra (quoted by Rosai et al.[81] and Kobayashi et al.[49]) believe the giant cells are epithelial and malignant since they can be found in blood vessels near the tumor and are present in metastatic sites.[31, 91] The nature of these cells remains unclear at present.

Although originally considered to be a somewhat less aggressive neoplasm,[91] subsequent studies have not borne this out.[20, 24, 31, 33, 61]

Associated Lesions. By light microscopy alone, it might be difficult to dogmatically categorize all these sarcoma-like lesions as carcinoma. Evidence which supports the epithelial nature of the sarcoma-like lesions includes the transition zones between the low and high grade lesions, finding epithelial nests in the spindle cells areas, and reticulin staining which outlines the epithelial pattern in the sarcomatous zones.[11, 46, 61]

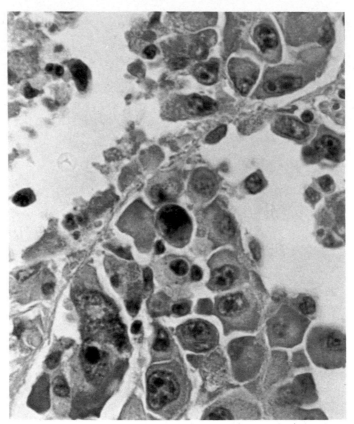

Figure 11–8. Markedly pleomorphic large cells reminiscent of melanoma, rhabdomyosarcoma, or malignant fibrous histiocytoma can occur. ×300, H & E.

Rare cases have been described wherein the anaplastic change occurs only in metastatic sites.[46, 66] The primary thyroid cancers are well differentiated papillary or follicular lesions; in some cases with which the present author is familiar, radioiodine therapy has been given to the differentiated metastases many months or years before "transformation" occurs.

If adequate tissue is available for study from the primary, at the periphery of many lesions well-differentiated lesions may be found.[3, 11, 54, 68, 81, 101, 108, 109] What do these patients have that corresponds to the goiter they frequently manifest? Histologically, this enlargement may represent adenomatous goiter, an adenomatous nodule (follicular adenoma), or a carcinoma of the well-differentiated type, e.g., papillary, follicular, or Hürthle cell. The incidence of cancer types has been variously quoted as "pure follicular," 88 percent, and papillary, 12 percent.[3, 42, 46, 71] In the present author's experience, the papillary cancers are as frequent or more frequent than pure follicular ones. (It is possible that some so-called follicular cancers in the above quoted percentages represent the follicular variant of papillary carcinoma. It is also possible, since follicular carcinoma is more commonly found in endemic goiter regions,[35] which also have a relatively larger number of anaplastic carcinomas, that follicular carcinomas do predispose to anaplastic transformation more frequently than papillary cancers.)[11, 54, 81]

Zones of transition between the low grade or benign lesion and the anaplastic ones can also be noted.[3, 11, 42, 46, 54, 71, 81] Some series have indicated that a significant percentage of anaplastic carcinomas are associated with or represent dedifferentiated medullary cancers.[59, 62, 70] However, others dispute this.[11, 54, 81] Thus, although one can find anaplastic, even giant cell areas in recognizable medullary thyroid carcinomas (MTC),[81] the recognition of the tumor as basically MTC is usually evident. If one examines classic anaplastic carcinomas for evidence of medullary carcinoma differentiation, i.e., calcitonin-containing cells, electron microscopic evidence of neurosecretory granules, etc., most authors find medullary features lacking.[81] Occasionally, case reports still suggest, however, that some undifferentiated thyroid cancers are associated with (derived from ?) tumors of combined follicular and medullary differentiation.[63, 74]

Electron Microscopic Studies. Such studies have indicated that almost all anaplastic thyroid tumors are indeed epithelial in nature. The cells contain many cytoplasmic organelles and dense bodies similar to those found in follicular epithelium (Figs. 11–12 and 11–13).[25, 27, 30, 37, 38, 43, 69, 81, 110] The neoplastic cells contain large, pleomorphic nuclei, prominent nucleoli, and abundant organelle-poor cytoplasm. All studies indicate that the tumor cells contain conspicuously folded rough endoplasmic reticulum and numerous free ribosomes. Variably present are lipid droplets, lysosomes, and microvilli. At least some cells show cell-cell junctions including desmosomes and tonofilaments; Jao and Gould stress that desmosomes are quite rare in the most anaplastic lesions, however.[43]

Newland et al. noted that one of the 10 cases they examined showed abundant cytoplasmic filaments consistent with keratin, indicating squamous differentiation.[69]

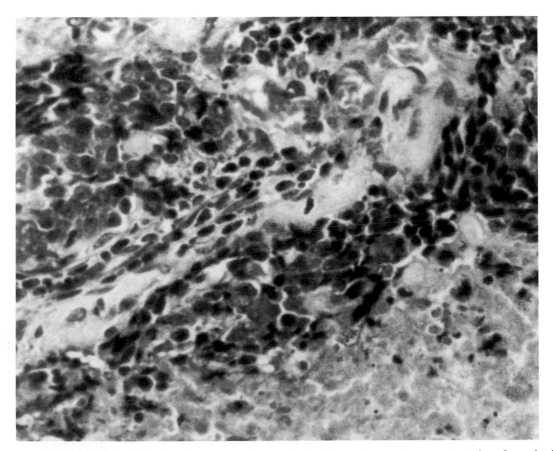

Figure 11–9. Islands of epithelial nests, often with central necrosis, can be seen in some examples of anaplastic carcinoma. × 250, H & E.

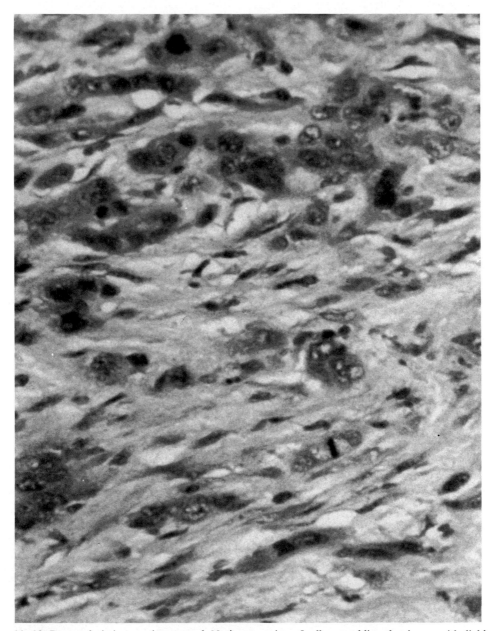

Figure 11–10. Desmoplasia is sometimes noted. Notice grouping of cells resembling that in an epithelial lesion and mitosis in lower half of picture. ×250, H & E.

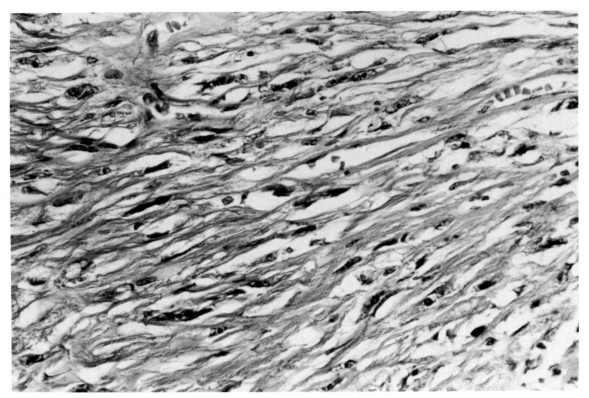

Figure 11–11. Occasional areas in anaplastic spindle cell tumors are paucicellular. Extensive fibrous tissue proliferation with few cells may not raise the suspicion of a high grade malignancy. However, spindle cells present are distinctly abnormal and pleomorphic. ×200, H & E.

Immunohistochemical Studies.[54, 64, 81, 87] These have also supported the epithelial nature of these tumors. Keratin has been found in 47 to 100 percent of these lesions[11, 41, 54, 81]; interestingly, even the obviously epithelial ones may not stain positively for keratin.[54]

The variability of staining for keratin may relate not only to methodologic and interpretation differences between laboratories, but also (and more likely) to antibodies used. Hence, using monoclonal antibodies directed against low molecular weight keratin gives positive staining in 50 to 100 percent of anaplastic thyroid tumors.[11, 36, 41, 54, 64, 67, 77, 81, 107] Antibodies to high molecular weight keratin stained only 17 percent of the cases in the series of Carcangiu et al., however.[11]

As more specific antikeratin antibodies are readily available, the percentage of anaplastic carcinomas which are immunohistologically stainable may increase. Future studies using different monoclonals to the various keratin subtypes may yield even higher percentages of positive in these tumors, providing further support for an epithelial origin.

In our anaplastic thyroid tumors, similar staining results were obtained with antiepithelial membrane antigen as for keratin.[54]

The practical value of vimentin immunostaining in distinguishing epithelial from mesenchymal anaplastic tumors has been questioned, since in some laboratories, including our own, coexpression of vimentin and keratin was recognized in about one-third of the lesions.[41, 54, 81]

If these tumors are epithelial, are they related to follicular or parafollicular cells? Most studies suggest the former[1, 11, 54, 64, 81]; ultrastructural evidence shows cells of these tumors resemble follicular cells.[25, 43] Immunohistologic studies suggest that some of these tumors may stain positively for thyroglobulin[11, 41, 54, 81]; however, a few studies suggest that a number of them represent medullary tumors and stain for calcitonin.[41, 59, 62, 70] In our own experience, none of the 29 cases we studied stained for calcitonin; a small number (27 percent) stained for thyroglobulin, but only primary tumors did so.[54] Indeed, it was found that those cases which did stain positively for thyroglobin did so only in areas which abutted upon preexisting thyroid or low grade thyroid tumor. This was interpreted as a diffusion phenomenon rather than actual production of thyroid hormone by the tumor cells.[11, 54, 81] However, other studies, including tissue culture work on isolated tumors, have shown that under certain conditions these undifferentiated tumors may indeed function and secrete thyroglobulin.[45, 47, 57, 65] In one study, 44 percent of the cases stained for thyroxine and/or triiodotyrosine.[41]

Differential Diagnostic Considerations

The histologic differential diagnosis of large cell anaplastic thyroid tumors includes large cell malignant lymphoma, true sarcomas of the thyroid and/or neck region, spindle cell medullary carcinoma, and Riedel's disease.

Large cell malignant lymphomas of diffuse type (i.e., diffuse histiocytic lymphomas) (see Chapter 14), can arise primarily in the thyroid, usually superimposed on thyroiditis. These tumors share clinical features with anaplastic cancers, but must be recognized as lymphomas, since the latter can be satisfactorily treated by modern radiotherapy and/or chemotherapeutic modalities.[56, 82]

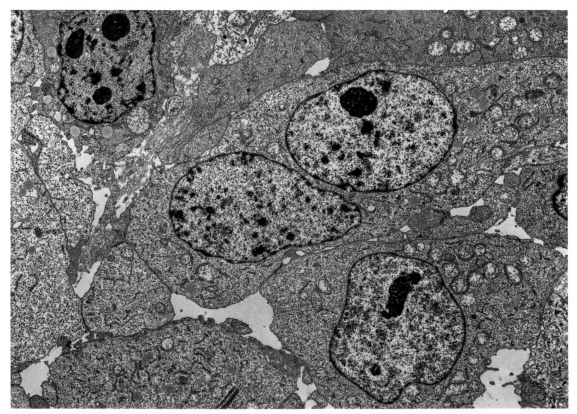

Figure 11–12. At the ultrastructural level, nesting of tumor cells is seen. Note abnormal nuclei and sparse cytoplasmic contents, chiefly mitochondria. ×8000.

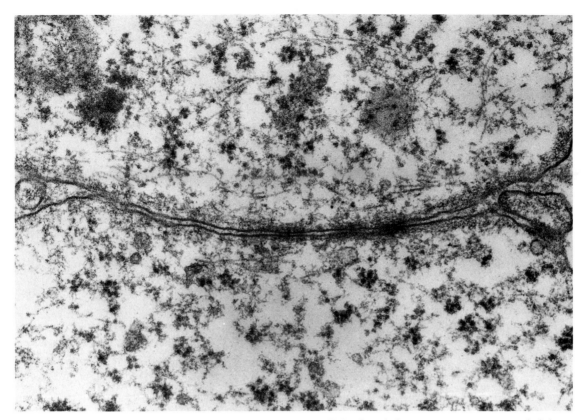

Figure 11-13. At higher power, cell junctions, including well-developed desmosomes, are present, helping to confirm the epithelial nature of this anaplastic thyroid tumor. ×60,000.

Immunohistologic stains can be extremely useful in distinguishing lymphoma from carcinoma: cell surface immunoglobulins may be helpful.[56] In fixed tissue the small battery of lymphoid markers, such as leukocyte common antigen and anticytokeratin, can be used in elucidating the type of tumor studied.

It seems to this author, however, that immunostains may be needed only as confirmation of a histologic diagnosis; the *education* of pathologists to the possibility of *primary* thyroid lymphoma usually allows the diagnosis of lymphoma to be rendered readily.

Ultrastructural studies can also distinguish lymphoma from carcinoma, but the need for appropriately prepared tissue and the expense involved often preclude the use of this technique.

True sarcomas of the thyroid (see below) are extremely rare. Most lesions so recorded in the world's literature probably represent spindle cell carcinomas. Clinical (historical) features, keratin immunostaining, and/or electron microscopy may be useful in the differential diagnosis. However, most of these tumors classified as sarcomas are associated with a dismal prognosis similar to that of anaplastic cancer; hence, for practical purposes, the distinction is academic.

Medullary carcinoma (MTC) of the spindle cell variety, especially if little amyloid is present, can occasionally be misinterpreted as anaplastic cancer. In the past, before the separation of MTC as a distinct pathologic entity, this diagnostic confusion was common. However, MTC does not usually show the pleomorphism, necrosis, and abnormal mitoses of anaplastic carcinoma. Immunolocalization for calcitonin is useful, of course. Some authors believe in the concept of anaplastic transformation of medullary carcinoma[59, 62, 70]; however, the experience of others, including the present author, does not support this concept.[81] (See above.)

Reidel's disease, discussed in Chapter 6, is a fibrous proliferation associated with inflammatory cells and vasculitis. It shares with anaplastic carcinoma the gross appearance of infiltration of extrathyroidal tissues; however, histologically, the proliferation in Riedel's disease is bland and necrosis is absent. Very rarely, anaplastic carcinomas will have paucicellular zones which superficially might be confused with a fibrosclerotic lesion (Fig. 11–11).

ANAPLASTIC TUMORS—SMALL CELL TYPE

The existence of small cell carcinoma primary in the thyroid has been called into question in recent years.[11, 54, 78, 81, 105] Indeed, about a quarter century ago, small cell carcinoma was included as a subtype of anaplastic carcinoma of the thyroid.

Meissner and Warren[61] described two histologic patterns in small cell carcinoma: compact and diffuse.[61] Table 11–2 outlines these patterns and what they may represent.

Epithelial Varieties of Small Cell Carcinoma. If primary, these include medullary thyroid carcinoma usually with no amyloid[11, 54, 81] and the so-called insular variant of thyroid cancer, which is follicular derived.[12]

1. Medullary carcinoma is distinguished by immunohistochemical studies localizing calcitonin or by ultrastructural studies showing characteristic granules; see Chapter 10.

2. The insular variant of thyroid carcinoma[12, 81] is a thyroglobulin-containing tumor which has a variety of histologic patterns, including solid, resembling medullary tumors, follicular, trabecular, and occasionally papillary (see Chapter 15).

3. Autopsy studies indicate that small (oat) cell carcinoma of the lung can metastasize to the thyroid in about 20 percent of cases.[86] The finding of metastatic small cell carcinoma in surgical material is distinctly unusual but may occur.

4. True small cell epithelial carcinoma of the thyroid may, in fact, exist, but is exceedingly rare. The tumors are presumably analogous to small cell lung cancer and may indeed represent totally dedifferentiated medullary cancer. Ultrastructural studies have appeared in the literature which show an epithelial nature to small cell tumors of the thyroid. The case of Luna et al. showed some areas of papillary carcinoma and may have represented an insular carcinoma.[55] Cameron et al. studied three small cell tumors, one of which was an epithelial lesion.[10] In the author's experience, one tumor has been studied which fits into this category. This was seen in a 36-year-old woman who presented with a neck mass extending from the thyroid into the extrathyroidal soft tissues. Immunostaining showed neither thyroglobulin nor calcitonin; electron microscopic study failed to show

Table 11–2. Small Cell Carcinoma of the Thyroid

Epithelial (compact) variety
    Medullary thyroid carcinoma with little or no amyloid
    Insular variant of thyroid carcinoma (follicular derived)
    Metastatic small cell carcinoma (lung)
    True small cell carcinoma ?
Diffuse pattern
    Small cell malignant lymphoma of *or* in the thyroid

neurosecretory granules. The patient had no known lung tumor. Chemotherapy for small cell lung cancer was given with excellent short-term results.

Diffuse Small Cell Tumors

Although the report by Meissner and Phillips in 1962 described the diffuse patterned small cell "carcinoma" of the thyroid, they noted that some of their cases showed cells with "lymphoblastic" or "plasmacytic" features. Even their illustrations showed "plasmacytoid" features to the tumor cells.[60] These tumors most probably all represented malignant lymphomas of the thyroid or involving the thyroid.[9, 10, 58, 67, 77, 81, 86, 99] Recently, numerous studies showing lack of immunostaining for epithelial markers (keratin, etc.) but presence of lymphoid markers (leukocyte common antigen, etc.) indicate that the overwhelming majority of diffuse small cell carcinomas of the thyroid indeed represent lymphoma. (See also Chapter 14.)

Prognosis for small cell anaplastic tumors varies depending on the subtype involved. Malignant lymphomas of the small cell type, although often of high stage, are indolent tumors, and these patients may survive for many years. Local symptoms may be readily controlled by radiation. In fact, in the era before immunostaining availability, the response of a thyroid small cell tumor to radiation was used as a therapeutic and a diagnostic measure: thus, if the tumor shrank with radiation, it was declared a lymphoma!

On the other hand, small cell medullary carcinomas and insular tumors have significant mortality, with distant and regional metastases occurring in 50 to 69 percent of cases. The five year survival rates range from 20 to 35 percent,[12, 81] and some patients succumb to tumor after five years. However, even these dismal figures can be appreciated as good when compared to the miserable survival rates of patients with giant cell carcinomas (<5 percent at five years).

SARCOMAS OF THE THYROID

Before 1969, the European literature indicated that about 20 percent of thyroid tumors represented sarcoma. Hedinger reviewed the European experience and noted that when modern diagnostic criteria are applied, the overwhelming majority of these tumors represented anaplastic carcinoma.[35] True thyroid sarcomas are very, very rare. Fibrosarcomas, schwannomas, osteosarcomas, and chondrosarcomas have all been described.[19, 35, 53, 79, 89, 94, 95, 96] In many of these reports, however, modern immunologic or ultrastructural studies are lacking; it is therefore possible that some of these tumors represented anaplastic epithelial tumors.[81]

The one truly well-documented sarcoma which does arise in the thyroid is the angiosarcoma or hemangioendothelioma.[17, 18, 22, 23, 75] Occurring in disproportionate numbers in certain geographic regions of the world, this lesion has been most commonly described as from the alpine regions of Europe. Clinically, the affected patients resemble those with anaplastic carcinoma: older individuals, with long histories of goiter and recent growth. The tumors are usually huge and often the gross appearance is that of a hemorrhagic and partially cystic mass. Microscopically, they resemble angiosarcoma of soft tissue,[17, 18, 23, 75, 83, 97] with interanastomosing vascular channels lined by pleomorphic malignant cells. Such areas can occasionally be recapitulated in anaplastic carcinomas, but these occur focally in the latter and compose the great majority of the tumor in the true angiosarcoma.[17, 18, 23, 63, 75, 83, 97] At the ultrastructural level there are Weibel-Palade bodies present and no epithelial structures.[83] Immunologic studies clinch the diagnosis: thus both

Factor VIII related antigen and Ulex lectin can be localized to the tumor cells.[83, 97] Keratin stains are negative.

Mills et al. reported a case of "angiomatoid" anaplastic carcinoma which had features of follicular *and* medullary differentiation as well as foci of "angiosarcomatous" appearance.[63] However, this lesion did not contain Weibel-Palade bodies by electron microscopic study, and immunostaining for Factor VIII related antigen and Ulex lectin (two endothelial cell markers) was negative. Mills et al. caution that Factor VIII positive areas in neoplasms with extensive vascular invasion be interpreted with caution.[63]

CARCINOSARCOMA

Just as sarcomas of the thyroid are very rare, tumors classified as carcinosarcomas are also unusual. Most such tumors represent anaplastic carcinomas with mesenchymal metaplasias, usually cartilage or bone.[4, 81] In this aspect they resemble metaplastic breast carcinomas.[2, 39, 104] The topic of carcinosarcoma of the thyroid was reviewed by Donnell et al.,[21] who identified 14 acceptable cases, including one of their own. Of these 14 cases, five had carcinoma associated with fibrosarcoma; seven had osteosarcoma, and two showed osteo- and chondrosarcoma. Donnell et al. noted that the epithelial component always showed follicular, not papillary, differentiation. The current author has had the opportunity to study three such lesions, each showing chondroid and osseous areas in intimate association with spindle cell anaplastic carcinoma. In two of these three cases, "lower grade" carcinomas were also seen—follicular in one case and Hürthle cell in the other.

These three patients and those reported in the literature share clinical and prognostic features with anaplastic carcinomas in general, i.e., elderly individuals with fast-growing, rapidly fatal malignancies.[21] I believe for therapeutic purposes these lesions can be categorized as anaplastic carcinoma.

POORLY DIFFERENTIATED CARCINOMA[12, 85, 98] OF THE THYROID

This is a term which has been applied to any or all of the following lesions:
• Insular carcinoma
• Mucoepidermoid carcinoma
• Tall or pink cell variant of papillary cancer
• Columnar cell variant of papillary carcinoma (Evans)
• "Poorly differentiated" solid areas in well-differentiated or follicular carcinomas

These lesions are discussed in detail in Chapter 15. Here it is sufficient to mention them and to recognize that although these lesions are associated with a more guarded prognosis than ordinary papillary or follicular carcinoma, the survival rates of patients with these lesions is measurable in years and thus differ significantly from those of anaplastic carcinoma (large cell type). Such tumors should be expected to occur in the thyroid since, in comparing thyroid primary tumors with those arising in other organs, there were two ends of the spectrum of thyroid cancer in terms of survival—the well-differentiated tumors were associated with prolonged survivals in terms of decades, and the anaplastic carcinomas were associated with survivals in months. Hence, as Carcangiu et al. point out,[12] the existence of intermediate malignancy was to be predicted.

REFERENCES

1. Albores-Saavedra, J., Nadjii, M., et al.: Thyroglobulin in carcinoma of the thyroid: An immunohistochemical study. Hum. Pathol. *14*:62–66, 1983.
2. Agnantis, N. T., and Rosen, P. P.: Mammary carcinoma with osteoclast like giant cells. Am. J. Clin. Pathol. *72*:383–389, 1979.
3. Aldinger, K. A., Samaan, N. A., et al.: Anaplastic carcinoma of the thyroid: a review of 84 cases of spindle and giant cell carcinoma of the thyroid. Cancer *41*:2267–2275, 1978.
4. Arean, V. M., and Schildecker, W. W.: Carcinosarcoma of the thyroid gland: Report of two cases. So. Med. J. *57*:446–451, 1964.
5. Baker, H. W.: Anaplastic thyroid cancer twelve years after radioiodine therapy. Cancer *23*:885–890, 1969.
6. Bakri, K., Smimaoka, K., et al.: Adenosquamous carcinoma of the thyroid after radiotherapy for Hodgkin's disease. Cancer *52*:465–470, 1983.
7. Borg-Grech, A., Morris, J. A., and Eyden, B. P.: Malignant osteoclastoma-like giant cell tumor of the renal pelvis. Histopathology *11*:415–425, 1987.
8. Buckwalter, J. A., and Meredith, L. K.: Small cell carcinoma of the thyroid gland of youth. Pediatrics *15*:317–321, 1955.
9. Burt, A. D., Kerr, D. J., et al.: Lymphoid and epithelial markers in small cell anaplastic thyroid tumours. J. Clin. Pathol. *38*:893–896, 1985.
10. Cameron, R. G., Seemayer, T. A., et al.: Small cell malignant tumors of the thyroid: a light and electron microscopic study. Hum. Pathol. *6*:731–740, 1975.
11. Carcangiu, M. L., Steeper, T., et al.: Anaplastic thyroid carcinoma: a study of 70 cases. Am. J. Clin. Pathol. *83*:135–158, 1985.
12. Carcangiu, M. L., Zampi, G., and Rosai, J.: Poorly differentiated ("insular") thyroid carcinoma. Am. J. Surg. Pathol. *8*:655–668, 1984.
13. Case Records of the M. G. H. Case 29–1975. N. Engl. J. Med. *293*:186–193, 1975.
14. Case Records of the M. G. H. Case 2–1977. N. Engl. J. Med. *206*:94–100, 1977.
15. Case Records of the M. G. H. Case 37–1979. N. Engl. J. Med. *301*:600–605, 1979.
16. Casterline, P. F., Jaques, D. A., et al.: Anaplastic giant and spindle cell carcinoma of the thyroid: a different therapeutic approach. Cancer *45*:1689–1692, 1980.
17. Chan, Y. F., Ma, L., et al.: Angiosarcoma of the thyroid. An immunohistochemical and ultrastructural study of a case in a Chinese patient. Cancer *57*:2381–2388, 1986.
18. Chesky, V. E., Dreese, W. C., and Hellwig, C. A.: Hemangioendothelioma of the thyroid. J. Clin. Endocrinol. Metab. *13*:801–808, 1953.
19. Chesky, V. E., Hellwig, C. A., and Welch, J. W.: Fibrosarcoma of the thyroid gland. Surg. Gynecol. Obstet. *111*:767–770, 1960.
20. Cibull, M. L., and Gray, G. F.: Ultrastructure of osteoclastoma like giant cell tumor of thyroid. Am. J. Surg. Pathol. *2*:401–405, 1978.
21. Donnell, C. A., Pollock, W. J., and Sybers, W. A.: Thyroid carcinosarcoma. Arch. Pathol. Lab. Med. *111*:1169–1172, 1987.
22. Eckert, F., Schmid, U., et al.: Evidence of vascular differentiation in anaplastic tumours of the thyroid—an immunohistological study. Virch. Arch. Pathol. Anat. A. *412*:203–215, 1986.
23. Egloff, B.: The hemangioendothelioma of the thyroid. Virch. Arch. Pathol. Anat. *400*:119–142, 1983.
24. Esmaili, H. J., Hafez, G. R., and Warner, T. F. C. S.: Anaplastic carcinoma of the thyroid with osteoclastoma-like giant cells. Cancer *52*:2122–2128, 1983.
25. Fisher, E. R., Gregorio, R., et al.: The derivation of so-called giant cell and spindle cell undifferentiated thyroid neoplasm. Am. J. Clin. Pathol. *61*:680–689, 1974.
26. Frantz, V. K., and Yannopoulos, K.: Carcinoma of the thyroid: A clinicopathologic study of 216 cases with a ten-year followup. Adv. Thyroid Res. *9*:377–384, 1961.
27. Gaal, J. M., Horvath, E., and Kovacs, K.: Ultrastructure of two cases of anaplastic giant cell tumor of the human thyroid gland. Cancer *35*:1273–1279, 1975.
28. Getaz, P. E.: Shimaoka, K., and Rao, U.: Anaplastic carcinoma of the thyroid following external irradiation. Cancer *43*:2248–2253, 1979.
29. Goldman, J. M., Goren, E. N., et al.: Anaplastic thyroid carcinoma: long term survival after radical surgery. J. Surg. Oncol. *14*:389–394, 1980.
30. Graham, H., and Daniel, C.: Ultrastructure of anaplastic carcinoma of the thyroid. Am. J. Clin. Pathol. *61*:690–696, 1974.
31. Gubetta, L.: Undifferentiated carcinoma of the thyroid with spindle cells and giant cells of osteoclastic aspects. Pathologica *68*:271–276, 1976.
32. Harada, T., Ito, K., et al.: Fatal thyroid carcinoma: anaplastic transformation of adenocarcinoma. Cancer *39*:2588–2596, 1977.
33. Hashimoto, H., Koga, S., et al.: Undifferentiated carcinoma of the thyroid gland with osteoclast-like giant cells. Acta Pathol. Jpn. *30*:323–334, 1980.
34. Hayashi, Y., and Tokuoka, S.: Anaplastic carcinoma of the thyroid gland. Acta Pathol. Jpn. *29*:119–133, 1979.
35. Hedinger, C. E.: Sarcoma of the thyroid gland. In: Hedinger, C. E. (ed.): Thyroid Cancer. Heidelberg, Springer-Verlag, 1969, p. 47.

36. Henzen-Logmans, S. C., Mullink, H., et al.: Expression of cytokeratins and vimentin in epithelial cells of normal and pathologic thyroid tissue. Virch. Arch. Anat. Pathol. A. *410*:347–354, 1987.

37. Hiasa, Y., Ita, N., et al.: Ultrastructure of an anaplastic giant-cell carcinoma found 8 years after operation on a papillar carcinoma of the thyroid. Acta Pathol. Jpn. *28*:737–644, 1978.

38. Hofstadter, F.: Electron microscopic investigations about the differentiation of thyroid carcinoma. Pathol. Res. Pract. *169*:304–322, 1980.

39. Holland, R., and Vanhaelst, U. J. G. M.: Mammary carcinoma with osteoclast-like giant cells. Cancer *53*:1963–1973, 1984.

40. Huang, T. Y., and Assor, D.: Primary squamous cell carcinoma of the thyroid gland. Am. J. Clin. Pathol. *55*:93–98, 1971.

41. Hurlimann, J., Gardiol, D., and Scazziga, B.: Immunohistology of anaplastic thyroid carcinoma. A study of 43 cases. Histopathology *11*:567–580, 1987.

42. Hutter, R. V. P., Tollefsen, H. R., et al.: Spindle and giant cell metaplasia in papillary carcinomata of the thyroid. Am. J. Surg. *110*:660–668, 1965.

43. Jao, W., and Gould, V. E.: Ultrastructure of anaplastic (spindle and giant cell) carcinoma of the thyroid. Cancer *35*:1280–1292, 1975.

44. Jereb, B., Stjernsward, J., and Lowhagen, T.: Anaplastic giant-cell carcinoma of the thyroid: a study of treatment and prognosis. Cancer *35*:1293–1295, 1975.

45. Jones, G. W., Simkovic, D., et al.: Human anaplastic thyroid carcinoma in tissue culture. Proc. Soc. Exp. Biol. Med. *126*:426–428, 1967.

46. Kapp, D. S., LiVolsı, V. A., and Sanders, M. M.: Anaplastic carcinoma following well-differentiated thyroid cancer: etiological considerations. Yale J. Biol. Med. *55*:521–528, 1982.

47. Karnauchow, P. N., and Wall, C. B.: A functioning pleomorphic carcinoma of the thyroid. Canad. Med. Assoc. J. *115*:41–43, 1976.

48. Kim, J. H., and Leeper, R. D.: Treatment of anaplastic giant and spindle cell carcinoma of the thyroid gland with combination adriamycin and radiation therapy. Cancer *52*:954–957, 1983.

49. Kobayashi, S., Yamadori, I., et al.: Anaplastic carcinoma of the thyroid with osteoclast-like giant cells. Acta Pathol. Jpn. *37*:807–815, 1987.

50. Komorowski, R. A., Hanson, G. A., and Garancis, J. C.: Anaplastic thyroid carcinoma following low-dose irradiation. Am. J. Clin. Pathol. *70*:303–307, 1978.

51. Kyriakides, G., and Sasin, H.: Anaplasic carcinoma of the thyroid. Ann. Surg. *179*:295–299, 1974.

52. Lev, R., Judd, E. S., et al.: Anaplastic carcinoma of the thyroid: Evaluation of postoperative results. J. Clin. Endocrinol. Metab. *14*:1355–1361, 1954.

53. Livingstone, D. J., and Sandison, A. T.: Osteogenic sarcoma of thyroid. Br. J. Surg. *50*:291–293, 1962.

54. LiVolsi, V. A., Brooks, J. J., and Arendash-Durand, B.: Anaplastic thyroid tumors: Immunohistology. Am. J. Clin. Pathol. *87*:434–442, 1987.

55. Luna, M. A., Mackay, B., et al.: Malignant small cell tumor of the thyroid. Ultrastruct. Pathol. *1*:265–270, 1980.

56. Macaulay, R. A. A., Dewar, A. E., et al.: Cell receptor studies on six anaplastic tumours of the thyroid. J. Clin. Pathol. *31*:461–468, 1978.

57. MacGregor, C. A., Ham, D. P.: Hormonal dependent anaplastic thyroid carcinoma. A case report. Surgery *71*:56–59, 1972.

58. Mambo, N. C., and Irwin, S. M.: Anaplastic small cell neoplasms of the thyroid: an immunoperoxidase study. Hum. Pathol. *15*:55–60, 1984.

59. Martinelli, G., Bazzocchi, F., et al.: Anaplastic type of medullary thyroid carcinoma. An ultrastructural and immunohistochemical study. Virch. Arch. Pathol. Anat. *400*:61–67, 1983.

60. Meissner, W. A., and Phillips, M. J.: Diffuse small cell carcinoma of the thyroid. Arch. Pathol. *74*:291–297, 1962.

61. Meissner, W. A., and Warren, S.: Tumors of the Thyroid Gland. Atlas of Tumor Pathology, second series, fascicle 4. Washington, D.C., Armed Forces Institute of Pathology, 1969.

62. Mendelsohn, G., Bigner, S. H., et al.: Anaplastic variants of medullary thyroid carcinoma. Am. J. Surg. Pathol. *4*:333–341, 1980.

63. Mills, S. E., Stallings, R. G., and Austin, M. B.: Angiomatoid carcinoma of the thyroid gland: Anaplastic carcinoma with follicular and medullary features mimicking angiosarcoma. Am. J. Clin. Pathol. *86*:674–678, 1986.

64. Miettinen, M., Franssila, K., et al.: Expression of intermediate filament proteins in thyroid gland and thyroid tumors. Lab. Invest. *50*:262–270, 1985.

65. Monaco, F., Carducci, C., et al.: Human undifferentiated thyroid carcinoma synthesizes and secretes 19s thyroglobulin. Cancer *54*:79–83, 1984.

66. Moore, J. H., Bacharach, B., and Choi, H. Y.: Anaplastic transformation of metastatic follicular carcinoma of the thyroid. J. Surg. Oncol. *29*:216–221, 1985.

67. Myskow, M. W., Krajewski, A. S., et al.: The role of immunoperoxidase techniques on paraffin embedded tissue in determining the histogenesis of undifferentiated thyroid neoplasms. Clin. Endocrinol. *243*:335–341, 1986.

68. Nel, C. J. C., van Heerden, J. A., et al.: Anaplastic carcinoma of the thyroid: a clinicopathologic study of 82 cases. Mayo Clin. Proc. *60*:51–58, 1985.

69. Newland, J. R., Mackay, B., et al.: Anaplastic thyroid carcinoma: An ultrastructural study of 10 cases. Ultrastruct. Pathol. 2:121–129, 1981.
70. Nieuwenhuijzen-Kruseman, A. C., Bosman, F. T., et al.: Medullary differentiation of anaplastic thyroid carcinoma. Am. J. Clin. Pathol. 77:541–547, 1982.
71. Nishiyama, R. H., Dunn, E. L., and Thompson, W. W.: Anaplastic spindle cell and giant cell tumors of the thyroid gland. Cancer 30:113–127, 1971.
72. Oppenheim, A., Miller, M., et al.: Anaplastic thyroid cancer presenting with hyperthyroidism. Am. J. Med. 75:702–704, 1983.
73. Orvoine, R. H., Cantin, M., et al.: Dedifferentiation of a transplantable papillary thyroid carcinoma over a 15-year period. Cancer 52:1720–1727, 1983.
74. Parker, L. N., Killin, J., et al.: Carcinoma of the thyroid with a mixed medullary, papillary, follicular, and undifferentiated pattern. Arch. Intern. Med. 145:1507–1509, 1985.
75. Pfaltz, M., Hedinger, C., et al.: Malignant hemangioendothelioma of the thyroid and factor VIII-related antigen. Virch. Arch. Pathol. Anat. 401:177–184, 1983.
76. Rafla, S.: Anaplastic tumors of the thyroid. Cancer 23:668–677, 1969.
77. Ralfkiaer, N., Gatter, K. C., et al.: The value of immunocytochemical methods in the differential diagnosis of anaplastic thyroid tumours. Br. J. Cancer 52:167–170, 1985.
78. Rayfield, E. J., Nishiyama, R. H., and Sisson, J. C.: Small cell tumors of the thyroid: a clinicopathologic study. Cancer 28:1023–1030, 1971.
79. Roberts, C.: Sarcomata of the thyroid gland: A report of 2 cases. J. Pathol. Bacteriol. 95:537–540, 1968.
80. Rogers, J. D., Lindberg, R. D., et al.: Spindle and giant cell carcinoma of the thyroid: a different therapeutic approach. Cancer 34:1328–1332, 1974.
81. Rosai, J., Saxen, E. A., and Woolner, L.: Undifferentiated and poorly differentiated carcinoma. Sem. Diag. Pathol. 2:123–136, 1985.
82. Rossi, R., Cady, B., et al.: Prognosis of undifferentiated carcinoma and lymphoma of the thyroid. Am. J. Surg. 135:589–596, 1978.
83. Ruchti, C., Gerber, H. A., and Schaffner, T.: Factor VIII-related antigen in malignant hemangioendothelioma of the thyroid: additional evidence for the endothelial origin of this tumor. Am. J. Clin. Pathol. 82:474–477, 1984.
84. Saito, R., and Sharma, K.: Fine structure of a diffuse undifferentiated small cell carcinoma of the thyroid. Am. J. Clin. Pathol. 65:623–630, 1976.
85. Sakamoto, A., Kasai, N., and Sugano, H.: Poorly differentiated carcinoma of the thyroid. A clinicopathologic entity for a high risk group of papillary and follicular carcinomas. Cancer 52:1849–1855, 1983.
86. Schmid, K. W., Kröll, M., et al.: Small cell carcinoma of the thyroid. A reclassification of cases originally diagnosed as small cell carcinoma of the thyroid. Pathol. Res. Pract. 181:540–543, 1986.
87. Schroder, J., Dockhorn-Dworniczak, B., et al.: Intermediate filament expression in thyroid gland carcinoma. Virch. Arch. Pathol. Anat. A. 409:751–766, 1986.
88. Shimaoka, K., Getaz, P. E., and Rao, U.: Anaplastic carcinoma of the thyroid: Radiation associated. N. Y. S. J. Med. 79:874–877, 1979.
89. Shin, W. Y., Aftalion, B., et al.: Ultrastructure of a primary fibrosarcoma of the human thyroid gland. Cancer 44:584–591, 1979.
90. Shrikhande, S. S., and Sirsat, M. V.: Anaplastic carcinoma of the thyroid: With special reference to the histological types and their biological behaviour. Indian J. Cancer 11:305–312, 1974.
91. Silverberg, S. G., and DeGiorgi, L. S.: Osteoclastoma-like giant cell tumor of the thyroid. Cancer 31:621–625, 1973.
92. Spanos, G. A., Wolk, D., et al.: Preoperative chemotherapy for giant cell carcinoma of the thyroid. Cancer 50:2252–2256, 1982.
93. St. Cyr, J. A., Shearen, J., Delaney, J. P.: New therapeutic approach for mixed anaplastic carcinoma of the thyroid. Minn. Med. 68:893–896, 1985.
94. Syrjänen, K. J.: An osteogenic sarcoma of the thyroid gland (Report of a case and survey of the literature). Neoplasma 26:623–628, 1979.
95. Syrjänen, K. J.: Fine needle aspiration cytology of the thyroid osteosarcoma. Report of a case. J. Cancer Res. Clin. Oncol. 93:319–323, 1980.
96. Tamada, A., Makimoto, K., et al.: Radiation-induced fibrosarcoma of the thyroid. J. Laryngol. Otol. 98:1063–1066, 1984.
97. Tanda, F., Massarelli, G., et al.: Angiosarcoma of the thyroid: a light, electron microscopic and immunohistological study. Hum. Pathol. 19:742–745, 1988.
98. Thomas, C. G., Jr., and Buckwalter, J. A.: Poorly differentiated neoplasms of the thyroid gland. Ann. Surg. 177:632–642, 1973.
99. Tobler, A., Maurer, R., and Hedinger, Chr. E.: Undifferentiated thyroid tumors of diffuse small cell type. Histological and immunohistochemical evidence of their lymphomatous nature. Virch. Arch. (Pathol. Anat.) 404:117–126, 1984.
100. Trepeta, R. W., Mathur, B., et al.: Giant cell tumor (osteoclastoma) of the pancreas: A tumor of epithelial origin. Cancer 48:2022–2028, 1981.
101. Tollefson, H. R., DeCosse, J. J., and Hutter, R. V. P.: Papillary carcinoma of the thyroid. A clinical and pathological study of 70 fatal cases. Cancer 17:1035–1044, 1964.

274 UNDIFFERENTIATED OR ANAPLASTIC CARCINOMA OF THE THYROID

bibliography
102. Ueda, G., and Furth, J.: Sarcomatoid transformation of transplanted thyroid carcinoma. Similarity to anaplastic human thyroid carcinoma. Arch. Pathol. *83*:3–12, 1967.
103. Voisin, M., Fawil, E., et al.: Epithelioma anaplastique de la thyroïde 6 ans aprés irradiation cervicale pour lymphome malin. Canad. Med. Assoc. J. *113*:648–652, 1975.
104. Volpe, R., Carbone, A., et al.: Cytology of a breast carcinoma with osteoclast-like giant cells. Acta Cytol. *27*:184–187, 1983.
105. Walt, A. J., Woolner, L. B., and Black, M. B.: Small-cell malignant lesions of the thyroid gland. J. Clin. Endocrinol. *17*:45–60, 1957.
106. Walts, A. E.: Osteoclast-type giant cell tumor of the pancreas. Acta Cytol. *27*:500–504, 1983.
107. Wilson, N. W., Pambakian, H., et al.: Epithelial markers in thyroid carcinoma: An immunoperoxidase study. Histopathology *10*:815–829, 1986.
108. Woolner, L. B.: Thyroid carcinoma: Pathologic classification with data on prognosis. Semin. Nucl. Med. *1*:481–515, 1971.
109. Wychulis, A. R., Beahrs, O. H., and Woolner, L. B.: Papillary carcinoma with associated anaplastic carcinoma in the thyroid gland. Surg. Gynecol. Obstet. *120*:28–34, 1965.
110. Yamana, K., Nakano, R., et al.: Ultrastructure of anaplastic carcinoma (spindle and giant cell type) with large calcification in the thyroid gland. Acta Pathol. Jpn. *34*:585–592, 1984.

HÜRTHLE CELL LESIONS

12

The Hürthle cell is a cell in the thyroid which has been associated with debate and confusion. The debate surrounds several aspects of the cell, including its origin, its functional state, and the clinical implications of nodules composed of these cells. The confusion derives from these considerations as well as from its name.

THE HÜRTHLE CELL ITSELF

The cell, described by Hürthle in 1894,[43] is now believed to represent the parafollicular cell.[61] Indeed, the eosinophilic cell, oncocyte, or oxyphilic cell that bears the Hürthle name was first described in 1898 by Askanazy.[3, 61] Unfortunately, the term Hürthle cell is so ingrained in the literature of pathology and clinical medicine that it would be virtually impossible to reeducate the scientific readership in the light of historical validity. Hence, the title of this chapter and the following discussion and descriptions of eosinophilic, oncocytic, or oxyphilic cell lesions of the thyroid will use the misnomer, Hürthle cell.

What is a so-called Hürthle cell? It is a cell derived from follicular epithelium, possessing the capacity (albeit somewhat limited) to produce thyroglobulin. It is characterized morphologically by its large size, square shape, distinct cell borders, voluminous granular cytoplasm, large nucleus, and prominent nucleolus[29, 61] (Fig. 12–1). The hyperchromatic nucleus may show folds or crenations. The cytoplasm, which is granular, stains intensely pink with eosin.

Ultrastructural studies have shown that the cytoplasmic granularity is produced by huge mitochondria filling the cell[7, 24, 56, 58, 65, 67] (Figs. 12–2 and 12–3). The studies of Nesland et al.[58] and Sobrinho-Simoes et al.[67] describe similar ultrastructural findings in Hürthle cells, whether they are derived from nonneoplastic lesions or from benign or malignant neoplasms. Thus, by transmission electron microscopy, the nuclei of these cells contain prominent nuclei. The most striking feature, however, is the cytoplasm, which is stuffed with mitochondria, many of which display abnormalities of shape, size, and content. Dense core granules are seen in the mitochondria[19, 58] and are believed to be a reaction to injury; filamentous inclusions probably are derived from the cristae. It is unclear why Hürthle cells have abundant and abnormal mitochondria.[58] Do they represent overproduction or insufficient or defective breakdown or both of these processes? Nesland et al. point out that the biochemical counterparts to the ultrastructural organelles remain unknown.[58]

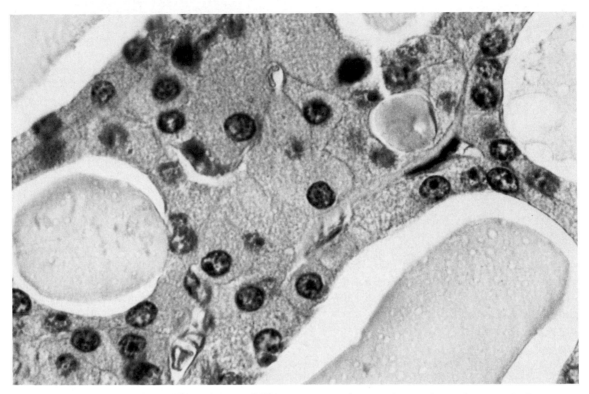

Figure 12–1. Close-up of oxyphilic cells lining follicles. Note granular cytoplasm and prominent nucleoli. × 1000 (oil), H & E. (Reproduced by permission of Field and Wood, Inc., Publishers, Ref. 14.)

Scanning electron microscopy shows smooth-surfaced cells intermixed with cells having abundant microvilli. These "bald" cells may represent transition forms between follicular cells and Hürthle cells, although this remains speculative.[58, 76] Bocker et al. distinguished among oxyphils (Hürthle cells), mitochondrion-rich cells, and ergastoplasm-rich cells by electron microscopy and immunohistology.[7] They noted in the ergastoplasm-rich cell an abundance of rough endoplasmic reticulum, absent intrafollicular colloid, and markedly positive staining for thyroglobulin. The distinction between Hürthle (oxyphil) cells and mitochondrion-rich cells is less pronounced, with the latter having fewer mitochondria and more prominent thyroglobulin staining. Whether these ultrastructural and immunostaining differences indicate three different cells or a spectrum of one cell in varying stages of functional activity remains unclear, although Nesland et al. favor the latter view.[58]

Studies by Tremblay and Harcourt-Webster and Stott[36, 72, 73] have shown that these cells contain high levels of oxidative enzymes; thus, although some authors consider these cells to be degenerative elements,[29, 40] their cytoplasmic and biochemical make-up belies this conclusion.[19, 58, 72, 73, 76]

Several lines of evidence suggest that Hürthle cells can function. These include the variety and abundance of oxidative enzymes identified histochemically,[36, 72, 73] the immunohistochemical localization of thyroglobulin in these cells,[1, 6, 51, 58, 59] and the in vitro studies which indicate functional capacity.[17, 20, 76]

Immunohistochemical (chiefly immunoperoxidase) studies have shown that Hürthle cells contain thyroglobulin, but lack calcitonin.[1, 14, 44, 51] Some authors, but not all, have shown carcinoembryonic antigen in these cells.[14, 44, 58]

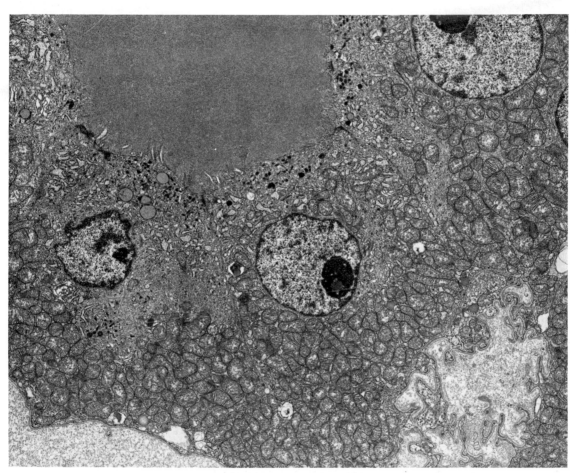

Figure 12–2. Lower power electron micrograph shows follicle lined by large Hürthle cells. Note cytoplasm stuffed with mitochondria. × 7500. (Electron photomicrograph kindly supplied by Dr. R. V. Iozzo.)

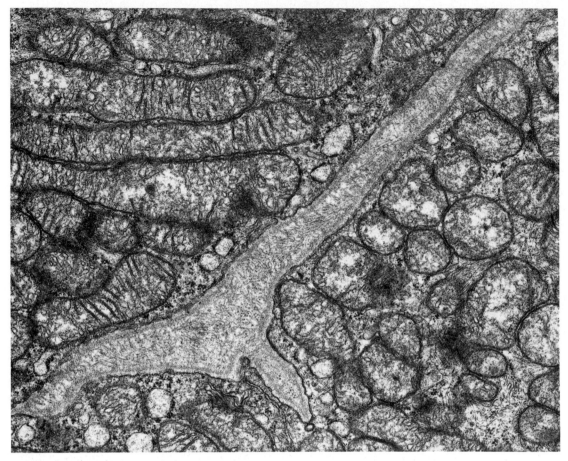

Figure 12–3. Higher power view of one cell in Figure 12–2. Note mitochondria. × 36,000. (Electron photomicrograph kindly supplied by Dr. R. V. Iozzo.)

SIGNIFICANCE OF THE HÜRTHLE CELL

What is the meaning of Hürthle cells in the thyroid? These elements are found in a wide variety of conditions affecting the gland and therefore they cannot be considered specific for any disease entity[4, 29, 46–50, 52, 75] (Table 12–1). Thus, individual cells, follicles, or groups of follicles may show Hürthle cell cytology in nodular goiter, "nonspecific" chronic thyroiditis, in the thyroids of elderly persons, especially women, and in thyroids of patients who have received head and neck irradiation or systemic chemotherapy.[29, 50] In addition, the thyroids of patients with longstanding hyperthyroidism (Graves' disease, or toxic nodular goiter (in fact, Askanazy originally described this cell from cases of thyrotoxicosis[3]) may show focal or diffuse Hürthle cell change.

In the above listed conditions, the oncocytes are found as isolated cells or lining one to a few follicles; in some cases, especially in nodular goiter, an entire nodule may be composed of oncocytes. However, the classic thyroid disorder in which Hürthle cells are prominent is chronic lymphocytic thyroiditis (Hashimoto's disease) (Fig. 12–4). In virtually all cases of classic and fibrosing variants of chronic lymphocytic thyroiditis, most or all of the follicular epithelium has taken on a Hürthle cell cytology. In juvenile thyroiditis, the oncocytic change is less pronounced.[50] It is rare to identify these cells in acute or subacute thyroiditis,

Table 12–1. Occurrence of Hürthle Cells

Hürthle cells found:
    In chronic lymphocytic thyroiditis and variants
    In nodular goiter
    In diffuse toxic goiter
    Post-radiation
    Post-chemotherapy
    As aging process

suggesting the possibility that the alteration in the follicular epithelium requires some chronic stimulation.

What is the nature of the Hürthle cell? Most authors suggest that this cell represents a degenerative or metaplastic phenomenon—damaged follicular epithelium (damaged by inflammatory or immunologic means) undergoes this change. In most tissues where metaplasia occurs commonly (uterine cervix, bronchus) the process is one of reversion of specialized epithelium to a simpler type (mucinous to squamous—see also Chapter 13). In the thyroid, the Hürthle cell is certainly not morphologically simpler than the follicular cell; hence, although it may be functionally less active, its morphology and enzymatic makeup is more complex. Is this then truly metaplasia? It is certainly not degeneration. Indeed, some patients develop hyperthyroidism after a long history of hypothyroidism; they may have had histologically documented chronic lymphocytic thyroiditis with oxyphil cells lining the follicles. Yet these follicles can overproduce thyroid hormone.[23, 53]

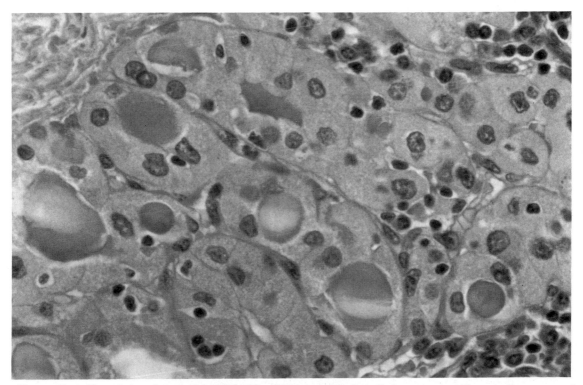

Figure 12–4. Chronic lymphocytic thyroiditis. The follicles are lined totally by oncocytes. Note small amounts of colloid and scattered plasma cells and lymphocytes in and around follicles. × 400, H & E.

HÜRTHLE CELL NODULES AND NEOPLASMS

Some Hürthle cell neoplasms of the thyroid represent papillary carcinomas in which the malignant cells exhibit an oncocytic cytology; these are carcinomas which behave as papillary tumors and are discussed further below and in Chapter 8.

The lesions which are important to distinguish and which have produced debate among pathologists are those oncocytic masses that show a follicular or solid pattern. These, then, are the lesions to which everyone refers as Hürthle cell tumors and form the basis for the following discussion.

Nodules of Hürthle cells are not all neoplastic. In fact, the majority of these represent Hürthle cell change of preexisting follicular adenomatous nodules in goiters or thyroiditis. Even if the nodule is encapsulated, it may still be nonneoplastic.[14] The definition of Hürthle cell nodules as Hürthle cell neoplasms has produced confusion with regard to the clinical importance of true neoplasms composed of these cells. The literature abounds with statistics about the incidence of such tumors, their multicentricity, and their malignant potential.[2, 10, 11, 14, 15, 16, 25–28, 30–35, 37, 41, 42, 44, 55, 57, 58, 60, 62–64, 66, 68, 70, 71, 77] Given that nonneoplastic nodules of Hürthle cells are so common, the definition of the true Hürthle cell neoplasm has become a confusing issue, as has the clinical importance of reported true neoplasms composed of Hürthle cells. Obviously if one is not careful to exclude the common nonneoplastic nodules found in nodular goiters or thyroiditis, then the vast majority of reported Hürthle cell neoplasms will be biologically benign.[11, 14]

Thus the data suggest that a gamut of clinical behavior is possible for such lesions: some authors cite that 80 percent or more of these lesions are benign, while others consider all such lesions malignant.[11, 34, 69] Are these "tumors" either epidemiologically and/or geographically heterogeneous? I prefer another explanation: that is, I believe the heterogeneity stems from the nonuniform pathologic interpretation of these tumors in the literature. Hence, those reports that include multiple Hürthle cell nodules found in a background of nodular goiter or Hashimoto's thyroiditis, regardless of encapsulation as "neoplasms," indicate that the majority of such tumors are benign.[2, 10, 11, 16, 32, 33, 41, 62] Conversely, those studies which carefully exclude such nodules and report the results of solitary encapsulated nodules of the thyroid composed of Hürthle cells indicate a significant percentage of malignant lesions—around 30 to 67 percent.[14, 34, 69]

Is there anything unusual about the Hürthle cell neoplasm? Yes, there is. The present author believes that these lesions may be classified as a subtype of follicular neoplasm: the criteria for distinguishing benign from malignant are the same and include the identification of invasion.[14, 70, 77] However, the pathologic criteria for malignancy are met more frequently for tumors composed of Hürthle cells than for their non-Hürthle counterparts. Thus, whereas 2 to 3 percent of solitary encapsulated follicular tumors of the thyroid show invasive characteristics, somewhere between 30 and 40 percent of such lesions showing Hürthle cell cytology will show such features. In addition, whereas true follicular carcinomas of the thyroid rarely metastasize embolically to lymph nodes, if ever, about 30 percent of Hürthle cell carcinomas do.[14, 77]

Do these differences warrant a separate category of thyroid neoplasms for the Hürthle cell group? In the opinion of the present author they do not until and unless further study brings to light other differences of biologic and/or clinical relevance. They should, however, be recognized as a variant of follicular tumor.[27]

Pathology of Hürthle Cell Neoplasms

Gross Pathology. Most Hürthle cell neoplasms of the thyroid are solitary mass lesions, which show complete or partial encapsulation. They are distinguished from the surrounding thyroid by their distinctive brown to mahogany color.[40, 42] Their size ranges from one to many centimeters; larger tumors may extend grossly beyond the thyroid. Occasionally small cystic areas may be noted. Hemorrhage and/or necrosis may be found in lesions over 3 centimeters. Rarely, a Hürthle cell neoplasm may undergo spontaneous infarction; the central portion of such a lesion is composed of totally necrotic material and only the capsule and subcapsular rim of the tumor are viable. The presence of infarction does not equate with malignancy, however, since benign lesions may display this gross feature. A recent study discloses that those thyroid tumors most likely to undergo infarction following fine needle aspiration biopsy are those composed of Hürthle cells[49]; so-called spontaneous regression of Hürthle cell tumors may also result from such spontaneous infarction.[5]

Microscopic Pathology. The histologic appearance of Hürthle cell tumors is variable. Basic patterns include macrofollicular, microfollicular, trabecular/solid, and pseudopapillary (Figs. 12–5 and 12–6). The trabecular and microfollicular patterns are most commonly encountered. Combinations of several patterns may be seen.[27, 42]

Trabecular Hürthle cell tumors show an appearance reminiscent of hepatic cords, with neoplastic cells arranged in elongated cords and lined laterally by delicate capillaries. Microfollicular lesions show Hürthle cells arranged in circular

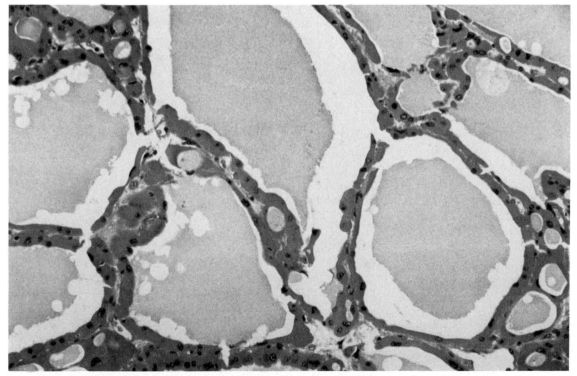

Figure 12–5. Macrofollicular nodule. Each dilated follicle is lined by oncocytes. × 200, H & E. (Reproduced by permission of Field and Wood, Inc., Publishers, Ref. 14.)

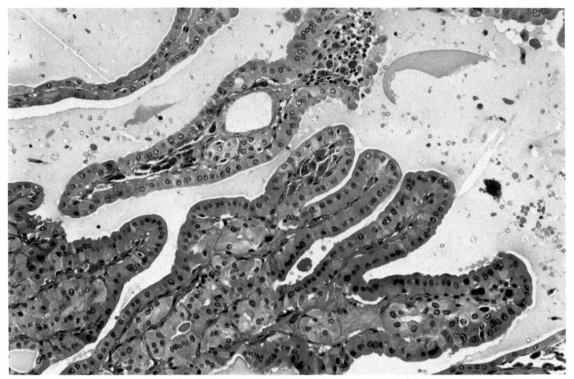

Figure 12–6. Pseudopapillary area in Hürthle cell nodule. × 200, H & E. (Reproduced by permission of Field and Wood, Inc., Publishers, Ref. 14.)

or elliptical fashion around a small central "lumen" containing a scant amount of colloid. The macrofollicular pattern is reminiscent of the large follicles seen in adenomatous goiter and is rarely found as the sole pattern. In the macrofollicular areas, however, one may occasionally find the pseudopapillary pattern, wherein the follicles appear to have disrupted or collapsed and result in a papillary appearance.[14]

Not all Hürthle neoplasms are composed exclusively of these cells: in some examples, follicles lined by non-Hürthle cells are found, usually in a microfollicular pattern. It has been my practice to diagnose lesions as Hürthle cell tumors if the predominant cytologic pattern (>75 percent) is oncocytic.

Biology of Hürthle Cell Neoplasms

Thompson et al. in 1974 claimed that all Hürthle cell neoplasms should be considered malignant or potentially malignant, even in the face of histologic benignity[69]; these authors modified their original recommendations regarding treatment for these lesions by suggesting that tumors greater than 2.0 cm. should all be considered malignant, but smaller ones might behave in a benign fashion.[34] Many additional studies from the U.S. and Europe have appeared in the literature which dispute the claim of the Michigan studies[10, 11, 14, 32, 41, 42, 62, 66, 70, 77] (Table 12–2). In these studies, careful pathologic definitions of these tumors refute the argument that the results are confounded by the inclusion of nonneoplastic proliferative nodules. Hence, true Hürthle cell neoplasms exist which behave in a benign fashion. Size in and of itself is not predictive of behavior, although larger

Table 12–2. Literature Summary: Recurrence in Histologic Carcinomas and Adenomas

	Recurrence			
	Cancer		*Benign*	
Author	N	(%CA)	N	(%Ad)
Thompson-Gundry[69, 34]	20	(57%)	3	(12%)
Heppe[41]	—	—	—	—
Gonzalez-Campora[32]	5	(42%)	—	—
Savino[66]	8	(53%)	—	—
Bronner-LiVolsi[14]	5	(31%)	—	—
Arganini[2]	2	(14%)	1	(3%)
Rosen[62]	—	—	—	—
Bondeson[10, 11]	2	(25%)	—	—
Caplan[16]	1	(33%)	—	—
Gosain[33]	1	(25%)	—	—
Watson[77]	10	(34%)	NA	NA
Tollefsen[70]	10	(29%)	NA	NA
Har-el[37]	7	(41%)	NA	NA
Total	71/207	(34%)	4/309	(1%)

(N = number, CA = carcinoma, Ad = adenoma, NA = not applicable). Note that the overall recurrence rate for so-called histologically benign tumors is only 1% (4/309 reported cases). Reprinted by permission of Field and Wood, Inc., Publishers (Ref. 14).

lesions tend to behave more aggressively than smaller ones.[11, 14] It has become clear that pathologic criteria for malignancy (vascular invasion, transcapsular penetration, destructive capsular invasion) can predict the clinical behavior of these tumors.[11, 14] Nuclear atypia, multinucleation, cellular pleomorphism, mitoses, or histologic pattern of the lesion does not affect the prognosis and therefore should not be used as diagnostic criteria for malignancy.[9, 14, 30, 32] Explanations for the data from the Michigan group abound, but it appears that the results may have been due mainly to the referral patterns existing in that institution. Of great interest is that more recent reports from the Michigan group regarding cytofluorometric and other studies indicate a spectrum of biologic behavior for Hürthle cell neoplasm treated at this institution.[25, 44]

In our own material, we identified a subgroup of Hürthle cell neoplasms which contained marked nuclear atypia, mitoses, spontaneous infarction, necrosis, or hemorrhage (these lesions had not been aspirated preoperatively), and/or trapping of tumor cells within the lesion's capsule. We designated this subgroup as "atypical Hürthle cell adenoma"; such criteria have been used in the past[39] to define as atypical certain follicular tumors. (However, such diagnostic criteria have not been rigorously applied in recent series of Hürthle cell tumors.) Our data, including long-term follow-up (average 10 to 13 years), indicates that even these atypical Hürthle cell tumors behave in a biologically benign fashion; all the cases in our material which we designated as simple Hürthle cell adenomas also were benign clinically.[14]

In conclusion, then, it is our belief that the category of neoplastic Hürthle cell lesions includes adenomas and atypical adenomas which are clinically benign and carcinomas which are malignant.[14, 31, 70, 77] The distinction among these three groups is made by the pathologic evaluation of the mass, applying strict criteria, as noted above for non-Hürthle follicular tumors. *In the absence of invasion, a Hürthle cell thyroid tumor should be considered benign.* Hence, histologic assessment can predict biologic behavior; therefore, therapy can be individualized according to the diagnosis. Total thyroidectomy is not needed for all Hürthle cell neoplasms.[10, 11, 14]

Unusual locations or settings for Hürthle cell tumors have been reported: mediastinum,[56] thyroglossal duct,[71] and in identical twins.[57]

Hürthle cell carcinomas do behave in a somewhat unusual way when compared to follicular carcinomas, in that metastases to regional lymph nodes do occur[14]; many of these cancers, however, metastasize hematogenously as well. Sites of metastasis most often encountered include lungs, bone, and liver.[14, 18, 77] The survival rates for Hürthle cell carcinomas vary and depend on whether the tumor was grossly infiltrative or encapsulated. Survival rates for histologically proven carcinomas range from about 50 to 60 percent at five years[12, 77]; however, late recurrences and metastases are not rare.

In addition, anaplastic transformation may occur in a metastatic site. Some Hürthle cell tumors, probably encapsulated carcinomas but perhaps adenomas, may be found in association with anaplastic carcinomas. This association has led to the speculation that Hürthle cell neoplasms can behave in a manner similar to low grade papillary and follicular cancers, i.e., they can undergo transformation to high grade malignancies. (See also Chapter 11.) The frequency of this occurrence is unknown.[27]

As is discussed in greater detail in Chapter 18, flow cytometric analysis of series of Hürthle cell tumors indicates that this technique cannot discriminate between benign and malignant Hürthle cell neoplasms, since adenomas may show aneuploidy and cancers may be diploid.[8, 9, 13, 22, 25, 54, 60, 63] However, in the histologically defined carcinomas, flow cytometric data may provide prognostic aid—carcinomas that show an aneuploid pattern histologically may behave more aggressively than those that are diploid.[22, 54, 60] Kinetic data obtained by this technique may also be helpful in this regard, although further work is necessary to define this.[9, 13, 25]

Differential Diagnosis of Hürthle Cell Tumors

Medullary Carcinoma. Some medullary thyroid carcinomas are composed of large cells with finely granular cytoplasm; superficial study can suggest a Hürthle cell lesion. However, the nuclear characteristics are different, since most medullary carcinomas have uniform, small nuclei unlike the pleomorphic ones in the Hürthle cell tumors. The cytoplasmic granularity is less pronounced in medullary lesions, and the latter rarely demonstrate intense eosinophilia. In any questionable case, of course, immunohistochemical staining for calcitonin and thyroglobulin will aid in reaching the correct diagnosis.

Papillary Carcinoma, Hürthle Cell Type. Unusual cases of obviously and overtly papillary cancers of the thyroid will show focally or totally Hürthle cell cytology.[21, 27] These lesions should not cause concern as to their biologic nature since most of them are overtly infiltrative. The diagnosis of carcinoma is not difficult. The clinical behavior of these lesions is similar to that of non-Hürthle cell lesions of similar size and stage. On occasion, Hürthle cell tumors of mixed papillary and follicular pattern which are encapsulated will be found; such lesions, usually occurring in young individuals, behave in an extremely indolent fashion.

Papillary Carcinoma, Tall Cell Variant, Pink Cell Variant. This unusual tumor of the thyroid was originally separated as a subtype of papillary carcinoma by Hawk and Hazard in 1976.[38] These authors noted that in their series of papillary cancers, this variant represented about 12 percent. They found that it often was a tumor of large size, extending extrathyroidally, and showed a propensity for vascular invasion. These tumors occurred in an older subset of their population. Tscholl-Ducommun and Hedinger described these tumors as eosinophilic variants of papillary carcinomas and classified them as of moderate biologic behavior.[74] Johnson et al. reported a group of these tumors and compared to age and sex matched controls.[45] In the latter series the tall cell subtype appeared to behave in a more clinically virulent fashion. (See Chapter 8.)

The cells in this type of tumor are described as tall, i.e., their height is at least twice their width; most of them have an eosinophilic cytoplasm. However, these cells are less granular than Hürthle cells and do not exhibit the marked nuclear atypia of the latter cells. In the few cases that have been examined ultrastructurally, these cells have increased numbers of mitochondria but not the abundant or abnormal ones characteristic of true Hürthle cells. It is possible that the eosinophilia in the tall cells is due to intermediate filaments. (All cases studied have been strongly positive for cytokeratin—LiVolsi, unpublished observations.) The tall cell papillary carcinoma is frequently associated with prominent lymphocytic thyroiditis which may be found near the tumor or in the entire gland. In addition, lymphocytes frequently expand and infiltrate the stroma of the papillae. In the present author's experience, these tumors are aggressive lesions; indeed, the majority of fatal papillary carcinomas I have seen have been of this particular histologic subtype. (See also Chapter 8.)

Relationship between Hürthle Cells and Clear Cells. Clear cells occur in the thyroid and can cause diagnostic dilemmas when they occur as tumors. This problem will be discussed in Chapter 15. However, isolated cells or cell groups which exhibit a clear cytoplasm may be found lining follicles in thyroiditis (Fig. 12–7). In some examples, the clear cells abut upon Hürthle cells, suggesting that the former may be derived from the latter. One unusual case of papillary

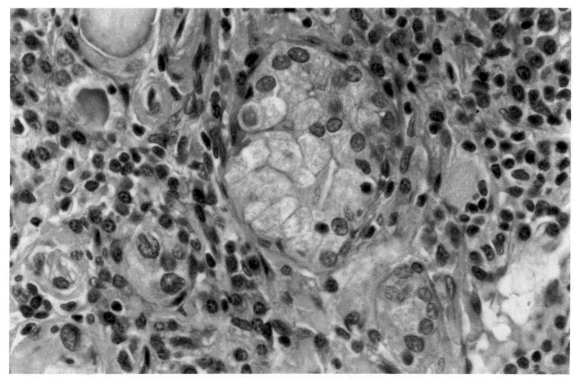

Figure 12–7. In this case of Hashimoto's thyroiditis, the central follicle is lined by cells undergoing clear cell change. This was a focal finding; nearby follicles were lined by Hürthle cells. These types of changes suggest a relationship between Hürthle and clear cells. × 400, H & E.

carcinoma composed of oxyphils and clear cells has been reported.[21] Certainly clear cell tumors of the thyroid are follicular cell derived since they can contain (? produce) thyroglobulin. Therefore, it seems likely that clear cell change (? metaplasia) may occur side by side with Hürthle cell metaplasia or as a further change, i.e., through Hürthle cell metaplasia first.

SUMMARY

This chapter has reviewed Hürthle cell lesions affecting the thyroid. Emphasis has been placed on neoplasms composed of these cells. The controversies have been presented and opinions and current views stressed.

REFERENCES

1. Albores-Saavedra, J., Nadji, M., et al.: Thyroglobulin in carcinoma of the thyroid: an immunohistochemical study. Hum. Pathol. 14:62–66, 1983.
2. Arganini, M., Behar, R., et al.: Hürthle cell tumors: a twenty-five year experience. Surgery 100:1108–1114, 1986.
3. Askanazy, M.: Pathologisch-anatomische Beitrage zur Kenntiss des Morbus Basedowii, insbesondere uber die dabei auftretende Muskelerkrankung. Dtsch. Arch. Klin. Med. 61:118–186, 1898.
4. Bastenie, P. A., and Ermans, A. M.: Thyroiditis and Thyroid Function: Clinical, Morphological and Physiopathological Studies. Oxford, Pergamon Press, 1972.
5. Bauman, A., and Strawbridge, H. T. G.: Spontaneous disappearance of an atypical Hürthle cell adenoma. Am. J. Clin. Pathol. 80:399–402, 1983.
6. Bocker, W., Dralle, H., et al.: Immunohistochemical analysis of thyroglobulin synthesis in thyroid carcinomas. Virch. Arch. Pathol. Anat. 385:187–200, 1980.
7. Bocker, W., Dralle, H., et al.: Immunohistochemical and electron microscope analysis of adenomas of the thyroid gland. Virch. Arch. Pathol. Anat. 380:205–220, 1978.
8. Bondeson, L., Azavedo, E., et al.: Nuclear DNA content and behavior of oxyphil thyroid tumors. Cancer 58:672–675, 1986.
9. Bondeson, L., Bondeson, A. G., et al.: Morphometric studies on nuclei in smears of fine needle aspirates from oxyphilic tumors of the thyroid. Acta Cytol. 27:437–440, 1983.
10. Bondeson, L., Bondeson, A. G., and Ljungberg, O.: Treatment of Hürthle cell neoplasms of the thyroid. Arch. Surg. 118:1453, 1983.
11. Bondeson, L., Bondeson, A. G., et al.: Oxyphil tumors of the thyroid. Followup of 42 surgical cases. Ann. Surg. 194:677–680, 1981.
12. Bosadjieva, E., Georgieva, S., et al.: Localized pretibial myxedema and thyroid acropachy in a case of Hürthle cell adenocarcinoma. Intl. J. Dermatol. 10:170–174, 1971.
13. Bronner, M. P., Clevenger, C. V., et al.: Flow cytometric analysis of DNA content in Hürthle cell adenomas and carcinomas of the thyroid. Am. J. Clin. Pathol. 89:764–769, 1988.
14. Bronner, M. P., and LiVolsi, V. A.: Oxyphilic (Askanazy/Hürthle cell) tumors of the thyroid: Microscopic features predict biologic behavior. Surg. Pathol. 1:137–150, 1988.
15. Bruni, F., Batsakis, J. G., et al.: Hürthle cell tumors of the thyroid gland. ASCP Abstract P45, 1987.
16. Caplan, R. H., Abellera, M., and Kisken, W. A.: Hürthle cell tumors of the thyroid gland: A clinicopathologic review and long-term follow-up. J.A.M.A. 251:3114–3117, 1984.
17. Clark, O. H., and Gerend, P. L.: Thyrotropin receptor-adenylate cyclase system in Hürthle cell neoplasms. J. Clin. Endocrinol. Metab. 39:719–723, 1985.
18. Cummings, C. W., Weymuller, E., and Goodman, M. L.: Follicular carcinoma of Hürthle cell type as cause of hemoptysis. Ann. Otol. 84:182–186, 1975.
19. David, R., and Kim, K. M.: Dense-core matrical mitochondrial bodies in oncocytic adenoma of the thyroid. Arch. Pathol. Lab. Med. 107:178–182, 1983.
20. DeKeyser, L., Layfield, L., et al.: Biochemical and immunohistochemical characterization of proteins in Hürthle cell carcinoma. J. Endocrinol. Invest. 7:449–453, 1984.
21. Dickersin, G. R., Vickery, A. L., and Smith, S. B.: Papillary carcinoma of the thyroid, oxyphil cell type, "clear cell" variant. A light and electron microscopic study. Am. J. Surg. Pathol. 4:501–509, 1980.
22. El-Naggar, A. K., Batsakis, J. G., et al.: Hürthle cell tumors of the thyroid: a flow cytometric DNA analysis. Arch. Otolaryngol. Head Neck Surg. 114:520–521, 1988.
23. Fatourechi, V., McConahey, W. M., and Woolner, L. B.: Hyperthyroidism associated with histologic Hashimoto's thyroiditis. Mayo Clin. Proc. 46:682–690, 1971.

24. Feldman, P. S., Horvath, E., and Kovacs, K.: Ultrastructure of three Hürthle cell tumors of the thyroid. Cancer *30*:1279–1285, 1972.

25. Flint, A., Davenport, R. D., et al.: Cytophotometric measurements of Hürthle cell tumors of the thyroid gland: correlation with pathologic features and clinical behavior. Cancer *61*:110–113, 1988.

26. Franssila, K. O.: Prognosis in thyroid carcinoma. Cancer *36*:1138–1146, 1975.

27. Franssila, K. O., Ackerman, L. V., et al.: Follicular carcinoma. Sem. Diag. Pathol. *2*:101–122, 1985.

28. Frazell, E. L., and Duffy, B. J.: Hürthle cell cancer of the thyroid: a review of forty cases. Cancer *4*:952–956, 1951.

29. Friedman, N. B.: Cellular involution in thyroid gland; significance of Hürthle cells in myxedema, exhaustion atrophy, Hashimoto's disease and reaction to irradiation, thiouracil therapy and subtotal resection. J. Clin. Endocrinol. *9*:874–882, 1949.

30. Galera-Davidson, H., Bibbo, M., et al.: Correlation between automated DNA ploidy measurements of Hürthle cell tumors and their histopathologic and clinical features. Analyt. Quant. Cytol. Histol. *8*:158–167, 1986.

31. Gardner, L. W.: Hürthle cell tumors of the thyroid. Arch. Pathol. *59*:372–381, 1955.

32. Gonzalez-Campora, R., Herrero-Zapatero, A., et al.: Hürthle cell and mitochondrion-rich cell tumors: a clinicopathologic study. Cancer *57*:1154–1163, 1986.

33. Gosain, A. K., and Clark, O. H.: Hürthle cell neoplasms: malignant potential. Arch. Surg. *119*:515–519, 1984.

34. Gundry, S. R., Burney, R. E., et al.: Total thyroidectomy for Hürthle cell neoplasm of the thyroid. Arch. Surg. *118*:529–532, 1983.

35. Hamperl, H.: Onkocytes and the so-called Hürthle cell tumor. Arch. Pathol. *49*:563–567, 1950.

36. Harcourt-Webster, J. N., and Stott, N. C. H.: Histochemical study of oxidative and hydrolytic enzymes in the human thyroid. J. Pathol. Bacteriol. *80*:353–361, 1960.

37. Har-el, G., Hadar, T., et al.: Hürthle cell carcinoma of the thyroid gland: a tumor of moderate malignancy. Cancer *57*:1613–1617, 1986.

38. Hawk, W. A., and Hazard, J. B.: The many appearances of papillary carcinoma of the thyroid. Cleve. Clin. Quart. *43*:207–216, 1976.

39. Hazard, J. B., and Kenyon, R.: Atypical adenoma of the thyroid. Arch. Pathol. *58*:554–563, 1954.

40. Heimann, P., Ljunggren, J. G., et al.: Oxyphilic adenoma of the human thyroid: a morphological and biochemical study. Cancer *31*:246–254, 1973.

41. Heppe, H., Armin, A., et al.: Hürthle cell tumors of the thyroid gland. Surgery *98*:1162–1165, 1985.

42. Horn, R. C.: Hürthle cell tumors of the thyroid. Cancer *7*:234–244, 1954.

43. Hürthle, K.: Beitrage zur Kenntiss der Secretionsvorgangs in der Schilddruse. Arch. Gesamte Physiol. *56*:1–44, 1894.

44. Johnson, T. L., Lloyd, R. V., et al.: Hürthle cell thyroid tumors: an immunohistochemical study. Cancer *59*:107–112, 1987.

45. Johnson, T. L., Lloyd, R. V., et al.: Prognostic implications of the tall cell variant of papillary thyroid carcinoma. Am. J. Surg. Pathol. *12*:22–27, 1988.

46. Katz, S. M., and Vickery, A. L.: The fibrosing variant of Hashimoto's thyroiditis. Hum. Pathol. *5*:161–170, 1974.

47. Kendall, C. H., McCluskey, E., and Naylor, J.: Oxyphil cells in thyroid disease: a uniform change? J. Clin. Pathol. *39*:908–912, 1986.

48. Kennedy, J. S., and Thomson, J. A.: The changes in the thyroid gland after irradiation with I[131] or partial thyroidectomy for thyrotoxicosis. J. Pathol. *112*:65–82, 1974.

49. Kini, S. R., Miller, J. M., et al.: Post fine needle aspiration biopsy infarction in thyroid nodules. Mod. Pathol. *1*:48A, 1988. (Abstract).

50. LiVolsi, V. A., and LoGerfo, P.: Thyroiditis. Boca Raton, CRC Press Inc., 1981.

51. LoGerfo, P., LiVolsi, V. A., et al.: Thyroglobulin production in thyroid cancers. J. Surg. Res. *24*:1–4, 1978.

52. Mauras, N., Zimmerman, D., and Goellner, J. R.: Hashimoto thyroiditis associated with thyroid cancer in adolescent patients. J. Pediatr. *106*:895–898, 1985.

53. McDermott, M. T., Kidd, G. S., et al.: Case Report: Hyperthyroidism following hypothyroidism. Am. J. Med. Sci. *291*:194–198, 1986.

54. McLeod, M. K., Thompson, N. W., et al.: Flow cytometric measurements of nuclear DNA and ploidy analysis in Hürthle cell neoplasm of the thyroid. Arch. Surg. *123*:849–854, 1988.

55. Miller, R. H., Estrada, R., et al.: Hürthle cell tumors of the thyroid gland. Laryngoscope *93*:884–888, 1983.

56. Mishriki, Y. Y., Lane, B. P., et al.: Hürthle cell tumor arising in the mediastinal ectopic thyroid and diagnosed by fine needle aspiration: light microscopic and ultrastructural features. Acta Cytol. *27*:188–192, 1983.

57. Nagamachi, Y., Nakamura, T., and Yamada, T.: Hürthle cell adenoma of the thyroid in identical twins with 13 year follow-up. Jpn. J. Surg. *3*:212–217, 1973.

58. Nesland, J. M., Sobrinho-Simoes, M. A., et al.: Hürthle cell lesions of the thyroid: a combined study using transmission electron microscopy, scanning electron microscopy and immunocytochemistry. Ultrastructural Pathol. *8*:269–290, 1985.

59. Permanetter, W., Nathrata, W. B. J., and Lohrs, U.: Immunohistochemical analysis of thyroglobulin and keratin in benign and malignant thyroid tumors. Virch. Arch. Pathol. Anat. [A] *398*:221–228, 1982.
60. Rainwater, L. M., Farrow, G. M., et al.: Oncocytic tumours of the salivary gland, kidney, and thyroid: Nuclear DNA patterns studied by flow cytometry. Br. J. Cancer *53*:799–804, 1986.
61. Roediger, W. E. W.: The oxyphil and C cells of the human thyroid gland. Cancer *36*:1758–1770, 1975.
62. Rosen, I. B., Luk, S., and Katz, I.: Hürthle cell tumor behavior: Dilemma and resolution. Surgery *98*:777–783, 1985.
63. Ryan, J. J., and Hay, I. D.: Flow cytometric DNA measurements in follicular and parafollicular thyroid malignancies. Presented at ACLIPS Meeting, Spring 1987.
64. Saull, S. C., and Kimmelman, C. P.: Hürthle cell tumors of the thyroid gland. Otolaryngol. Head Neck Surg. *93*:58–62, 1985.
65. Satoh, M., and Yagawa, K.: Electron microscopic study on mitochondria in Hürthle cell adenoma of thyroid. Acta Pathol. Jpn. *31*:1079–1087, 1981.
66. Savino, D., Sibley, R. K., and Hatton, S.: Significance of Hürthle cells in thyroid neoplasms: Reexamination of an old but persistent problem. Lab. Invest. *44*:59A, 1981 (Abstract).
67. Sobrinho-Simoes, M. A., Nesland, J. M., et al.: Hürthle cell and mitochondrion-rich papillary carcinomas of the thyroid gland: an ultrastructural and immunocytochemical study. Ultrastructural Pathol. *8*:131–142, 1985.
68. Tan, P. B. K., Van der Vis-Melsen, M. J. E., et al.: Hürthle cell tumours of the thyroid gland. Netherlands J. Med. *28*:509–515, 1985.
69. Thompson, N. W., Dunn, E. L., et al.: Hürthle cell lesions of the thyroid gland. Surg. Gynecol. Obstet. *139*:555–560, 1974.
70. Tollefson, H. R., Shah, J. P., and Huvos, A. G.: Hürthle cell carcinoma of the thyroid. Am. J. Surg. *130*:390–394, 1975.
71. Tovi, F., Fliss, D. M., and Inbar-Yanai, I.: Hürthle cell adenoma of the thyroglossal duct. Head and Neck Surg. *10*:346–349, 1988.
72. Tremblay, G.: Histochemical study of cytochrome oxidase and adenosine triphosphatase in Askanazy cells (Hürthle cells) of the human thyroid. Lab. Invest. *11*:514–517, 1962.
73. Tremblay, G., and Pearse, A. G. E.: Histochemistry of oxidative enzyme systems in the human thyroid with special reference to Askanazy cells. J. Pathol. Bacteriol. *80*:353–358, 1960.
74. Tscholl-Ducommun, J., and Hedinger, C. E.: Papillary thyroid carcinomas—morphology and prognosis. Virch. Arch. Pathol. Anat. [A] *396*:19–39, 1982.
75. Valdeserri, R. O., and Borochovitz, D.: Histologic changes in previously irradiated thyroid glands. Arch. Pathol. Lab. Med. *104*:150–152, 1980.
76. Valenta, L. J., Michel-Bechet, M., et al.: Human thyroid tumors composed of mitochondrion-rich cells: electron microscopic and biochemical findings. J. Clin. Endocrinol. Metab. *39*:719–733, 1974.
77. Watson, R. G., Brennan, M. D., et al.: Invasive Hürthle cell carcinoma of the thyroid: Natural history and management. Mayo Clin. Proc. *59*:851–855, 1984.

13

SQUAMOUS LESIONS OF
THE THYROID

Squamous cells can be identified in the thyroid in a variety of conditions, including developmental rests, inflammatory processes, and neoplasms (Table 13–1).

The term "squamous," when used in the context of thyroidal lesions, describes two major types of cells: true squamous elements as well as "epidermoid" nonkeratinizing cells. True squamous cells are recognized by their characteristic abundant eosinophilic glassy cytoplasm, keratin formation, and intercellular bridges. The "epidermoid" elements, on the other hand, consist of spindled or elongated cells with adequate but not voluminous cytoplasm; keratin is not seen by light microscopy and intercellular connections are less easily discernible. This latter group of cells resembles so-called squamous morules seen in endometrial metaplasia or pelvic Walthard rests.

This chapter reviews those thyroid lesions in which squamous or squamous-like cells are present, illustrates some of these, and attempts to explain the known or theoretical significance of these cells.

SQUAMOUS CELLS IN DEVELOPMENTAL RESTS

Three embryologic remnants may give rise to squamous cells in the thyroid: thymic epithelium, thyroglossal duct remnants,[40] and rests of ultimobranchial body (solid cell nests SCN).[23, 26, 64]

Thymic Remnants. These may be found in the thyroid since the thymus, derived from the third pharyngeal pouch, descends with the thyroid during fetal life. Occasionally thymic epithelium, consisting of small nests of spindled cells, and, rarely, identifiable Hassall's corpuscles are found; these are associated with lymphocytes, recapitulating the histology of the normal thymus. In this author's experience, it is more common to find thymic remnants abutting the thyroid capsule, i.e., extraglandular, rather than within the thyroid itself. These remnants are usually found in the lateral aspects of the gland.[9, 18, 28, 31, 39]

Remnants of the Thyroglossal Duct. These are usually found in the central portion of the thyroid, in the isthmus. Not infrequently, these elements will appear as small cystic lesions lined by nonkeratinizing squamous epithelium. Rarely, other types of epithelium, such as respiratory epithelium, are noted lining the cyst (Fig. 13–1). Most of these remnants are microscopic findings; rare examples of grossly evident cysts representing thyroglossal duct rests are reported.[18, 60]

Table 13–1. Squamous Cells in the Thyroid

Developmental Rests
   thymic rests
   thyroglossal rests
   ultimobranchial rests
Inflammatory
   nodular goiter
   post biopsy
   chronic thyroiditis
Tumors
   papillary carcinoma
   mucoepidermoid carcinoma
   adenoacanthoma; adenosquamous carcinoma
   squamous cell carcinoma and variants
      primary
      metastatic
Teratoma

Ultimobranchial Body Rests (Solid Cell Nests). These can be identified in about 20 to 30 percent of carefully sectioned thyroids; they are found in the lateral aspects of the lobes (Fig. 13–2). This location is expected if these structures do represent remnants of the ultimobranchial body, as most studies conclude.[1, 9, 22–24, 31, 47, 60, 65] The ultimobranchial body, which represents the end of the fourth or the entire fifth pharnygeal pouch (fourth-fifth pouch complex—see Chapter 1), descends near the thyroid in fetal life and presumably fuses with the median thyroid anlage.[60] The ultimobranchial body is theoretically the source of the parafollicular cells, which are also found predominantly in the lateral aspects of the thyroid lobes.

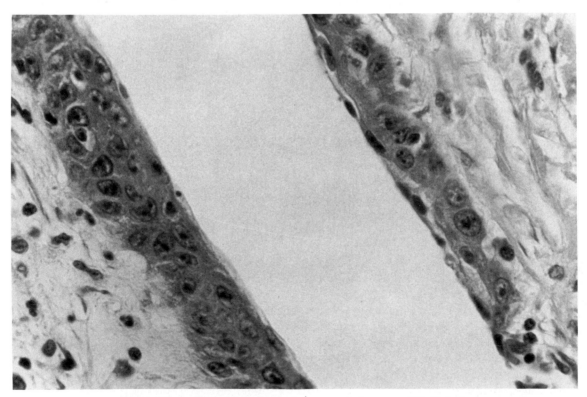

Figure 13–1. Lining of thyroglossal duct cyst is shown. × 150, H & E.

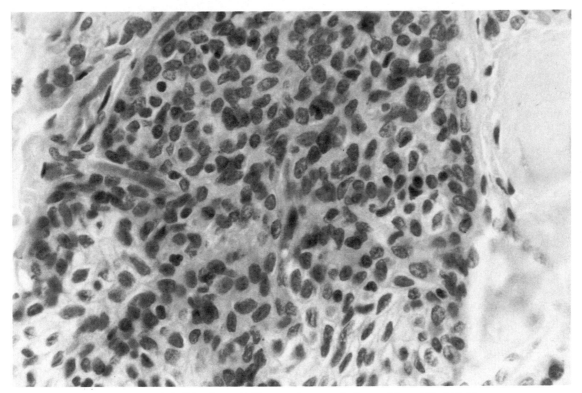

Figure 13–2. Solid cell nest is illustrated; note spindly nuclei. × 150, H & E.

In the postnatal thyroid the ultimobranchial body rests can be recognized by their interfollicular location. The remnants are composed of small usually solid nests of bland spindled cells; occasionally central cystic spaces may be seen, and these often contain mucin. The cells lining these mucin-filled cysts may be large and contain mucin as well; it has been postulated by Harach that these types of ultimobranchial body rests give rise to rare mucoepidermoid carcinomas of the thyroid[23-27] (see below). Vollenweider and Hedinger suggest that solid cell nests rather than metaplasia of follicular epithelium are the source of "squamous" cells in chronic thyroiditis.[64]

The solid cell nests may be associated with lymphoid tissue; distinguishing solid cell nests with abundant lymphocytes from thymic remnants may be difficult if not impossible unless mucin can be demonstrated.

Several immunohistologic studies of solid cell nests have been recently reported.[1, 22, 23, 25, 26, 32, 47] These indicate keratin and calcitonin positive cells either within the nests themselves or closely associated with them. The presence of calcitonin has been cited as supportive evidence for the relationship of these rests to parafollicular cells.[1, 22, 23, 32, 47] Harach has also identified thyroglobulin in or near solid cell nests[23, 25, 26]; this author suggests the ultimobranchial body may also give rise to some follicles. Harach postulates further that recently described mixed tumors of the thyroid (calcitonin- and thyroglobulin-producing lesions) may be histogenetically related to the solid cell nests,[22-25] as can thyroid mucoepidermoid cancers.[23-27] Autelitano et al., however, failed to find immunoreactive thyroglobulin or thyroxine in solid cell nests.[1]

METAPLASTIC SQUAMOUS LESIONS OF THE THYROID

Inflammatory or destructive processes that are associated with reparative phenomena can give rise to squamous cells in the thyroid. It is believed that most of these represent metaplasia of follicular epithelium.

Metaplasia in general is a very common process in pathology, but is incompletely understood. Several recent reviews and studies have attempted to clarify and classify metaplastic processes.[33, 41, 55]

Metaplasias of various types have been described, including epithelial and mesenchymal metaplasias, i.e., squamous metaplasia in the endocervix, and spindle cell metaplasia in breast carcinoma. Lugo and Putong postulated several pathways for the metaplastic process to occur.[41] *Stem cell metaplasia,* probably the most common type, involves undifferentiated "basal" cells, which, in response to trauma and/or inflammation, proliferate and replace the "normal" preexisting cells with a new and different cell type. Rarer types of metaplasia include the *direct type* (in which mature cells of one type transform into mature cells of another type) and the *indirect type* (in which mature cells proliferate and then differentiate into another type of mature element).[41]

Squamous metaplasia, the most common epithelial metaplasia, probably proceeds from proliferation of the stem cells toward the squamous phenotype. ^{3}H-thymidine-labelling studies of Schaefer et al. have shown that the occurrence of squamous metaplasia requires mitoses; these authors concluded that the origin of squamous metaplastic cells is from stem cells rather than direct transformation.[55]

The requirement of substratum or stromal matrix for support of the metaplastic process has been proved in rabbit tracheal epithelium by Jetten et al.[33] Specific

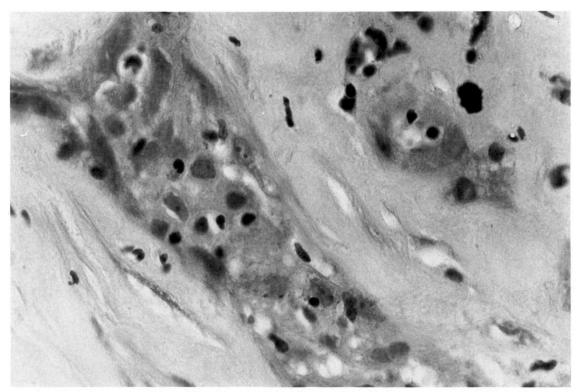

Figure 13–3. Reactive squamous metaplasia in nodular goiter; area of hemorrhage was nearby; note fibrosis around metaplastic cells. × 150, H & E.

types of collagen matrix are needed for tracheal cells grown *in vitro* to differentiate toward squamous lines.

It appears that squamous metaplasia in the thyroid results from stem-cell differentiation of inflamed or reparative follicular epithelium toward squamous type (Figs. 13–3 and 13–4). Occasional examples of squamous cells abutting upon recognizable follicular cells make one consider the possibility of direct metaplasia. Neither theory has been tested in the thyroid, however. Ultrastructural studies indicate that these histologically "squamous" cells do contain features of follicular and squamous epithelium[20]; indeed, "hybrid" cells have been described.[34, 62] In addition, keratin proteins are found in cells of the normal gland and in proliferative and neoplastic lesions.[15]

The role of the substrate or stroma is unclear, although of interest is that squamous metaplasia in the thyroid is most frequently associated with fibrotic areas in the gland.[13, 35]

Squamous metaplasia of the inflammatory type is found in the thyroid in nodular goiter and in chronic thyroiditis.[13, 31, 39] In nodular goiter, squamous foci are often found in areas of hemorrhage and fibrosis; obvious squamous features can be seen, including keratin pearls (Figs. 13–3 and 13–4). In chronic thyroiditis, the most marked squamous metaplasia is seen in the fibrosing variant of Hashimoto's thyroiditis or in fibrous atrophy (myxedema)[5, 35, 56]; as noted above, some authors believe these structures are closely related to solid cell nests and not metaplasia of follicular cells.[64] Although occasional keratin pearl formation can be identified, most examples of this type of metaplasia resemble endometrial "morules" (Figs. 13–5 to 13–7). The importance of recognizing these metaplastic foci is to realize that they represent merely a morphologic manifestation of thyroiditis.

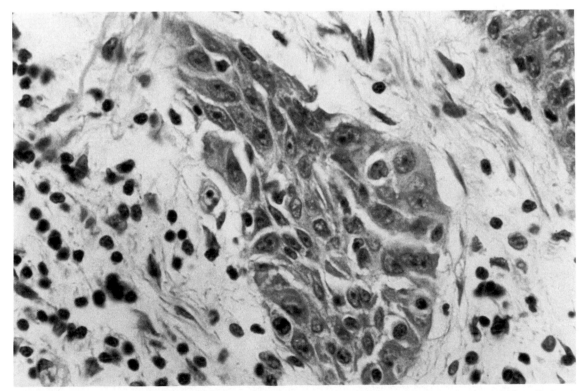

Figure 13–4. Another metaplastic focus in nodular goiter. Here the tendency toward squamous differentiation is better developed. Note scattered inflammatory cells. × 250, H & E.

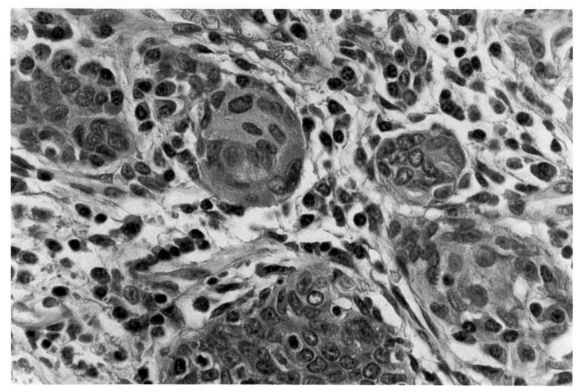

Figure 13–5. Squamous metaplasia in chronic lymphocytic thyroiditis. × 150, H & E.

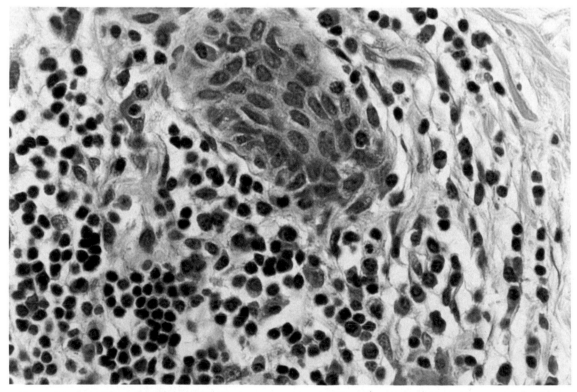

Figure 13–6. Another area of thyroiditis. Here metaplastic cells resemble endometrial morular metaplasia. × 150, H & E.

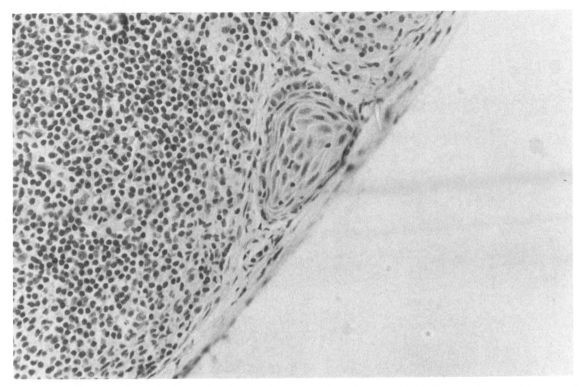

Figure 13–7. Edge of gland affected by chronic thyroiditis. Extensive lymphoid infiltrate obscured this area of thyroid such that original examiner felt this was a lymph node with subcapsular metastasis of squamous carcinoma. × 100, H & E.

SQUAMOUS CELLS IN THYROID NEOPLASMS

Mahoney et al. proposed a classification of thyroid cancers containing squamous elements.[42] These include:
- papillary or mixed papillary–follicular cancers with small benign metaplastic squamous components;
- adenoacanthoma, which is similar to the preceding, but in which the benign squamous element is prominent;
- adenosquamous carcinoma, in which the squamous elements are malignant;
- squamous cell carcinoma; and
- malignant teratoma.

I would add to this classification:
- mucoepidermoid carcinoma,
- metastatic squamous carcinoma, and
- metaplasia in benign nodules.

Adenomas: Adenomatoid Nodules

Squamous metaplasia is rare in benign adenomatous nodules. In the present author's experience, such changes have been seen in nodules that have been aspirated or subjected to biopsy. The mechanism for the metaplasia is probably similar to that in nodular goiter, i.e., postinflammatory.[42]

Papillary Carcinoma

Squamous or squamoid areas can be found focally in about 16 to 40 percent of ordinary papillary cancers[37, 43] (Figs. 13–8 and 13–9). Franssila did not note any

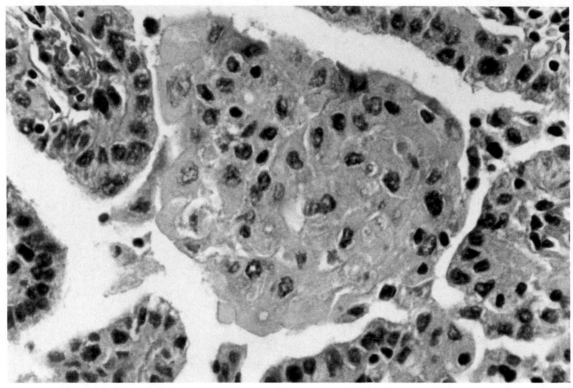

Figure 13–8. Area of squamous change in center of a papillary carcinoma. Note papillae surrounding this focus. × 200, H & E.

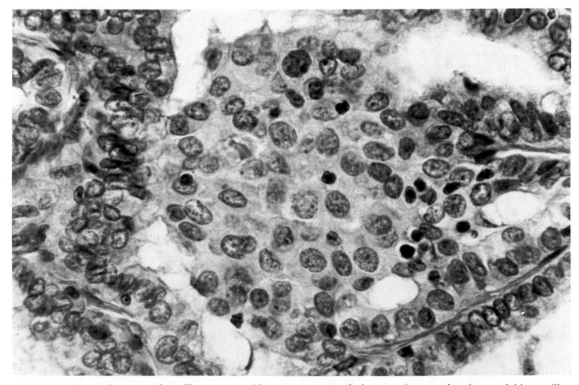

Figure 13–9. Another case of papillary cancer with squamous metaplasia; note clear overlapping nuclei in papillae. × 200, H & E.

prognostic significance to this focal finding.[16] Meissner and Warren concur.[43] Ultrastructural studies indicate that, although the squamous component appears histologically benign, the metaplastic cells indeed represent derivatives of the follicular, i.e., malignant, epithelium (not unlike a similar situation in endometrial cancers).[19, 34, 38, 62]

Diffuse Sclerosis Variant of Papillary Carcinoma. This unusual variant of papillary carcinoma is characterized by diffuse, often bilateral, involvement of the thyroid by a papillary tumor, with many psammoma bodies and prominent squamous metaplasia.[6, 11, 63] Hazard,[29] Vickery et al.,[63] and Carcangiu et al.[6] considered such lesions as more locally aggressive than ordinary papillary cancer, with a tendency to occur in young individuals, including children. This entity is quite rare, and further clinicopathologic studies of it are needed to define its prognosis.

Solid Variant of Papillary Carcinoma. Tsholl-Ducommun and Hedinger described a subtype of papillary carcinoma with solid epidermoid sheets[61]; this tumor behaved in a clinically aggressive fashion. These authors considered these lesions among the moderately differentiated papillary thyroid neoplasms.[61]

Anaplastic Carcinoma

Although some authors prefer to classify primary squamous cell carcinomas of the thyroid as a separate group, many authors include such tumors among the anaplastic carcinoma group.[8, 51] Pure squamous cell carcinoma of the thyroid does share certain clinical features with anaplastic cancer, but since the former can be recognized histologically as as epithelial neoplasm, and can be morphologically subtyped, the present author prefers to separate it (see below).

Mucoepidermoid Carcinoma

This rare but distinctive variant of thyroid carcinoma was first described as an entity by Rhatigan et al. in 1977.[49] These authors could not prove a histogenesis for this tumor, but postulated origin from intrathyroidal ectopic salivary gland rests.

Mucoepidermoid carcinoma of thyroid origin is composed of solid masses of squamoid cells and mucin-producing cells, sometimes forming glands[17, 27, 45] (Figs. 13–9 and 13–10). Central necrosis in the solid squamoid nests is often seen. The nuclei may on occasion show a ground-glass appearance; psammoma bodies may be found. Although some authors consider this lesion as a variant of papillary carcinoma, absence of thyroglobulin or thyroxine by immunostaining and biochemical analysis makes a straightforward follicular histogenesis unlikely.[17]

Franssila et al.[17] and Harach et al.[26, 27] suggested origin from vestiges of ultimobranchial body (solid cell nests). Harach indicates that solid cell nests can contain epidermal keratin, mucin and calcitonin-containing cells[26, 27]; mucoepidermoid carcinoma of the thyroid can contain similar elements. These observations present a strong argument for the proposed histogenesis of this unusual neoplasm from solid cell nests.[17, 26, 27] In the cases so far reported, no evidence of a primary salivary gland tumor has been found.

The prognosis of thyroid mucoepidermoid carcinoma is quite good. Of the six cases reported, five patients are alive without disease following therapy at intervals of 18 months to 11 years; one of these five patients developed nodal metastases.[17]

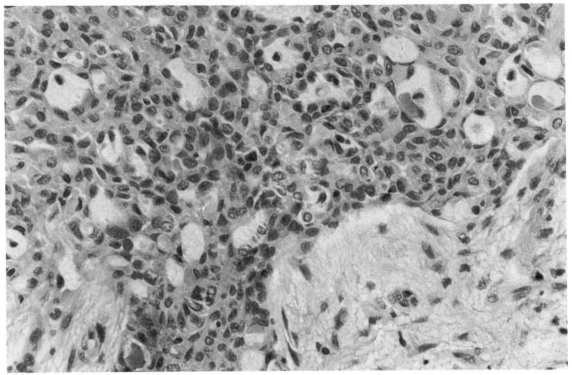

Figure 13–10. Mucoepidermoid carcinoma of thyroid. Note resemblance to salivary gland neoplasms. × 150, H & E.

One of the patients reported by Franssila et al. died of recurrent neck tumor at 13 months.[17]

In one case of thyroid mucoepidermoid cancer seen by the current author, regional nodal metastases developed 12 years after initial thyroidectomy.

Studies of larger numbers of patients with these rare lesions are needed to assess the true biology of these tumors.

Adenoacanthoma and Adenosquamous Carcinoma

The literature describing these tumors remains confused, since some authors designate thyroid cancers as adenoacanthoma without consideration of the benign or malignant appearance of the squamous epithelium.[12, 21, 52, 57, 58]

A few tumors apparently of primary thyroid origin have contained areas of recognizable papillary or mixed papillary-follicular cancer admixed with zones of benign-appearing metaplastic squamous epithelium: Mahoney et al.[42] accepted only three cases of this tumor from the literature and added one other case.[12, 14, 21] The clinical behavior of these tumors is similar to that of the malignant component alone, and the metaplastic squamous elements do not alter the prognosis.[42]

More common, but still quite rare, are mixed tumors showing combinations of papillary (or papillary and follicular) neoplasms with overtly malignant squamous areas. These adenosquamous carcinomas are aggressive tumors, usually occurring in late-middle-aged or elderly patients. Their biologic behavior closely resembles that of "pure" squamous cell cancers of the thyroid.[3, 30, 52]

Squamous Cell Carcinoma of the Thyroid

Primary squamous cell carcinoma of the thyroid is very rare. In the Huang and Assor review,[30] only 50 cases were accepted; these authors added four new cases. Recently, Simpson and Carruthers recorded eight new cases.[59]

Thyroid squamous cancer occurs in elderly patients who have histories of goiter.[2, 4, 19, 30, 48, 53, 54] The tumors resemble squamous carcinomas of other organs and range from well to poorly differentiated lesions, with or without keratinization. Origin in abnormal thyroids is common and, as such, these tumors clinically and pathologically share features with anaplastic thyroid cancers. Indeed, Carcangiu et al.[8] and Rosai et al.[51] group squamous cell carcinoma among the anaplastic group. The prognosis is also similar; these tumors are radioresistant and often rapidly fatal.

In the current author's view, the presence of a recognizable histologic pattern of squamous carcinoma deserves a separate subcategory. The histogenesis of these lesions remains unclear. They do not contain thyroglobulin,[44] but most authors consider that they derive from metaplasia and subsequent transformation of the follicular epithelium.

Clear cell change has been noted focally in many types of thyroid cancer, including squamous carcinoma.[7, 15] Such clear cell features have been reported in squamous neoplasms from other sites, notably lung.[36]

Squamous Carcinoma in Fibrosing Hashimoto's Thyroiditis. Rosai et al. recently described four cases of a squamous thyroid cancer arising in chronic thyroiditis.[50] These tumors were well-differentiated keratinizing neoplasms in which the tumor stroma showed prominent eosinophilic leukocyte infiltration. This lesion was believed to derive from the metaplastic squamous epithelium in chronic thyroiditis. Although the tumors in two of the four patients had grossly extended outside the thyroid, no metastases or deaths were reported in these individuals. It is important to distinguish these very unusual tumors from pure squamous or adenosquamous carcinoma, in which the prognosis is guarded.

Metastatic Squamous Carcinoma in the Thyroid. Far more common than the primary tumors, metastatic squamous cell carcinoma can involve the thyroid.[30, 39] Direct extension from laryngeal or esophageal primaries is probably encountered most often. Hematogenous metastases from lung or other primary sites also occur. (These latter are often noted at autopsy; thyroid dysfunction is rare.) Metastatic squamous cell carcinomas usually present as multiple nodules grossly; if microscopic foci only are found, they may often be found within thyroid stromal lymphatics.

The present author has studied an extremely instructive case in this regard. A middle-aged woman had a thyroidectomy for follicular carcinoma. Several years later, local recurrence necessitated radiation therapy and tracheostomy. About five years following this, she died of widespread metastases. Some of the metastases were obviously follicular thyroid cancer (immunostaining for thyroglobulin was positive); other metastases appeared as keratinizing squamous cell cancer (thyroglobulin stain negative). Although initially considered a metaplastic change in the thyroid cancer possibly related to radiotherapy, reexamination of the tracheostomy stomal site disclosed *in situ* and invasive squamous carcinoma of tracheal origin. A case similar to this has been reported[10]; in that instance, squamous metaplasia had been noted in the primary thyroid tumor and the subsequent squamous carcinoma was considered of thyroid origin.

Collision Tumors. An unusual case of two separate and co-synchronous thyroid tumors has been described by Motoyama and Watanabe.[46] A squamous cell carcinoma was present in one lobe, whereas the opposite lobe contained a papillary cancer. Both tumors were present in the isthmus.

Teratomas. Squamous epithelium, including keratin, can be found in thyroid teratomas. For discussion, see Chapter 15.

SUMMARY

This chapter has reviewed lesions of the thyroid in which squamous or squamoid cells are found. These include developmental and postinflammatory conditions as well as squamous differentiation in thyroid tumors. The significance of these morphologic changes is discussed.

REFERENCES

1. Autelitano, F., Santeusanio, G., et al.: Immunohistochemical study of solid cell nests of the thyroid gland found from an autopsy study. Cancer 59:477–483, 1987.
2. Bahuleyan, C. K., and Ramachandran, P.: Primary squamous cell carcinoma of thyroid. Indian J. Cancer 9:89–91, 1972.
3. Bakri, K., Simaoka, K., et al.: Adenosquamous carcinoma of the thyroid after radiotherapy for Hodgkin's disease. Cancer 52:465–470, 1983.
4. Budd, D. C., Fink, D. L., et al.: Squamous cell carcinoma of the thyroid. J. Med. Soc. N. J. 79:838–840, 1982.
5. Bullock, W. K., Hummer, G. J., and Kahler, J. E.: Squamous metaplasia of the thyroid gland. Cancer 5:966–974, 1952.
6. Carcangiu, M. L., Bianchi, S., and Rosai, J.: Diffuse sclerosing papillary carcinoma: report of 8 cases of a distinctive variant of thyroid malignancy. Lab. Invest. 56:10A, 1987 (abstract).
7. Carcangiu, M. L., Sibley, R. K., and Rosai, J.: Clear cell change in primary thyroid tumors. Am. J. Surg. Pathol. 9:705–722, 1985.
8. Carcangiu, M. L., Steeper, T., et al.: Anaplastic thyroid carcinoma. Am. J. Clin. Pathol. 83:135–158, 1985.
9. Carpenter, G. R., and Emery, J. L.: Inclusions in the human thyroid. J. Anat. 133:77–89, 1976.
10. Case records of the Massachusetts General Hospital No. 29–1975. N. Engl. J. Med. 29:186–193, 1975.
11. Chan, J. K. C., Tsui, M. S., and Tse, C. H.: Diffuse sclerosing variant of papillary carcinoma of the thyroid: a histological and immunohistochemical study of three cases. Histopathology 11:191–201, 1987.
12. Cocke, W. M., and Carrera, G. M.: Mixed squamous cell carcinoma and papillary adenocarcinoma (adenoacanthoma) of the thyroid gland. Am. J. Surg. 100:432–433, 1964.
13. Dube, V. E., and Joyce, T. G.: Extreme squamous metaplasia in Hashimoto's thyroiditis. Cancer 27:434–437, 1971.
14. Englisch, E., and Slany, A.: Ein ungewöhnliches epitheliales gewochs der schildrüse ('Adeno-Kankroid'–Operation, Hielung). Zentralblatt für Chirurgie 48:2830–2838, 1936.
15. Fisher, E. R., and Kim, W. S.: Primary clear cell thyroid carcinoma with squamous features. Cancer 39:2497–2502, 1977.
16. Franssila, K. O.: Value of histologic classification of thyroid cancer. Acta Pathol. Microbiol. Scand. Suppl. 225:5–76, 1971.
17. Franssila, K. O., Harach, H. R., and Wasenius, V. M.: Mucoepidermoid carcinoma of the thyroid. Histopathology 8:847–860, 1984.
18. Goldberg, H. M., and Harvey, P.: Squamous cell cysts of the thyroid. With special reference to the aetiology of squamous epithelium in the human thyroid. Br. J. Surg. 43:565–569, 1956.
19. Goldman, R. L.: Primary squamous cell carcinoma of the thyroid gland. Am. Surgeon 30:247–252, 1964.
20. Gould, V. E., Gould, N. S., and Benditt, E. P.: Ultrastructural aspects of papillary and sclerosing carcinomas of the thyroid. Cancer 29:1613–1625, 1972.
21. Halpert, B., and Thuss, W. G.: Columnar cell and squamous cell carcinoma (adenoacanthoma) of the thyroid gland. Surgery 28:1043–1046, 1950.
22. Harach, H. R.: Solid cell nests of the thyroid. Acta Anat. 122:249–253, 1985.
23. Harach, H. R.: Thyroid follicles with acid mucins in man: a second kind of follicles? Cell Tissue Res. 242:211–215, 1985.

24. Harach, H. R.: A study on the relationship between solid cell nests and mucoepidermoid carcinoma of the thyroid. Histopathology 9:195–207, 1985.
25. Harach, H. R.: Histological markers of solid nests of the thyroid. Acta Anat. 124:111–116, 1985.
26. Harach, H. R.: Solid cell nests of the thyroid. J. Pathol. 155:191–200, 1988.
27. Harach, H. R., Day, E. S., and de Strizic, N. A.: Mucoepidermoid carcinoma of the thyroid. Medicina 146:213–216, 1986.
28. Harcourt-Webster, J. N.: Squamous epithelium in the human thyroid gland. J. Clin. Pathol. 19:384–388, 1966.
29. Hazard, J. B.: Nomenclature of thyroid tumors. In: Young, S., and Inman, D. R. (eds.): Thyroid Neoplasia. New York, Academic Press, 1968, pp. 3–37.
30. Huang, T. Y., and Assor, D.: Primary squamous cell carcinoma of the thyroid gland: A report of four cases. Am. J. Clin. Pathol. 55:93–98, 1971.
31. Jaffe, R. H.: Epithelial metaplasia of the thyroid gland. Arch. Pathol. 23:821–830, 1937.
32. Janzur, R. C., Weber, E., and Hedinger, C.: The relation between solid cell nests and C cells of the thyroid gland. Cell Tissue Res. 197:295–312, 1979.
33. Jetten, A. M., Brody, A. et al.: Retinoic acid and substratum regulate the differentiation of rabbit tracheal epithelial cells into squamous and secretory phenotype. Lab. Invest. 56:654–664, 1987.
34. Johannesson, J. V., Gould, V. E., and Jao, W.: The fine structure of human thyroid cancer. Hum. Pathol. 9:385–400, 1978.
35. Katz, S. M., and Vickery, A. L.: The fibrous variant of Hashimoto's thyroiditis. Hum. Pathol. 5:161–170, 1974.
36. Katzenstein, A. A., Prioleau, P. G., and Askin, F. B.: The histologic spectrum and significance of clear-cell change in lung carcinoma. Cancer 45:943–947, 1980.
37. Klinck, G. H., and Menk, K. F.: Squamous cells in the human thyroid. Milit. Surg. 109:406–414, 1951.
38. Klinck, G. H., Oertel, J. E., and Winship, T.: Ultrastructure of normal human thyroid. Lab. Invest. 22:2–22, 1970.
39. LiVolsi, V. A., and Merino, M. J.: Squamous cells in the human thyroid gland. Am. J. Surg. Pathol. 2:133–140, 1978.
40. LiVolsi, V. A., Perzin, K. A., and Savetsky, L.: Carcinoma arising in median ectopic thyroid (including thyroglossal duct tissue). Cancer 34:1303–1315, 1974.
41. Lugo, M., and Putong, P. B.: Metaplasia: an overview. Arch. Pathol. Lab. Med. 108:185–189, 1984.
42. Mahoney, J. P., Saffos, R. O., and Rhatigan, R. M.: Follicular adenoacanthoma of the thyroid gland. Histopathology 4:547–557, 1980.
43. Meissner, W. A., and Warren, S.: Tumors of the thyroid gland. In: Atlas of Tumor Pathology. Fascicle 4. Washington, D.C., Armed Forces Institute of Pathology, 1969.
44. Miettinen, M., Franssila, K., et al.: Expression of intermediate filament proteins in thyroid gland and thyroid tumors. Lab. Invest. 50:262–270, 1984.
45. Mizukami, Y., Matsubara, F., et al.: Primary mucoepidermoid carcinoma in the thyroid gland. Cancer 53:1741–1745, 1984.
46. Motoyama, T., and Watanabe, H.: Simultaneous squamous cell carcinoma and papillary adeno-carcinoma of the thyroid. Hum. Pathol. 14:1009–1010, 1983.
47. Nadig, J., Weber, E., and Hedinger, C.: C-cells in vestiges of the ultimobranchial body in human thyroid glands. Virch. Arch. B 27:189–191, 1978.
48. Prakash, A., Kukreti, S. C., and Sharma, M. P.: Primary squamous cell carcinoma of the thyroid gland. Intl. Surgery 50:538–541, 1968.
49. Rhatigan, R. M., Roque, J. L., and Bucher, R. L.: Mucoepidermoid carcinoma of the thyroid gland. Cancer 39:210–214, 1977.
50. Rosai, J., Albores Saavedra, J., and Battifora, H.: A sclerosing squamous tumor of the thyroid with eosinophilic infiltration arising in Hashimoto's thyroiditis. Report of 4 cases of a distinctive tumor entity. Lab. Invest. 56:66A, 1987 (abstract).
51. Rosai, J., Saxen, E. A., and Woolner, L.: Undifferentiated and poorly differentiated carcinoma. Sem. Diagn. Pathol. 2:123–136, 1985.
52. Ross, R. C.: Mixed squamous cell carcinoma and papillary adenocarcinoma (adenoacanthoma) of the thyroid gland. Arch. Pathol. 44:192–197, 1947.
53. Saito, K., Kuratomi, Y., et al.: Primary squamous cell carcinoma of the thyroid associated with marked leucocytosis and hypercalcemia. Cancer 48:2080–2083, 1981.
54. Saxen, E.: Squamous metaplasia in the thyroid gland and histogenesis of epidermoid carcinoma of the thyroid. Acta Pathol. Microbiol. Scand. 28:55–60, 1951.
55. Schaefer, F. V., Custer, R. P., and Sorof, S.: Induction of squamous metaplasia: requirement for cell multiplication and competition with lobuloalveolar development in cultured mammary glands. Differentiation 25:185–192, 1983.
56. Sclare, G.: The thyroid in myxoedema. J. Pathol. Bacteriol. 85:263–273, 1963.
57. Segal, K., Sidi, J., et al.: Pure squamous cell and mixed adenosquamous cell carcinoma of the thyroid gland. Head and Neck Surg. 6:1035–1042, 1984.
58. Shimaoka, K., and Tsukada, Y.: Squamous cell carcinomas and adenosquamous carcinomas originating from the thyroid gland. Cancer 46:1833–1842, 1980.

59. Simpson, W. J., and Carruthers, J.: Squamous cell carcinoma of the thyroid gland. Am. J. Surg. *156*:44–46, 1988.
60. Sugiyama, S.: The embryology of the human thyroid gland including ultimobranchial body and others related. Adv. Anat. Embryol. Cell Biol. *44*:1–111, 1971.
61. Tsholl-Ducommun, J., and Hedinger, C. D.: Papillary thyroid carcinoma: morphology and prognosis. Virch. Arch. (A) *396*:19–39, 1982.
62. Valenta, L. J., and Michel-Bechet, M.: Ultrastructure and biochemistry of thyroid carcinoma. Cancer *40*:284–300, 1977.
63. Vickery, A. L., Carcangiu, M. L., et al.: Papillary carcinoma. Sem. Diagn. Pathol. *2*:90–100, 1985.
64. Vollenweider, I., and Hedinger, C.: Solid cell nests (SCN) in Hashimoto's thyroiditis. Virch. Arch. Pathol. Anat. *412*:357–363, 1988.
65. Yamaoka, Y.: Solid cell nests (SCN) of the human thyroid gland. Acta Pathol. Jpn. *23*:493–506, 1973.

Chapter

14

LYMPHOID AND HEMATOPOIETIC LESIONS

Nonepithelial neoplasms that affect the thyroid include lymphoid and rare hematopoietic and mesenchymal tumors. This chapter reviews those lesions of the thyroid that are lymphocytic or hematopoietic. (Mesenchymal lesions are discussed in Chapters 11 and 15.)

LYMPHOCYTIC LESIONS AFFECTING THE THYROID

Lymphocytes are seen commonly in a variety of thyroid lesions; among these are:

1. nodular goiter, toxic and nontoxic;
2. thyroiditides;
3. peritumoral (epithelial tumor) infiltrates;
4. lymphoproliferative disorders and frank malignant lymphomas.

It is likely that any lymphocytic infiltration of the gland reflects an abnormality[94]; indeed, all such infiltration most likely signifies a response to inflammation (nontoxic nodular goiter) or, more frequently, a manifestation of an immunologic derangement. (See also Chapter 5.) The benign lymphoid infiltrates of the thyroid are seen most often in autoimmune thyroid diseases. Both T and B cells are present in these glands. In chronic thyroiditis and autoimmune hyperthyroidism, follicular centers, i.e., B cells, are prominent; in fact, lymphoid cells within the thyroid in these diseases show ratios that vary from the normal circulating T to B cell ratios. This predominance of B lymphocytes supports the finding by immunophenotyping that most primary thyroid lymphomas are B-cell tumors (see below).

Malignant Lymphoma

Malignant lymphoma may involve the thyroid as part of systemic lymphoma (secondary lymphoma) or may arise primarily in the thyroid.

"Secondary" Lymphoma. It is estimated from the older literature that about 20 percent of patients dying of generalized malignant lymphoma will show thyroid involvement at autopsy.[80] Rarely is thyroid replacement extensive enough to produce clinical hypothyroidism.[129] These reports predate the use of modern therapies for lymphoma. Many patients dying of lymphoma nowadays die of

infectious and/or hemorrhagic complications, and residual tumor is not frequently found at autopsy. In those cases in which secondary lymphomatous involvement is seen, the thyroid contains one or more discrete nodules of tumor, which are often partly necrotic. In most patients with secondary lymphoma, the remaining thyroid tissue appears histologically normal.

Primary Malignant Lymphoma of the Thyroid. Malignant lymphoma initially or solely presenting in extranodal sites constitutes between 10 and 25 percent of all malignant lymphomas.[34, 58] A small number of these (estimated at less than 5 percent) arise primarily in the thyroid. Of all thyroid malignancies, 1 to 3.5 percent are malignant lymphomas[35, 107]; in some areas of the world where thyroiditis is very common, up to 10 percent of thyroid malignancies are lymphoma.[107, 117]

Usually (in 25 to 100 percent of cases) lymphoma arises in an immunologically abnormal gland, often one affected by chronic lymphocytic thyroiditis.[1, 2, 4, 6, 13, 16, 22, 24, 26, 29, 32, 35, 37, 38, 40, 41, 44, 48, 53, 55, 57, 72, 78, 83, 85, 93, 102, 107, 111, 112, 126, 128, 129] Kato et al. identified a risk factor of 80 for thyroid lymphoma in patients with chronic thyroiditis when compared to controls.[55] Fujimoto et al. found levels of thyroid autoantibodies in patients with thyroid lymphoma to be as high as in individuals with Hashimoto's disease.[35]

Clinically, thyroid lymphoma affects women more frequently than men (ratio 2.5 to 8.4:1). Most patients are elderly (ages 50 to 80). The mass, often arising in a patient with goiter, is rapidly growing and may extend outside the gland. The rapidity of the growth and its extent may produce dysphagia, hoarseness, and respiratory difficulties.[2, 4, 11, 16, 24, 26, 29, 32, 41, 53, 93, 102, 111, 129]

The clinical presentation (Table 14–1) of a rapidly growing mass in an elderly patient with a history of goiter leads to a clinical suspicion of anaplastic thyroid carcinoma. There has been confusion in the pathologic distinction of these entities as well. It is of great importance, however, that the differential diagnosis between lymphoma and anaplastic carcinoma be made, since successful therapeutic options exist for the former, and the prognosis is far from dismal.[2, 4, 16, 22, 38, 41, 94, 100, 117, 129]

The presence of abnormal thyroid function, usually hypothyroidism, has been documented historically in a minority of reported cases.[2, 4, 32, 41, 92, 94, 129] In most of these cases, hypothyroidism is caused by preexisting chronic thyroiditis. Hypothyroidism resulting from the lymphomatous replacement of the gland is rare; usually the mass presents the most significant clinical problem. Very rarely hyperthyroidism may be noted; in these cases the mechanism postulated is similar to the hyperthyroidism found in subacute thyroiditis, i.e., rapid destruction of follicles with attendant release of colloid and stored thyroid hormone into the circulation.[36, 51]

The *histogenesis* of primary thyroid lymphoma has elicited a great deal of discussion and research. When sufficient uninvolved nontumoral thyroid tissue has been examined in cases of primary thyroid lymphoma, the majority show

Table 14–1. Clinical Features of Thyroid Lymphoma

Age	50–80 (average 63–64)
Sex	F > M (2.6–8.4:1)
Presentation	Goiter, often rapid growth; sometimes stridor, hoarseness
Thyroid Function	Minority hypothyroid
Stage	Majority localized initially
Associated Lesions	Chronic thyroiditis historically in a few
	Propensity for gastrointestinal lymphoma
Survival	~50%, depends on stage

evidence of lymphocytic thyroiditis. In addition, a few series reporting long-term follow-up studies of patients with clinically and serologically documented autoimmune thyroiditis indicate that a disproportionate number of neoplasms occurring in such individuals are malignant lymphoma.[2, 4, 6, 16, 24, 26, 32, 37, 41, 53, 55, 93, 102, 129]

These histologic and clinical observations indicate that an immunologically abnormal tissue produces the background for lymphoma development. Thyroid lymphomas share with lymphomas arising in other extranodal sites a propensity to occur in an already abnormal tissue setting.[14, 45, 47, 48, 50, 102] However, primary thyroid lymphoma is rare; Fujimoto et al. found that 3.7 percent of the thyroid malignancies in their institution were malignant lymphomas.[35] When this is compared to the incidence of thyroiditis, which, depending on the definition used and the population studied, can range from 5 to 54 percent of the population, the rarity of lymphoma can be appreciated.[2, 4, 84, 93, 129] Hence, it is important not to view autoimmune thyroiditis as a premalignant condition[30, 31] as some authors have.[23, 47, 97] Recently Ben-Ezra et al. found no evidence of monoclonality in the lymphoid infiltrate of glands involved by Hashimoto's thyroiditis.[9] Hence this abnormal tissue is not of itself neoplastic. The case of Matsubayashi et al.[77] suggests, however, that some patients with florid thyroiditis may develop a clonal lesion, which over many years may progress to full-blown lymphoma. This event must be very rare.

Some reports indicate that carcinoma of the thyroid occurs more frequently in patients with thyroiditis[23, 30, 47, 97]; these studies have often confused localized peritumoral lymphoid infiltrates with chronic thyroiditis. Serologic, clinical, and pathologic evidence to support this opinion is lacking. The consideration of chronic thyroiditis as a premalignant state, and its corollary, i.e., all such thyroids should be surgically removed,[97] is to be condemned.[30]

Various reports of extranodal lymphoma, in general, have discussed the relationship of immune aberration and lymphoid neoplasia. Burke indicates that some "immunologically mediated" extranodal proliferations may predispose to the development of lymphoma.[15] Whether this is due to loss of T suppressor cells or results from neoplastic transformation following chronic antigenic stimulation is unclear. It is known that most extranodal lymphomas, and certainly the majority of those apparently arising primarily in the thyroid, are of B-cell origin[7, 15, 48, 85]; most of the latter are of large cell type (older classifications: diffuse histiocytic lymphoma; reticulum cell sarcoma). Rare cases of T-cell lymphoma have been recorded.[86]

The concept of MALT (mucosa associated lymphoid tissue) proposed by Isaacson and his colleagues[49, 50] and others [78, 79] fits well with the ideas regarding the development of thyroid lymphoma. The MALT concept refers to foregut-derived lymphoid tissue (such as that of the gastrointestinal tract, Waldeyer's ring, thyroid) which can serve as a target for autoimmune disease.[2, 49, 50, 78] The latter can become the substrate for the development of lymphoma. MALT organ lymphomas share certain histologic and clinical features.

A common histologic finding is the so-called "lymphoepithelial lesion" (Figs. 14–1 and 14–2). In the thyroid, this consists of thyroid follicles stuffed with neoplastic lymphoid cells—sometimes the latter partially or totally replace the follicular epithelium. This finding is not seen in reactive lymphoid lesions, even in florid thyroiditis.[2, 93] Another histologic clue to MALT lymphomas is plasma cell differentiation of the neoplastic clone. Isaacson and Wright believe this reflects the normal response of MALT to antigenic stimulation, i.e., B cells differentiating toward plasma cells.[49]

Plasmacytic differentiation suggests well-differentiated lymphomas and, indeed,

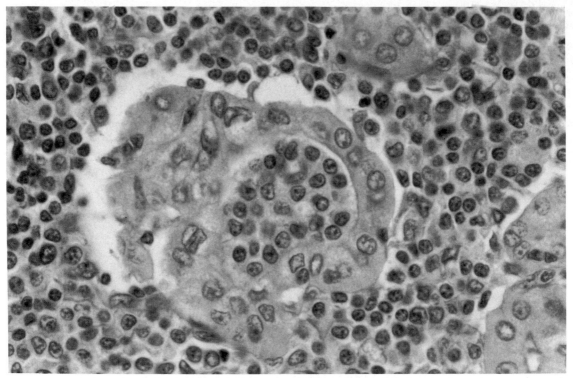

Figure 14–1. Lymphoepithelial lesion in thyroid lymphoma. Note "stuffing" of follicle. × 250, H & E.

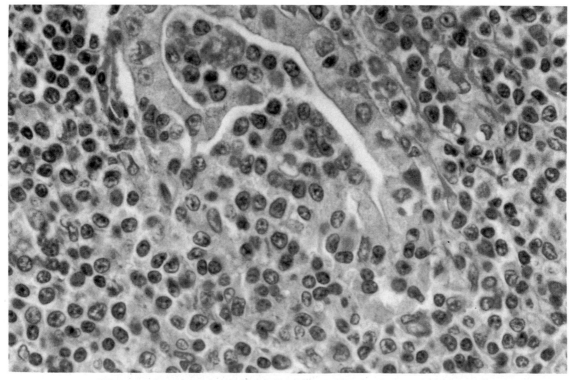

Figure 14–2. Another lymphoepithelial lesion is illustrated. × 250, H & E.

lesions in this group tend to behave in an indolent fashion.[2] (Of course, not all MALT or thyroid lymphomas are well differentiated.)

From the clinical standpoint, differences between nodal and extranodal (thyroidal) lymphomas are found.[2] Whereas node-based lymphomas often are high stage lesions at presentation, MALT lymphomas tend to be localized. Anscombe and Wright believe this finding reflects the "limited circulation pathways" of these MALT lymphocytes between mucosal and epithelial surfaces and regional lymph nodes.[2] Of course, localized disease can be treated less aggressively than generalized lymphoma (see below).

Another clinically important finding in patients with thyroid lymphoma is the relatively high incidence of concomitant or metasynchronous involvement of other MALT organs, especially in the gastrointestinal tract. As noted in the series reported by Brewer and Orr,[13] Metcalfe and Sclare,[83] Stone et al.,[114] and Woolner et al.,[129] gastrointestinal and thyroid lymphoma occur too frequently in the same patient to be considered fortuitous (considering the relative rarity of extranodal lymphoma). (Smithers[112] and Compagno and Oertel[26] did not find this association in their material, however.) Anscombe and Wright in their series of 76 thyroid lymphomas noted gastrointestinal involvement histologically in five and clinically in an additional two patients (total 10 percent of the series).[2]

Pathology

Grossly, most thyroid lymphomas appear as large fleshy tan to gray masses, often extending outside the thyroid capsule. Infiltration of the residual thyroid tissue may be seen. The nontumoral thyroid may show the gross appearance of lymphocytic thyroiditis, with beige color, fibrosis, and lobular accentuation, although the findings often depend upon the amount of thyroid tissue uninvolved by the tumor[2, 4, 26, 93, 129] (Table 14–2).

The *microscopic* appearance of thyroid lymphomas resembles that of lymphoma occurring in other sites. The gamut of small, intermediate, and large cell lesions is found; sometimes nodular areas are noted, although a diffuse pattern is more common. The most common histologic subtype is large cell diffuse malignant lymphoma (Figs. 14–3 and 14–4).[16, 42, 63, 103, 107] (See Table 14–3.) Some tumors demonstrate a plasmacytoid appearance (Fig. 14–5); others show features of immunoblastic sarcoma. In occasional tumors, a pleomorphic cell population is noted; a few of these latter lesions have been shown to type as T cell tumors.

The tumors often disclose areas of zonal necrosis (Fig. 14–4). This feature is more frequently encountered in large cell lymphomas.

Infiltration of surrounding thyroid is seen. It is common to see infiltration of

Table 14–2. Pathologic Features of Thyroid Lymphoma

Gross
Fleshy, firm tumor
Often extrathyroidal
Gray to tan-gray; occasional necrosis
Surrounding gland pale, lobulated—thyroiditis

Histology
Effaced architecture
May be nodular; usually diffuse
Usually lymphocytic thyroiditis background
Tumor cells among and in between preexisting follicles
"Lymphoepithelial" lesions
Plasmacytic differentiation common

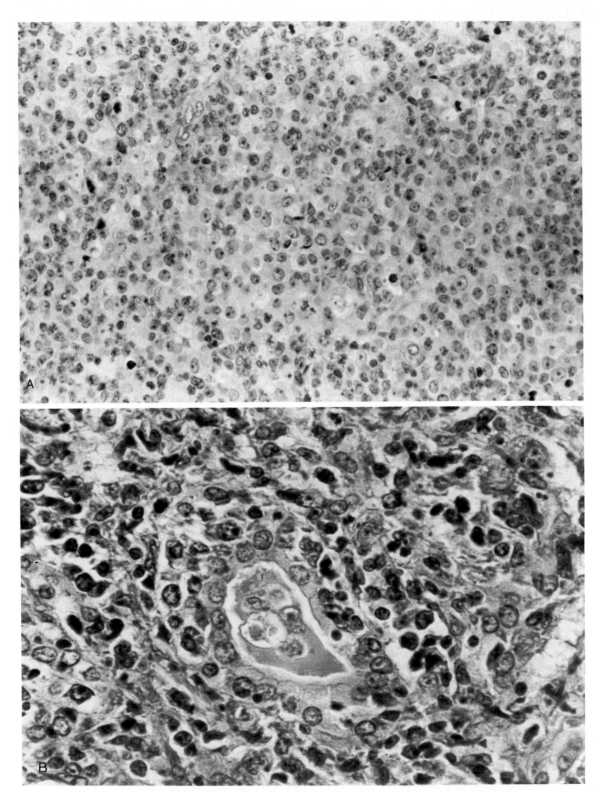

Figure 14–3. *A,* Large cell diffuse malignant lymphoma. This is from a thyroid tumor but resembles lymphomas arising elsewhere. × 150, H & E.
B, Here a large cell lymphoma surrounds a residual thyroid follicle. × 250, H & E.

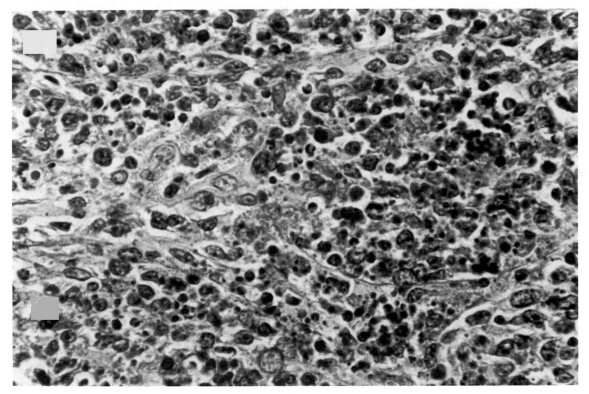

Figure 14–4. Necrosis as seen here is common in large cell lymphomas. × 250, H & E.

lymphocytes into residual thyroid follicles; sometimes the malignant cells replace the follicular epithelium. In the older literature, the latter phenomenon had been equated with an epithelial origin for the tumor, since the tumor "produced" follicles.[2, 93] Invasion beyond the thyroid itself, into surrounding strap muscles and soft tissue, is seen in 50 to 60 percent of cases.[2, 16, 93, 129] Some series indicate that this finding is associated with a poor prognosis.[16, 129]

Table 14–3. Primary Lymphoma of the Thyroid: Subtypes

	Percentage
Large cell lymphoma (histiocytic lymphoma) including immunoblastic sarcoma	70–80
Intermediate grade lymphoma (poorly differentiated lymphoma; and mixed cell lymphoid-histiocytic)	5–10
Low grade lymphoma—small cell lymphoma, with or without plasmacytoid features	10–12
Signet cell lymphoma	Very rare
Intermediate lymphocytic lymphoma	Rare to 20 (see text)
Hodgkin's disease	Very rare
Diffuse	80–90
Nodular	10–20
B-cell	>95
T-cell	<5

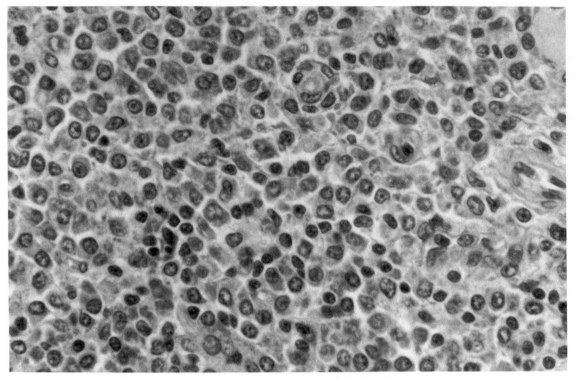

Figure 14–5. Malignant lymphoma, B-cell type of thyroid. Smaller cells compose the lesion; some plasmacytoid features are seen. Note thyroid follicle in upper right corner. × 250, H & E.

Vascular invasion is common.[93] Oertel and Heffess noted this finding in 25 percent of their cases. These authors indicate that infiltration of the vascular intima by neoplastic lymphocytes is a finding not seen in reactive lymphoid proliferations.[93] In addition, prominent vascular proliferation can be noted at the invasive edges of the tumor. Proliferated plump endothelial cells may mimic epithelial structures: again such structures may be confused with epithelial differentiation of the neoplasm (Fig. 14–6).[2, 83]

Transitions from chronic lymphocytic thyroiditis to marked lymphoid hyperplasia to lymphoma can be seen.[15] The reactive hyperplasia is usually found abutting upon the overt lymphoma.

The *differential diagnosis* of thyroid lymphoma is listed in Table 14–4. In small and intermediate cell lymphomas, especially those that are focally nodular, distinction from reactive hyperplasia may be difficult. Of use in this differential are the monotony of the cell population, cytologic atypia, especially nuclear irregularities, absence of true reactive follicular centers, and architectural destruction—all features shared by extranodal lymphomas in general.[15, 103] In small cell lymphoid thyroid lesions, other useful histologic clues for a diagnosis of malignancy include a sheet-like growth pattern and replacement of residual thyroid follicles by the lymphoid cells—"lymphoepithelial lesion" (Figs. 14–1 and 14–2).[2, 49, 50, 93]

The differential diagnosis of small cell lymphoma lies chiefly with small cell carcinoma; however, true small cell carcinoma of the thyroid, if it exists, is exceedingly rare[82, 93, 101, 118] (Chapter 11). Small cell medullary carcinoma may contain cells that occasionally show plasmacytic features.[71, 74, 81] Immunohistologic stains (calcitonin; leukocyte common antigen) are helpful in this distinc-

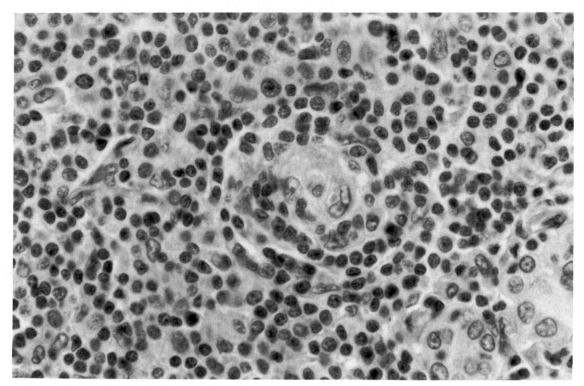

Figure 14–6. Malignant lymphoma with reactive vessel in center. Note red cell within it. This nest may resemble an epithelial structure. Such structures should not be misconstrued as evidence of epithelial differentiation of a small cell thyroid tumor. × 250, H & E.

tion.[17, 63, 75, 88, 98, 106] Large cell lymphomas similarly need to be differentiated from anaplastic carcinomas. This distinction is usually easily made on the basis of histology alone (once the pathologist recognizes that lymphoma can occur as a primary thyroid tumor!). Marked individual cell pleomorphism and spindle and giant cells are rare in lymphomas. However, for confirmation of the diagnosis, immunostains for leukocyte common antigen and cytokeratins will be useful.[17, 20, 44, 63, 71, 75, 88, 95, 98, 106, 118]

Special nonimmunostains are of little use in defining lymphoid from epithelial tumors in the thyroid.[82] Reticulin stains to distinguish epithelial nests rarely help in undifferentiated thyroid neoplasms. Periodic acid–Schiff (PAS) stains to detect

Table 14–4. Distinction between Lymphoma and Mimickers in the Thyroid

Lesion	Mimicker	Distinguish Between	Helpful Hint
Large cell lymphoma; immunoblastic sarcoma	Anaplastic carcinoma	Large cell lymphoma and carcinoma	Immunostaining keratin; leukocyte common antigen
Small cell lymphoma	Medullary carcinoma "Insular" carcinoma "Small cell carcinoma" Florid thyroiditis	Small cell lymphoma and carcinoma	Same; also stains for thyroglobulin and calcitonin
		Small cell lymphoma and florid thyroiditis	Lymphoepithelial lesions; monoclonality by immunomarkers
Plasmacytoma	Medullary carcinoma	Plasmacytoma and medullary carcinoma	Immunostaining for calcitonin and immunoglobulin light chains

colloid are of little help since, as noted above, lymphomas can replace follicular cells and colloid can still be present; the PAS positivity, therefore, does not prove the epithelial nature of the tumor!

Immunohistology. As indicated previously, antibodies to leukocyte common antigen, which can be used successfully in fixed, paraffin-embedded tissue, are often helpful in distinguishing lymphoma from carcinoma.[75, 95] Staining for epithelial keratins is also helpful.[17, 63, 71, 74, 98, 118] Combinations of panels of antibodies strengthen the diagnostic confidence; it is therefore our practice to evaluate immunostains for both cytokeratin and leukocyte antigens in most cases. Confirmatory evidence of clonality can occasionally be demonstrated in fixed tissue by immunostaining for immunoglobulin light chains. Thus, if the neoplastic cells all contain lambda *or* kappa, clonality is established.[42, 58–61, 69, 78] Not all malignant lymphomas contain stainable cytoplasmic immunoglobulins, however; hence, a negative result is meaningless.[2]

If fresh tumor tissue is available, panels of monoclonal antibodies to various B, T, and pre-B cell antigens, and immunoglobulins (heavy and light chains) can be used to define the lymphoma further, i.e., its monoclonal neoplastic nature and its cell type. (One note of caution appears warranted, however.[2, 4, 6, 7, 17, 42, 58–61, 69, 78] Confusion in interpretation of clonality may occur, especially if the lymphoproliferative lesion is closely associated with residual thyroiditic gland. However, looking at these stains may show pockets of clonality in areas that are histologically monotonous even when the immunophenotype is heterogeneous in the entire population. In these cases, immunotyping alone may be insufficient to prove clonality; modern techniques such as DNA analysis for gene rearrangement may be needed to prove the clonal origin of the proliferating cells.[2] Small clonal populations in patients with immunologic abnormalities need to be interpreted with some caution, however, if they constitute the sole malignant criterion; correlation with morphology is essential.)

Ultrastructure. Ultrastructural studies have been reported by several authors who have examined cases of thyroidal lymphomas.[19, 70, 91, 101] Epithelial features such as desmosomes and tonofilaments are absent. Features suggesting lymphoma, including some cases showing rich endoplasmic reticulum characteristic of plasma cell differentiation, have been reported. With the current availability of immunoperoxidase staining, which can be successfully applied to fixed tissue, electron microscopy is of limited utility in the definition of thyroid lymphomas.

Associations. Between 25 and 100 percent of primary thyroid lymphomas reported apparently arise upon a background of lymphocytic thyroiditis.[2, 4, 6, 16, 23, 26, 32, 37, 41, 53, 55, 93, 100, 111, 129] This may be noted by history, prior biopsy, serologic studies, or, most commonly, by histologic examination of the residual nontumorous thyroid (Figs. 14–7 to 14–9). This immunologically abnormal tissue then provides the setting for the origin of the lymphoma.[2, 49, 50] The definition of chronic lymphocytic thyroiditis is probably responsible for the considerable variation in the percentages noted above; some pathologists require all the features of so-called Hashimoto's thyroiditis to include a case of lymphoma as arising in a background of thyroiditis. However, since virtually all lymphoid infiltration of the thyroid reflects an abnormality and most are immunologic abnormalities, it seems that, if such cases of "nonspecific lymphocytic thyroiditis" are included, the percentage of lymphomas arising in immunoderanged tissue is very high and approaches 100 percent.[2, 84] Additionally, the percentage range may reflect the fact that in many cases sufficient nontumor thyroid tissue is lacking for accurate pathologic assessment for preexisting thyroid pathology.[2, 16, 93, 129]

A rare case of lymphoma arising in a thyroid affected by Graves' disease

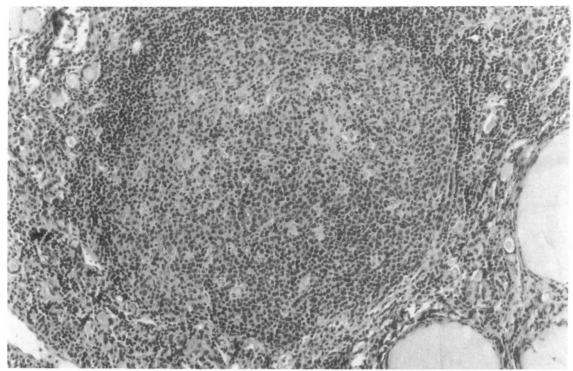

Figure 14–7. Chronic lymphocytic thyroiditis. Well-developed germinal center is visible. × 100, H & E.

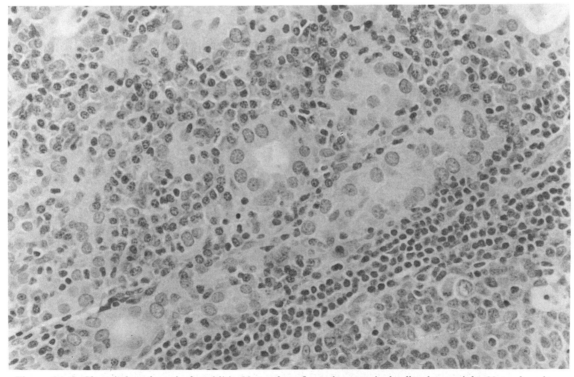

Figure 14–8. Chronic lymphocytic thyroiditis. Note edge of reactive germinal cell at lower right. Note also plasma cells and the lymphoid and plasma cells abutting on and, rarely, in follicle. × 150, H & E.

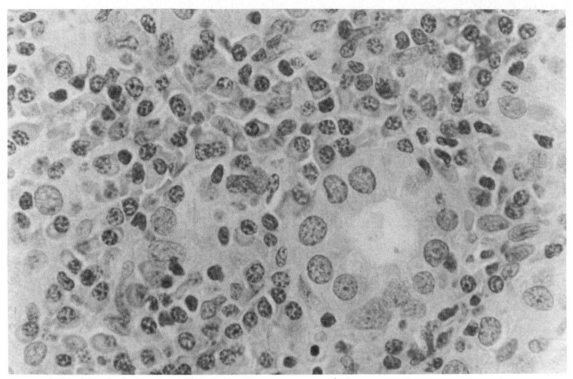

Figure 14–9. Higher power of Figure 14–7. Contrast with lymphoepithelial lesions in Figures 14–1 and 14–2. ×
300, H & E.

provides further evidence of lymphoma originating in immunologically abnormal
tissue.[132]

Thyroid lymphoma has been documented to arise in a patient with history of
prior neck irradiation.[12]

An unusual case of thyroid malignant lymphoma has been reported in a
genetically abnormal patient who had 14/21 translocation.[65]

A small number of primary thyroid lymphomas arise in nonthyroiditic glands,
such as in nodular goiter (although the immune abnormalities associated with
some of these cases remain to be evaluated[93]).

Diagnosis, Therapy, and Prognosis

The diagnosis of thyroid lymphoma can be established by fine needle aspiration
or large bore needle biopsy.[41, 67, 125] These techniques are especially effective in
large cell lymphomas or immunoblastic sarcomas. If appropriately directed biopsies are performed, i.e., biopsies of a dominant mass or nodules rather than of
nonnodular gland, the diagnosis of lymphoma can be rendered. In small cell
lymphoma, large bore needle biopsy or even open surgical biopsy may be necessary
to evaluate the diffuse nature of the infiltrate and distinguish it from thyroiditis.
In some cases, surgical wedge biopsy may be needed to obtain sufficient tissue for
immunostaining or DNA analysis to establish clonality and thus the neoplastic
nature of the process. These studies require saving a portion of tissue fresh at
time of biopsy. If the diagnosis can be established with minimally invasive methods,
radiotherapy can be instituted rapidly.[41]

When a diagnosis of thyroid lymphoma is made, careful clinical staging of the
disease is warranted. Radiologic assessment of the mediastinum, abdomen, and

retroperitoneum, as well as bone marrow biopsy, should be performed. In some cases, more widespread disease will be found. Of interest, as discussed above, lymphoma in other extranodal sites may be discovered. A peculiar propensity for gastric or small bowel involvement has been noted.[2, 13, 114, 129] Saul and Kapadia noted a similar strong association of malignant lymphoma of Waldeyer's ring and gastrointestinal disease.[104, 105]

Treatment for thyroid lymphoma depends upon the staging results. If the disease is widespread, chemotherapy is the choice; on the other hand, if the tumor is localized to the gland only and/or the regional lymph nodes, radiotherapy with or without adjuvant chemotherapy appears warranted.[100, 117, 120, 121] The role of surgery, beyond decompression of the trachea and obtaining sufficient tissue for diagnosis and immunophenotyping, appears limited.[41, 93, 100] Rasbach et al. suggested a larger role for surgical excision if the tumor is confined to the thyroid.[100]

The prognosis for localized thyroid lymphoma is excellent. Over 50 percent of affected patients survive 10 years. In recently reported series, survival rates have improved for localized thyroid lymphoma; Tennvall et al. noted a 77 percent survival rate.[117] These authors attributed this result to more intensive staging procedures which defined truly localized disease. It has been noted by several authors that plasmacytic differentiation of the tumor portends an even better survival.[2, 26, 93] This may reflect the low proliferative activity in well-differentiated lesions.[2] Zirkin et al. suggested that determination of ploidy in thyroidal lymphoma may have prognostic import.[133] (See also Chapter 18.)

Of course, if staging procedures disclose disseminated lymphoma, the prognosis is less good.[100, 117, 120]

ATYPICAL LYMPHOPROLIFERATIVE LESIONS

Florid reactive hyperplasia associated with chronic thyroiditis can on occasion cause diagnostic concern for the histopathologist. Distinguishing such lesions from malignant lymphoma (usually the confusion arises with small cell lymphoma) requires attention to the presence of reactive follicular centers, absence of lymphoepithelial lesions and confinement of the lesion within the thyroid.[2, 26, 93] In doubtful cases studies searching for monoclonal proliferation by immunophenotyping or for gene rearrangement[61] may have to be done in order to define the precise nature of a particular lesion.

PLASMA CELL LESIONS

Plasmacytoma

Infiltration of the thyroid gland is rare in patients with systemic myeloma: anywhere from 0 to 2.6 percent of patients in large series of cases of multiple myeloma show thyroid involvement.[52, 54, 127] Extramedullary plasma cell tumors have been reported to occur in the thyroid; through 1986, 30 cases had been described.[5, 8, 10, 18, 21, 28, 39, 43, 56, 62, 64, 68, 73, 76, 87, 96, 108–110, 115, 119, 122, 127, 131] In a few cases, a serum immunoelectrophoresis showed an immunoglobulin spike.[5, 64, 73, 76, 108, 119] In five of these (four gamma, one alpha[119]),[64, 76, 96, 108, 119] the tumor was associated with production of heavy chain disease. Resection of the tumor in two of these cases resulted in disappearance of the abnormal serum paraprotein.[76, 96] Aozasa et al. considered the possibility that some of their cases represented benign inflammatory lesions—so-called plasma cell granulomas.[5] However, immunophenotyping disclosed the monoclonal nature of these proliferations, and thus these tumors were classified as neoplasms.

In the cases in which adequate peritumoral thyroid was available for histologic examination, chronic thyroiditis was found in the majority.[73]

Microscopically, the lesion consists of sheets of mature plasma cells replacing thyroid. Capsular extension and/or penetration can be seen.[5, 73, 76] In at least three cases, areas of the tumor showed histologic evidence of large cell lymphoma.[3, 5, 18] One of these was reported as a composite lymphoma and plasmacytoma by Aozasa et al.[3]

It is likely that thyroidal plasmacytoma represents a mature B-cell neoplasm similar to low grade lymphoma arising in the thyroid.

The question of whether extramedullary thyroid plasmacytoma indicates the initial manifestation of systemic myeloma is not easily answered from the literature, but at least in one of the cases reported by More et al.,[87] the thyroid lesion preceded the diagnosis of myeloma. Bone marrow examination performed at the time of diagnosis of the thyroid tumor has been reported in about 30 percent of cases and has been within normal limits.[5, 73] Therapy has consisted of various combinations of surgery, radiation, and chemotherapy.[5, 73] Most reported cases have relatively short periods of follow-up (15 months to 10 years).[5, 73] However, in several cases, local intrathyroidal or cervical recurrences were documented[43, 87]; in one case, lung recurrence was noted two years following thyroid lobectomy.[28] (See Table 14–5.)

Plasma Cell Granuloma. Three reports of polyclonal plasma cell proliferations affecting the thyroid are published.[25, 46, 130] All patients were women and two had hypothyroidism. In each instance, a mass composed of mature plasma cells was described; polyclonality was established by immunostaining in each case. Follow-up showed a normal bone marrow in Holck's patient, but further follow-up was absent.[46] In the case of Chan et al. no serum abnormalities were apparent but follow-up was only two months.[25] In the case reported by Yapp et al.,[130] the patient had a bone marrow plasmacytosis of 15 percent and a small diclonal serum gammopathy; however, the patient was otherwise well 10 years after thyroidectomy. Each of these cases is considered an example of plasma cell granuloma of the thyroid.

Other. A unique case of plasmacytoma involving the thyroid cartilage in a patient with myeloma has been described by Sporn and O'Donnell.[113]

OTHER LYMPHOID LESIONS

Mycosis Fungoides. In autopsies of 45 patients with mycosis fungoides (cutaneous T cell lymphoma), Rappaport and Thomas identified extracutaneous involvement in 71 percent.[99] Of the latter, 13 of 31 individuals demonstrated thyroid infiltration by the tumor. Grossly tumoral nodules or diffuse infiltration was found. Histologically, atypical mononuclear cells, often showing nuclear irregularity and infoldings, are seen. Differing from secondary involvement of the thyroid by more usual types of malignant lymphoma, mycosis often grows around preexisting normal structures and produces little destruction.

Chronic Lymphocytic Leukemia (CLL). In cases of CLL in which tissue involvement is found, thyroidal infiltration may be seen. In late stages, distinction from secondary involvement of the thyroid by systemic lymphoma is not possible.

Table 14–5. Plasmacytoma of the Thyroid

Total reported	30 cases
Age range	37–77 years
Sex ratio M/F	3:2
Extrathyroidal extension	occasionally
Surrounding thyroiditis	if studied, ~80 percent
Paraproteinemia	7 cases
Systemic plasma cell neoplasms	~20 percent
Follow-up	1 month–10 years
Survival rate	85 percent

Special Types of Lymphoma

Intermediate Lymphocytic Lymphoma. Aozasa et al. described four patients (three women, one man) who developed rapidly growing thyroid masses.[6] The three females had had documented autoimmune thyroiditis from two to 20 years. The authors discuss the difficulty in histologic diagnosis of these lymphomas since they are composed of small cells surrounding nonneoplastic follicles in the thyroiditic gland. (These authors and others stress the difficulty in diagnosing such lesions in lymph nodes also.[6, 123, 124]) By immunostaining, clonality was established in these cases, however. Aozasa et al. suggest that, prior to routine immunostaining of lymphoid lesions of the thyroid, cases such as they report may have been considered reactive hyperplasia.[6] In Japan, at least, these lymphomas constitute about 20 percent of thyroid lymphomas.[6]

Signet Ring Cell Lymphoma. Allevato et al. reported one unusual and so far unique case of a signet ring cell lymphoma arising in the thyroid of a 53-year-old woman with Hashimoto's disease.[1] (This case was also one of the series initially reported by Hamburger et al.[41]) The authors stressed the unusual features of this B-cell neoplasm in which cytoplasmic PAS-positive material (really immunoglobulin) gives the appearance of signet ring cells. Such a lesion may be mistaken for metastatic carcinoma if appropriate stains for mucin and lymphocyte lineage are not evaluated.

Hodgkin's Disease. Although rarely reported as primary in the thyroid, Hodgkin's disease can involve the gland.[33, 89] Naylor indicated a 7 percent incidence of secondary thyroidal involvement in patients with Hodgkin's disease.[89] Oertel and Heffess noted that they have examined cases of Hodgkin's disease apparently presenting initially as thyroid tumors; however, they point out that in each case, at least one cervical lymph node was also affected.[93] The literature also indicates that cases of Hodgkin's disease presenting initially in the thyroid always have cervical lymph node involvement[33]; this differs from non-Hodgkin's lymphoma, which can, of course, be confined to the gland.

In the present author's experience, one case of Hodgkin's disease, nodular sclerosis type, was seen in the thyroid. The patient had had a history of cervical and mediastinal node-based Hodgkin's disease for over 10 years; the thyroid mass proved to be the initial site of recurrent disease.

HEMATOPOIETIC LESIONS OF THE THYROID

Chloroma. Granulocytic sarcoma, or chloroma, is a mass lesion composed of immature granulocytes. Most of these lesions occur in patients with known acute myelogenous leukemia or a known myeloproliferative disorder.[90] Occasionally, granulocytic sarcoma will arise in patients with no known hematologic disorder, and in these the tumor may represent the first manifestation of acute leukemia. In the series of 61 patients reported by Neiman et al., 25 percent had no known preexisting blood or marrow disease.[90] The tumors usually occur in bone, soft tissue, skin and nodes but any organ may be affected. The present author has seen a granulocytic sarcoma occurring in the thyroid in a patient previously treated for endometrial carcinoma with radiation and chemotherapy.

The histologic diagnosis of granulocytic sarcoma may be difficult, especially in patients without a preexisting marrow disease. It can be confused microscopically with lymphoma or undifferentiated carcinoma; the histopathologist must keep this diagnosis in mind; appropriate stains, including chloroacetate esterase for myeloid granules or immunoperoxidase staining for lysozyme, can clinch the diagnosis.[90]

Nonlymphoid Leukemia. Just as chronic lymphocytic leukemia can infiltrate organs (including thyroid) in its tissue invasive phase, various types of acute and chronic leukemias of granulocytic lineage can involve the gland, especially in terminal phases. This type of involvement is usually found only at autopsy.[89]

HISTIOCYTOSIS

Histiocytosis X. A few cases of histiocytosis X involving the thyroid have been recorded.[27, 116] Teja et al. reported hypothyroidism in a 27-month-old male infant with suspected histiocytosis.[116] Biopsy showed the characteristic histiocytes involving the interstitium and follicles with follicular destruction. Therapy directed at the histiocytosis and thyroxine supplements relieved the symptoms. The patient reported by Coode and Shaikh was a 27-year-old woman in whom the histiocytosis involved the thyroid clinically and pathologically mimicked carcinoma.[27] The recognition of characteristic histiocytes and ultrastructural confirmation corrected the diagnosis.

Sinus Histiocytosis with Massive Lymphadenopathy. An apparently unique case of subclinical hypothyroidism and painful goiter in a 26-year-old woman was reported by Larkin et al.[66] Clinically, the thyroid disease was considered subacute thyroiditis, but biopsies of lymph nodes and thyroid showed a histiocytic infiltrate with lymphophagocytosis. The disease in this patient apparently remitted without specific therapy.

SUMMARY

This chapter has reviewed lymphoid and hematopoietic tumors affecting the thyroid: clinical and pathologic features were discussed. The importance of recognizing these lesions and distinguishing them from epithelial tumors (undifferentiated carcinomas) is stressed.

REFERENCES

1. Allevato, P. A., Kini, S. R., et al.: Signet ring cell lymphoma of the thyroid: a case report. Hum. Pathol. _16_:1066–1068, 1985.
2. Anscombe, A. M., and Wright, D. H.: Primary malignant lymphoma of the thyroid—a tumour of mucosa-associated lymphoid tissue: Review of seventy-six cases. Histopathology _9_:81–97, 1985.
3. Aozasa, K., Inoue, A., et al.: Plasmacytoma and follicular lymphoma in a case of Hashimoto's thyroiditis. Histopathology _10_:735–740, 1986.

4. Aozasa, K., Inoue, A., et al.: Malignant lymphomas of the thyroid gland. Analysis of 79 patients with emphasis on histologic prognostic factors. Cancer *58*:100–104, 1986.

5. Aozasa K., Inoue, A., et al.: Plasmacytoma of the thyroid gland. Cancer *58*:105–110, 1986.

6. Aozasa, K., Inoue, A., et al.: Intermediate lymphocytic lymphoma of the thyroid. An immunologic and immunohistologic study. Cancer *57*:1762–1767, 1986.

7. Aozasa, K., Ueda, T., et al.: Immunologic and immunohistologic analysis of 27 cases with thyroid lymphomas. Cancer *60*:969–973, 1987.

8. Barton, F. E., and Farmer, D. A.: Plasmacytoma of the thyroid gland. Ann. Surg. *132*:304–309, 1949.

9. Ben-Ezra, J., Wu, A., and Sheibani, K.: Hashimoto's thyroiditis lacks detectable clonal immunoglobulin and T cell receptor gene rearrangements. Hum. Pathol. *19*:1444–1448, 1988.

10. Bevilacqua, G.: Il plasmacytoma primitivo delle tiroide. Arch. de Vecchi Anat. Pathol. Med. Clin. *41*:385–392, 1981.

11. Billie, J. D., Wetzel, W. J., and Suen, J. Y.: Thyroid lymphoma with adjacent nerve paralysis. Arch. Otolaryngol. *108*:517–519, 1982.

12. Bisbee, A. C., and Thoeny, R. H.: Malignant lymphoma of the thyroid following irradiation. Cancer *35*:1296–1299, 1975.

13. Brewer, D. B., and Orr, J. W.: Struma reticulosa: a reconsideration of the undifferentiated tumours of the thyroid. J. Pathol. Bacteriol. *65*:193–208, 1953.

14. Burek, C. L., and Rose, N. R.: Cell mediated immunity in autoimmune thyroid disease. Hum. Pathol. *17*:246–253, 1986.

15. Burke, J. S.: Histologic criteria for distinguishing between benign and malignant extranodal lymphoid infiltrates. Semin. Diagn. Pathol. *2*:152–162, 1985.

16. Burke, J. S., Butler, J. J., and Fuller, L. M.: Malignant lymphomas of the thyroid. Cancer *39*:1587–1602, 1977.

17. Burt, A. D., Kerr, D. J., et al.: Lymphoid and epithelial markers in small cell anaplastic thyroid tumors. J. Clin. Pathol. *38*:893–896, 1985.

18. Buss, D. H., Marshall, R. B., et al.: Malignant lymphoma of the thyroid gland with plasma cell differentiation (plasmacytoma). Cancer *46*:2671–2675, 1980.

19. Cameron, R. G., Seemayer, T. A., et al.: Small cell malignant tumors of the thyroid: a light and electron microscopic study. Hum. Pathol. *6*:731–740, 1975.

20. Carcangiu, M. L., Steeper, T., et al.: Anaplastic thyroid carcinoma. A study of 70 cases. Am. J. Clin. Pathol. *83*:135–158, 1985.

21. Cascinelli, N., and Veronesi, U.: Plasmacitoma solitario della tirode. Tumori *52*.151–154, 1966.

22. Case Records of Massachusetts General Hospital: Case 15–1987. N. Engl. J. Med. *316*:931–938, 1987.

23. Catz, B., Perzik, S. L., et al.: Association of lymphocytic thyroiditis with other lesions of the thyroid. Surg. Gynecol. Obstet. *136*:47–48, 1973.

24. Chak, L. Y., Hoppe, R. T., et al.: Non-Hodgkin's lymphoma presenting as thyroid enlargement. Cancer *48*:2712–2716, 1981.

25. Chan, K. W., Poon, G. P., and Choi, C. H.: Plasma cell granuloma of the thyroid. J. Clin. Pathol. *39*:1105–1107, 1986.

26. Compagno, J., and Oertel, J. E.: Malignant lymphoma and other lymphoproliferative disorders of the thyroid gland: A clinicopathologic study of 245 cases. Am. J. Clin. Pathol. *74*:1–11, 1980.

27. Coode, P. E., and Shaikh, M. U.: Histiocytosis X of the thyroid masquerading as thyroid carcinoma. Hum. Pathol. *19*:239–241, 1988.

28. Corwin, J., and Lindberg, R. D.: Solitary plasmacytoma of bone vs. extramedullary plasmacytoma and their relationship to multiple myeloma. Cancer *43*:1007–1013, 1979.

29. Cox, M. T.: Malignant lymphoma of the thyroid. J. Clin. Pathol. *17*:591–601, 1964.

30. Crile, G.: Struma lymphomatosa and carcinoma of the thyroid. Surg. Gynecol. Obstet. *147*:350–352, 1978.

31. Crile, G., and Hazard, J. B.: Incidence of cancer in struma lymphomatosa. Surg. Gynecol. Obstet. *115*:101–103, 1962.

32. Devine, R. M., Edis, A. J., and Banks, P. M.: Primary lymphoma of the thyroid. A review of the Mayo Clinic experience through 1978. World J. Surg. *5*:33–38, 1981.

33. Feigin, G. A., Buss, D. H., et al.: Hodgkin's disease manifested as a thyroid nodule. Hum. Pathol. *13*:774–776, 1982.

34. Freeman, C., Berg, J. W., and Cutler, S. J.: Occurrence and prognosis of extranodal lymphomas. Cancer *29*:252–260, 1972.

35. Fujimoto, Y., Suzuki, H., et al.: Autoantibodies in malignant lymphoma of the thyroid gland. N. Engl. J. Med. *276*:380–383, 1967.

36. Gavin, L. A.: The diagnostic dilemmas of hyperthyroxinemia and hypothyroxinemia. Adv. Intern. Med. *33*:185–204, 1988.

37. Goudie R. B., and Angouridakis, C. E.: Autoimmune thyroiditis associated with malignant lymphoma of thyroid. J. Clin. Pathol. *23*:377, 1970 (abstract).

38. Grimley, R. P., and Oates, G. D.: The natural history of malignant thyroid lymphomas. Br. J. Surg. *67*:475–477, 1980.

39. Guerrier, Y., Mirouze, J., et al.: Goitre kalherian solitaire. Ann. Endocrinol. (Paris) *24*:637–641, 1963.

40. Habeshaw, J. A.: The immune system and lymphoma. La Ricerca Clin. Lab. *17*:87–109, 1987.
41. Hamburger, J. I., Miller, J. M., and Kini, S. R.: Lymphoma of the thyroid. Ann. Intern. Med. *99*:685–693, 1983.
42. Harris, N. J., and Bhan, A. K.: B-cell neoplasms of the lymphocytic, lymphoplasmacytoid and plasma cell types: Immunohistologic analysis and clinical correlation. Hum. Pathol. *16*:829–837, 1985.
43. Hazard, J. B., and Schildecker, W. W.: Plasmacytoma of the thyroid. Am. J. Clin. Pathol. *25*:819–820, 1949.
44. Hermann, R., Vannineuse, A., and DeSloover, C.: Malignant lymphomas and undifferentiated small cell carcinoma of the thyroid: a clinicopathologic review in light of the Kiel classification of malignant lymphomas. Histopathology *2*:201–213, 1978.
45. Hernandez, J. A., and Sheehan, W. W.: Lymphomas of the mucosa-associated lymphoid tissue. Signet ring cell lymphomas presenting in mucosal lymphoid organs. Cancer *55*:592–597, 1985.
46. Holck, S.: Plasma cell granuloma of the thyroid. Cancer *48*:830–832, 1981.
47. Holmes, H., Kreutner, A., and O'Brien, P. H.: Hashimoto's thyroiditis and its relationship to other thyroid diseases. Surg. Gynecol. Obstet. *144*:887–890, 977.
48. Hyjek, E., and Isaacson, P. G.: Primary B cell lymphoma of the thyroid and its relationship to Hashimoto's thyroiditis. Hum. Pathol. *19*:1315–1326, 1988.
49. Isaacson, P., and Wright, D. H.: Malignant lymphoma of mucosa-associated lymphoma tissue. A distinctive type of B-cell lymphoma. Cancer *52*:1410–1416, 1983.
50. Isaacson, P., and Wright, D. H.: Extranodal malignant lymphoma arising from mucosa-associated lymphoid tissue. Cancer *53*:2515–2524, 1984.
51. Jennings, A. S., and Saberi, M.: Thyroid lymphoma in a patient with hyperthyroidism. Am. J. Med. *76*:551–552, 1984.
52. Kapadia, S. B.: Multiple myeloma: A clinicopathologic study of 62 consecutively autopsied cases. Medicine *59*:380–392, 1980.
53. Kapadia, S. B., Dekker, A., et al.: Malignant lymphoma of the thyroid gland: A clinicopathologic study. Head Neck Surg. *4*:270–280, 1982.
54. Kapadia, S. B., Desai, U., and Cheng, V. A.: Extramedullary plasmacytoma of the head and neck: a clinicopathologic study of 20 cases. Medicine *61*:317–329, 1982.
55. Kato, I., Tajima, K., et al.: Chronic thyroiditis as a risk factor for B-cell lymphoma in the thyroid gland. Jpn. J. Cancer Research (Gann) *76*:1085–1090, 1985.
56. Kawanishi, H., Ushio, H., et al.: Primary plasmacytoma of the thyroid. Geka-Chiryo *21*:1237–1241, 1979.
57. Kenyon, R., and Ackerman, L. V.: Malignant lymphoma of the thyroid apparently arising in struma lymphomatosa. Cancer *8*:964–969, 955.
58. Knowles, D. M.: The extranodal lymphoid infiltrate: a diagnostic dilemma. Semin. Diagn. Pathol. *2*:147–151, 1985.
59. Knowles, D. M., Halper, J. P., and Jakobiec, F. A.: The immunologic characterization of 40 extranodal lymphoid infiltrates: usefulness in distinguishing between benign pseudolymphoma and malignant lymphoma. Cancer *49*:2321–2335, 1982.
60. Knowles, D. M., II, and Jakobiec, F. A.: Cell marker analysis of extranodal lymphoid infiltrates: To what extent does the determination of mono- or polyclonality resolve the diagnostic dilemma of malignant lymphoma vs. pseudolymphoma in an extranodal site? Semin. Diagn. Pathol. *2*:163–168, 1985.
61. Korsmeyer, S. J.: B-lymphoid neoplasms: immunoglobulin genes as molecular determinants of clonality, lineage, differentiation and translocation. Adv. Intern. Med. *33*:1–16, 1988.
62. Koyama, H. Y., Takahashi, K., et al.: Plasmacytoma of the thyroid gland. Geka-chiryo *48*:119–121, 1983.
63. Kurtin, P. J., and Pinkus, G. S.: Leukocyte common antigen—a diagnostic discriminant between hematopoietic and nonhematopoietic neoplasms in paraffin sections using monoclonal antibodies: Correlation with immunologic studies and ultrastructural localization. Hum. Pathol. *16*:353–365, 1985.
64. Kyle, R. A., Griepp, R. P., and Banks, P.: The diverse picture of gamma heavy chain disease; report of seven cases and review of literature. Mayo Clin. Proc. *56*:439–451, 1981.
65. Langlands, A. O., and Maclean, N.: Lymphoma of the thyroid. An unusual clinical course in a patient possessing a 14/21 translocation. Cancer *38*:259–264, 1976.
66. Larkin, D. F. P., Dervan, P. A., et al.: Sinus histiocytosis with massive lymphadenopathy simulating subacute thyroiditis. Hum. Pathol. *17*:321–324, 1986.
67. Limanova, Z., Neuwirtova, R., and Smejkal, V.: Malignant lymphoma of the thyroid. Exp. Clin. Endocrinol. *90*:113–119, 1987.
68. Lopez, M., Lauro, L. D., et al.: Plasmacytoma of the thyroid gland. Clin. Oncol. *19*:61–66, 1983.
69. Lukes, R. J., and Collins, R. D.: Immunologic characterization of human malignant lymphomas. Cancer *34*:1488–1503, 1974.
70. Luna, M. A., Mackay, B., et al.: The quarterly case: Malignant small cell tumor of the thyroid. Ultrastruct. Pathol. *1*:265–270, 1980.
71. Macauley, R. A. A., Dewar, A. E., et al.: Cell receptor studies on six anaplastic tumours of the thyroid. J. Clin. Pathol. *31*:461–468, 1978.
72. Maceri, D. R., Sullivan, M. J., and McClatchney, K. D.: Autoimmune thyroiditis: pathophysiology and relationship to thyroid cancer. Laryngoscope *96*:82–86, 1986.

73. Macpherson, T. A., Dekker, A., and Kapadia, S. B.: Thyroid gland plasma cell neoplasms (plasmacytoma). Arch. Pathol. Lab. Med. *105*:570–572, 1981.

74. Mambo, N. C., and Irwin, S. M.: Anaplastic small cell neoplasms of the thyroid: An immunoperoxidase study. Hum. Pathol. *15*:55–60, 1984.

75. Marder, R. J., Variakojis, D., et al.: Immunohistochemical analysis of human lymphomas with monoclonal antibodies and Ia antigens reactive in paraffin sections. Lab. Invest. *52*:497–504, 1985.

76. Matsubayashi, S., Tamai, H., et al.: Extramedullary plasmacytoma of the thyroid gland producing gamma heavy chain. Endocrinol. Jpn. *32*:427–433, 1985.

77. Matsubayashi, S., Tamai, H., et al.: Thyroid prelymphoma. J. Endocrinol. Invest. *11*:211–214, 1988.

78. Maurer, R., Taylor, C. R., and Terry, R.: Non-Hodgkin lymphomas of the thyroid. A clinicopathological review of 29 cases applying the Lukes-Collins classification and an immunoperoxidase method. Virch. Arch. Path. [A] *383*:293–317, 1979.

79. McDermott, M. R., and Bienenstock, J.: Evidence for a common mucosal immunologic system. J. Immunol. *122*:1892–1898, 1979.

80. Meissner, W. A.: Surgical Pathology. In: Sedgwick, C. E. (ed.): Surgery of the Thyroid Gland. Philadelphia, W. B. Saunders Company, 1974, pp. 24–40.

81. Meissner, W. A., and Phillips, M. J.: Diffuse small cell carcinoma of the thyroid. Arch. Pathol. *74*:291–297, 1962.

82. Meissner, W. A., and Warren, S.: Tumors of the Thyroid Gland. Fasc. 4, second series. Washington, D.C., Armed Forces Institute of Pathology, 1969.

83. Metcalfe, W. J., and Sclare, G.: Primary lymphosarcoma of the thyroid. Br. J. Surg. *48*:541–549, 1961.

84. Mitchell, J. D., Kirkham, N., and Mackin, D.: Focal lymphocytic thyroiditis in Southampton. J. Pathol. *144*:269–273, 1984.

85. Mithilesh, C., Saxena, H. M. K., et al.: Primary B cell lymphoma of thyroid gland with coexisting Hashimoto's disease. Indian J. Pathol. Microbiol. *27*:263–267, 1984.

86. Mizukami, Y., Matsubara, F., et al.: Primary T-cell lymphoma of the thyroid. Acta Pathol. Jpn. *37*:1987–1995, 1987.

87. More, J. R. S., Dawson, D. W., et al.: Plasmacytoma of the thyroid. J. Clin. Pathol. *21*:661–667, 1968.

88. Myskow, M. W., Krajewski, A. S., et al.: The role of immunoperoxidase techniques on paraffin embedded tissue in determining the histogenesis of undifferentiated thyroid neoplasms. Clin. Endocrinol. *24*:335–341, 1986.

89. Naylor, B.: Secondary lymphoblastomous involvement of the thyroid gland. Arch. Pathol. *67*:432–438, 1959.

90. Neiman, R. S., Barcos, M., et al.: Granulocytic sarcoma: a clinicopathologic study of 61 biopsied cases. Cancer *48*:1426–1437, 1981.

91. Newland, J. R., Mackay, B., et al.: Anaplastic thyroid carcinoma: An ultrastructural study of 10 cases. Ultrastruct. Pathol. *2*:121–129, 1981.

92. Noguchi, M., Mori, N., et al.: A case report of malignant lymphoma with Hashimoto's thyroiditis. Am. J. Clin. Pathol. *83*:650–655, 1985.

93. Oertel, J. E., and Heffess, C. S.: Lymphoma of the thyroid and related disorders. Semin. Oncol. *14*:333–342, 1987.

94. Oertel, J. E., and LiVolsi, V. A.: Pathology of the Thyroid. In: Ingbar, S., and Braverman, L. E. (eds.): Werner's The Thyroid, 5th ed. Philadelphia, J. B. Lippincott Co., 1986, pp. 651–686.

95. Okon, E., Felder, B., et al.: Monoclonal antibodies reactive with B-lymphocytes and histiocytes in paraffin sections. Cancer *56*:95–104, 1985.

96. Otto, S., Peter, I., et al.: Gamma chain heavy chain disease with primary thyroid plasmacytoma. Arch. Pathol. Lab. Med. *110*:893–896, 1986.

97. Pollock, W. F., and Sprong, D. H.: The rationale for thyroidectomy for Hashimoto's thyroiditis. West. J. Surg. Obstet. Gynecol. *66*:17–20, 1958.

98. Ralfkaier, N., Gatter, K. C., et al.: The value of immunocytochemical methods in the differential diagnosis of anaplastic thyroid tumors. Br. J. Cancer *52*:167–170, 1985.

99. Rappaport, H., and Thomas, L. B.: Mycosis fungoides: The pathology of extracutaneous involvement. Cancer *34*:1198–1229, 1974.

100. Rasbach, D. A., Mondschein, M. S., et al.: Malignant lymphoma of the thyroid gland: a clinical and pathologic study of twenty cases. Surgery *98*:1166–1170, 1985.

101. Rayfield, E. J., Nishiyama, R. H., and Sisson, J. C.: Small cell tumors of the thyroid: a clinicopathologic study. Cancer *28*:1023–1030, 1971.

102. Rigaud, C., Bogomoletz, W. V., and Delisle, M. J.: Lymphomes malin (primitifs et secondaires) de la thyroide. Bull. Cancer (Paris) *72*:210–219, 1985.

103. Saltzstein, S. L.: Extranodal malignant lymphomas and pseudolymphomas. Pathol. Annu. *4*:159–184, 1969.

104. Saul, S. H., and Kapadia, S. B.: Primary lymphoma of Waldeyer's ring: clinicopathologic study of 68 cases. Cancer *56*:157–166, 1985.

105. Saul, S. H., and Kapadia, S. B.: Secondary lymphoma of Waldeyer's ring. Am. J. Otolaryngol. *7*:34–41, 1986.

106. Schmid, K. W., Kroll, M., et al.: Small cell carcinoma of the thyroid: a reclassification of cases originally diagnosed as small cell carcinoma of the thyroid. Pathol. Res. Pract. *181*:540–543, 1986.
107. Schwarze, E. W., and Papadimitriou, C. S.: Non-Hodgkin's lymphoma of the thyroid. Pathol. Res. Pract. *167*:346–362, 1980.
108. Seligman, M., Mihaesco, E., et al.: Heavy chain disease: current findings and concepts. Immunol. Rev. *48*:145–167, 1979.
109. Shaw, R. C., and Smith, F. B.: Plasmacytoma of the thyroid gland. Arch. Surg. *40*:646–657, 1940.
110. Shimaoka, K., Gailani, S., and Tsukada, Y.: Plasma cell neoplasm involving the thyroid. Cancer *41*:1140–1146, 1978.
111. Sirota, D. K., and Segal, R. L.: Primary lymphomas of the thyroid gland. J.A.M.A. *242*:1743–1746, 1979.
112. Smithers, D. W.: Malignant lymphoma of the thyroid. *In:* Smithers, D. (ed.): Tumours of the Thyroid Gland. Edinburgh, E. and S. Livingstone, 1970, pp. 141–154.
113. Sporn, J. R., and O'Donnell, J. F.: Plasmacytoma of the thyroid: cartilage airway obstruction in a patient with myeloma. Am. J. Med. Sci. *293*:390–392, 1987.
114. Stone, C. W., Slease, R. B., et al.: Thyroid lymphoma with gastrointestinal involvement: report of three cases. Am. J. Hematol. *21*:357–365, 1986.
115. Takamatsu, O., Furukawa, N., et al.: Primary and solitary plasmacytoma of the thyroid. Geka-Chiryo *10*:1619–1622, 1968.
116. Teja, K., Sabio, H., et al.: Involvement of the thyroid gland in histiocytosis X. Hum. Pathol. *12*:1137–1139, 1981.
117. Tennvall, J., Cavallin-Stahl, E., and Akerman, M.: Primary localized non-Hodgkin's lymphoma of the thyroid: A retrospective clinicopathological review. Eur. J. Surg. Oncol. *13*:297–302, 1987.
118. Tobler, A., Maurer, R., and Hedinger, C. E.: Undifferentiated thyroid tumors of diffuse small cell type: Histological and immunohistochemical evidence for their lymphomatous nature. Virch. Arch. [Pathol. Anat.] *404*:117–126, 1984.
119. Tracy, R. P., Kyle, R. A., and Leitch, J. M.: Alpha heavy chain disease presenting as goiter. Am. J. Clin. Pathol. *82*:336–339, 1984.
120. Tupchong, L., Hughes, F., and Harmer, C. L.: Primary lymphoma of the thyroid: clinical features, prognostic factors, and results of treatment. Int. J. Radiat. Oncol. Biol. Phys. *12*:1813–1821, 1986.
121. Vigliotti, A., Kong, J. S., et al.: Thyroid lymphomas stages IE and IIE: comparative results for radiotherapy only, combination chemotherapy only, and multimodality therapy. Int. J. Radiat. Oncol. Biol. Phys. *12*:1807–1812, 1986.
122. Voegt, H.: Extramedulläre plasmacytome. Virchows Arch. Pathol. Anat. *302*:497–508, 1938.
123. Weisenberger, D. D., Linder, J., et al.: Intermediate lymphocytic lymphoma. Hum. Pathol. *18*:781–790, 1987.
124. Weisenberger, D. D., Nathwani, B. N., et al.: Malignant lymphoma, intermediate lymphocytic type: A clinicopathologic study of 42 cases. Cancer *48*:1415–1425, 1981.
125. Willems, J. S., and Lowhagen, T.: The role of fine needle aspiration cytology in the management of thyroid disease. Clin. Endocrinol. Metab. *10*:267–273, 1981.
126. Williams, E. D.: Malignant lymphoma of the thyroid. Clin. Endocrinol. Metab. *10*:379–389, 1981.
127. Wiltshaw, E.: The natural history of extramedullary plasmacytoma and its relation to solitary myeloma of bone and myelomatosis. Medicine *55*:217–238, 1976.
128. Woolner, L. B., McConahey, W. M., and Beahrs, O. H.: Struma lymphomatosa (Hashimoto's thyroiditis) and related thyroidal disorders. J. Clin. Endocrinol. Metab. *19*:53–83, 1959.
129. Woolner, L. B., McConahey, W. M., and Beahrs, O. H.: Primary malignant lymphoma of the thyroid. Review of forty-six cases. Am. J. Surg. *111*:502–523, 1966.
130. Yapp, R., Linder, J., et al.: Plasma cell granuloma of the thyroid. Hum. Pathol. *16*:848–850, 1985.
131. Yoshioka, M., Yumoto, T., et al.: A case report of primary plasmacytoma of the thyroid. Cancer Clin. *24*:831–835, 1978.
132. Zeki, K., Eto, S., et al.: Primary malignant lymphoma of the thyroid in a patient with long-standing Graves' disease. Endocrinol. Jpn. *32*:435–440, 1985.
133. Zirkin, T. A., Baybick, J. H., et al.: Flow cytometric analysis of DNA ploidy in lymphomas of the thyroid. Head Neck Surg. *10*:324–329, 1988.

15

UNUSUAL TUMORS AND TUMOR-LIKE CONDITIONS OF THE THYROID

In this chapter, unusual tumors of, or presenting in, the thyroid are described. These lesions, most of which represent neoplastic growths, may produce diagnostic difficulties since their appearance is different from the main categories of papillary, follicular, or medullary tumors usually encountered in the gland. Some of these lesions have already been discussed in the chapters on anaplastic tumors (Chapter 11), squamous lesions (Chapter 13), and lymphoid lesions (Chapter 14). In the following discussion, some of the points iterated in these chapters are reemphasized and embellished; in addition, other rare entities are covered. Table 15–1 lists the lesions discussed in this chapter.

CLEAR CELL TUMORS

Four diagnostic possibilities need to be considered when faced with a thyroid neoplasm composed wholly or in part of clear cells:[23, 34, 36, 46, 91, 103, 105, 160, 163, 167, 176, 184, 185, 190, 192]

1. A primary follicular-derived tumor (whether papillary, follicular, solid, or trabecular in pattern);
2. The rare clear cell medullary carcinoma;
3. Parathyroid tumors;
4. Metastatic renal cell cancer.

Primary Clear Cell Thyroid Tumors

Follicular cells in the thyroid may undergo a variety of metaplastic changes: squamous, oncocytic, and occasionally clear cell. The latter change can be identified in nonneoplastic conditions, especially congenital disorders of thyroid metabolism[13] and chronic lymphocytic thyroiditis. In this author's experience, clear cell change in cases of thyroiditis is often closely associated with oncocytic metaplasia. In thyroid nodules and neoplasms with clear cell cytology, an association with oncocytic change has also been described. The cases reported by Civantos et al.,[36]

Table 15–1. Unusual Lesions of the Thyroid

1. Clear cell tumor
   a. Primary lesions—follicular, papillary, medullary, anaplastic
   b. Metastatic clear cell tumors
   c. Parathyroid lesions
2. Signet ring cell tumors
3. Tumors with fat
4. Tumors with mucin; mucoepidermoid tumors
5. Metastatic tumors
6. Small cell tumors
7. Poorly differentiated carcinoma
8. Thymoma
9. "Paraganglioma"
10. Mixed follicular and parafollicular tumors
11. Teratomas, hamartomas; mixed tumors
12. Sarcomas; "carcinosarcomas"
13. Other mesenchymal lesions
14. Amyloid goiter
15. Atypical pseudoneoplastic lesions
16. Other

Dickersin et al.,[46] and Variokojis et al.,[192] as well as many of the lesions described by Carcangiu et al.,[23] fall into this group.

Although most primary clear cell tumors of the thyroid display a follicular, usually microfollicular or trabecular, histology (Figs. 15–1 and 15–2), sometimes a papillary carcinoma will demonstrate clear cell cytology wholly or in part.[46, 87, 91, 103] On occasion, zones of clear cell change can be found in anaplastic carcinomas; these lesions not infrequently will also show a squamous or squamoid pattern in surrounding zones.[23, 54] Fisher and Kim indicate that the ultrastructural finding of tonofibrils and keratohyaline granules in the clear cell thyroid tumor they studied suggested squamous differentiation.[54] These authors claim that such features are absent in clear cell tumors of renal and parathyroid origin.

Why are the cells in these lesions clear? Carcangiu et al.[23] and Schroder and Bocker[163] have suggested four reasons for this phenomenon: the formation of intracytoplasmic vesicles from mitochondria; glycogen accumulation; fat accumulation; and deposition of intracellular thyroglobulin.

In primary follicular-derived tumors, especially those with oncocytic or Hürthle cell cytology, the cytoplasmic clearing is predominantly due to vesicle formation from enlarged mitochondria.[23] In some of these, glycogen and thyroglobulin are also present. In nononcocytic tumors, especially those having a papillary pattern, glycogen accumulation in the cytoplasm can be responsible for the clear cell change. In clear cell thyroid tumors described by Valenta and Michel-Bechet[190] and Fisher and Kim,[54] the cytoplasm of the neoplastic cells was distended with glycogen.

Lipid has been identified either by special stains or by electron microscopic study in some clear cell thyroid tumors[23, 54, 163, 166]; Schroder and Bocker found three lipid-rich carcinomas in their series of primary thyroid clear cell tumors and likened them to lipid-rich breast carcinomas.[163]

The presence of intracellular thyroglobulin is responsible for cytoplasmic clearing in a few of these clear cell lesions; this finding is particularly prevalent in the so-called signet ring cell adenomas.[5, 15, 39, 62, 124, 154, 162] The finding of immunostainable thyroglobulin is an essential diagnostic clue for defining the tumor as one of thyroid origin.[23, 36] Carcangiu et al. indicate that although thyroglobulin localization in the tumor cells is critical in proving thyroid origin and distinction from metastatic renal carcinoma, the staining may be very focal, may be found

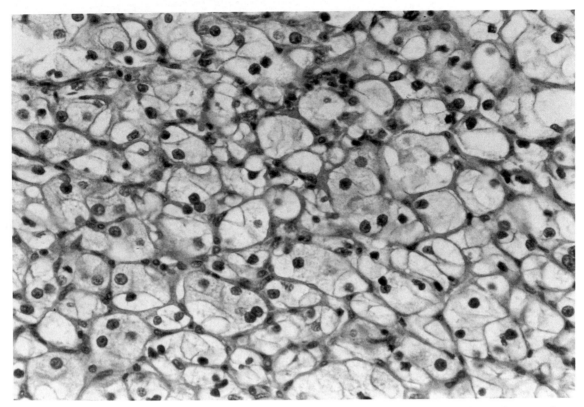

Figure 15–1. Clear cell follicular tumor of thyroid. Note lack of follicle formation and voluminous clear cytoplasm. × 150, H & E.

only in extracellular "colloid" or nonclear areas of the tumor, and extensive search may be needed to locate staining.[23] On the other hand, occasionally thyroglobulin positivity may be found in metastatic tumors, including renal lesions; the positive stain may result from trapping of preexisting normal follicles within the tumor or from "osmosis" wherein neoplastic cells adsorb hormone and give falsely positive results.[23, 114]

From the above, it must be concluded that clear cell neoplasms of thyroid follicular cell origin do exist and that these form part of a spectrum of tumors—some papillary, some follicular, and some anaplastic. Often oncocytic cells are found in close association with the clear cells. It appears unnecessary to designate a separate classification of "clear cell tumors," however.[23]

The question then arises: are all clear cell tumors of the thyroid malignant? If a primary thyroid neoplasm shows papillary differentiation but is partly or completely composed of clear cells, it is still a papillary cancer. If an anaplastic thyroid tumor contains clear cell areas, it is still carcinoma. However, those clear cell neoplasms that display a follicular, microfollicular, or trabecular pattern need to be separated into benign and malignant groups, based on the application of criteria for malignancy in usual follicular tumors, e.g., invasion. Based upon these considerations, then, it may be stated that some clear cell follicular tumors are benign, i.e., a clear cell follicular adenoma does exist.[23]

Although sufficient data are not yet available, it appears likely that follicular tumors of clear cell type exhibit a range of biologic behavior.[163] In a series of 17 cases, Carcangiu et al. found two with obvious invasion, seven that were encapsulated and considered benign, and eight that were indeterminate because of

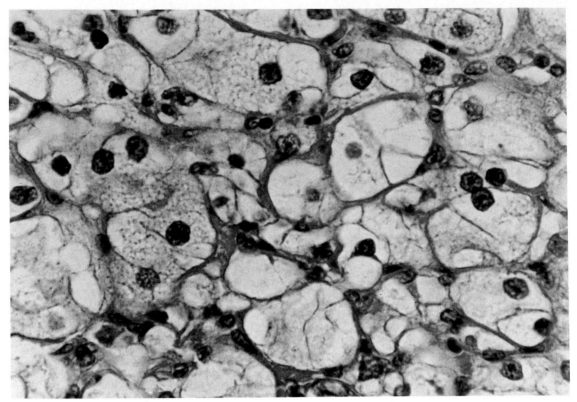

Figure 15–2. Higher power view of specimen shown in Figure 15–1. Thyroglobulin stain was positive. × 400, H & E.

irregular capsules or impingement into tumor capsule.[23] (It is noteworthy that oncocytic tumors with clear cell change more often demonstrate malignant characteristics, i.e., invasion, than do Hürthle cell tumors without clear cells.[23])

Some authors have speculated as to the reason for the clear cell change. Civantos et al.[36] and Kniseley and Andrews[103] indicate that thyrotropin (TSH) stimulation of a tumor may provoke clear cell change. Hence, hypertrophy and dilation of mitochondria or hypertrophy of Golgi apparatuses[46, 190] may be caused by TSH stimulation and lead to clear cytoplasm. Indeed, in the two patients described by Kniseley and Andrews an increased ability to concentrate radioiodine was associated with clear cell change.[103] In fact, in one of these cases, thyroid supplementation after total thyroidectomy was associated with reversion of the clear cell cytology in the tumor. It is possible that the TSH effect on certain thyroid tumors involves a change in thyroglobulin produced so that it is more preferentially stored intracytoplasmically or is ineffectively released.[23, 36]

Clear Cell Medullary Carcinoma

Landon and Ordonez described one case of a clear cell thyroid tumor that contained calcitonin.[105] This patient was a 43-year-old woman with no family history or personal stigmata of multiple endocrine neoplasia, who underwent resection of a 4.5 cm cold thyroid nodule. Histologically, the lesion was composed of nests of large polygonal cells with clear cytoplasm and distinct cell borders. Focally spindled cells were seen; neither papillary nor follicular structures were noted. Stromal amyloid was identified. Immunostaining for thyroglobulin and parathyroid hormone was negative, whereas calcitonin was localized in the lesion. Ultrastructural examination disclosed the presence of dense core granules. Follow-up in this patient showed the presence of bony and lung metastases occurring at six years after the initial diagnosis. The metastatic tumor in the bone showed an immunostaining pattern identical to the primary. These authors concluded that the immunostaining and electron microscopic findings in this case confirm this tumor as a medullary carcinoma and expand the variations of this group of lesions to include a clear cell variant.

Parathyroid Tumors

Embryologic considerations, discussed in detail in Chapter 1 of this monograph, explain the occasional occurrence of intrathyroidal parathyroid glands. Various authors estimate the occurrence of true intrathyroidal parathyroid tissue (as distinguished from parathyroid tissue abutting against the thyroid capsule) as 0.2 percent.[2, 27] On rare occasions such glands may be affected by hyperplasia or neoplasia; hyperparathyroidism may result.[2, 3, 27, 66, 176, 184] Sometimes these tumors are cystic and only small quantities of diagnostic material are present.[197] If the tumor is solid it may exhibit a clear cell cytology and be confused with a primary thyroid neoplasm. (The older literature contains reference to primary clear cell thyroid tumors; these lesions were termed "parastruma," indicating the belief that they were derived from misplaced parathyroid remnants.[23, 34])

In contrast to primary clear cell thyroid tumors, parathyroid tumors that occur in the thyroid contain a more delicate vascular pattern, and the nesting pattern is more pronounced. The individual cells are smaller and the trabeculae of a parathyroid tumor are generally thinner than those seen in primary or metastatic clear cell neoplasms in the thyroid. The presence of clinical hypercalcemia is helpful in diagnosis; stains for thyroglobulin or parathyroid hormone may be very useful in problematic cases.

Metastatic Clear Cell Carcinoma

Metastases to the thyroid gland are discussed in a more general fashion below. However, the differential diagnostic dilemma faced by the pathologist is most critical in the distinction between primary clear cell thyroid tumors and metastatic renal carcinoma. Many reports, some cited in the references in this chapter, have described and discussed this problem.[19, 31, 37, 42, 49–52, 58, 59, 61, 67, 81, 82, 107–109, 118, 119, 122, 132, 133, 142, 147, 152, 167, 169, 170, 172, 181–183, 185, 194, 200, 201]

A survey of the literature will show that the frequency of solitary renal cancer metastases to the thyroid seems disproportionate to the frequency of kidney carcinoma. Reasons for the affinity of this tumor to spread to the thyroid are unknown and may be spurious, reflecting the difficulties in distinguishing metastases from primary thyroid lesions, and hence spawning a flurry of interesting case reports.

From the clinical standpoint, renal tumor metastases to the thyroid are interesting.[19, 31, 42, 43, 49, 59, 61, 92, 107, 109, 118, 119, 122, 132, 142, 169, 185] Three important facts need to be stressed: first, the thyroid metastasis may be the initial manifestation of the kidney neoplasm; second, the thyroid metastasis may be solitary and represent the only spread of the disease; and third, in patients with a history of kidney cancer, the time interval between the initial renal neoplasm resection and the thyroid metastasis may be many years. There are several well-documented cases in the literature as well as anecdotal accounts among endocrinologists and surgeons of resection of a thyroid metastasis from a kidney cancer and subsequent long-term survival.[169] The present author is aware of a case of a woman who manifested a solitary thyroid metastasis from a clear cell renal carcinoma 16 years after resection of the primary; following thyroidectomy, she was well without evidence of tumor for seven years.

The histopathologic distinction between a clear cell thyroid tumor and a renal cancer metastasis in the thyroid may be quite difficult. Carcangiu et al. indicate that kidney cancers tend to show more hemorrhage and the "follicles" formed contain blood rather than colloid[23]; however, this is not always evident (Fig. 15–3). Special stains for glycogen may be misleading, since, although kidney tumors usually contain glycogen, some thyroid lesions may also.[23] Fat stains that require non-embedded tissue (which is often not available) may not be helpful. Several authors have indicated that, although renal tumors almost always contain lipid, some thyroid clear cell tumors do also.[23, 54] Stains for immunoreactive thyroglobulin, if positive, are very helpful; however, one must remember that the staining may be weak or equivocal in a primary thyroid tumor, and may be falsely positive because of diffusion in a metastatic lesion.[23, 114]

SIGNET RING CELL TUMORS OF THE THYROID

Another group of thyroid lesions that may cause diagnostic confusion are the rare cases described as signet ring cell adenomas. Such tumors are solitary

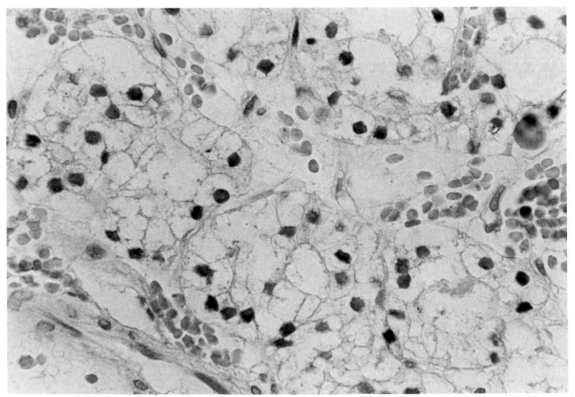

Figure 15–3. Renal cell carcinoma metastatic to thyroid. Note "follicles." × 150, H & E.

encapsulated nodules, which, histologically, are composed of nests and microfollicles made up of signet ring cells (Figs. 15–4 and 15–5). These cells resemble those of signet ring cancers in other sites and have an eccentric nucleus and a prominent cytoplasmic "inclusion." Ultrastructural studies of signet ring cell tumors have shown that the cytoplasm may contain intracytoplasmic lumina.

Special stains demonstrate the presence of both thyroglobulin and mucin in the cytoplasm. In the original case studied by Mendelsohn,[124] a dual differentiation of endocrine and "acinar" was suggested to explain the unusual staining reactions. However, Gherardi, in his detailed histochemical studies of two cases,[62] presented convincing evidence that altered or abnormal thyroglobulin could produce the unusual staining results. Gherardi reported that signet ring cell adenomas stain strongly for immunoreactive thyroglobulin, contain diastase resistant PAS positivity, and focal sialidase sensitive positivity, as seen with alcian blue stain at pH 2.5. Normal thyroglobulin is a glycoprotein containing sialic acid; as such, PAS positivity and evidence of acid mucins would be expected. However, when the thyroglobulin is bound in the colloid, the material responsible for positive mucin staining is unavailable. Sialidase digestion can "unmask" the sialic acid residues and mucin staining can be found in normal thyroid. Gherardi postulated that in the signet cell tumors, alterations in the thyroglobulin produced by these neoplastic follicular cells result in "unmasking" of the sialic acid residues, and hence mucicarminophilia.[62] At the same time, apparently the immunoreactive portion of the thyroglobulin molecule is unaffected.

Of the ten cases reported of signet ring cell adenoma,[5, 15, 23, 62, 124, 154, 162] all have behaved in a benign fashion (Table 15–2A). Schroder and Bocker did include in their series three carcinomas that showed signet ring features[162]; these tumors

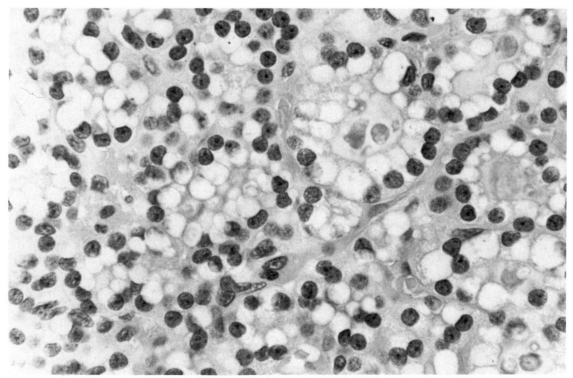

Figure 15–4. Signet ring cell adenoma of thyroid. Note follicles lined by cells mimicking signet cells. × 200, H & E.

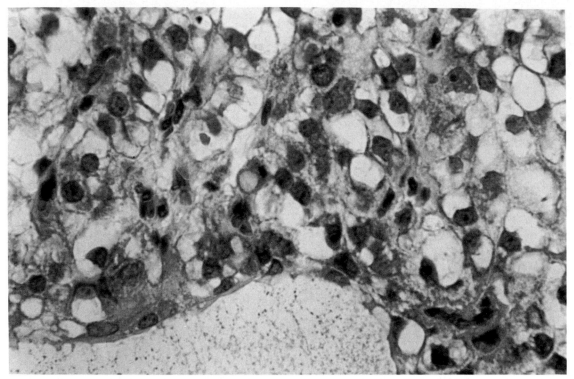

Figure 15–5. Another area of tumor shown in Figure 15–4. Note signet cell with intracellular mucin droplet to left of center. × 250, H & E.

were all follicular-derived. One of these was diagnosed as a minimally invasive follicular carcinoma, another as an oxyphilic cancer, and the third as focally a squamous carcinoma. The latter was associated with metastases and a fatal outcome (Table 15–2B).

In addition, Schroder and Bocker described one patient in whom signet ring cell adenomatous nodules were present in a hyperplastic goiter.[162] The present author has had the opportunity to study a case of multinodular goiter with many nodules composed of signet ring cells lining microfollicles. Table 15–2B lists the pertinent findings.

In summary, the results of all the reported cases of signet cell adenoma indicate that these lesions have an alarming cytologic appearance, but are histologically encapsulated and have a benign follow-up. The staining results include uniform immunoreactivity for thyroglobulin, confirming a follicular cell origin; when tested, stains for calcitonin, carcinoembryonic antigen, and keratin have been negative. Mucin has been identified in all cases; all have been PAS-positive and diastase-resistant; when tested the lesions have been weakly mucicarminophilic, and all but one have shown staining with alcian blue at pH 2.5. Histochemical assessment for mucin types has shown the presence of sialic acid and on occasion sulfomucins.[154] The latter finding, however, was questioned by Gherardi and needs further confirmation.

THYROID TUMORS WITH FAT

Fat in the thyroid can accumulate in follicular cells as a result of aging; in some series, oil red O stains for fat have been positive in 50 percent of normal thyroids.[93]

Table 15–2A. Signet Ring Thyroid Adenomas

Case	Age/Sex	Size	TG	Mucin	Follow-up
1 (Ref. 124)	39 F	1.8 cm	+	PAS + Mucicarmine + Colloidal iron +	Benign
2 (Ref. 154)	30 F	2 cm	+	PAS + Alcian blue pH 2.5 + Sulfomucin +	Benign
3 (Ref. 15)	33 F	4 cm	+	PAS + Alcian blue pH 2.5 + Mucicarmine + (weak)	Benign (incidental tiny papillary ca)
4 (Ref. 162)	29 F	3 cm	+	PAS +	Benign
5 (Ref. 162)	39 F	2.5 cm	+	PAS +	Benign
6 (Ref. 5)	61 M	4 cm	+	PAS + Colloidal iron + Alcian blue pH 2.5 −	Benign
7 (Ref. 62)	65 F	0.7 cm	+	PAS + Alcian blue pH 2.5 + Mucicarmine + Colloidal iron +	Benign
8 (Ref. 62)	53 M	0.4 cm	+	PAS + Alcian blue pH 2.5 + Mucicarmine + Colloidal iron +	Benign
9 (Ref. 23)	70 F	NA	+	NA	Benign
10 (Ref. 23)	50 F	NA	+	NA	Benign

M = male; F = female; TG = thyroglobulin.

The presence of adipose tissue in the thyroid gland is unusual, and in most cases it is found in a subcapsular location; most authors attribute this finding to inclusion of mesenchymal fat and sometimes muscle during embryologic development. Much rarer are tumors, or at least mass lesions, containing fat and thyroid tissue mixed together, sometimes surrounded by a fibrous capsule. Such lesions have been variously termed adenolipomas, thyrolipomas, or hamartomas.[11, 33, 44, 60, 84, 141, 164, 173, 186] Some authors consider them to represent developmental anomalies although the reported cases have been in adults. One very unusual case reported by Trites concerned a man who over many years had three distinctive fatty lesions develop—a pharyngeal lipoma, a thymolipoma, and a thyrolipoma.[186]

The origin of thyrolipoma is unclear; since there appears to be a proliferation of both fat and thyroid tissue, it may represent a hyperplasia of both the thyroid and mesenchymal tissue, or, conversely and less likely, the fat may represent a mesenchymal metaplasia. I believe the latter is unlikely since the cases reported indicate no associated fibrosis or inflammation, which is usual in fatty metaplasia in other organs, e.g., cystic fibrosis.

Some patients have been reported in whom amyloid goiter has been associated with fat.[60]

Table 15–2B. Signet Ring Thyroid Carcinomas

Case	Age/Sex	Size	TG	Mucin	Follow-up
1 (Ref. 162)	30 F	4.5 cm	+	PAS +	NED—3 yrs
2 (Ref. 162)	17 F	3.5 cm	+	PAS +	NED—2 yrs
3 (Ref. 162)	62 M	7 cm (areas squamous ca)	+	PAS −	DOD—1 yr

M = male; F = female; TG = thyroglobulin; NED = no evident of disease; DOD = died of disease.

A few cases of adipose tissue admixed with thyroid have been described in which the entire gland is affected; these lesions have been called hamartomatous adiposity,[44, 60] or adenolipomatosis.[33, 173] In virtually all reported cases, sufficient functioning thyroid tissue has been present so that hypothyroidism did not occur.

In most cases reported recently thyroglobulin immunostaining showed a positive reaction in the thyroid cells of the adenolipomas and in the lipid rich adenoma.[164, 166] This rules out the hypothesis that these tumors represent parathyroid lipoadenomas.

Whether thyroid adenolipomas represent adenomas with fatty infiltration as a result of obesity has been speculated upon; this does not appear to be the case.

An apparently unique case of lipid-rich thyroid adenoma was reported by Schroder et al.[166] This tumor was a 2 centimeter mass found at autopsy in a 64-year-old man who died of metastatic rectal carcinoma. The tumor was composed of follicles lined by cells containing large amounts of lipid. The authors compared this lesion to lipid-rich carcinomas of the breast and postulated that the tumor cells were overproducing lipid.

An extremely unusual tumor has been reported by Vestfrid[193]; this was a papillary thyroid carcinoma occurring in a 53-year-old woman. In many areas of the tumor the cores of the papillae were composed of mature adipose tissue.

The topic of fatty tissue in thyroid lesions has been reviewed by Gnepp et al;[63a] these authors identified fat in papillary cancers, follicular adenomas, and nodules, as well as thyroiditis, congenital goiter and atrophic thyroid. They confirmed the finding of fat in amyloid goiter also. Hence the spectrum of thyroid lesions containing adipose tissue is broader than previously thought; however, no cause for this finding is yet known.

TUMORS WITH MUCIN

The presence of mucin in thyroid tumors has been considered very rare. However, Mlynek et al. cite Mueller and Wegelin, who both reported the presence of mucinous substances in thyroid tumors, in 1871 and 1926 respectively.[131]

In addition to the signet ring cell adenomas described previously, carcinomas of the thyroid in which some or many of the neoplastic cells contained stainable mucin have been described. Some of these have been of follicular cell origin,[41, 45, 80, 130, 131] and some of presumed C cell derivation, i.e., medullary carcinomas.[65] The presence of mucin in medullary carcinomas was described by Zaatari et al.[203] and Fernandes et al.[53] In fact, about 8 percent of medullary carcinomas do contain intracellular mucin and 40 percent extracellular mucin.[53, 203]

The histogenesis of some mucin-containing tumors of the thyroid has been questionable. These tumors resemble mucoepidermoid carcinomas of salivary gland origin; some authors believe they arise from embryologic remnants of salivary gland tissue within the thyroid,[129, 151] but others consider them to originate from solid cell nests or ultimobranchial body remnants.[57, 73–77, 79, 195] Still others consider these unusual lesions to arise from follicular cells and believe that they represent variants of papillary carcinoma. Although some of these tumors have contained areas resembling the epidermoid components of salivary tumors, other cases have shown definite keratinizing squamous foci; these have been considered adenosquamous carcinomas.[80, 130] (These lesions have been discussed in detail in Chapter 13.)

A rare mucin-producing tumor of presumed thyroid origin was reported by Sobrinho-Simoes et al.[174]; this lesion contained mucin but neither thyroglobulin nor calcitonin. Its definite origin from thyroid was considered likely although the follow-up was short.

Mlynek et al. addressed the question of the frequency of finding mucin in primary thyroid neoplasms.[131] These authors studied 142 cases of thyroid cancer and identified mucin in 50 percent of papillary, 50 percent of medullary, 35 percent of follicular, and 21 percent of anaplastic tumors. The stains used were mucicarmine, alcian blue–PAS, and a modified Masson and alcian green stain, the Chesa stain. The results obtained using these various techniques were similar. The authors caution that mucin production by follicular and parafollicular derived tumors is more common than usually thought and that, in evaluation of metastatic carcinomas, the presence of mucin in the tumor cells cannot rule out a thyroid primary.[131] Similar results have been reported by Chan et al. for metastatic papillary cancer[29]; 17 percent of their cases contained stainable (mucicarmine; alcian blue) intracytoplasmic mucin.

METASTATIC TUMORS TO THE THYROID

Metastases to the thyroid may be found in two separate settings: at postmortem examination or in a surgical specimen.

At autopsy, about 1.9 to 26 percent of patients dying with disseminated malignancy will have metastases in the thyroid gland. The differences in incidence of metastases probably reflect two differences among reported series: the care with which the gland is examined at autopsy and whether the population studied is unselected autopsies of individuals or patients dying of malignancy.[122]

According to Gowing,[67] thyroid involvement by nonthyroid malignancies may arise in three ways:

1. Direct extension from tumors in adjacent structures;
2. Retrograde lymphatic spread; and
3. Hematogenous metastases.

Carcinomas of the larynx, pharynx, trachea, and esophagus may invade the thyroid directly.[67, 82, 90, 122, 194, 204] Harrison states that postcricoid and subglottic cancers most commonly extend into the thyroid via the thyroidal cartilages.[82] Most of the neoplasms involved in this group are squamous cell carcinomas, in which the primary site is known or is obvious. Often, multiple areas of the gland are involved; distinction from thyroid primary is usually not difficult.

Retrograde extension via lymphatic routes into the thyroid is unusual. In Gowing's experience, this type of spread is seen most frequently with breast carcinoma.[67] In theory, at least, any tumor involving cervical lymph nodes could extend into the thyroid by this mechanism.

Hematogenous metastases to the thyroid vary according to tumor type. In addition, differences can be noted between autopsy and surgical series that examine this issue.[49, 67, 92, 122, 133, 152, 170, 181, 182, 200] Differences exist between the types of tumors involved and the pattern of metastatic spread.

Virtually any malignant tumor may metastasize to the thyroid[165]; some of these may resemble primary lesions.[37] In autopsy series, the most commonly encountered primaries include breast, lung, kidney, and melanoma (Table 15–3A). The pattern

Table 15–3A. Metastatic Tumors to the Thyroid: Autopsy Data*

Primary Site	Percent
Breast	25.3
Lung	24.5
Melanoma	9.9
Kidney	9.5
GI tract	7.9

*Approximately 77 percent of metastases at autopsy are derived from common cancers, with breast and lung accounting for 50 percent of these tumors:[122] this differs considerably from results reported in surgical series.

of gland involvement is usually multiple nodules grossly noted; microscopically, many foci of tumor may be seen either in thyroid stroma or destroying parenchyma. Rarely, disturbances in thyroid function have been recorded.[170] Indeed, almost total destruction of the thyroid may occur without the development of clinical hypothyroidism.[170] Even more unusual is the association of hyperthyroidism with metastatic cancer to the thyroid.[52, 183] The mechanism for this phenomenon is purported to be similar to that for hyperthyroidism associated with anaplastic carcinoma (see Chapter 11), i.e., rapidly growing tumor destroying thyroid follicles.

From the viewpoint of the clinician and the surgical pathologist, the possibility that a solitary mass in the thyroid may represent a metastasis needs to be considered when the histology is unusual for a thyroid primary. Some patients may have a history of cancer elsewhere, but this is not always the case. The primary may have been diagnosed many years before, or it may have been forgotten by the patient, or the surgeon may fail to communicate the history to the pathologist.

In surgical series, carcinomas of the kidney and colon and melanoma are most commonly found[37, 49, 50, 58, 63, 81, 92, 122, 147, 181, 182, 201]; the incidence of these tumor types in thyroid metastases is disproportionate to the frequency of occurrence of these tumors. Grossly, such lesions are often solitary, circumscribed masses; they may appear quite compatible with a primary tumor. Histologically, the neoplasm may also be a single nodule. Resemblance to colonic adenocarcinoma, breast cancer, or pigmented melanoma reassures the pathologist that he or she is dealing with a metastasis. However, clear cell carcinoma of the kidney may present a problem; this has produced a flood of reports in the literature.[19, 31, 37, 42, 43, 49, 50, 58, 59, 61, 81, 87, 107–109, 118, 119, 132, 142, 165, 169, 185]

As discussed above, follicular derived clear cell primary thyroid tumors exist, and differentiating them from metastatic kidney cancer can be problematical (Fig. 15–3). Histochemical and electron microscopic studies may be helpful in distinguishing these lesions. The classic teaching has been that fat and large amounts of glycogen are found in renal tumors, but not in primary thyroid lesions[192]; however, both fat and glycogen can be found in primary thyroid tumors.[23, 162] Intracellular lipid, many mitochondria, and prominent microvilli are seen ultrastructurally in renal tumors,[192] but not in follicular thyroid lesions.[190] Staining for immunoreactive thyroglobulin may help, although this can be erroneous (see above).

Table 15–3B lists the types of carcinomas that present as surgical thyroid lesions and their relative frequencies.

The treatment of metastatic cancer to the thyroid is surgical removal of the

Table 15–3B. Metastatic Tumors to the Thyroid: Surgical Series

Primary Site	Percent
Kidney (usually clear cell)	20–70
Colon	12
Lung	12
Breast	12
Melanoma	4
Larynx, oropharynx, nasopharynx, esophagus (direct extension)*	~30
Other (cervix, bladder, meningioma, choriocarcinoma, etc.)	<2

*Many surgical series do not include tumors extending to the thyroid from nearby organs but rather stress hematogenous metastases.

lesion. Although most authors stress that the thyroid metastasis is often the manifestation of disseminated malignancy and the prognosis is poor, surgical removal may provide relief of symptoms of dysphagia or dyspnea. However, it must be remembered that, especially with renal cell carcinoma metastases, the thyroid mass may represent a solitary metastasis, and hence thyroidectomy or thyroid lobectomy may be associated with prolonged survival (?cure).[58, 122, 132]

SMALL CELL TUMORS

This confusing topic has been discussed in Chapter 11 on anaplastic tumors. However, it is worth reiterating here that true small cell carcinoma of the thyroid is a very rare lesion if it exists at all.[22, 117, 120, 123, 150, 158, 161] Small cell tumors of the thyroid may be conveniently divided into the groups shown in Table 15–4.

Small cell variants of medullary carcinoma resemble small cell neuroendocrine carcinomas of other organs, including lung and cervix. These tumors are discussed in more detail in Chapter 10. Most of these lesions contain demonstrable immunoreactive calcitonin, and no thyroglobulin.

The curious tumor termed "insular carcinoma" by Carcangiu et al.[24] consists of a small cell tumor of follicular histogenesis (thyroglobulin positive) which may contain small solid nests, microfollicles (Figs. 15–6 and 15–7), and occasionally papillae. Some examples contain zones with cells having ground glass nuclei. Necrosis is common and the viable tumors cells may be arranged around blood vessels in a peritheliomatous pattern.[24] This tumor may also contain zones of dense collagen reminiscent of amyloid. For this reason some of these tumors may have been diagnosed as medullary carcinomas; however, thyroglobulin is present and calcitonin is not.

These lesions probably all represent poorly differentiated papillary or mixed papillary follicular or pure follicular neoplasms. They should be recognized as such to differentiate them from medullary cancers on the one hand and anaplastic carcinoma on the other. The prognosis of these tumors is intermediate between well-differentiated follicular derived tumors (papillary and follicular) and anaplastic tumors; local recurrences and metastases are common (65 percent or greater). Both nodal and hematogenous metastases are seen. The insular lesions have a five-year survival rate of about 20 percent and as such can be considered intermediate grade cancers of the thyroid with a prognosis between the indolent usual "well-differentiated" papillary and follicular tumors and anaplastic cancer.[24, 56]

POORLY DIFFERENTIATED CARCINOMA

Sakamoto et al. described a group of thyroid tumors that they classified as poorly differentiated.[159] These lesions had areas of recognizable papillary or follicular cancer admixed with zones of solid or trabecular tumor, showing mitoses,

Table 15–4. Small Cell Thyroid Tumors

Epithelial pattern	Medullary carcinoma with little or no amyloid: "insular carcinoma"
Diffuse pattern	Malignant lymphoma
Other	Metastatic small cell carcinoma, especially lung primary

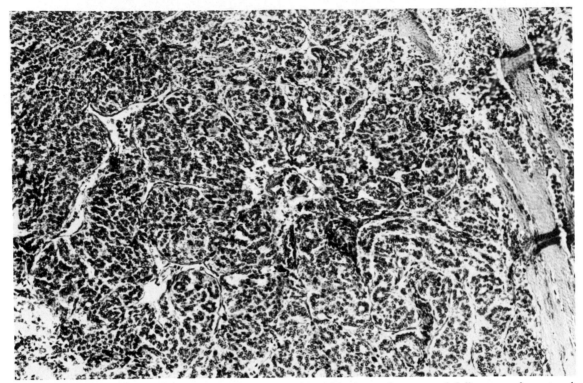

Figure 15–6. "Small cell carcinoma." Note microfollicle formation, nests of tumor, and delicate vascular network; this resembles the insular variant of thyroid carcinoma. × 100, H & E.

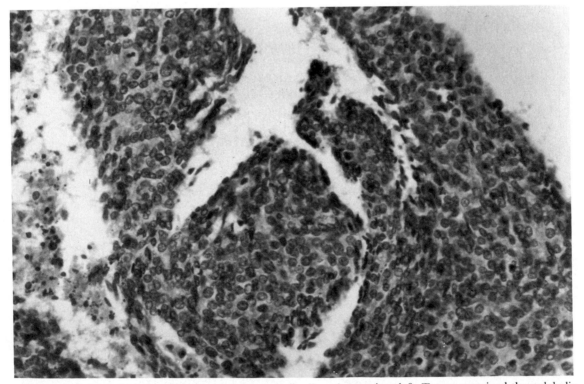

Figure 15–7. Higher power of Figure 15–6. Note small cells and necrosis at left. Tumor contained thyroglobulin but no calcitonin by immunostain. × 250, H & E.

necrosis or other features associated with more aggressive biologic behavior. Indeed, in this series the authors illustrate a survival rate halfway between well-differentiated thyroid tumors and anaplastic variants.[159] It is possible that included with these poorly differentiated thyroid neoplasms are examples of the insular carcinoma of Carcangiu et al.[24] Tscholl-Ducommun and Hedinger reported a series of papillary carcinomas with a less favorable prognosis than usual papillary cancer.[187] As discussed in Chapters 8 and 13, such tumors as the tall cell variant, the columnar cell variant, or the diffuse sclerosis variant of papillary carcinoma may behave in more malignant clinical fashion than expected in ordinary papillary carcinoma.

THYMOMA

Embryologic studies, as discussed in Chapter 1, offer an explanation for the finding of thymic rests or remnants in the neck above the level of the clavicles. According to Martin et al., the incidence of ectopic thymic tissue in the neck may be as high as 21 percent in fetuses and newborns.[121] On rare occasions, thymic tissue may be located intrathyroidally; Yamashita et al. found thymic tissue in 1.8 percent of thyroid glands from patients with Graves' disease.[202] More frequently, however, thymic rests are strewn very close to the thyroid gland capsule. Tumors may arise in these thymic rests; they can produce diagnostic problems for the clinician, radiologist, and pathologist if their location mimics an intrathyroidal mass.[10, 78, 128, 136]

The thymomas reported to arise in this location have been predominantly lymphoid types and have mimicked lymphoma. In some cases, the diagnosis of lymphoma or exuberant thyroiditis was suggested on fine needle aspiration biopsy. If the epithelial component is sparse or not recognized, the diagnosis of thymoma may not even be considered. In our own case, the epithelial cells were recognized only after immunostains for keratin were performed (Vengrove et al.: unpublished observations).

Martin et al. suggest that the incidence of cervical thymoma may be higher than the literature discloses since some of these tumors may have been histologically classified as lymphomas.[121] Conversely, these authors did not accept two cases recorded as cervical thymoma since in their opinion one of these represented an example of Castleman's giant lymph node hyperplasia,[153] and the other was a lesion that was not completely cervical in location and extended into the superior mediastinum.[14]

Several case reports of perithyroidal cervical thymomas have been published.[121] The present author has seen an additional case, bringing the number of acceptable cases to 13. The statistics on these cases are summarized in Table 15–5.

Table 15–5. Thyroidal or Perithyroidal Thymoma: 13 Cases*

Age	11 to 75
Sex ratio (F/M)	11/2
Cytologic diagnosis: lymphoma	2 cases
Histologic diagnosis:	
Benign thymoma	10
Malignant (invasive) thymoma	3
Follow-up	
Recurrence	1
Metastases	0

*See also References 10 and 128 for so-called "thymic carcinomas" of thyroid origin.

A few recent reports of predominantly epithelial tumors resembling poorly differentiated epidermoid carcinoma, but behaving clinically as indolent lesions, have appeared.[10, 128] These lesions stain for keratin but not thyroglobulin or calcitonin; it has been suggested that they represent thymomic carcinomas arising from intrathyroidal branchial remnants.[10]

The very unusual lesion described by Rosai et al. as "ectopic hamartomatous thymoma" occurs in the lower neck and supraclavicular area and should not be mistaken for a thyroid tumor.[155] These lesions, which show a mixture of spindle cells, epithelial islands and cysts, fat, and lymphocytes, were considered to represent hamartomatous proliferations involving branchial pouch remnants.

PARAGANGLIOMAS

Paragangliomas arise in areas where normal paraganglia are located. The occurrence of a normal paraganglion within the thyroid is not documented. Hence the diagnosis of paraganglioma of the thyroid must be questioned. Lesions of the thyroid that display the histologic appearance of paraganglioma have been described; their histologic pattern has been compared with some patterns seen in medullary carcinoma.[125] Such tumors have been variously termed "paraganglioma," "hyalinizing trabecular adenoma,"[25] and paraganglioma-like adenoma of the thyroid (PLAT).[16] These lesions have been studied both by electron microscopy (EM) and immunohistochemistry.[16, 25] EM shows dense core "neurosecretory" granules and numerous mitochondria. The cells of the tumors were in close proximity to capillaries. Amyloid was not seen; cells having the ultrastructural appearance of sustenacular cells were very rarely identified.[20, 69]

By immunostaining, these lesions were shown to contain thyroglobulin but not calcitonin. Neurofilament and S100 stains have been negative. In the past such lesions have been classified as atypical adenomas of the thyroid; this group of tumors has included follicular tumors with necrosis, mitoses, and pleomorphism but without invasion, medullary carcinomas that are encapsulated, and "paragangliomas." It is the author's current view that "paragangliomas" of the thyroid represent a peculiar variant of follicular lesion that is benign (Figs. 15–8 and 15–9). From our experience with such lesions and also that reported by Carney et al.,[25] we do not believe that they represent a peculiar papillary cancer, since the nuclear and cytologic features are different from ordinary papillary cancer and since none of the cases so far reported has behaved as malignant.

The case reported by Mitsudo et al. as malignant paraganglioma[127] may have represented a true paraganglioma, which arose outside the thyroid and invaded it. Similarly, the case of Kay et al.[96] was in the region of the thyroid, but not clearly of thyroid origin. For further discussion on atypical follicular adenoma and paraganglioma of the thyroid, see Chapter 9.

MIXED THYROID CARCINOMA: MEDULLARY-FOLLICULAR CARCINOMA

Over the past decade, a number of reports have appeared in the literature of thyroid tumors that show features of follicular and parafollicular differentiation. Initially, these papers described individual cases in which histologic or ultrastructural evidence of two types of differentiation was noted.[21, 72, 143, 191] However, more

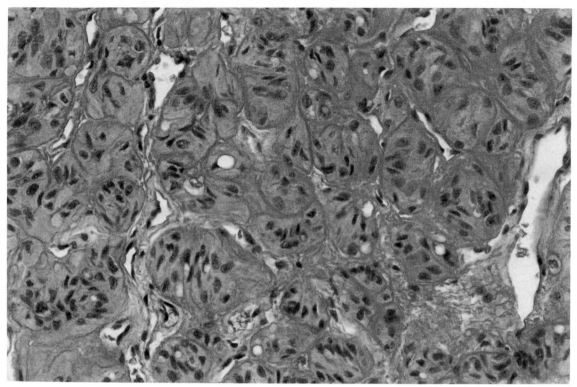

Figure 15–8. Paraganglioma-like thyroid adenoma. Note trabeculae of the lesion arranged amid delicate vascular framework. × 200, H & E.

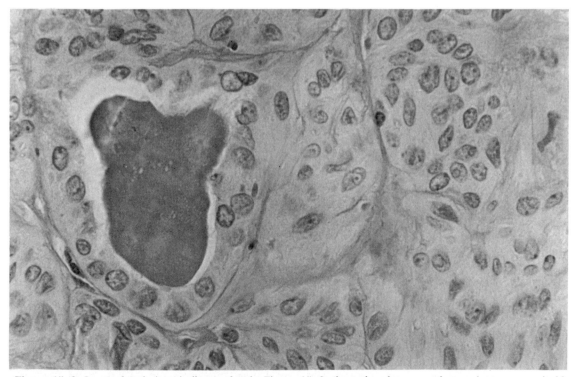

Figure 15–9. In another lesion similar to that in Figure 15–8, the trabecular areas abut against a recognizable follicle, found in the center of the lesion. × 300, H & E.

recently, series of such tumors have appeared in the literature. Electron microscopic and immunohistochemical evidence for the existence of such mixed tumors has been presented.[86, 143, 144] One may argue that the diagnosis of a mixed tumor in the thyroid cannot be proved because immunostaining results may be marred by diffusion of hormone into tumor cells, e.g., thyroglobulin, into the tumor cells of a medullary carcinoma. However, a few cases of dual hormone localization in distant metastases of a thyroid tumor belie this argument.[189]

The existence of dual hormone–producing thyroid tumors probably needs to be accepted. Questions still remaining to be answered include: how frequently do they occur; are there epidemiologic factors to explain their apparent geographic distribution; does the existence of such lesions necessitate a search for yet another cell in the thyroid that could serve a precursor; or are these tumors really follicular carcinomas that are producing calcitonin ectopically?[85, 86, 113, 115, 116, 137]

Examples of "mixed tumors" that the current author has personally studied have all been confined to the gland or to gland and regional nodes. In each instance, the dual staining could be explained by the diffusion effect; in the case with nodal metastases in which there was two-hormone staining in the primary tumor and the metastasis, it is possible to speculate that destruction of thyroid tissue by the growing tumor allowed for release of hormone and subsequent drainage and pickup in regional nodes. It is the belief of the present author that further studies of this subset of tumors, using molecular biologic techniques, are needed to fully prove the hypothesis that they exist.

TERATOMAS, HAMARTOMAS, PLEOMORPHIC ADENOMAS (MIXED TUMORS)

Some early reports indicated that a cervical teratoma may be classified as a thyroidal teratoma if the tumor receives its blood supply from the thyroid arteries. However, these midline lesions, the majority of which are found in the newborn period, all present in similar fashion and for practical purposes may be lumped as teratomas of the neck.[177] Many of these tumors do involve or replace portions of the thyroid.

Clinically, teratomas present in neonates or infants under the age of one year as huge midline neck masses. Often these tumors measure 10 centimeters or more.[71, 138, 148, 171, 177, 199] About 35 percent of these pregnancies are associated with polyhydramnios; this is especially noted in cases with tumors over 10 centimeters.[55, 71] A significant number of cases reported in series and reviews have been identified in stillborns.[12, 70, 71, 98] Many patients require emergency surgery because of respiratory compromise and stridor.[55, 71] Grossly, most of these tumors are predominantly or partially cystic. Histologically, the teratomas in newborns and young infants have contained elements of all three germ layers and have been benign; Hajdu et al. note that 70 percent have contained brain tissue.[71] In at least one case elevated serum alpha-fetoprotein has been documented.[148] Successful surgical removal has been associated with cure; in most cases sufficient thyroid tissue is present so that replacement medication is not needed.[55, 71, 171, 177] There does not appear to be an increased association of congenital abnormalities in these children.

Teratomas of the thyroid in adults differ from those in newborns, since they are more frequently malignant.[17, 18, 70, 99, 100, 101, 135, 140] These lesions develop in adult life in patients who had no congenital neck masses. (One patient apparently had a benign neck teratoma in infancy.[17]) Presumably, these tumors are derived from

Table 15–6. Adult Teratoma of the Neck (Thyroid)

Age	10 to 68
Sex (F/M)	10/4
Thyroidal	11
Malignant/Benign	12/1 /1?malignant
Survival	
Dead	8
Alive, free of tumor	4
Postmortem finding	1
Lost	1

midline misplaced germ cells, as are similar neoplasms arising in the thymus or pineal region. The histologic descriptions of these teratomatous lesions have varied and include some early literature reports of sarcomas arising in teratomas. It seems likely that these lesions conform to immature teratomas or malignant germ cell neoplasms arising in teratomas, as can occur in the gonads. In the review by Buckley et al. in 1986[17] a total of 14 adult cervical teratomas were accepted (one was reported twice). Table 15–6 lists the pertinent data about these lesions. Most were malignant lesions and were fatal.

A chondromatous hamartoma of the thyroid was reported in an 18-month-old boy by Chalal and Bhattacharjea[28]; it may have represented a benign teratoma since it was noted at birth. A pleomorphic adenoma resembling mixed tumor of the salivary gland has been reported to arise in the thyroid of a 65-year-old woman. Lange described this tumor as resembling benign mixed tumor of the salivary gland, considered it a unique example in the thyroid, and postulated its origin from developmental salivary gland rests.[106] The follow-up was benign.

SARCOMAS, CARCINOSARCOMAS

Sarcomas arising in the thyroid gland are extremely rare. Many examples of fibrosarcoma and spindle cell sarcoma of the thyroid were reported in the older literature before immunohistochemical or electron microscopic studies could be done on these tumors. It is likely that many of these lesions represented anaplastic carcinomas.[83, 102, 188] They share clinical features of anaplastic thyroid carcinoma in that they occur in elderly individuals, are rapidly growing, and are almost uniformly fatal.[35, 102, 114, 156] It must be remembered that, although current classifications include many spindle and giant cell tumors of the thyroid as carcinomas, immunostaining data sometimes do not support a specific origin for these neoplasms.[114] A recent report of leiomyosarcoma[95] appears valid, with electron microscopic evidence of mesenchymal origin.

Osteosarcoma and chondrosarcoma of the thyroid have been reported[4, 112, 139, 178, 179] (Fig. 15–10); some of these tumors, however, probably represent osseous and cartilaginous differentiation and/or metaplasia in anaplastic carcinomas; thus they are similar to lesions of this type that can occur in the female breast.[4] These neoplasms have been reported in the literature as either carcinosarcoma or malignant mixed tumors.[4, 9, 111]

The sarcoma that apparently does arise in the thyroid is angiosarcoma.[30, 32, 47, 48, 102, 145, 157, 180] This tumor shares clinical characteristics with anaplastic carcinoma, although its epidemiologic features are interesting. It occurs predominantly in the endemic goiter areas of Europe.[83, 104, 156] Recent reports have questioned the true nature of this tumor; Mills et al. describe an angiomatoid anaplastic carcinoma of

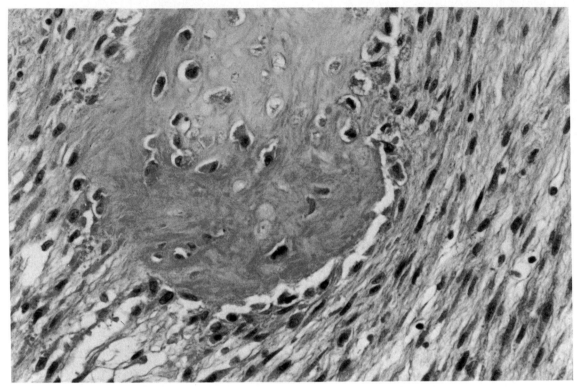

Figure 15–10. "Carcinosarcoma" of thyroid. This lesion was found in an elderly woman with a huge rapidly growing neck mass. Spindle cells and islands of cartilage and bone were found. Immunostain for cytokeratin was focally positive in spindle cell areas. × 150, H & E.

the thyroid and indicate that angiosarcoma may not arise in the thyroid.[126] These authors call into question immunostaining results in previous reports and suggest that all such neoplasms are indeed carcinomas. Pfaltz et al. attempted to address this issue by studying 36 cases of angiomatous thyroid tumors[145]; these authors found 20 of the 36 stained as angiosarcomas; 14 tumors gave equivocal results and could not be definitely classified as angiosarcoma or anaplastic carcinoma, and two were definitively proved to be anaplastic carcinomas. A more recent study by Hedinger's group from Switzerland indicates that some anaplastic carcinomas (7 of 16 cases) can contain endothelial markers, and conversely some angiosarcomas (3 of 4) contain keratin.[47] This study supports a related (?common) precursor for these lesions. It is possible that some cases classified as angiosarcoma indeed represent epithelial neoplasms, but it is also likely that at least some of these tumors are true angiosarcomas.[47, 126, 145]

Rare examples of tumors classified as hemangioendothelioma of the thyroid have been associated with hyperthyroidism[175]; the histologic evidence of malignancy in these cases and the possibility that the lesions were not of thyroid origin make their acceptance problematic. These patients each had a benign (up to 15 year) course[175]!

OTHER MESENCHYMAL LESIONS

Rare nonsarcomatous mesenchymal lesions of the thyroid form the basis of individual case reports. Pickleman et al. described a thyroid hemangioma in a 56-year-old man who presented with a cystic thyroid mass that histologically appeared to represent a hemangioma occurring within and around a thyroid adenoma.[146]

Delaney and Fry reported a neurilemoma of the thyroid,[40] whereas Goldstein et al. reported a schwannoma of the gland.[64] In each case the lesion presented as a thyroid mass in an adult without evidence of neurofibromatosis. Although immunostaining was not done in either case, the histologic descriptions and photographs are convincing. It is possible these tumors arose from autonomic nerve twigs within the gland.

Andrion et al. reported a leiomyoma and one neurilemoma of the thyroid with immunohistochemical and ultrastructural correlations.[7]

AMYLOID GOITER

Amyloid may be present in the thyroid as part of systemic amyloidosis, or in association with medullary thyroid carcinoma[94, 168]; in the former, if the lesion presents as a mass, it is known as amyloid goiter.

The amyloid associated with medullary thyroid carcinoma is discussed in Chapter 10. It is important to recognize that in those medullary carcinomas with extensive amyloid deposition, the cancer cells may be widely dispersed in the amyloid and difficult to find. Before assuming that such a lesion represents amyloid goiter, a careful search for neoplastic cells must be undertaken; on occasion, immunostaining for calcitonin or evaluation of further tissue sections from the tumor may be useful.

Systemic amyloidosis may affect any organ and the endocrine glands are no exception.[26] Usually associated with a plasma cell dyscrasia (primary A-L amyloid) or long history of chronic infection or inflammation (tuberculosis, rheumatoid arthritis—A-A amyloid), amyloid may deposit in the thyroid. In early stages it settles around vessel walls, but then extends to replace portions of the gland itself. In far advanced cases, hypothyroidism may result. (See Chapter 6.) The incidence of microscopic amyloid deposition in the thyroid in patients with generalized amyloidosis is high, averaging about 50 percent of such patients.[6, 8, 38]

Amyloid goiter is very rare, with approximately 80 acceptable cases in the world literature through 1982.[1, 6, 8, 68, 88, 94, 97, 134, 168, 196] These patients present with thyroid enlargement, but usually they will have evidence of other organ dysfunction (hepatic or renal most commonly) due to amyloid infiltration.[97] The case reported by Amado et al. was unusual since the amyloid goiter was the initial manifestation of systemic amyloidosis.[6] A recent report describes two patients with amyloid goiter and several episodes of illness resembling subacute thyroiditis.[89]

Grossly amyloid goiter presents as a solid white to beige mass replacing thyroid or streaks of abnormal tissue interdigitating normal gland. Histologically, masses of hyaline pink material with the appropriate staining characteristics are noted; in some cases and often at the edges of the mass lesions, streaks of amyloid spread through the surrounding thyroid follicles.[6] Calcification and foreign body giant cells can be found. Rare cases have shown fat admixed with the nodules of amyloid.[60]

The prognosis of amyloid goiter is that of the underlying systemic disease, i.e., it is poor. In virtually all reported cases, the goiter was believed to be a neoplasm and the diagnosis of amyloid goiter was not made preoperatively. Surgical treatment is advisable to relieve symptoms associated with the mass.[6]

Rare cases of amyloid in tumors other than medullary carcinoma have been described. A total of three cases have appeared in the literature that describe amyloid in the stroma of mixed papillary-follicular and follicular carcinomas.[110, 149, 191] The lesion reported by Valenta and Michel-Bechet bore some features suggesting medullary carcinoma.[191] The case of Polliack and Freund[149] contained stromal amyloid in the primary and prominent amyloid in the lymph node metatases. Liftin's[110] patient was a woman with longstanding rheumatoid arthritis and amyloid goiter; the amyloid apparently extended to involve a mixed papillary-follicular carcinoma that was present in the same thyroid. In the last case it seems possible that the patient suffered from systemic amyloidosis and this involved the thyroid which incidentally contained a carcinoma. The stromal amyloid in the case described by Polliack and Freund[149] is more difficult to explain, since the patient had no systemic illness and since amyloid is not known to result as a byproduct of thyroid hormone or thyroglobulin precipitation (in medullary carcinoma, the amyloid is believed to represent precipitated preprocalcitonin).

ATYPICAL PSEUDONEOPLASTIC LESIONS ASSOCIATED WITH RADIATION

In Chapter 6, the changes that occur in the morphology of the thyroid following low dose radiation were discussed. High doses of radiation given in the therapeutic range, usually for treatment of malignant lymphoma or epithelial neoplasms of the head and neck, may give rise to multinodular glands with a bizarre and frightening histologic appearance. In our experience,[25a] the changes include the presence of multiple highly cellular closely apposed nodules. Some of these nodules have fibrous capsules, although many do not. The nodules are all circumscribed, and in none of the cases we studied was there evidence of vascular or capsular invasion. The nodules, which were all follicular in pattern, contained a predominance of microfollicles; focally, Hürthle cell change was seen. Random cytologic atypia was a striking finding; this consisted of nucleomegaly with nuclear irregularity and prominent nucleoli. Occasionally multinucleated cells were noted. In a few cases, mild lymphocyte infiltration as well as stromal fibrosis was seen. No evidence of malignancy has been recognized in these cases,[25a] either histologic invasion or clinical metastasis.

OTHER TUMORS

An apparently unique thyroid tumor was reported by Ward et al.[198] This lesion, which was a circumscribed tumor, consisted of trabeculae of cells showing hyaline cells similar to those described for mixed tumors of the salivary gland. Some of these cells had plasmacytoid features. Immunostaining disclosed weakly positive reaction for thyroglobulin and strong staining for S100 protein; calcitonin stain was negative. Electron microscopic study showed accumulation of microfilaments in the cytoplasm of the tumor cells. The meaning of these immunologic and ultrastructural findings is unclear. The tumor was histologically and presumably clinically benign. Although this case was not published as a complete paper (at least, the current author cannot find reference to it), it is likely that this lesion may be similar to those tumors described by Carney et al.[25] and Bronner et al.[16] as the hyalinizing trabecular adenoma of the thyroid.

SUMMARY

As a guide to the reader confronted with an uncommon histologic pattern in a thyroid neoplasm, this chapter has reviewed a variety of unusual tumors affecting the thyroid.

REFERENCES

1. Abraham, S., Damordaran, V. N., and Sharma, V. N.: Amyloid goiter. Indian J. Chest Dis. 9:233–235, 1967.
2. Akerstrom, G., Malmaeus, J., and Bergstrom, R. Surgical anatomy of human parathyroid glands. Surgery 95:14–21, 1984.
3. Alagumalai, K., Avramides, A., et al.: Uptake of technetium pertechnetate in a parathyroid adenoma presenting as an iodine-131 "cold" nodule. Ann. Intern. Med. 90:204–205, 1979.
4. Al-Kaisi, N., and Mendelsohn, G.: Malignant mixed tumor (carcinosarcoma) of the thyroid gland with chondrosarcomatous and osteosarcomatous elements. ASCP Check Sample TD88–2, 1988.
5. Alsop, J. E., Yerbury, P. J., et al.: Signet ring cell microfollicular adenoma arising in a nodular ectopic thyroid. A case report. J. Oral Pathol. 15:518–519, 1986.
6. Amado, J. A., Palacios, S., et al.: Fast growing goitre as the first clinical manifestation of systemic amyloidosis. Postgrad. Med. J. 58:171–172, 1982.
7. Andrion, A., Bellis, D., et al.: Leiomyoma and neurilemoma: report of two unusual non-epithelial tumours of the thyroid gland. Virch. Arch. A. Pathol. Anat. 413:367–372, 1988.
8. Arean, V. M., and Klein, R. E.: Amyloid goiter. Am. J. Clin. Pathol. 36:343–355, 1961.
9. Arean, V. M., and Schildecker, W. W.: Carcinosarcoma of the thyroid gland: report of two cases. South. Med. J. 57:446–451, 1964.
10. Asa, S. L., Dardick, I., et al.: Primary thyroid thymoma: a distinct clinicopathologic entity. Hum. Pathol. 19:1463–1467, 1988.
11. Asirwatham, J. E., Barcos, M., and Shimaoka, K.: Hamartomatous adiposity of thyroid gland. J. Med. 10:197–206, 1979.
12. Bale, G. F.: Teratoma of the neck in the region of the thyroid gland. A review of the literature and report of four cases. Am. J. Pathol. 26:565–579, 1950.
13. Batsakis, J. G., Nishiyama, R. H., and Schmidt, R. W.: "Sporadic goiter syndrome": a clinicopathologic analysis. Am. J. Clin. Pathol. 39:241–251, 1963.
14. Bothra, R., Dahiya, S. L., et al.: Cervical thymoma. Int. Surgery. 60:301–302, 1975.
15. Brisigotti, M., Lorenzini, P., et al.: Mucin producing adenoma of the thyroid gland. Tumori 72:211–214, 1986.
16. Bronner, M., LiVolsi, V. A., and Jennings, T.: Paraganglioma-like adenomas of the thyroid. Surg. Pathol. 1:383–389, 1988.
17. Buckley, N. J., Burch, W. M., and Leight, G. S.: Malignant teratoma of the thyroid gland in an adult: A case report and a review of the literature. Surgery 100:932–937, 1986.
18. Buckwalter, J. A., and Layton, J. M.: Malignant teratoma in the thyroid gland of an adult. Ann. Surg. 139:218–223, 1954.
19. Burge, J. H., and Blalock, J. B.: Metastatic hypernephroma of the thyroid gland. Am. J. Surg. 113:387–389, 1967.
20. Buss, D. H., Marshall, R. B., et al.: Paraganglioma of the thyroid gland. Am. J. Surg. Pathol. 4:589–593, 1980.
21. Bussolati, G., and Monga, G.: Medullary carcinoma of the thyroid with atypical patterns. Cancer 44:1769–1777, 1979.
22. Cameron, R. G., Seemayer, T. A., et al.: Small cell malignant tumors of the thyroid: a light and electron microscopic study. Hum. Pathol. 6:731–740, 1975.
23. Carcangiu, M. L., Sibley, R. K., and Rosai, J. Clear cell change in primary thyroid tumors. Am. J. Surg. Pathol. 9:705–722, 1985.
24. Carcangiu, M. L., Zampi, G., and Rosai, J.: Poorly differentiated (insular) thyroid carcinoma. Am. J. Surg. Pathol. 8:655–668, 1984.
25. Carney, J. A., Ryan, J., and Goellner, J. R.: Hyalinizing trabecular adenoma of the thyroid gland. Am. J. Surg. Pathol. 11:583–591, 1987.
25a. Carr, R. F. and LiVolsi, V. A.: Morphologic changes in the thyroid after irradiation for Hodgkin's and non-Hodgkin's lymphoma. Cancer 64:825–829, 1989.
26. Case records of the Massachusetts General Hospital (Case 37451). Primary systemic amyloidosis, generalized. N. Engl. J. Med. 245:736–740, 1951.
27. Castleman, B., and Roth, S.: Tumors of the parathyroid glands. AFIP fascicle 14, second series. Washington, D.C., 1978.
28. Chalal, A. S., and Bhattacharjea, A. K.: Chondromatous hamartoma of the thyroid gland: Report of a case. Aust. N.Z. J. Surg. 45:30–31, 1975.
29. Chan, J. K. C., and Tse, C. C. H.: Mucin production in metastatic papillary carcinoma of the thyroid. Hum. Pathol. 19:195–220, 1988.
30. Chan, Y. F., Ma, L., et al.: Angiosarcoma of the thyroid. Cancer 57:2381–2388, 1986.
31. Chatzkel, S., Cole-Beuglet, C., et al.: Ultrasound diagnosis of a hypernephroma metastatic to the thyroid gland and external jugular vein. Radiology 142:165–166, 1982.
32. Chesky, V. E., Dreese, W. C., and Hellwig, C. A.: Hemangioendothelioma of the thyroid. J. Clin. Endocrinol Metab. 13:801–809, 1953.
33. Chesky, V. E., Dreese, W. C., and Hellwig, C. A.: Adenolipomatosis of the thyroid. Surgery 34:38–45, 1953.
34. Chesky, V. E., Hellwig, C. A., and Barbosa, E.: Clear cell tumors of the thyroid. Surgery 42:282–289, 1957.

35. Chesky, V. E., Hellwig, C. A., and Welch, J. W.: Fibrosarcoma of the thyroid gland. Surg. Gynecol. Obstet. *111*:767–770, 1960.
36. Civantos, F., Albores-Saavedra, J., et al.: Clear cell variant of thyroid carcinoma. Am. J. Surg. Pathol. *8*:187–192, 1984.
37. Czech, J. M., Lichtor, T. R., et al.: Neoplasms metastatic to the thyroid gland. Surg. Gynecol. Obstet. *155*:503–505, 1982.
38. Daoud, F. S., Nieman, R. E., and Vilter, R. W.: Amyloid goiter in a case of generalized primary amyloidosis. Am. J. Med. *43*:604–608, 1967.
39. Dayal, Y., Ucci, A. A., et al.: Thyroglobulin and clear cell tumors. Am. J. Surg. Pathol. *10*:70–72, 1986.
40. Delaney, W. E., and Fry, K. E.: Neurilemoma of the thyroid gland. Ann. Surg. *160*:1014–1016, 1964.
41. Deligdisch, L., Subhani, Z., and Gordon, R. E.: Primary mucinous carcinoma of the thyroid gland. Cancer *45*:2564–2567, 1980.
42. Dempsey, W. S., Crile, G., and Engel, W. J.: Clear cell carcinoma (hypernephroma) of the kidney with metastasis to the thyroid gland. J. Urol. *68*:576–578, 1952.
43. Denton, G. R., and McClintock, J. C.: Hypernephroma metastatic to the thyroid gland. Ann. Surg. *129*:399–403, 1949.
44. Dhayagude, R. G.: Massive fatty infiltration in a colloid goiter. Arch. Pathol. *33*:557–560, 1942.
45. Diaz-Perez, R., Quiroz, H., and Nishiyama, R. H.: Primary mucinous adenocarcinoma of the thyroid gland. Cancer *38*:1323–1325, 1976.
46. Dickersin, G. R., Vickery, A. L., and Smith, S. B.: Papillary carcinoma of the thyroid, oxyphil cell type, "clear cell" variant. Am. J. Surg. Pathol. *4*:501–509, 1980.
47. Eckert, F., Schmid, U., et al.: Evidence of vascular differentiation in anaplastic tumours of the thyroid—an immunohistological study. Virch. Arch. Pathol. Anat. *410*:203–215, 1986.
48. Egloff, B.: The hemangioendothelioma of the thyroid. Virch. Arch. Pathol. Anat. *400*:119–142, 1983.
49. Elliot, R. H. E., and Frantz, V. K.: Metastatic carcinoma masquerading as primary thyroid cancer: A report of authors' 14 cases. Ann. Surg. *151*:551–561, 1960.
50. Ericsson, M., Biorklund, A., et al.: Surgical treatment of metastatic disease in the thyroid gland. J. Surg. Oncol. *17*:15–23,
51. Erikson, A., and Gezelius, C.: Metastatic choriocarcinoma during normal pregnancy presenting as thyroid tumor. Arch. Gynecol. *236*:119–122, 1984.
52. Eriksson, M., Ajmani, S. K., and Mallette, L.: Hyperthyroidism from thyroid metastasis of pancreatic adenocarcinoma. J.A.M.A. *238*:1276–1278, 1977.
53. Fernandes, B. J., Bedard, Y. C., and Rosen, I.: Mucus-producing medullary cell carcinoma of the thyroid gland. Am. J. Clin. Pathol. *78*:536–540, 1982.
54. Fisher, E. R., and Kim, W. S.: Primary clear cell thyroid carcinoma with squamous features. Cancer *39*:2497–2502, 1977.
55. Fisher, J. E., Cooney, D. R., et al.: Teratoma of thyroid gland in infancy: review of the literature and two case reports. J. Surg. Oncol. *21*:135–140, 1982.
56. Flynn, S. D., Forman, B. H., et al.: Poorly differentiated ("insular") carcinoma of the thyroid: an aggressive subset of differentiated thyroid neoplasms. Surgery *104*:963–970, 1988.
57. Franssila, K., Harach, H. R., and Wasenius, V. M.: Mucoepidermoid carcinoma of the thyroid. Histopathology *8*:847–860, 1984.
58. Freund, H. R.: Surgical treatment of metastases to the thyroid gland from other primary malignancies. Ann. Surg. *162*:285–290, 1965.
59. Friberg, S., and Kinnman, J.: Renal adenocarcinoma with metastases to the thyroid gland. Acta Otolaryngol. *67*:552–562, 1969.
60. Fuller, R. H.: Hamartomatous adiposity with superimposed amyloidosis of thyroid gland. J. Laryngol. Otol. *77*:92–93, 1963.
61. Gault, E. W., Leung, T. H., and Thomas, D. P.: Clear cell renal carcinoma masquerading as thyroid enlargement. J. Pathol. *113*:21–25, 1974.
62. Gherardi, G.: Signet ring cell 'mucinous' thyroid adenoma: a follicle cell tumour with abnormal accumulation of thyroglobulin and a peculiar histochemical profile. Histopathol. *11*:317–326, 1987.
63. Gherardi, G., Scherini, P., and Ambrosi, S.: Occult thyroid metastasis from untreated uveal melanoma. Arch. Ophthal. *103*:689–691, 1985.
63a. Gnepp, D. R., Ogorzalek, J. M., and Heffers, C. S.: Fat-containing lesions of the thyroid gland. Am. J. Surg. Pathol. *13*:605–612, 1989.
64. Goldstein, J., Tovi, F., and Sidi, J.: Primary schwannoma of the thyroid gland. Int. Surg. *67*:433–434, 1982.
65. Golouh, R., Us-Krasovec, M., et al.: Amphicrine-composite calcitonin and mucin-producing carcinoma of the thyroid. Ultrastruct. Pathol. *8*:197–206, 1985.
66. Goodman, M. L., Egdahl, R. H., et al.: Hyperparathyroidism from intrathyroid parathyroid adenomas. Arch. Pathol. *87*:418–422, 1969.
67. Gowing, N. F. C.: The pathology and natural history of thyroid tumours. *In:* Smithers, D. (ed.): Tumours of the Thyroid Gland. Edinburgh, E. S. Livingstone, 1970. pp. 103–129.
68. Habbick, B. F., and McDicken, I. W.: Amyloid goitre in a patient with rheumatoid arthritis. Scot. Med. J. *12*:405–407, 1967.
69. Haegert, D. G., Wang, N. S., et al.: Nonchromaffin paragangliomatosis manifesting as a cold thyroid nodule. Am. J. Clin. Pathol. *61*:561–570, 1974.

70. Hajdu, S. I., and Hajdu, E. O.: Malignant teratoma of the neck. Arch. Pathol. *83*:567–570, 1967.
71. Hajdu, S. I., Faruque, A. A., et al.: Teratoma of the neck in infants. Am. J. Dis. Child. *111*:412–416, 1966.
72. Hales, M., Rosenau, W., et al.: Carcinoma of the thyroid with a mixed medullary and follicular pattern. Cancer *50*:1352–1359, 1982.
73. Harach, H. R.: Thyroid follicles with acid mucins in man: A second kind of follicles? Cell Tissue Res. *242*:211–215, 1985.
74. Harach, H. R.: Solid cell nests of the thyroid: An anatomical survey and immunohistochemical study for the presence of thyroglobulin. Acta Anat. *122*:249–253, 1985.
75. Harach, H. R.: A study on the relationship between solid cell nests and mucoepidermoid carcinoma of the thyroid. Histopathology *9*:195–207, 1985.
76. Harach, H. R.: Mixed follicles of the human thyroid gland. Acta Anat. *129*:27–30, 1987.
77. Harach, H. R., Day, E. S., and deStrizic, N. A.: Mucoepidermoid carcinoma of the thyroid. Medicina (Buenos Aires) *46*:213–216, 1986.
78. Harach, H. R., Day, E. S., and Franssila, K. O.: Thyroid spindle cell tumor with mucous cysts. An intrathyroidal thymoma? Am. J. Surg. Pathol. *9*:525–530, 1985.
79. Harach, H. R., and Wasenius, V. M.: Expression of 'visceral' cytokeratin and ultrastructural findings in solid cell nests of the thyroid. Acta Anat. *129*:289–292, 1987.
80. Harada, T., Shimaoka, K., et al.: Mucin-producing carcinoma of the thyroid gland—a case report and review of the literature. Jpn. J. Clin. Oncol. *14*:417–424, 1984.
81. Harcourt-Webster, J. N.: Secondary neoplasm of the thyroid presenting as a goitre. J. Clin. Pathol. *18*:282–287, 1965.
82. Harrison, D. F. N.: Thyroid gland in the management of laryngo-pharyngeal cancer. Arch. Otolaryngol. *97*:301–302, 1973.
83. Hedinger, C.: Sarcomas of the thyroid gland. *In*: Hedinger, C. (ed.): Thyroid Cancer. Heidelberg, Springer-Verlag, 1969, pp. 47–52.
84. Hjorth, L., Thomsen, L. B., and Nielsen, V. T.: Adenolipoma of the thyroid gland. Histopathology *10*:91–96, 1986.
85. Holm, R., Sobrinho-Simoes, M., et al.: Medullary thyroid carcinoma with thyroglobulin immunoreactivity. A special entity? Lab. Invest. *57*:258–268, 1987.
86. Holm, R., Sobrinho-Simoes, M., et al.: Concurrent production of calcitonin and thyroglobulin by the same neoplastic cells. Ultrastructural Pathol. *10*:241–248, 1986.
87. Horowitz, J. J., Fajardo, M. et al.: Clear cell carcinoma of the thyroid. Int. Surg. *45*:429–439, 1966.
88. Hunter, W. R., McDougall, C. D. M., and Evans, R. W.: Amyloid goitre. Br. J. Surg. *55*:885–887, 1968.
89. Ikenoue, H., Okamura, K., et al.: Thyroid amyloidosis with recurrent subacute thyroiditis-like syndrome. J. Clin. Endocrinol. Metab. *67*:41–45, 1988.
90. Ishihara, T., Yamazaki, S., et al.: Resection of the trachea infiltrated by thyroid carcinoma. Ann. Surg. *195*:496–500, 1982.
91. Ishimaru, Y., Fukuda, S., et al.: Follicular thyroid carcinoma with clear cell change showing unusual ultrastructural features. Am. J. Surg. Pathol. *12*:240–246, 1988.
92. Ivy, H. K.: Cancer metastatic to the thyroid: A diagnostic problem. Mayo Clin. Proc. *59*:856–859, 1984.
93. Jaffe, R. H.: Histologic studies on the fat content of normal human thyroid. Arch. Pathol. *3*:955–962, 1927.
94. James, P. D.: Amyloid goitre. J. Clin. Pathol. *25*:683–688, 1972.
95. Kawahara, E., Nakanishi, I., et al.: Leiomyosarcoma of the thyroid gland. Cancer *62*:2558–2563, 1988.
96. Kay, S., Montague, J. W., and Dodd, R. W.: Nonchromaffin paraganglioma (chemodectoma) of thyroid region. Cancer *36*:582–585, 1975.
97. Kennedy, J. S., Thomson, J. A., and Buchanan, W. M.: Amyloid in the thyroid. Quart. J. Med. *43*:127–143, 1974.
98. Keynes, W. M.: Teratoma of the neck in relation to the thyroid gland. Br. J. Surg. *46*:466–472, 1959.
99. Kier, R., Silverman, P. M., et al.: Malignant teratoma of the thyroid in an adult: CT appearance. J. Comp. Assist. Tomog. *9*:174–176, 1985.
100. Kimler, S. C., and Muth, W. F.: Primary malignant teratoma of the thyroid. Case report and literature review of cervical teratomas in adults. Cancer *42*:311–317, 1978.
101. Kingsley, D. P. E., Elton, A., and Bennett, M. H.: Malignant teratoma of the thyroid. Case report and review of the literature. Br. J. Cancer *22*:7–11, 19.
102. Klinck, G. H.: Hemangioendothelioma and sarcoma of the thyroid. *In:* Hedinger, C. (ed.): Thyroid Cancer. Heidelberg, Springer-Verlag, 1969, pp. 60–64.
103. Kniseley, R. M., and Andrews, G. A.: Transformation of thyroidal carcinoma to clear cell type. Am. J. Clin. Pathol. *26*:1427–1438, 1956.
104. Krisch, K., Holzner, J. H., et al.: Hemangioendothelioma of the thyroid gland—true endothelioma or anaplastic carcinoma? Pathol. Res. Pract. *170*:230–234, 1980.
105. Landon, G., and Ordonez, N. G.: Clear cell variant of medullary carcinoma of the thyroid. Hum. Pathol. *16*:844–947, 1985.

106. Lange, M. J.: Pleomorphic adenoma of the thyroid containing salivary gland cells with pseudo-cartilage and myoepithelial cells. Int. Surgery 59:178–179, 1974.
107. Lasser, A., Rothman, J. G., and Calamia, V. J.: Renal cell carcinoma metastatic to the thyroid. Aspiration cytology and histologic findings. Acta Cytol. 29:856–858,
108. Lehur, P. A., Cote, R. A., et al.: Thyroid metastasis of clear cell renal carcinoma. Canad. Med. Assoc. J. 128:154–156,
109. Linton, R. R., Barney, D., et al.: Metastatic hypernephroma of the thyroid gland. Surg. Gynecol. Obstet. 83:493–498, 1946.
110. Liftin, A. J.: Nonmedullary carcinoma of the thyroid gland in association with amyloid goiter: case report. Mt. Sinai J. Med. 52:225–227, 1985.
111. Lira, V., and Maranhao, E.: Malignant mixed tumour of the thyroid gland. J. Pathol. Bacteriol. 89:377–379, 1965.
112. Livingston, D. J., and Sandiston, A. T.: Osteogenic sarcoma of thyroid. Br. J. Surg. 50:291–293, 1962.
113. LiVolsi, V. A.: Mixed thyroid carcinoma: A real entity? Lab. Invest. 57:237–239, 1987.
114. LiVolsi, V. A., Brooks, J. J., and Arendash-Durand, B.: Anaplastic thyroid tumor: immunohistology. Am. J. Clin. Pathol. 87:434–442, 1987.
115. Ljungberg, O., Bondeson, L., and Bondeson, A. G.: Differentiated thyroid carcinoma, intermediate type. A new tumor entity with features of follicular and parafollicular cell carcinoma. Hum. Pathol. 15:218–228, 1984.
116. Ljungberg, O., Ericsson, U. B., et al.: A compound follicular-parafollicular cell carcinoma of the thyroid: A new tumor entity? Cancer 52:1053–1061, 1983.
117. Luna, M. A., Mackay, B., et al.: Malignant small cell tumor of the thyroid. Ultrastruct. Pathol. 1:265–270, 1980.
118. Madore, P., and Lan, S.: Solitary thyroid metastasis from clear cell renal carcinoma. Canad. Med. Assoc. J. 112:719–721, 1975.
119. Mailander, J. C., and Graves, V. B.: A thyroid nodule representing metastatic renal carcinoma. Clin. Nuclear Med. 10:650–652, 1985.
120. Mambo, N. C., and Irwin, S. M.: Anaplastic small cell neoplasms of the thyroid. An immunoperoxidase study. Hum. Pathol. 15:55–60, 1984.
121. Martin, J. M. E., Randhawa, G., and Temple, W. J.: Cervical thymoma. Arch. Pathol. Lab. Med. 110:354–357, 1986.
122. McCabe, D. P., Farrar, W. B., et al.: Clinical and pathologic correlations in disease metastatic to the thyroid gland. Am. J. Surg. 150:519–523, 1985.
123. Meissner, W. A., and Phillips, M. J.: Diffuse small cell carcinoma of the thyroid. Arch. Pathol. 74:291–297, 1962.
124. Mendelsohn, G.: Signet ring cell simulating microfollicular adenoma of the thyroid. Am. J. Surg. Pathol. 8:705–708, 1984.
125. Mendelsohn, G., and Oertel, J. E.: Encapsulated medullary carcinoma: Differentiation from "atypical" adenomas by calcitonin immunohistochemistry. Lab. Invest. 44:43A, 1981. (Abstract).
126. Mills, S. E., Stallings, R. G., and Austin, M. B.: Angiomatoid carcinoma of the thyroid gland: Anaplastic carcinoma with follicular and medullary features mimicking angiosarcoma. Am. J. Clin. Pathol. 86:674–678, 1986.
127. Mitsudo, S. M., Grajower, M. M., et al.: Malignant paraganglioma of the thyroid gland. Arch. Pathol. Lab. Med. 111:378–380, 1987.
128. Miyauchi, A., Kuma, K., et al.: Intrathyroidal epithelial thymoma: an entity distinct from squamous cell carcinoma of the thyroid. World J. Surg. 9:128–135, 1985.
129. Mizukami, Y., Matsubara, S., et al.: Primary mucoepidermoid carcinoma in the thyroid gland. Cancer 53:1741–1745, 1984.
130. Mizukami, Y., Matsubara, F., et al.: Primary mucin-producing adenosquamous carcinoma of the thyroid gland. Acta Pathol. Jpn. 37:1157–1164, 1987.
131. Mlynek, M. K., Richter, H. J., and Leder, L. D.: Mucin in carcinomas of the thyroid. Cancer 56:2647–2650, 1985.
132. Moore, G. E., and Walker, W. W.: Metastatic hypernephroma of the thyroid gland with subsequent thyroidectomy, nephrectomy and resection of pulmonary metastases. Surgery 27:929–934, 1950.
133. Mortenson, J. D., Woolner, L. B., and Bennett, W. A.: Secondary malignant tumors of the thyroid gland. Cancer 9:306–309, 1956.
134. Mosmans-Smits, A. H., and Van Der Meer, J. W.: Amyloid goiter. Neth. J. Med. 17:115–120, 1974.
135. Murao, T., Nakanishi, M., et al.: Malignant teratoma of the thyroid gland in an adolescent female. Acta Pathol. Jpn. 29:109–117, 1979.
136. Neill, J.: Intrathyroidal thymoma. Am. J. Surg. Pathol. 10:660–661, 1986.
137. Nesland, J. M., Sobrinho-Simoes, M. A., et al.: Organoid tumor in the thyroid gland. Ultrastruct. Pathol. 9:65–70, 1985.
138. Newstedt, J. R., and Shirkey, H. C.: Teratoma of the thyroid region. Am. J. Dis. Child. 107:88–95, 1964.
139. Ohbu, M., Kameya, T., et al.: Primary osteogenic sarcoma of the thyroid gland. Surg. Pathol. 2:1989 (in press).

140. O'Higgins, N., and Taylor, S.: Malignant teratoma in the adult thyroid gland. Br. J. Clin. Pract. *29*:237–238, 1975.
141. Pages, A., and Tiraskis, B.: Deux cas de thyro-lipome. Ann. Pathol. *5*:283–286, 1985.
142. Pemberton, J. D., and Bennett, R. J.: Hypernephroma of the thyroid gland: A report of the literature and a report of two cases. Surg. Clin. N. Amer. *14*:593–599, 1934.
143. Perrone, T.: Mixed medullary-follicular thyroid carcinoma. Am. J. Surg. Pathol. *10*:362–363, 1986.
144. Pfaltz, M., Hedinger, C., and Muhlethaler, J. P.: Mixed medullary and follicular carcinoma of the thyroid. Virch. Arch. Pathol. Anat. *400*:53–59, 1983.
145. Pfaltz, M., Hedinger, C., et al.: Malignant hemangioendothelioma of the thyroid and factor VIII-related antigen. Virch. Arch. Pathol. Anat. *401*:177–184, 1983.
146. Pickleman, J. R., Lee, J. F., et al.: Thyroid hemangioma. Am. J. Surg. *129*:331–336, 1975.
147. Pillay, S. P., Angorn, I. B., and Baker, L. W.: Tumour metastasis to the thyroid gland. So. Afr. Med. J. *51*:509–512, 1977.
148. Pinelli, V., Pierro, V., et al.: Dysontogenetic neoplasms of the thyroid gland in infancy. Int. J. Pediatr. Otorhinolaryngol. *10*:101–110, 1985.
149. Polliack, A., and Freund, U.: Mixed papillary and follicular carcinoma of the thyroid with stromal amyloid. Am. J. Clin. Pathol. *53*:592–595, 1970.
150. Rayfield, E. J., Nishiyama, R. H., and Sisson, J. C.: Small cell tumors of the thyroid: a clinicopathologic study. Cancer *28*:1023–1030, 1971.
151. Rhatigan, R. M., Roque, J. I., and Bucher, R. L.: Mucoepidermoid carcinoma of the thyroid gland. Cancer *39*:210–214, 1977.
152. Rice, C. O.: Microscopic metastases in the thyroid gland. Am. J. Pathol. *10*:407–412, 1934.
153. Ridenhour, C. E., Henzel, J. H., et al.: Thymoma arising from undescended cervical thymus. Surgery *67*:614–619, 1970.
154. Rigaud, C. M., Peltier, F., and Bogomoletz, W.: Mucin-producing microfollicular adenoma of the thyroid. J. Clin. Pathol. *38*:277–280, 1985.
155. Rosai, J., Limas, C., and Husband, E. M.: Ectopic hamartomatous thymoma: A distinctive benign lesion of the lower neck. Am. J. Surg. Pathol. *8*:501–513, 1984.
156. Rosai, J., Saxen, E. A., and Woolner, L.: Undifferentiated and poorly differentiated carcinoma. Sem. Diagn. Pathol. *2*:123–136, 1985.
157. Ruchti, C., Gerber, H. A., and Schaffner, T.: Factor VIII-related antigen in malignant hemangioendothelioma of the thyroid: additional evidence for the endothelial origin of this tumor. Am. J. Clin. Pathol. *82*:474–480, 1984.
158. Saito, R., and Sharma, K.: Fine structure of a diffuse undifferentiated small cell carcinoma of the thyroid. Am. J. Clin. Pathol. *65*:623–630, 1976.
159. Sakamoto, A., Kasai, N., and Sugano, H.: Poorly differentiated carcinoma of the thyroid. A clinicopathologic entity for a high risk group of papillary and follicular carcinomas. Cancer *52*:1849–1855, 1983.
160. Schaub, C. R., and Mendelsohn, G.: The spectrum of clear cell thyroid tumors. Am. J. Clin. Pathol. *84*:561, 1985 (abstract).
161. Schmid, K. W., Kroll, M., et al.: Small cell carcinoma of the thyroid. A reclassification of cases originally diagnosed as small cell carcinoma of the thyroid. Pathol. Res. Pract. *181*:540–543, 1986.
162. Schroder, S., and Bocker, W.: Signet ring cell thyroid tumors: a follicle cell tumor with arrest of folliculogenesis. Am. J. Surg. Pathol. *9*:619–629, 1985.
163. Schroder, S., and Bocker, W. L.: Clear cell carcinoma of thyroid gland: a clinicopathological study of 13 cases. Histopathology *10*:75–89, 1986.
164. Schroder, S., Bocker, W., et al.: Adenolipoma (thyrolipoma) of the thyroid gland: report of two cases and review of the literature. Virch. Arch. (Pathol. Anat.) *404*:99–103, 1984.
165. Schroder, S., Burk, C. G., and de Heer, K.: Metastasen in der Schilddruse-morphologie und Klinik von 25 sekundaren Schilddrusen-Geschwulsten. Langenbecks Arch. Chir. *370*:25–35, 1987.
166. Schroder, S., Husselmann, H., and Bocker, W.: Lipid rich adenoma of the thyroid gland. Report of a peculiar thyroid tumor. Virch. Arch. (Pathol. Anat.) *404*:105–108, 1984.
167. Segal, K., Har-el, G., et al.: Clear cell carcinoma of the thyroid gland. Head & Neck Surg. *8*:313–319, 1986.
168. Shapiro, S. T., Kohut, R. I., and Potter, J. M.: Amyloid goiter. Arch. Otolaryngol. *93*:203–208, 1971.
169. Shima, H., Mori, H., et al.: A case of renal cell carcinoma solitarily metastasized to thyroid 20 years after the resection of primary tumor. Pathol. Res. Pract. *179*:666–670, 1985.
170. Shimaoka, K., Sokal, J. E., and Pickren, J. W.: Metastatic neoplasms in the thyroid. Cancer *15*:557–565, 1962.
171. Silberman, R., and Mendelson, I. R.: Teratoma of the neck. Arch. Dis. Child. *35*:159–170, 1960.
172. Silverberg, S., and Vidone, R.: Metastatic tumors in the thyroid. Pacif. Med. Surg. *74*:175–180, 1966.
173. Simha, M. R., and Doctor, V. M.: Adenolipomatosis of the thyroid gland. Indian J. Cancer *20*:215–217, 1983.
174. Sobrinho-Simoes, M. A., Nesland, J. M., and Johannessen, J. V.: A mucin-producing tumor in the thyroid gland. Ultrastructural Pathol. *9*:277–281, 1985.

175. Spaulding, S. W., and Burrow, G. N.: Hemangioendothelioma of the thyroid and concurrent hyperthyroidism. Am. J. Med. 57:831–835, 1974.
176. Spiegel, A. M., Marx, S. J., et al.: Intrathyroidal parathyroid adenoma or hyperplasia: An occasionally overlooked cause of surgical failure in primary hyperparathyroidism. J.A.M.A. 234:1029–1033, 1975.
177. Stone, H. H., Henderson, W. D., and Guidio, F. A.: Teratomas of the neck. Am. J. Dis. Child. 113:222–224, 1967.
178. Syrjanen, K. J.: An osteogenic sarcoma of the thyroid gland. Neoplasma 26:623–628, 1979.
179. Syrjanen, K. J.: Fine needle aspiration cytology of the thyroid osteosarcoma. J. Cancer Res. Clin. Oncol. 96:319–323, 1980.
180. Tanda, F., Massarelli, G., et al.: Angiosarcoma of the thyroid: a light electron microscopic and histoimmunological study. Hum. Pathol. 19:742–745,
181. Thomson, J. A., Kennedy, J. S., et al.: Secondary carcinoma of the thyroid gland. Br. J. Surg. 62:692–693, 1975.
182. Thorpe, J. D.: Metastatic cancer in the thyroid gland. West. J. Surg. Obstet. Gynecol. 62:574–576, 1954.
183. Tibaldi, J. M., Shapiro, L. E., and Mahadevia, P. S.: Thyroiditis mimicked by metastatic carcinoma to the thyroid. Mayo Clin. Proc. 61:399–400, 1986.
184. Tolstedt, G. E., Cammock, E. E., and Bell, J. W.: Hyperparathyroidism associated with intrathyroidal parathyroid glands. Am. J. Surg. 100:757–760, 1960.
185. Treadwell, T., Alexander, B. B., et al.: Clear cell renal carcinoma masquerading as a thyroid nodule. South. Med. J. 74:878–879, 1981.
186. Trites, A. E. W.: Thyrolipoma, thymolipoma and pharyngeal lipoma: A syndrome. Canad. Med. Assoc. J. 95:1254–1259, 1966.
187. Tscholl-Ducommun, J., and Hedinger, C.: Papillary thyroid carcinoma. Morphology and prognosis. Virchows Arch. Pathol. Anat. A. 396:19–39, 1982.
188. Ueda, G., and Furth, J.: Sarcomatoid transformation of transplanted thyroid carcinoma. Arch. Pathol. 83:3–12, 1967.
189. Uribe, M., Grimes, M., et al.: Medullary carcinoma of the thyroid gland: clinical, pathological and immunohistochemical features with review of the literature. Am. J. Surg. Pathol. 9:577–594, 1985.
190. Valenta, L. J., and Michel-Bechet, M.: Electron microscopy of clear cell thyroid tumors. Arch. Pathol. Lab Med. 101:140–144, 1977.
191. Valenta, L. J., Michel-Bechet, M., et al.: Microfollicular thyroid carcinoma with amyloid rich stroma, resembling the medullary carcinoma of the thyroid. Cancer 39:1573–1586, 1977.
192. Variokojis, D., Getz, M. L., et al.: Papillary clear cell carcinoma of the thyroid gland. Hum. Pathol. 6:384–389, 1975.
193. Vestfrid, M. A.: Papillary carcinoma of the thyroid gland with lipomatous stroma: report of a peculiar histological type of thyroid tumor. Histopathology 10:97–100, 1986.
194. Vitug, A. C., Lopchinsky, R. A., et al.: Tracheal carcinoma presenting as a thyroid cyst. Arch. Otolaryngol. 111:340–341, 1985.
195. Vollenweider, I., and Hedinger, C.: Solid cell nests (SCN) in Hashimoto's thyroiditis. Virch. Arch. Pathol. Anat. 412:357–363, 1988.
196. Walker, G. A.: Amyloid goiter. Surg. Gynecol. Obstet. 75:374–378, 1942.
197. Wang, C., Vickery, A. L., and Maloof, F.: Large parathyroid cysts mimicking thyroid nodules. Ann. Surg. 175:448–453, 1972.
198. Ward, J. V., Murray, D., et al.: Hyaline cell tumor of thyroid with massive accumulation of cytoplasmic microfilaments. Lab. Invest. 46:88, 1982. (Abstract).
199. Weitzner, S.: Benign teratoma of the neck in an infant. Am. J. Dis. Child. 107:84–87, 1964.
200. Willis, R. A.: Metastatic tumours in the thyroid gland. Am. J. Pathol. 7:187–208, 1931.
201. Wychulis, A. R., Beahrs, O. H., and Woolner, L. B.: Metastases of carcinoma to the thyroid gland. Ann. Surg. 160:169–177, 1964.
202. Yamashita, H., Murakami, N., et al.: Cervical thymoma and incidence of cervical thymus. Acta Pathol. Jpn. 33:189–194, 1983.
203. Zaatari, G. S., Saigo, P. E., and Huvos, A. G.: Mucin production in medullary carcinoma of the thyroid. Arch. Pathol. Lab. Med. 107:70–74, 1984.
204. Zirkin, H. J., and Tovi, F.: Tracheal carcinoma presenting as a thyroid tumor. J. Surg. Oncol. 26:268–271, 1984.

Chapter

16

THYROID LESIONS IN UNUSUAL PLACES

The embryology of the thyroid has been reviewed in Chapter 1 of this monograph. In this chapter, pathologic lesions arising in the ectopic thyroid tissue are discussed, with the major emphasis on tumors arising in aberrantly located thyroid (Table 16–1).

Normally the precursor of the median thyroid is located at the foramen cecum of the tongue. During the first two months of fetal life, the thyroid anlage descends caudally until it comes to rest in the anterior neck in front of the trachea. Developmental anomalies may lead to thyroid tissue remnants being present anywhere along the path of descent. These sites include base of tongue (so-called lingual thyroid), thyroglossal duct thyroid, and thyroid tissue extending into superior mediastinum, or even within the heart.

Thyroid tissue located lateral to the jugular veins, so-called lateral aberrant thyroid, has been discussed in Chapter 1. In summary, thyroid tissue, even if normal in appearance, found in lateral lymph nodes signifies a metastatic papillary thyroid carcinoma. Normal appearing thyroid tissue unassociated with lymph nodes may occur in the lateral neck in patients who have undergone prior neck surgery (implantation of thyroid tissue) or in individuals who have large goiters

Table 16–1. Ectopic Thyroid Tissue and Its Lesions

Median Ectopias
Lingual thyroid
Thyroglossal duct associated thyroid
Intratracheal/intralaryngeal thyroid
Mediastinal thyroid
Cardiac thyroid
Medial node associated thyroid
Lateral Aberrant Thyroid
Ovarian Thyroid
Nonneoplastic
Neoplastic
Papillary carcinoma
Malignant lymphoma
Strumal carcinoid
Strumatosis
Other Locations
Vaginal thyroid
Sella turcica

due to adenomatous goiter or chronic thyroiditis. In the latter two situations, nodules of thyroid unattached to the main gland may be found.[44]

The presence of thyroid tissue within teratomas of ovarian origin, i.e., struma ovarii, will be reviewed. Lesions affecting this type of thyroid tissue, including neoplasms, will be discussed.

Other unusual locations of thyroid tissue in which neoplasms have been reported to arise will be mentioned.[47, 85]

LINGUAL THYROID

Thyroid tissue located at the base of the tongue, i.e., lingual thyroid, is considered a developmental anomaly in which the median thyroid anlage fails to descend. Although clinically significant lingual thyroid is an unusual disorder ranging from 1 in 4500 to 1 in 100,000 patients,[30, 68] microscopic remnants of thyroid tissue have been described in 9.8 percent of tongues examined at autopsy.[2]

When clinically evident, lingual thyroid presents as a mass with associated dysphagia or occasionally bleeding. If the lingual thyroid is large in the perinatal period, severe respiratory compromise may occur.[48, 77] Females are affected more often than males [2, 34, 36, 38, 68, 88, 104]; some authors have speculated that hormonal influences may produce this sex difference. Most cases of clinically significant lingual thyroid are diagnosed in teenagers and young adults, probably reflecting enlargement of the thyroid tissue due to increased demand for thyroid hormone associated with growth.[36, 68]

In the group of patients who present with this disorder, the lingual thyroid represents the *only* thyroid tissue in 70 to 100 percent of cases.[36, 65, 68, 104] About 10 percent of such patients are hypothyroid at initial evaluation[68]; rarely, hyperfunction has been documented.[46] Patients with lingual thyroid rarely have thyroid tissue in a normal pretracheal location; if these individuals do have additional thyroid tissue, it is often located in a perihyoid or suprahyoid region.[36, 68, 102] A significant family history of thyroid disease or of thyroglossal duct cysts is found in many of the affected patients.[68]

Grossly, lingual thyroid appears as a mass at the base of the tongue; it is usually solid in consistency. Rarely, ulceration of the overlying mucosa may be noted.[34, 48]

Histologic examination discloses normal-appearing thyroid follicles interdigitating with skeletal muscle fibers. No capsule is present.[59, 68, 101] This resembles thyroid tissue which intermingles with normal skeletal muscle in the neck. The differences between this finding and invasive cancer include the totally normal appearance of the thyroid (lack of papillae, clear nuclei, etc.) and, most importantly, the lack of a stromal tissue response, i.e., there is no desmoplasia. In some cases, changes simulating adenomatous goiter are seen; focal areas of hyperplasia with scalloped colloid may be noted.[65, 68] Inflammatory cell infiltration is not uncommon and may mimic thyroiditis.[2, 68, 97]

Rare cases of thyroid carcinoma arising in lingual thyroid are recorded. Three reviews of the literature, including those of Mill et al.,[56] Smithers,[94] and Fish and Moore,[20] culled about 24 cases through 1970. Potdar and Desai reported one additional case.[75] The reviews of lingual thyroid carcinoma have stressed the lack of clinical and histologic evidence of malignancy in many of the reported cases[68, 94]; as noted by Nienas et al.,[68] the normal histologic pattern of lingual thyroid is interdigitation with skeletal muscle fibers of the tongue—this must not be equated with carcinoma. Of the 25 cases reported in the literature, only 10 have documented recurrences of tumor, metastases, or death caused by tumor[94]; the others either have no significant follow-up recorded or have behaved in a clinically benign fashion.[68, 94]

The literature on lingual thyroid carcinoma indicates that the disease affects women more frequently than men (about 1.5:1); ages of patients ranged from 12 to 86 years. Of the reported cases in women, two became symptomatic during pregnancy.[56, 94] Only one patient was a child (age 12); this case, reported by Potdam and Desai, was diagnosed as follicular carcinoma. However, the photomicrographs are inconclusive and the diagnosis in this author's opinion is doubtful. The follow-up was reportedly benign. The pathologic diagnoses in other cases include "malignant struma," "adenocarcinoma," or just "carcinoma" in most cases. A few tumors were diagnosed as "undifferentiated" or "poorly differentiated."[94]

Since the few cases reported have appeared over a period of about 80 years, therapy has varied widely. Most of the tumors were primarily treated surgically. The patient of Mill et al. also received radioiodine.[56]

CARCINOMA ARISING IN ASSOCIATION WITH THYROGLOSSAL DUCT

The thyroglossal duct represents the connection between the median anlage of the thyroid at the foramen cecum and the descended thyroid gland. In the normal postfetal condition, the duct atrophies[53, 66]; however, in some individuals it persists and may become cystic. It may also become inflamed and even infected. In these cases, the lesion will present clinically as a mass lesion in the midline of the neck above the thyroid isthmus.

In the normal noninflamed state the thyroglossal duct is lined by columnar epithelium; occasionally squamous epithelium will line parts of the duct. When the duct is inflamed, however, the lining epithelium becomes squamous; if the inflammatory reaction is severe, the lining may be totally destroyed. Normal thyroid tissue can be found in association with the duct in over 60 percent of cases.[53] (Recent studies by deMello et al. indicate that midline cervical cysts may contain, in addition to thyroid in their wall, skin and other derivatives suggesting teratomatous lesions.[15] These authors postulated a histogenetic reason for these findings: because both ectodermal and endodermal derivatives are present in the region of the foramen cecum during fetal life, the thyroglossal duct could contain cells capable of differentiating along various cell lines. However, since preoperatively the distinction between teratomatous and thyroglossal cysts cannot be made, therapy for both is identical[15].)

Neoplasms arising in association with the thyroglossal duct might be expected to be squamous carcinomas, but these are extremely rare [12, 33, 58, 86, 87, 91]; indeed, most tumors occurring in this setting have been thyroid carcinomas, and most are described as papillary or mixed papillary and follicular.[31, 32, 41, 45, 51, 53, 54, 70, 98, 99, 109] Nussbaum et al. described one case of anaplastic carcinoma apparently arising in thyroglossal duct remnants.[69] Medullary carcinoma has not been described; since the parafollicular cells are not found in the median thyroid, this is not unexpected.[53] Tovi et al. reported a Hürthle cell adenoma occurring in thyroglossal duct associated thyroid.[105]

Thyroglossal duct associated carcinoma is rare and constitutes fewer than 1 percent of all thyroid cancers[106]; over 100 cases have been documented in the English literature (Tables 16-2 and 16-3).[31, 32, 37, 41, 45, 49, 51, 53, 67, 70, 87, 93, 98, 106, 109, 115] The sex ratio favors females (1.5:1); this is interesting since benign thyroglossal cysts are more common in males.[28] Most patients are adults, although a few cases

Table 16–2. Thyroglossal Duct Associated Carcinoma I

		(109 cases)	
Histology:	Papillary carcinoma	99	(94%)
	(of which 7 were mixed pap-follicular)		
	Adenocarcinoma, NOS	2	
	Malignant struma	1	
		(102)	
F:M	60:41 (1 unknown)		
Age	6 to 75 years (usually young adults)		
Thyroid gland:			
	Grossly normal	52	
	Microscopically examined	28	
	Carcinoma	5	(16% of histologically examined glands)
Metastases			
	Lymph node metastases	15	
	Other metastases	2	
Recurrences		7	(plus 2 possible)
Died of tumor		2	
History of neck radiation		3	

have been diagnosed in children under age 10.[31, 53] The symptoms consist of a midline neck swelling; the mass has been noted by the patient from days to "many years." Most of the tumors measure between 2 and 3 cm., although lesions as large as 12 cm. have been reported.[31, 32, 41, 51, 53, 67, 70, 87, 93, 98, 106, 109, 115] A history of prior head and neck irradiation has been noted in some cases.[54, 98]

The clinical presentation of thyroglossal duct carcinoma is identical to that of benign thyroglossal duct cysts, i.e., a swelling in the anterior neck.[111] Grossly, the lesions are usually cystic, but portions of the cyst may be occupied by solid or even obviously papillary tissue.[31, 32, 41, 49, 53, 70] On occasion, gritty material has been noted either in the cyst lining or in fluid present within the cyst.[53, 98] The cyst fluid has been described as brown to clear and is usually serous in nature. Microscopically, the most common tumor type is papillary carcinoma; these lesions make up about 95 percent of thyroglossal duct carcinomas. (Indeed, to be precise, these tumors are not strictly of thyroglossal duct origin but are arising from thyroid tissue in the duct wall.) The pattern of these tumors resembles that of usual thyroid papillary carcinomas, with some showing significant areas of follicular differentiation.[54] Psammoma bodies are often seen; the characteristic ground glass nuclei are usually present. Not uncommonly, normal-appearing thyroid follicles will be seen in the surrounding tissue.[31, 53] Invasion of the hyoid bone has been described in some cases.

Tumors arising in this area which have not been described as papillary have been diagnosed as "malignant struma," "adenocarcinoma," or "follicular carcinoma"; most of these cases were reported in the older literature and probably all represent variants of papillary cancer.

Table 16–3. Thyroglossal Duct Associated Carcinoma II

		(109 cases)	
Histology:	Squamous cell carcinoma	7	(6%)
F:M	6:1		
Age	28 to 81 years		
Thyroid gland:	Grossly normal	3	
	Metastases	0	
	Recurrences	3	
	Died of tumor	1	

Seven cases of squamous or epidermoid carcinoma have been reported[12, 33, 58, 86, 87, 91, 114]; these probably are the only tumors which arise from the duct itself, i.e., the lining epithelium. Six squamous cancers have occurred in women ranging in age from 28–81 years. Recurrences were found in three of these women at one to thirteen years after diagnosis. One of these patients died of tumor.[91] In the case of White and Talbert, transition between benign squamous cyst lining and squamous cancer was demonstrated.[114]

One case of anaplastic carcinoma has been recorded[69]; this tumor apparently arose in a benign or ?low-grade malignant follicular thyroid tumor present in thyroglossal duct associated thyroid tissue.

The diagnosis of papillary carcinoma in thyroglossal cysts is rendered after review of the pathology since the clinical suspicion of a tumor is rare in these patients. Fine needle biopsy of the cyst may produce a preoperative diagnosis, however.[41, 93] Therapy is similar to that for benign thyroglossal duct cyst, i.e., the Sistrunk procedure, which involves removal en bloc of the cyst and the hyoid bone.[31, 33, 53, 83] (Indeed, as Hoffman and Schuster indicate,[29] about 8 percent of benign thyroglossal duct cysts have outpouchings which need to be included as part of the surgical excision of the duct to prevent recurrence.)

When the diagnosis of thyroglossal cyst associated thyroid cancer is made, the question of its origin arises: does this tumor represent a metastasis from a primary lesion in the gland, or is the primary site in the region of the cyst? This question has been addressed by many authors. Some consider all thyroglossal duct associated papillary carcinoma as cystic metastases from a thyroid primary.[33, 37] Such authors claim that only squamous cell carcinoma would be expected to arise in the duct itself. Further doubts expressed include the fact that papillary carcinoma is overwhelmingly the most common tumor type (>85 percent) encountered in these thyroglossal remnants; if these are primary in the thyroglossal remnants, why should not the spectrum of thyroid carcinomas be seen, these authors ask. The case of anaplastic cancer reported by Nussbaum et al. certainly partially answers this issue.[69] In addition, since no parafollicular cells would be expected to be present in this midline thyroid, the existence of medullary carcinoma would not be reasonable.[53, 69]

In some reports (about 50 percent of the cases), the thyroid has been examined by scan or grossly at surgery. In 28 (one quarter of the total) cases, thyroidectomy has been performed or the gland was examined microscopically at autopsy.[8–10, 31, 32, 53, 54, 67, 69, 78, 95, 98, 106, 113, 115] In only five of these cases were areas of papillary carcinoma found in the gland; most of these were microscopic foci; however, exhaustive sectioning of the gland was carried out in many cases.[31, 53, 78, 113] The conclusion reached by most of the authors studying this problem has been that the thyroglossal lesion was indeed a primary tumor arising in remnants of thyroid associated with the duct; in those few cases where intrathyroidal tumor has been found, this was considered a separate primary.[31, 53] (On this last point, Katz and Hachigian disagree, considering the thyroid as the primary site and recommending total thyroidectomy.)[37] Most authors thus suggest that therapy should be directed at the midline primary site and that total thyroidectomy is unwarranted in most cases; evaluation of the gland by scan is recommended to rule out gross malignancy.[53]

The behavior of thyroglossal duct associated papillary carcinoma resembles that of thyroid papillary cancer in general. Metastases to lymph nodes have been documented in 15 cases.[3, 8, 20, 31, 39, 53, 67, 78, 98, 106] However, following removal of these nodes, the prognosis has been excellent. Only two patients have died as a result of tumor; each of these had widespread extracervical metastases.[32, 39] Follow-up periods for the reported cases have been significant, ranging from months to more than 20 years; hence it appears that an indolent biologic behavior is characteristic of thyroglossal duct papillary carcinomas.[31, 53, 83, 98] The patient reported by Nussbaum et al. died of her anaplastic thyroid carcinoma.[69]

INTRATRACHEAL AND INTRALARYNGEAL THYROID CARCINOMA

As has been described in Chapter 1, thyroid tissue may occasionally be found within the trachea or larynx.[6, 64, 79] Indeed, Waggoner defined two types of intratracheal thyroid tissue: "false" aberrant thyroid that arises in prenatal or neonatal life and is contiguous with the thyroid and "true" aberrant thyroid, which is isolated thyroid tissue apparently arising early in the embryo.[110]

It is estimated that normal thyroid tissue rests make up between 6 and 7 percent of primary tracheal "tumors."[6]

Carcinoma arising in this ectopic location is very rare. (Tracheal invasion by thyroid cancer is obviously more common.[17]) Fish and Moore[20] quote the report of Waggoner,[110] but underscore doubts about the documentation in this case. Dowling et al. indicate in their review[18] that malignancy occurring primarily in this tissue does occur; these authors reviewed 12 cases previously reported. They accepted five as probably carcinoma (these invaded surrounding tissues, metastasized to nodes, or recurred) and two sarcomas. Pathologic details and documentation in some of these cases was questionable, however. An additional case of "follicular carcinoma" that arose in the trachea and invaded tracheal wall and thyroid cartilage was reported by Donegan and Wood.[17] No pathologic photographs are shown, however.

MEDIASTINAL THYROID CARCINOMA

Although thyroid tissue has been described as an intracardiac tumor, the tissue present in these cases was histologically benign.[35, 72] In addition, nodules of benign thyroid tissue have presented as esophageal masses; none of these has behaved in a malignant fashion.[73, 74]

Thyroid carcinoma apparently arising within substernal or retrosternal goiters has been reported, although most mediastinal goiters are benign.[89] Often this thyroid tissue is connected to the main gland in the neck. However, the mass lesion is present in the mediastinal location. One case each of papillary carcinoma and malignant lymphoma in retrosternal goiter were documented by deSouza and Smith in their review of goiter in this site.[16] Two mediastinal Hürthle cell carcinomas (one diagnosed by fine needle biopsy) were reported by Mishriki et al.[57] and Shin et al.[92] The present author has seen two cases of follicular carcinoma and one case of a Hürthle cell cancer arising in large goiters with mediastinal extension; in each of these the neoplasm was present in (? arose in) the substernal portion of the gland.

Normal thyroid tissue occurring within the capsule of medially located perithyroidal lymph nodes has given rise to debate. It is the belief of the present author and others[5] that such benign-appearing tissue in the nodal capsule does indeed represent developmental rests and does not indicate metastatic thyroid carcinoma. This finding may be equated with so-called benign nevus cells in lymph node, which can be found in cervical, axillary, or inguinal nodes. Of course, if the thyroid shows papillary configuration, ground glass nuclei, or psammoma bodies, or if the thyroid tissue replaces portions of the node itself, then the diagnosis of metastatic tumor must be made.[22, 43, 53, 55, 84]

LATERAL ABERRANT THYROID

This topic, also discussed in Chapter 1 of this monograph, needs to be laid to rest. The presence of thyroid tissue, whether normal in appearance or showing features of papillary thyroid carcinoma, within a lymph node that is located lateral to the jugular vein indicates metastatic thyroid carcinoma.[5, 7, 11, 21, 50, 53, 61, 112] Finding normal thyroid in these nodes does not mean developmental anomaly! Finding a papillary tumor in these nodes does not mean that tumor arose in this area; a primary papillary thyroid cancer is virtually always found in the main gland in these cases. The intrathyroidal lesion may be minute and careful examination of many sections may be required to define it, but it is there!

On the other hand, the presence of thyroid tissue that is normal or goitrous in appearance but which is *not associated with lymph nodes* in the lateral neck may represent a benign process. As noted in Chapter 1, this may occur following neck trauma or surgery, or may be found in patients with large nodular goiters or goiters due to chronic thyroiditis. As described elegantly by Kraemer, these thyroid remnants may or may not be connected to the main gland.[44] They are always histologically benign; clinical follow-up indicates they are biologically benign also.[1]

OVARIAN THYROID

Not strictly a developmental anomaly, ovarian thyroid represents differentiation in a teratoma. The presence of normal-appearing thyroid tissue in an ovarian teratoma is common and the incidence of this finding depends on the care with which ordinary cystic teratomas of the ovary are examined histologically. Estimates of incidence range from 0.2 to 1.3 percent of all ovarian tumors.[117] Bilaterality is noted in 5 to 6 percent of cases.[62, 117] Functional abnormalities are found in 5 percent.[82, 117]

The diagnosis of "struma ovarii" should be reserved for those teratomas in which a considerable portion of the lesion is composed of thyroid tissue; various authors indicate anywhere from 50 to 100 percent of the teratoma should consist of thyroid before the designation of struma ovarii can be made.[62, 117] The gross lesion usually shows solid brown shiny tissue resembling nodular goiter.[40] Thyroid in these lesions usually appears normal or more often shows features suggesting colloid goiter, with large dilated macrofollicles and extensive colloid storage.[40, 117] Thyroglobulin similar biochemically and immunohistologically to that of the normal gland is present.[40, 52]

A rare case of ovarian thyroid showing changes of Hashimoto's thyroiditis has been described by Erez et al.[19]

Most struma ovarii presents as an ovarian mass; evidence of hyperfunction is very rare.[40] However, hyperthyroidism has been reported and has been apparently caused by the ovarian lesion. Benign struma ovarii may also be associated with ascites and clinically raise the suspicion of ovarian carcinoma.[40]

Neoplasms arising in struma ovarii are very rare[23, 24, 27, 40, 82, 116, 118] and many form the basis of case reports. Malignancy has been reported in up to 5 percent of struma ovarii.[82, 118] However, some of these cases represent poorly circumscribed follicular nodules called carcinoma, but behaving in a totally benign fashion. In addition, other cases may represent strumal carcinoid (see below). Documented metastasis of a recognizable thyroid carcinoma in struma ovarii is very unusual. Pardo-Minian et al.[71] noted 45 reported cases of "histologically" malignant struma ovarii, but only 17 of these had metastasized. These authors believe, and the present author concurs, that tumors arising in struma ovarii behave in a biologically aggressive fashion only if the tumor is clearly invasive or has metastasized.

We have recently had the opportunity to review the topic of papillary carcinoma arising in ovarian thyroid.[82] In some of the reported cases, histologic proof of carcinoma is lacking; in others, the photomicrographs are not convincing—papillary hyperplastic foci have been interpreted as carcinoma or the lesions are follicular nodules with encroachment of the tumor "capsule." However, some cases indeed show features of thyroid papillary cancer, including nuclear features and psammoma bodies; some of the tumors have metastasized, as did the case we had the opportunity to study. In our case, microscopic metastases of papillary tumor were present in the superficial cortex of the contralateral ovary; immunoperoxidase staining of these foci for thyroglobulin showed strong reactivity, proving the thyroid histogenesis of this tumor.

The biologic behavior of thyroid cancer arising in struma ovarii is difficult to assess because of the few cases reported and because therapy has varied widely over the years. A few cases have been fatal, with metastases to the peritoneum, liver, brain, and other organs.[40, 117] Some reported long-term survivals following surgery and radiotherapy are known, but late metastases are seen, with survival rates of eight to 20 years having been reported before tumor recurrence. So-called "benign strumatosis," i.e., benign-appearing thyroid follicles in the peritoneum, reflects metastases of a low-grade thyroid carcinoma from a struma ovarii and is not benign.

The question of what to do with the cervical thyroid always is raised in these patients; if the gland is normal by palpation and scan, it probably can be left in place.[82] However, if metastases are to be treated with radioiodine, thyroid ablation would be needed. In the case reported by Rosenblum et al., the ascites fluid contained metastatic tumor, as did the opposite ovary; treatment with intraperitoneal radioactive phosphorus was chosen with apparent success.[82]

One unique case of malignant lymphoma arising in struma ovarii has been reported.[90]

The topic of ovarian thyroid would remain incompletely addressed without the mention of so-called strumal carcinoid tumors. These neoplasms are composed of recognizable thyroid follicles admixed with tissue that resembles carcinoid arranged in a trabecular pattern. Over 120 documented cases are reported.[4, 13, 14, 26, 42, 60, 63, 76, 80, 96, 100, 103, 107, 108] Patients with strumal carcinoid range in age from 21 to 77 years,[80, 96, 103] although the majority are postmenopausal women. The usual presentation is that of an ovarian mass, although one case of carcinoid syndrome is known.[108] Occasional cases of hyperestrogenic symptoms (endometrial hyperplasia, uterine bleeding) have been described, but these effects have been attributed to associated ovarian stromal luteinization near the tumors.[80]

Grossly, strumal carcinoids may appear in three forms: pure strumal carcinoid; within a dermoid cyst; or associated with another neoplasm.[80] When pure, the tumors are solid yellow to tan homogeneous masses ranging in size from 1 to 20 centimeters. Occasional areas resembling colloid-filled follicles can be seen. When arising in association with a dermoid cyst, the strumal carcinoid is usually a solid nodule of yellow tissue attached to the cyst wall; sizes range from 4 to 20 centimeters. Those strumal carcinoid tumors associated with other ovarian tumors can show an appearance similar to the above, but the associated ovarian neoplasm may be a solid mature teratoma or a mucinous cystic neoplasm.[80]

Histologically, the thyroid and carcinoid tissue are always admixed, although one or another component may predominate. The carcinoid is usually of the trabecular variety; the thyroid tissue resembles normal gland, including the presence of calcium oxalate crystals within the colloid.[80, 103] The cells of the carcinoid component may contain argentaffin granules, which by ultrastructural study correspond to neurosecretory granules.[80] Occasionally intracellular acid mucin is found.[96] Rarely, amyloid has been identified in the tumor stroma.[60] Immunohistochemical studies have shown the presence of thyroglobulin[25] and thyroxine[108] in the thyroid tissue; calcitonin, serotonin, and other peptide hormones have been localized to the carcinoid.[4, 13, 14, 25, 42]

The prognosis for strumal carcinoids is excellent. Most patients appear cured following excision of the tumor. One patient in the large series of Robboy and Scully[80] showed extension beyond the ovary; however, that patient also was cured by surgery. One woman died of metastatic disease.[80] The literature recommends bilateral oophorectomy and hysterectomy in the older patient and unilateral salpingo-oophorectomy in the younger woman.[103]

The question of the histogenetic classification of this tumor has been debated. Some authors felt that the tissue that appeared to be thyroid was part of the carcinoid[26, 76]; the presence of thyroglobulin and thyroxine in the tumor negated this theory. Some authors believe that strumal carcinoid represents a medullary thyroid carcinoma arising in ovarian thyroid tissue; support for this view has come from the occasional presence of amyloid in the stroma, the presence of calcitonin in the tumor, and the presence of calcitonin-containing cells in and around nearby thyroid follicles.[4, 13, 25, 26, 60, 108] However, as Stagno et al. point out,[100] the carcinoid cells can grow to replace the following epithelium, leading to a pattern reminiscent of C-cell hyperplasia in the thyroid. Furthermore, no case of strumal carcinoid so far tested has contained immunoreactive CEA, whereas virtually all medullary thyroid carcinomas do.[100] Recent studies seem to support a common cell origin for the thyroid and carcinoid components, i.e., a derivation from the endodermal germ cell precursors of the teratoma.[42, 96, 103]

OTHER LOCATIONS

Kurman and Prabha reported a case of a vaginal tumor in a 3-year-old girl which was composed of thyroid and parathyroid tissue.[47] These authors postulated a teratomatous origin for this finding. The tissue was histologically benign.

Ruchti et al. reported an apparently unique case of a thyroglobulin-containing follicular tumor in the region of the sella turcica in a 71-year-old woman.[85] The tumor was initially diagnosed on clinical grounds as a chordoma; the lesion was evaluated pathologically at autopsy because of the patient's sudden death. Careful examination of thyroid gland and the ovaries failed to disclose a primary site and the authors postulated an origin in ectopic thyroid in the region of the sella. Although they indicate that an embryologic explanation is difficult to define since thyroid tissue should not be found as a developmental rest above the level of the tongue, the authors could find no other reasonable explanation for their patient's tumor. The possibility of a tumor originating in a teratoma in this region was considered, but no evidence of teratoma was identified.[85]

The recent description by Rosen and Scott of cystic hypersecretory carcinoma of the breast[81] needs to be mentioned for completeness, since this lesion may resemble well-differentiated thyroid follicles within the breast. Cystic secretory hyperplasia and carcinoma represent an unusual type of breast duct proliferation in which the dilated ducts contain eosinophilic material histologically resembling colloid. In Rosen's cases immunoperoxidase staining for thyroglobulin failed to localize this hormone in any case. Hence, it appears that these unusual breast proliferations represent a peculiar histologic pattern unrelated to thyroid tissue.

SUMMARY

This chapter has reviewed lesions occurring in thyroid tissue located in areas other than the lower anterior neck region. It has stressed the neoplasms which can be encountered at these sites. The literature review has discussed debates and issues still unresolved, especially regarding thyroglossal duct associated carcinoma and ovarian strumal carcinoid.

REFERENCES

1. Asp, A., Hasbargen, J., et al.: Ectopic thyroid tissue on thallium/technetium parathyroid scan. Arch. Intern. Med. 147:595–596, 1987.
2. Baughman, R. A.: Lingual thyroid and lingual thyroglossal tract remnants. Oral Surg. 34:781–799, 1972.
3. Bhagaven, B. S., Govinda, D. R., and Weinberg, T.: Carcinoma of thyroglossal duct cyst. Surgery 67:281–292, 1970.
4. Blaustein, A.: Calcitonin secreting strumal-carcinoid of the ovary. Hum. Pathol. 10:222–228, 1979.
5. Block, M. A., Wylie, J. H., et al.: Does benign thyroid tissue occur in the lateral part of the neck? Am. J. Surg. 112:476–481, 1966.
6. Bone, R. C., Biller, H. F., and Irwin, T. M.: Intralaryngotracheal thyroid. Ann. Otol. 81:424–428, 1972.
7. Butler, J. J., Tulinius, H., et al.: Significance of thyroid tissue in lymph nodes associated with carcinoma of the head, neck or lung. Cancer 20:103–112, 1967.
8. Choy, F. J., Ward, R., and Richardson, R.: Carcinoma of the thyroglossal duct. Am. J. Surg. 108:361–369, 1964.
9. Clawson, J., and Kimball, H.: Papillary adenocarcinoma of the thyroglossal duct cyst. Ariz. Med. 19:80–82, 1962.
10. Coon, W. W.: Thyroid carcinoma—three unusual problems in diagnosis and management. Am. J. Surg. 109:629–632, 1965.
11. Dalgaard, J. G., and Wetteland, P.: Lateral cervical thyroid metastases: A followup study of 30 cases. Acta Chir. Scand. 111:431–443, 1956.
12. Dalgaard, J. B., and Wetteland, P.: Thyroglossal anomalies: A followup study of 58 cases. Acta Chir. Scand. 111:444–455, 1956.
13. Dayal, Y., Tashjian, A. H., and Wolfe, H. J.: Immunocytochemical localization of calcitonin-producing cells in a strumal carcinoid with amyloid stroma. Cancer 43:1331–1338, 1979.
14. DeMaurizi, M., Bondi, A., et al.: Strumal carcinoid of the ovary: an immunohistochemical and electron microscopic study. Tumori 69:261–267, 1983.
15. deMello, D. E., Lima, J. A., and Liapis, H.: Midline cervical cysts in children; thyroglossal anomalies. Arch. Otolaryngol. Head Neck Surg. 113:418–420, 1987.
16. deSouza, F. M., and Smith, P. E.: Retrosternal goiter. J. Otolaryngol. 12:393–396, 1983.
17. Donegan, J. O., and Wood, M. D.: Intratracheal thyroid—familial occurrence. Laryngoscope 95:6–8, 1985.
18. Dowling, E. A., Johnson, I. M., et al.: Intratracheal goiter: A clinicopathologic review. Ann. Surg. 156:258–267, 1962.
19. Erez, S. E., Richart, R. M., and Shettles, L. B.: Hashimoto's disease in a benign cystic teratoma of the ovary. Am. J. Obstet. Gynecol. 92:273–274, 1965.
20. Fish, J., and Moore, R. M.: Ectopic thyroid tissue and ectopic thyroid carcinoma. Ann. Surg. 157:212–222, 1963.
21. Frantz, V. K., Forsythe, R., et al.: Lateral aberrant thyroids. Ann. Surg. 115:161–183, 1942.
22. Gerard-Marchant, R.: Thyroid follicle inclusions in cervical lymph nodes. Arch. Pathol. 77:633–637, 1964.

23. Gonzalez-Angulo, A., Kaupman, R. H., et al.: Adenocarcinoma of thyroid arising in struma ovarii (malignant struma ovarii). Obstet. Gynecol. *21:*567–576, 1963.
24. Gould, S. F., Lopez, R. L., and Speers, W. C.: Malignant struma ovarii. J. Reprod. Med. *28:*415–419, 1983.
25. Greco, M. A., LiVolsi, V. A., et al.: Strumal carcinoid of the ovary; An analysis of its components. Cancer *43:*1380–1388, 1979.
26. Hart, W. R., and Regezi, J. A.: Strumal carcinoid of the ovary: Ultrastructural observations and long-term followup study. Am. J. Clin. Pathol. *69:*356–359, 1978.
27. Haselton, P. S., Kelehan, P., et al.: Benign and malignant struma ovarii. Arch. Pathol. Lab. Med. *102:*180–184, 1978.
28. Hawkins, D. B., Jacobsen, B. E., and Klatt, E. C.: Cysts of the thyroglossal duct. Laryngoscope *92:*1254–1258, 1982.
29. Hoffman, M. A., and Schuster, S. R.: Thyroglossal duct remnants in infants and children: Reevaluation of histopathology and methods for resection. Ann. Otol. Rhinol. Laryngol. *97:*483–486, 1988.
30. Jain S. N.: Lingual thyroid. Int. Surg. *52:*320–325, 1969.
31. Jaques, D. A., Chambers, R. G., and Oertel, J. E.: Thyroglossal tract carcinoma: A review of the literature and addition of eighteen cases. Am. J. Surg. *120:*439–446, 1970.
32. Joseph, T. J., and Komorowski, R. A.: Thyroglossal duct carcinoma. Hum. Pathol. *6:*717–729, 1975.
33. Judd, E. S.: Thyroglossal duct cysts and sinuses. Surg. Clin. North Am. *43:*1023–1032, 1963.
34. Kansal, P., Sakati, N., et al.: Lingual thyroid. Arch. Intern. Med. *147:*2046–2048, 1987.
35. Kantelip, B., Lusson, J. R., et al.: Intracardiac ectopic thyroid. Hum. Pathol. *17:*1293–1296, 1986.
36. Kaplan, M., Kauli, R., et al.: Ectopic thyroid tissue: A clinical study of 30 children and review. J. Pediatr. *92:*205–209, 1978.
37. Katz, A. D., and Hachigian, M. P.: Thyroglossal duct cysts: A thirty year experience with emphasis on occurrence in older patients. Arch. Surg. *155:*741–743, 1988.
38. Katz, A. D., and Zager, W. J.: The lingual thyroid: Its diagnosis and treatment. Arch. Surg. *102:*582–585, 1971.
39. Keeling, J. H., and Ochsner, A.: Carcinoma in thyroglossal duct remnants. Cancer *12:*596–600, 1959.
40. Kempers, R. D., Dockerty, M. B. et al.: Struma ovarii—ascitic, hyperthyroid and asymptomatic syndromes. Ann. Intern. Med. *72:*883–893, 1970.
41. Kimberley, B., Cohen, J., and Posalsky, I.: Papillary thyroid carcinoma within a thyroglossal duct cyst. Arch. Otolaryngol. Head Neck Surg. *113:*206–208, 1987.
42. Kimura, N., Sasano, N., and Tsuneo, N.: Evidence of hybrid cell of thyroid follicular cell and carcinoid cell in strumal carcinoid. Int. J. Gynecol. Pathol. *5:*269–277, 1986.
43. Klopp, C. T., and Kirson, S. M.: Therapeutic problems with ectopic noncancerous follicular thyroid tissue in the neck. Ann. Surg. *163:*653–664, 1966.
44. Kraemer, B. B.: Thyroid. *In:* Silva, E., and Kraemer, B. B. (eds.): Intraoperative Pathologic Diagnosis. Baltimore, Williams and Wilkins Co., 1987, pp. 51–69.
45. Kristensen, S., Juul, A., and Moesner, J.: Thyroglossal cyst carcinoma. J. Laryngol. Otol. *98:*1277–1280, 1984.
46. Kuehn, P. G., Newell, R. C., and Reed, J. F.: Exophthalmos in a woman with lingual, subhyoid and lateral lobe thyroid glands. N. Engl. J. Med. *274:*652–654, 1966.
47. Kurman, R. J., and Prabha, A. C.: Thyroid and parathyroid glands in the vaginal wall. Am. J. Clin. Pathol. *59:*503–507, 1973.
48. Larochelle, D., Arcand, P., et al.: Ectopic thyroid tissue—a review of the literature. J. Otolaryngol. *8:*523–530, 1979.
49. LaRouere, M. J., Drake, A. F., et al.: Evaluation and management of carcinoma arising in a thyroglossal duct cyst. Am. J. Otolaryngol. *8:*351–355, 1987.
50. Lester, I. A.: Two cases of lateral aberrant thyroid. Med. J. Australia *1:*1117–1118, 1966.
51. Liu, A. H. F., and Littler, E. R.: Thyroid carcinoma originating in thyroglossal cyst. Am. Surg. *36:*546–548, 1970.
52. LiVolsi, V. A., LoGerfo, P., and Feind, C.: Thyroglobulin in struma ovarii. J. Surg. Res. *25:*12–14, 1978.
53. LiVolsi, V. A., Perzin, K. H., and Savetsky, L.: Carcinoma arising in median ectopic thyroid (including thyroglossal duct tissue). Cancer *34:*1303–1315, 1974.
54. McGuirt, W. F., and Marshall, R. B.: Postirradiation carcinoma in a thyroglossal duct remnant: Follicular variant of papillary thyroid carcinoma. Head Neck Surg. *2:*420–424, 1980.
55. Meyer, J. S., and Steinberg, L. S.: Microscopically benign thyroid follicles in cervical lymph nodes. Cancer *24:*302–311, 1969.
56. Mill, W. A., Gowing, N. F., et al.: Carcinoma of the lingual thyroid treated with radioactive iodine. Lancet *1:*76–79, 1959.
57. Mishriki, Y. Y., Lane, B. P., et al.: Hürthle cell tumor arising in the mediastinal ectopic thyroid and diagnosed by fine needle aspiration. Acta Cytol. *27:*188–192, 1983.
58. Mobini, J., Krouse, T. B., and Klinghoffer, J. F.: Squamous cell carcinoma arising in a thyroglossal duct cyst. Am. Surg. *40:*290–294, 1974.

59. Monroe, J. B., and Fahey, D.: Lingual thyroid: Case report and review of the literature. Arch. Otolaryngol. *101*:574–576, 1975.
60. Morgan, K., Wells, M., and Scott, J. S.: Ovarian strumal carcinoid tumor with amyloid stroma—report of a case with 20-year followup. Gynecol. Oncol. *22*:121–128, 1985.
61. Moses, D. C., Thompson, N. W., and Nishiyama, R. H.: Ectopic thyroid tissue in the neck. Benign or malignant? Cancer *38*:361–365, 1976.
62. Mulligan, R. M.: Pathogenesis of teratoid tumors of the ovary and testis. Pathol. Annu. *10*:271–298, 1975.
63. Murayama, H., Kikuchi, M., and Imai, T.: Ovarian carcinoid composed of argyrophil and argentaffin cells. Am. J. Surg. Pathol. *5*:77–84, 1981.
64. Myers, E. N., and Pantangco, I. P.: Intratracheal thyroid. Laryngoscope *85*:1833–1840, 1975.
65. Myerson, M., and Smith, H. W.: Lingual thyroid—A review. Conn. Med. *30*:341–344, 1966.
66. Nachlas, N. E.: Thyroglossal duct cysts. Ann. Otorhinol. Larynx *59*:381–390, 1950.
67. Nathanson, S.: Carcinoma in thyroglossal duct cysts—a review. Trans. Am. Acad. Ophthalmol. Otolaryngol. *82*:571–575, 1976.
68. Nienas, F. W., Gorman, C. A., et al.: Lingual thyroid: Clinical characteristics of 15 cases. Ann. Intern. Med. *79*:205–210, 1973.
69. Nussbaum, M., Buchwald, R. P. et al.: Anaplastic carcinoma arising from median ectopic thyroid (thyroglossal duct remnants). Cancer *48*:2724–2728, 1981.
70. Page, C. P., Kemmerer, W. T., et al.: Thyroid carcinomas arising in thyroglossal ducts. Ann. Surg. *180*:799–803, 1974.
71. Pardo-Mindan, F. J., and Vazquez, J. J.: Malignant struma ovarii. Cancer *51*:337–343, 1983.
72. Pollice, L., and Caruso, G.: Struma cordis: Ectopic thyroid goiter in the right ventricle. Arch. Pathol. Lab. Med. *110*:452–453, 1986.
73. Porto, G.: Esophageal nodule of thyroid tissue. Laryngoscope *70*:1336–1338, 1960.
74. Postlewait, R. W., and Detman, D. E.: Ectopic thyroid nodule in the esophagus. Ann. Thor. Surg. *19*:98–100, 1975.
75. Potdar, G. G., and Desai, P. B.: Carcinoma of the lingual thyroid. Laryngoscope *81*:427–429, 1971.
76. Ranchod, M., Kempson, R. L., and Dorgeloh, J. R.: Strumal carcinoid of the ovary. Cancer *37*:1913–1922, 1976.
77. Reaume, C. E., and Sofie, V. L.: Lingual thyroid: Review of the literature and report of a case. Oral Surg. *45*:841–845, 1978.
78. Rees, C. E., and Brown, M. J.: Cysts of the thyroglossal duct. Am. J. Surg. *85*:597–599, 1953.
79. Richardson, G. M., and Assor, D.: Thyroid tissue within the larynx. Laryngoscope *81*:120–125, 1975.
80. Robboy, S. J., and Scully, R. E.: Strumal carcinoid of the ovary: An analysis of 50 cases of a distinctive tumor composed of thyroid tissue and carcinoid. Cancer *46*:2019–2034, 1980.
81. Rosen, P. P., and Scott, M.: Cystic hypersecretory duct carcinoma of the breast. Am. J. Surg. Pathol. *8*:31–41, 1984.
82. Rosenblum, N. G., LiVolsi, V. A., et al.: Malignant struma ovarii. Gynecol. Oncol. *32*:224–227, 1989.
83. Roses, D. F., Snively, S. L., et al.: Carcinoma of the thyroglossal duct. Am. J. Surg. *145*:266–269, 1983.
84. Roth, L. M.: Inclusions of nonneoplastic thyroid tissue within cervical lymph nodes. Cancer *128*:105–111, 1965.
85. Ruchti, C., Balli-Antunes, M., and Gerber, H. A.: Follicular tumor in the sellar region without primary cancer of the thyroid. Am. J. Clin. Pathol. *87*:776–780, 1987.
86. Ruppman, E., and Georgsson, G.: Squamous carcinoma of the thyroglossal duct. Ger. Med. Monthly *11*:442–445, 1966.
87. Saharia, P. C.: Carcinoma arising in thyroglossal duct remnant: Case reports and review of the literature. Br. J. Surg. *62*:689–691, 1975.
88. Sauk, J. J.: Ectopic lingual thyroid. J. Pathol. *102*:239–242, 1970.
89. Salvatore, M., and Gallo, A.: Accessory thyroid in the anterior mediastinum. J. Nucl. Med. *16*:1135–1136, 1975.
90. Seifer, D. B. Weiss, L. M., and Kempson, R. L.: Malignant lymphoma arising within thyroid tissue in a mature cystic teratoma. Cancer *58*:2459–2461, 1986.
91. Shepard, G. H., and Rosenfeld, G.: Carcinoma of thyroglossal duct remnants. Am. J. Surg. *115*:125–130, 1968.
92. Shin, C. S., Bakst, A. A., and Levowitz, B. S.: Intrathoracic goiter located in the posterior mediastinum. N. Y. State J. Med. *72*:1723–1727, 1972.
93. Silverman, P. M., Degesys, G. E., et al.: Papillary carcinoma in a thyroglossal duct cyst. CT findings. J. Comp. Asst. Tomog. *9*:806–808, 1985.
94. Smithers, D. W.: Carcinoma associated with thyroglossal duct anomalies. *In:* Smithers, D. (ed.): Tumours of the Thyroid Gland. Edinburgh, E. & S. Livingstone, 1970, pp. 155–165.
95. Snedecor, P. A., and Groshong, L. E.: Carcinoma of the thyroglossal duct. Surgery *58*:969–978, 1965.

96. Snyder, R. R., and Tavassoli, F. A.: Ovarian strumal carcinoid: Immunohistochemical, ultrastructural and clinicopathologic observations. Int. J. Gynecol Pathol. *5:*187–201, 1986.
97. Soames, J. V.: A review of the histology of the tongue in the region of the foramen cecum. Oral Surg. *36:*220–224, 1973.
98. Sohn, N., Gumport, S. L., and Blum, M.: Thyroglossal duct carcinoma. N.Y. State J. Med. *74:*2004–2005, 1974.
99. Stanley, D. G., and Robinson, F. W.: Thyroid carcinoma in thyroglossal duct cysts. Am. Surg. *36:*581–582, 1970.
100. Stagno, P. A., Petra, R. E., and Hart, W. R.: Strumal carcinoids of the ovary: An immunohistologic and ultrastructural study. Arch. Pathol. Lab. Med. *111:*440–446, 1987.
101. Steinwald, O. P., Muehrcke, R. C., and Economou, S. G.: Surgical correction of complete lingual ectopia of the thyroid gland. Surg. Clin. North Am. *50:*1177–1186, 1970.
102. Strickland, A. L., Macfie, J. A., et al.: Ectopic thyroid glands simulating thyroglossal duct cysts. J.A.M.A. *208:*307–310, 1969.
103. Talerman, A.: Carcinoid tumors of the ovary. J. Cancer Res. Clin. Oncol. *107:*125–135, 1984.
104. Talib, H.: Lingual thyroid. Br. J. Clin. Pract. *20:*322–323. 1966.
105. Tovi, F., Fliss, D. M., and Inbar-Yania, I.: Hürthle cell adenoma of the thyroglossal duct. Head Neck Surg. *10:*346–349, 1988.
106. Trail, M. L., Zeringue, G. P., and Chicola, J. P., Carcinoma in thyroglossal duct remnants. Laryngoscope *87:*1685–1691, 1977.
107. Tsubura, A., and Sasaki, M.: Strumal carcinoid of the ovary. Acta Pathol. Jpn. *36:*1383–1390, 1986.
108. Ulbright, T. M., Roth, L. M., and Ehrlich, C. E.: Ovarian strumal carcinoid: An immunocytochemical and ultrastructural study of two cases. Am. J. Clin. Pathol. 77:622–631, 1982.
109. Villet, W. T., and Kemp, C. B.: Thyroglossal duct carcinoma. S. Afr. Med. J. *60:*795–796, 1981.
110. Waggoner, L. G.: Intralaryngeal intratracheal thyroid. Ann. Otol. Rhinol. Laryngol. *67:*61–71, 1958.
111. Wampler, H. W., Krolls, S. O., and Johnson, R. P.: Thyroglossal tract cyst. Oral Surg. *45:*32–38, 1978.
112. Ward, R.: Relation of tumors of lateral aberrant thyroid tissue to malignant disease of the thyroid gland. Arch. Surg. *40:*606–615, 1940.
113. Weber, A. O.: Carcinoma of the thyroglossal duct. Calif. Med. *108:*127–129, 1968.
114. White, I. L., and Talbert, W. M.: Squamous cell carcinoma arising in thyroglossal duct remnant cyst epithelium. Otolaryngol. Head Neck Surg. *90:*25–31, 1982.
115. Widstrom, A., Magnusson, P., et al.: Adenocarcinoma originating in thyroglossal ducts. Ann Otol. Rhinol. Laryngol. *85:*286–290, 1976.
116. Willemse, P. H. B., Oosterhuis, J. W., et al.: Malignant struma ovarii treated by ovariectomy, thyroidectomy and ^{131}I administration. Cancer *60:*178–182, 1987.
117. Woodruff, J. D., Rauh, J. T., and Markley, R. L.: Ovarian struma. Obstet. Gynecol. *27:*194–202, 1966.
118. Yannopoulos, D., Yannopoulos, K., and Ossowski, R.: Malignant struma ovarii. Pathol. Annu. *11:*403–413, 1976.

III

Special Diagnostic Techniques in Thyroid Pathology

In this final part of the monograph, the topics of special techniques as they apply to thyroid disease diagnosis will be discussed. These techniques include cytology, large bore needle biopsy, and frozen sections which are described in Chapter 17; electron microscopy, flow cytometric analysis, and immunohistochemistry which are discussed in Chapter 18. A brief mention of recent developments, such as oncogenes in thyroid neoplasms, is also included.

Chapter 19, entitled "All You Wanted to Know About Thyroid Pathology But Were Afraid to Ask," has engendered some debate among my close colleagues because of its title. Some have suggested that this chapter's title may appear capricious. However, this title is indeed accurate, since in this brief chapter I discuss the ten most frequently asked questions (hence reflecting the ten most commonly encountered problems in thyroid morphologic pathology). Therefore, despite mixed reviews about the title appearing facetious, I have decided to retain it.

17

CYTOLOGY AND NEEDLE BIOPSY

The diagnostic approach to the patient with the clinically evident thyroid nodule has changed dramatically in recent years. Whereas in the days before the availability of aspiration and large needle biopsy, patients with solitary and/or dominant thyroid nodules underwent numerous costly diagnostic tests (radioiodine or other nuclide scans, ultrasonographic examinations, or suppression trials), in the modern era the initial approach to such a patient is often a needle biopsy.[1, 3, 4, 7, 9, 16, 18, 20, 26, 32, 41, 53, 57, 62, 72, 81, 94, 95, 97, 98, 102, 104, 107, 110, 116] Miller et al. summarized the reported experience on sensitivity and specificity data for these various diagnostic modalities in evaluating thyroid nodules (Table 17–1).[88]

It has become the practice in many large centers that the initial and only approach to the patient with a thyroid nodule is a needle aspiration biopsy. This cost-effective diagnostic and screening technique has replaced the use of radionuclide scans and ultrasonography. Silverman et al.[109] and Miller et al.[83] indicate that the yearly cost saving on the U.S. national health care bill would be about 15 million dollars if fine needle biopsy were used on all thyroid nodules. This approach avoids the costs of many radiologic and laboratory tests and the costs associated with surgery.

Some authors caution, however, that the patient with the hyperfunctioning nodule may undergo surgery since the cytologic diagnosis of hypercellular nodule may thus be made.[9, 104] In addition, ultrasound may pick up multiple small nodules in a gland which clinically contains a solitary and hence suspicious lesion, leading to unnecessary biopsy and possibly surgery.[9] However, the ease, cost effectiveness, and patient acceptance of the fine needle aspiration biopsy has overcome these concerns; the use of scans and ultrasound for evaluation of thyroid nodules is virtually becoming obsolete. Franklyn et al. noted that the number of technetium[m99] scans plummeted from 77 in 1984 to three in 1986 in their hospital once the reliability of aspiration biopsy was appreciated.[33] Diagnostic surgical procedures for thyroid nodules have decreased by more than 50 percent[15, 47]; the percentage of malignant lesions surgically removed (i.e., "necessary surgery") has tripled.[47, 83, 97]

Table 17–1. Techniques Used in Thyroid Nodule Evaluation (Miller et al.[88])

	FNA	LNB	Clinical Exam	Ultrasound
Sensitivity	66–93%	98–99%	98%	89–100%
Specificity	47–95%	45–100%	13%	33–52%

Fine needle aspiration biopsy generates a cytologic sample and often a histologic preparation, i.e., a cell block. The use of larger bore needles (14–18 gauge; Tru-cut, Vim-Silverman) yields tissue samples which are processed in routine manner for generating histologic slides. Either of these techniques can be useful in diagnosing thyroid lesions and/or in providing guidance as to which nodules should be surgically removed.[3, 7, 9–11, 15, 18, 23–26, 29–31, 34, 39, 40, 43, 46, 47, 49, 54, 69, 72, 76, 77, 80–83, 85, 88, 91, 92, 94–96, 98, 99, 101, 102, 108, 109, 114, 116–122, 124, 125] The two biopsy methods have different yields and different complications. Thus, fine needle aspiration biopsy is associated with virtually no mortality, minimal morbidity and has never been proved to result in needle track seeding.[45] The diagnostic accuracy of this test, however, is excellent for papillary and anaplastic and less so for medullary carcinomas; however, in the current author's opinion, fine needle aspiration biopsy provides limited information regarding follicular neoplasms since the periphery of the lesion, i.e., the presence or absence of invasion, cannot be assessed. In addition, a cellular hyperplastic (adenomatous or adenomatoid) nodule may be difficult to distinguish from a true neoplasm by cytologic criteria.

On the other hand, the larger bore needle biopsy can be associated with a greater although still acceptable morbidity (usually bleeding)[10, 29]; on rare occasions needle track seeding of cancer has been documented.[121] In many cases, since the sample obtained is larger than with fine needle aspiration biopsy, diagnosis can be rendered more readily; on occasion since the larger cutting needle can sample the nodule's capsule, evidence of invasion may be identified and the diagnosis of follicular carcinoma may be made (although this is rare[86]).

This chapter will summarize some of the extensive experience with needle biopsy diagnosis of thyroid lesions; since this is a rapidly proliferating field and newer series appear in the literature constantly, this review cannot be all-inclusive. The references listed include the initial, seminal, or major review articles and chapters on the topic of needle biopsy. I will attempt to list the major diagnostic criteria utilized for the diagnosis of the major nonneoplastic and neoplastic thyroid lesions. (The reader is referred to original articles for further discussion and illustration of diagnostic criteria.) I will also tabulate, using major large case series, the diagnostic yields, correlations with histologic diagnoses, and false positive and false negative rates. In addition, I will attempt to document some of the diagnostic pitfalls and dilemmas that can be common enough to cause real problems for the pathologist.

CYTOLOGY OF NORMAL THYROID

The histology of the normal thyroid is recapitulated in its cytology. The follicles can be seen in cross section, or en face. In the former case, one sees a circlet of bland-appearing cells surrounding central colloid; in the latter, one sees a lattice work or honeycomb formation,[63] consisting of a monolayer sheet composed of uniform cells with defined cell boundaries and central nuclei.

CYTOLOGY OF NONNEOPLASTIC INFLAMMATORY CONDITIONS OF THE THYROID

Nodular Goiter. Cytologic features similar to those of normal thyroid are noted in nodular goiter, since here the proliferation is of bland follicles, and irregularities of outline and nuclear features are not seen. Of course, in nodular goiter, superimposed degenerative changes, such as hemorrhage, fibrosis, and calcification, may be noted. However, in the usual case, the epithelial changes are cytologically bland. Kini,[63] Miller et al.[82, 86] and others [33, 106, 111, 130] have described the cytologic features of nodular goiter as consisting of colloid and benign follicular cells. Depending upon the stage of the goiter, colloid may be scant or abundant; if the latter, the colloid stained with Romanowsky stain appears as an acellular material with retraction artifact resembling cracks on the slide. With other stains, colloid appears as large chunks of blue-green to orange amorphous material. Within the colloid, small groups of follicular cells may be found. In hyperplastic areas of a goiter, the follicles predominate; the cellularity of the specimen may be marked. There is a gradual increase in nuclear size from colloid nodules through hypercellular ones to follicular neoplasms; in an individual lesion, however, the distinctions may be difficult.[63, 114]

The cytologic counterparts of the degenerative changes in nodular goiter include reactive changes in the follicular cells, such as the finding of prominent nucleoli, vacuolated cytoplasm, and phagocytized hemosiderin. Histiocytes, lymphocytes, and foreign body giant cells may be found, as can calcium fragments and stromal cells. Obviously the cytologic appearance will depend upon the stage of the goiter and the degree of secondary changes.[33, 63, 86, 106, 111, 130]

Thyroiditis. In acute thyroiditis, the cytologic preparation shows the features of acute suppuration, including granulocytes and debris. Organisms may be visible or may be discernible with the use of special stains.[63, 86, 93, 115]

In subacute thyroiditis, macrophages, giant cells, and degenerative changes in the follicular epithelium are seen.[55, 63, 86, 93] Epithelioid granulomas may be noted.[93]

In chronic lymphocytic thyroiditis, the cytologic picture often depends on the degree of fibrosis in the gland. In classic cases, in which the fibrosis is not marked, the aspirate will show lymphocytes of various types (reflecting the germinal centers characteristic of this disease), plasma cells, some multinucleated giant cells, and associated follicular epithelium, which may show oncocytic (Hürthle cell) change.[65] The epithelial cells often occur in cohesive fragments or singly. Colloid is usually scant or absent.[6, 36, 44, 58, 63, 86, 93] In the fibrous variants of this disease, the aspirate yields scanty material; in Reidel's disease the aspirate is basically a "dry tap."[63, 93, 125]

The problems associated with the cytologic diagnosis of chronic lymphocytic thyroiditis fall into three major categories: the distinction of thyroiditis from Hürthle cell neoplasm; the distinction of thyroiditis from malignant lymphoma; and the recognition of epithelial neoplasms, which may coexist with thyroiditis.[44, 63–65]

The problem of distinguishing Hürthle cell neoplasms from Hürthle cell nodules in chronic thyroiditis is very real. If the patient clinically presents with a solitary or dominant nodule, which is then the portion of the gland that is aspirated, the cytologic smears and even cell block preparations may show only groups and clusters of Hürthle cells. Even if the antibody titers are significantly high, the absence of accompanying lymphocytic background may lead the cytopathologist to a diagnosis of Hürthle cell neoplasm.[64] It has been our practice to suggest reaspiration in the clinical setting of a dominant nodule in a patient with serologic evidence of thyroiditis if the cytology shows Hürthle cells only. In some of these cases, aspirates of thyroid near the nodule will disclose thyroiditis and surgery can be avoided. In some cases, large bore needle biopsy may be helpful in establishing the correct diagnosis and avoiding operation. Guarda and Baskin noted that in their two cases of Hürthle cell nodule overdiagnosed as neoplasm, a mild lymphocytic infiltrate was admixed with the Hürthle cells.[44] This may be an extremely valuable clue to the correct diagnosis.

The problem of distinguishing thyroiditis from lymphoma can also be quite difficult.[44, 63, 79, 86] However, in the case of large cell lymphoma the monotonous nature of the lymphoid cells, their atypia, and the commonly found background of necrotic debris should prove useful in diagnosis.[44, 51, 63, 64, 79, 86]

In small cell lymphomas, the problem is much more difficult. The monotony of the population without the polymorphism characteristic of germinal centers might be a helpful clue. The absence of epithelial elements is also suspicious. However, the pathologist must be aware of the exuberant lymphocytic reaction that can occur in some cases of chronic thyroiditis and thus caution is advised before rendering a diagnosis of small cell lymphoma on cytology alone. If appropriately prepared material is available for immunophenotyping, then the diagnosis may rest on firmer criteria. Since once the diagnosis of malignant lymphoma of the thyroid is made, radiotherapy or chemotherapy is begun without further documentation of the diagnosis, this author believes caution should be exercised in small cell lymphocytic lesions. In large cell lymphomas, the diagnosis is more readily rendered with confidence.

The association of epithelial tumors of the thyroid with thyroiditis must be viewed from two aspects: an epithelial neoplasm arising in a patient with known or serologically documented thyroiditis or a patient presenting with a nodule in which the thyroid immediately adjacent to the nodule contains many lymphocytes.[44, 63–65] In the latter instance, the cytologic diagnosis can usually be adequately rendered based upon the features of the epithelial cellular component in the specimen, e.g., papillary carcinoma. In the case of a thyroiditic gland in which an epithelial tumor arises, the features of the neoplasm and thyroiditis are usually both present in the smears of the aspirated sample; in experienced hands and with adequate and representative material, the coexistent diagnoses should be readily made.[44, 63, 64]

CYTOLOGY OF THYROID NODULES

Papillary Carcinoma (Table 17–2, A). This tumor, the most common epithelial neoplasm of the thyroid, can be relatively easily diagnosed by fine needle aspiration cytology. The cytologic features of this tumor include the formation of papillae, the characteristic nuclei and, on occasion, the presence of psammoma bodies.[84]

The smears from a papillary cancer are often quite cellular and contain tissue fragments which may show actual papillary configuration; alternatively, the cellular sample may contain monolayered sheets of lesional cells.

The papillae when present may show complex branching with a smooth outer contour; rarely, a central vascular core may be identified.[63, 67, 86]

The nuclei of papillary carcinoma represent the most characteristic feature of this tumor. They are especially helpful in diagnosis and may be the best clue in predominantly follicular variants of this neoplasm.[22, 27, 63, 67] The nuclei are enlarged, round to oval and show a pale ground-glass appearance (Fig. 17–1). Nuclear ridges or grooves are often seen.[27, 63] In addition, as in histologic preparations there is overlapping of nuclei in the follicular, papillary, or monolayer groups. Intranuclear cytoplasmic invaginations are also seen often; they can, of course, be identified in histologic sections as well, but appear more readily recognizable in cytologic preparations.[22, 63, 86, 128] These inclusions differ from the ground-glass nuclei which often appear in every cell; inclusions are usually seen in occasional cells scattered throughout the sample.[63] Nuclear grooves (as discussed in Chapter 8) can also be helpful in cytologic preparations.

Table 17–2. Features of Thyroid Tumors Seen in Fine Needle Biopsy

A. **Papillary Carcinoma** (Refs. 22, 27, 63, 67, 77)
   Cellular aspirate
   Papillary fronds; monolayer sheets
   Dusty nuclear chromatin
   Intranuclear inclusions
   Nuclear grooves
   Psammoma bodies
   Multinucleated giant cells

B. **Medullary Carcinoma** (Refs. 38, 63, 68, 77)
   Individual cells or groups
   Spindle and polygonal cells; some plasmacytoid
   Eccentric nuclei
   Intranuclear inclusions common
   Amyloid

C. **Hürthle Cell Tumors** (Refs. 12, 63, 65, 89)
   Large cells, often in sheets
   Granular cytoplasm
   Eccentric nuclei
   Binucleation
   Prominent nucleoli
   Possible follicle formation

D. **Anaplastic Carcinoma** (Refs. 63, 77, 86, 105)
   Large pleomorphic cells, in sheets or singly
   Bizarre nuclei
   Spindle cells often
   Necrotic background

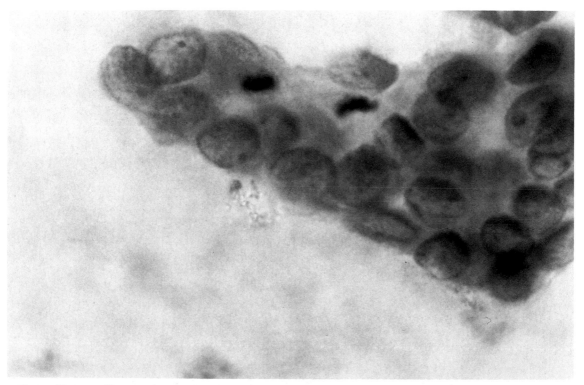

Figure 17–1. Papillary carcinoma. Papillary cluster contains cells with large nuclei and dusty nuclear chromatin. Rare micronucleoli are seen. × 630, Pap stain.

Psammoma bodies (described in detail in Chapter 8), if present, are very helpful in establishing the diagnosis of papillary cancer. Although they have rarely been described in nontumoral thyroids such as in diffuse toxic goiter, nodular goiter, and thyroiditis, their presence in an aspirate of a thyroid nodule should be considered almost diagnostic of papillary cancer; surgery should be recommended in these cases.[28]

The cytologic differential diagnosis of papillary carcinoma includes medullary cancer, follicular neoplasms, and benign lesions.[63, 86] Papillary carcinoma shares with medullary carcinoma the presence of intranuclear inclusions; however, the overall configuration of the sample, the absence of colloid in the latter, and the coarser nuclei of medullary cancer should be helpful in distinguishing the two.[63, 68, 73, 86] Papillary cancer can be confused with follicular lesions; the follicular variant of papillary carcinoma is indeed a type of this tumor and shares the nuclear characteristics. Other benign follicular lesions such as nodules in goiter or solitary nodules may contain areas of papillary hyperplasia and papillary change secondary to degeneration, causing diagnostic confusion. Here, attention to the nuclear features will be most useful.[22, 27, 63, 86]

False negative diagnosis in papillary thyroid cancer is usually due to inadequate sampling of the lesion or improper preparatory techniques, which obscure the cytologic features. Cystic lesions may also produce false negative results.[42, 90, 100] Muller et al. reported a 45 percent false negative rate in their series of 11 cystic papillary cancers.[90] These authors and others caution that if an apparently cystic nodule does not entirely disappear after fine needle aspiration (as determined by clinical examination or ultrasonogram), further biopsy (fine needle or large bore needle) or excision should be considered.[42, 63, 90, 100, 103]

False positive results in papillary carcinoma may occur in Hashimoto's thyroiditis or nodular goiter, in which a few cells may show considerable atypia. However, as Kini warns, the minimum criteria need to be seen for definitive diagnosis to be rendered.[63] Thus, atypia and occasional clear nuclei are insufficient evidence on which to base a diagnosis.

According to Kini, the minimum criteria for a diagnosis of papillary carcinoma in a cytologic aspirate include a high degree of cellularity and syncytial tissue fragments that show the typical nuclei (containing dusty clear or powdery chromatin, nuclear ridges or grooves, and intranuclear inclusions).[63, 67] The background in these smears may contain many foreign body multinucleated giant cells. (It is interesting to me that, before the cytologists made a point of teaching us the frequency of giant cells in papillary carcinoma, these cells were ignored in histologic preparations. If one traverses the gap from the cytologic slides to the histologic ones, the giant cells are easily found in the latter.) In addition, in many examples of papillary cancer, the background contains many lymphocytes; this again reflects the changes noted in histologic slides of these tumors, especially at the invasive edges of these lesions.

Follicular Tumors. Follicular nodules, a few of which represent true neoplasms (see Chapter 9), are the most frequently seen lesions in fine needle aspirates, since these represent the most common thyroid "tumor."

Nodules from goiters and colloid nodules contain varying amounts of cellular material and often abundant colloid. The aspirate often shows well-formed follicles, usually with uniform cells and nuclei. However, it is not uncommon to observe some degree of variation in the sizes of the nuclei. In large goiters or large solitary nodules, degenerative changes, including hemorrhage and fibrosis, may occur; the background in the smears may reflect these changes.[63, 86, 106]

Solitary follicular nodules may range from colloid rich ("macrofollicular type") to very cellular lesions with microfollicles and little to absent colloid. The latter when aspirated will show extremely cellular samples with syncytia of cells; the nuclear features may be bland or may show enlargement and small nucleoli. Some of these lesions can raise the suspicion of malignancy.[114]

Can the cytology alone predict the histologic diagnosis in follicular thyroid nodules? Kini and others[63, 66, 81, 86, 87, 113] indicate that, with increasing experience in the interpretation of needle aspiration cytology of thyroid follicular lesions, diagnostic accuracy increases; Kini claims that 70 to 75 percent of follicular carcinomas can be diagnosed in cytologic samples.[63] This author indicates that "alterations in structural patterns of the tissue fragments and nuclear enlargement" allow for the distinction between benign and malignant follicular nodules.

Debate about the diagnostic use of fine needle aspirate in follicular lesions continues at present[5]; some cytologists claim that a diagnosis of follicular carcinoma of the thyroid can be given on a fine needle aspirate sample. These authors cite nuclear size and cellularity differences between benign and malignant follicular nodules.[63, 66, 81, 86, 87] As will be discussed more fully in Chapter 18, the adjuvant use of flow cytometric analysis for the presence of aneuploidy or nondiploid cell populations in the aspirated samples has been cited as a useful diagnostic criterion; image analysis on aspirates from follicular lesions has also been reported as diagnostically useful.[13, 14, 71, 129]

However, it seems to the present author that these arguments do not support the use of cytology alone as a *diagnostic* technique in follicular thyroid tumors. (I recognize fully the use of this tool as diagnostic in follicular variants of papillary cancer, as discussed above.) Most if not all pathologists require that, for a diagnosis of follicular carcinoma of the thyroid, it is necessary to identify *invasion* into or through the capsule of the lesion or into capsular or pericapsular veins. How can a needle aspirate of the center of a nodule supply this type of information necessary for the diagnosis?

In addition, nuclear atypia (including nucleomegaly and hyperchromatism) can be found in a wide range of benign thyroid lesions (nodular and diffuse goiter, thyroiditis, adenomatous nodules, adenomas); how can atypia in and of itself be diagnostic? Aneuploid and nondiploid cell populations can be identified in follicular nodules that are histologically and clinically benign. (See Chapter 18.) In addition, Luck et al. indicate that in their studies image analysis cannot successfully separate benign from cancerous follicular tumors.[78] Hence, to the present author at least, the use of fine needle aspiration of follicular nodules is for *screening—not for diagnosis.*[56, 76, 125, 126]

Follicular lesions showing a microfollicular, trabecular, or solidly cellular pattern, with or without nuclear atypia, should be considered candidates for surgical removal. It is from this subgroup of follicular lesions that follicular carcinomas will be found; however, not all these lesions will be histologically or by clinical behavior malignant. (It is estimated that about 20 percent will be.[75]) It, of course, can be argued that these cellular, atypical, and/or nondiploid follicular nodules are carcinomas (? in-situ carcinoma), and that surgical removal of these lesions was curative. It is impossible to effectively counter this argument; we just don't know.

Those authors who advocate diagnosis of well-differentiated follicular carcinoma from a cytologic sample claim that false positive results are acceptable since cellular follicular adenomas, atypical adenomas and follicular carcinomas all should be surgically removed. In institutions where the surgical therapy of all three lesions in similar, i.e., unilateral thyroid lobectomy, this approach seems sensible to me.

However, the claim of diagnostic accuracy in follicular tumors of the thyroid by fine needle aspirate can lead to a knee-jerk response on the part of treating physicians at some institutions, i.e., proceeding to total thyroidectomy based on a diagnosis of cancer; this appears totally unjustified. Clinician-cytopathologist interaction is stressed to avoid inappropriate therapy; this approach, while invaluable, ignores the pragmatic aspects of the practice of pathology in general, unfortunately.

My approach has been and continues to be to utilize cytology as a screening tool for well-differentiated follicular lesions, not as a diagnostic modality! (It is recognized that poorly differentiated follicular tumors can be identified by cytology as malignant. Some of these samples will show necrosis, marked pleomorphism, and mitoses.)

Medullary Carcinoma. (Table 17–2, B). The cytologic features of medullary carcinoma are variable, reflecting the histology of the different subtypes of this neoplasm. In the classical case, however, the aspirate sample shows single cells or small groups without a follicular pattern (Fig. 17–2). Often the cells are spindle-shaped; round to oval cells can also be found. In many examples, the tumor cells have a plasmacytoid appearance; in some cases, the spindle-shaped cells appear to contain cytoplasmic processes.[38, 63, 68, 73, 86] The nuclei of the tumor cells are round to oval and range from quite uniform to pleomorphic. (In some cases, giant cells may be identified.) Multiple nuclei may be seen in the tumor cells. Kini points out that the nuclei in medullary cancer are always eccentrically located in relationship to the cytoplasm.[63]

The background of the smears may show clumps of extracellular material, often staining pale orange or light green with Papanicolaou stain; this material is

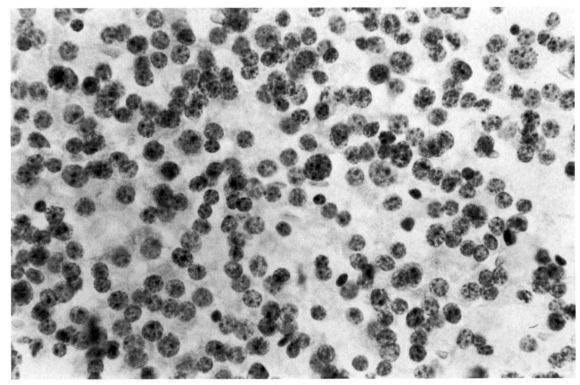

Figure 17–2. Medullary carcinoma. This extremely cellular aspirate contains cells with poorly defined cytoplasmic borders and a range of nuclear sizes. However, the nuclei are quite round. Histology confirmed a diagnosis of medullary carcinoma. × 400, Pap stain.

amyloid. In order to confirm the tumor as medullary, immunostaining for calcitonin is necessary.[63] (See also Chapters 10 and 18.)

The differential diagnosis of medullary carcinoma includes Hürthle cell tumors, follicular tumors, papillary cancer, and even anaplastic carcinoma. Hürthle cell lesions usually contain voluminous amounts of cytoplasm, and their nuclei are often quite irregular and contain prominent nucleoli. Follicular tumors may be difficult to distinguish from medullary, since some medullary cancers contain follicles and amyloid may be absent; conversely, follicular lesions may show few if any follicles. The presence of intranuclear inclusions and the finding of spindle cells may be useful in the distinction.[63, 68, 86] Papillary carcinomas contain papillae, sometimes psammoma bodies, and peculiar clear nuclei; medullary cancers can show papillary areas, can contain calcification, and do show intranuclear inclusions. The clear nuclei with their dusty chromatin are useful. Most anaplastic carcinomas are so pleomorphic that the diagnosis should not be difficult. However, some medullary carcinomas do contain many multinucleated giant tumor cells and many spindle-shaped cells; these features may produce diagnostic problems; however, extensive areas of necrosis are rare in medullary tumors. As with all difficult cases, one may need to resort to immunostaining to differentiate among these lesions.

Hürthle Cell Tumors. (Table 17–2 C). Hürthle cells can be found in numerous conditions which affect the thyroid. (See Chapter 12.) However, the solitary thyroid nodule composed of Hürthle cells produces an especially difficult problem. If an aspirate shows only oncocytes, and there is no background of lymphocytes or clinical suspicion of thyroiditis, then the diagnosis of Hürthle cell neoplasm is justified. Since a large percentage (20 to 62 percent) of such tumors fulfill the histologic criteria for malignancy, it is prudent to recommend surgical removal of all such lesions.

The cytologic features of Hürthle cell tumors include the presence of small groups of monomorphic cells. The cells are large oval or polygonal with abundant granular cytoplasm (Fig. 17–3). Nuclei may be multiple, but characteristically contain a prominent nucleolus. The background is usually clear; colloid is rarely present.[12, 63, 86, 89] Distinguishing benign from malignant Hürthle cell lesions presents the same type of difficulty as does the distinction of benign from malignant follicular nodules in general (see above). (Of course, if the theory that all Hürthle cell tumors are malignant is followed, then even attempts at cytologic, or for that matter histologic, differentiation are futile.)

The major diagnostic dilemma facing the cytopathologist in the evaluation of an aspirate from a Hürthle cell nodule is whether the nodule represents a part of a nodular goiter or lymphocytic thyroiditis.[44, 63, 64] The clinical information regarding thyroid function and serology is of course extremely useful; in the absence of such data, the presence of lymphocytic infiltrates among the Hürthle cells or in the background is very helpful. Such findings will tend to favor the diagnosis of a benign Hürthle cell proliferation rather than a neoplasm. A helpful clue is the paucity of nucleoli in oncocytic changes in goiter, whereas these are usually seen in neoplasms.

Anaplastic Tumors. (Table 17–2, D). The diagnostic question faced by the cytologist evaluating an aspirate from a thyroid mass is usually: Is the lesion benign or malignant? In anaplastic carcinoma, the issue is simple. These lesions yield markedly pleomorphic cellular aspirates with necrotic debris, obviously from a malignant neoplasm. In most instances, the diagnosis is so obvious that there are no other considerations.[63, 105, 127] On occasion, the tumor will be extremely fibrous and the cellular sample will be sparse and inadequate.[56, 61] The rare case

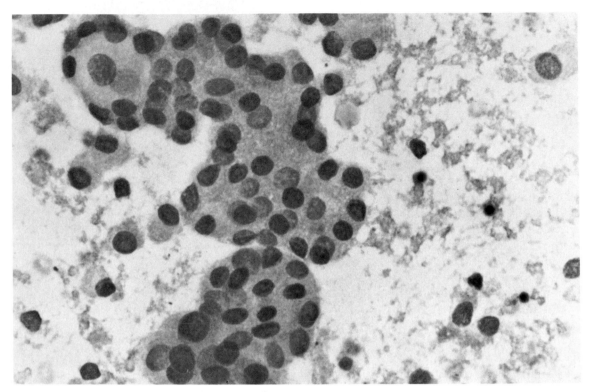

Figure 17–3. Hürthle cell nodule. This group of cells shows a follicular pattern. There is voluminous granular cytoplasm and some variability of nuclear size. No lymphoid cells were seen; there was no history of thyroiditis. Surgery disclosed a Hürthle cell adenoma. × 400, Pap stain.

of medullary carcinoma with giant cells may raise some diagnostic problems, but this is unusual.

Malignant Lymphoma. This lesion, discussed above, should not present diagnostic difficulties in the usual case of a large cell lymphoma. In those instances of small cell lymphoid lesions, or those with extensive plasmacytic differentiation, distinction from florid lymphocytic thyroiditis may be impossible on an aspirate sample.[44, 63] In some cases, if sufficient appropriately prepared material is available, immunostaining for immunoglobulins in attempts to define monoclonality may be useful.[79] (See Chapter 14.)

Other Tumors. A number of case reports or small series of cases have appeared describing the cytologic features of metastatic tumors to the thyroid.[21, 112, 123] In some instances (pigmented melanoma, for example) the diagnosis is clear. In cases of renal carcinoma metastatic to the gland, the differential diagnosis of primary thyroid tumor must be considered. (See Chapter 15.) Immunostaining for thyroglobulin may be useful in these cases.[2, 37, 130] Other metastases, such as breast or lung cancer, may not be definitively diagnosed without appropriate historical information; the aspirate will be diagnosed as showing carcinoma, but the primary site may be impossible to define. When faced with an aspirate that is malignant but does not fit into one of the previously discussed categories of primary tumors, one should always question the possibility of metastasis; unnecessary surgery may be avoided.

The fine needle aspiration cytology of parathyroid adenomas mimicking thyroid lesions has been described.[35]

On occasion the aspiration will cause necrosis of the nodule it entered[60]; this is most often found in Hürthle cell lesions. The infarct-like necrosis and accompanying inflammation may make definitive histologic diagnosis very difficult or impossible.

Another unusual change the present author has noted in nodules resected after aspiration (usually within two to four weeks of the aspiration procedure) is squamous metaplasia of follicular epithelium; metaplastic cells contain abundant eosinophilic cytoplasm and often assume spindle shapes not unlike regenerative squamous epithelium abutting a cervical or esophageal ulcer.

The Problem of Adequacy. Many studies have addressed the question of an adequate sample in thyroid needle aspirates. When the experience with this technique was limited, samples which would now be considered inadequate would be diagnosed as negative or benign; hence the false negative rate was considerable. In addition, the question of who should perform the biopsy (endocrinologist, surgeon, pathologist) remained to be settled; it now appears that any of these individuals can do the aspiration, given the right equipment and training. A variety of authors expound on the preferred method of handling the sample—direct smears, fixed or air-dried smears, fixation in carbowax, etc.[59, 76, 125] It apparently matters little which technique is utilized so long as the individual interpreting the smears is familiar with the vagaries of it.

Hamburger has recently summarized his group's large experience with thyroid aspirates.[48] He found that to consider a specimen adequate requires (a) six aspirates from the nodule, therefore sampling several areas; (b) at least two of the smears must each contain six clusters of benign epithelial cells and no malignant cells. If these criteria are adhered to, the false negative rate declines as does the need for further biopsy. Many cytologists believe these adequacy criteria are excessive. If a cytologist performs the aspiration or is present, a rapid assessment of the aspirate may be given after each pass of the needle, thus limiting the number of passes and still obtaining sufficient material.

Obviously, if a sample contains diagnostic material (papillae and psammoma bodies, for example) but falls below the limit of adequacy as defined above, the cytopathologist should still render a diagnosis on such a case!

The Indeterminate Specimen. What does one do with a sample that has some but not all of the criteria on which to render a definitive diagnosis? Some samples are indeterminate because there are extensive degenerative changes or fibrosis in the nodule. In this author's opinion, a definitive diagnosis should not be given unless all criteria are met. It is important to honestly assess what is available and only that.

It is possible to suggest reaspiration within a short period of time; conversely, if the clinical suspicion of malignancy is great, the decision to proceed to surgery may be correct.[8, 40]

Large Bore Needle Biopsy. The ease which physicians have in performing it and its acceptance by patients have made fine needle aspiration biopsy the technique most widely used for the minimally invasive diagnosis of thyroid disease. However, the large bore needle biopsy which yields a histologic specimen can be utilized with success in specific instances. The morphologic diagnosis of thyroiditis can be more readily established with this technique. In some cases, because at least theoretically the large needle can obtain samples from the capsule of a follicular lesion, the possibility of noting capsular and/or vascular invasion exists; hence in a small number of cases a definitive diagnosis of follicular cancer may be rendered.[86]

In those cases wherein immunostaining may be helpful in defining the nature of a lesion (lymphoid lesions, medullary carcinoma), large needle biopsy can supply an adequate sample for that procedure. However, immunostaining can be performed on smears of the aspirate if sufficient material is available.

The diagnostic accuracy of large bore needle biopsy is about 89 percent.[117] Many series in the literature indicate that fine needle and large needle biopsies are complimentary to each other[10, 11, 17, 29, 30, 51, 52, 74, 75, 82, 86, 91]—though in some reports, one method is somewhat better than the other for certain lesions. Most reports indicate that the large needle biopsy may give better yields in follicular neoplasms of the thyroid (91 percent versus 86 percent for fine needle).[10, 11, 17, 75]

Complications with large needle biopsy are slightly more frequent than with fine needle aspiration; these complications include bleeding and rare needle track implantation of tumor.[29, 122]

Use of the Cell Block. I believe this chapter would be incomplete if I did not allude to the technique of using some of the aspirated material, especially in cystic lesions,[42, 46] obtained with the fine needle method to produce a cell block, i.e., a histologic slide of the lesion. In some instances this method may prove useful, since, for example, it allows for the application of immunostaining. In some cases, it may make unnecessary the large bore needle biopsy, saving the patient another procedure.

Of course, the cell block can be prepared only if the aspirate is delivered to the laboratory in some medium such as carbowax[59]; it cannot be used if all the aspirated material is immediately smeared onto slides. An alternative approach involves rinsing the needle itself in carbowax or saline after the smears have been prepared. In samples containing neoplasms (often highly cellular specimens) there is usually enough material for cell block preparations.

Frozen Section Diagnosis and the Thyroid. Before the advent of fine and large bore needle biopsy, the method most used in diagnosis of thyroid nodules was intraoperative frozen section. The nodule, or preferably the thyroid lobe, was excised and a representative portion (preferably encompassing nodule-capsule-thyroid interface) was prepared for frozen section and intraoperative interpretation by a pathologist. In those cases in which the diagnosis of papillary, medullary, or anaplastic cancer was given, appropriate surgery was immediately undertaken.

Even with frozen section, however, despite recommendations of sampling two or even four different areas, the diagnosis of follicular carcinomas was notoriously difficult.[70] In many cases, the diagnosis rendered is "follicular lesion—diagnosis deferred to permanent sections." Our experience is similar to that reported in the literature; the diagnosis of follicular lesions on frozen sections is usually completely benign or is deferred. For the cases in which the diagnosis is deferred, most are benign when evaluated by permanent sections; rarely, we have identified a follicular variant of papillary cancer or a true follicular carcinoma, minimally invasive type, after further histologic evaluation.

Several studies have evaluated frozen section and fine needle aspirate diagnostic results for thyroid nodules.[19, 50, 61, 70] Although frozen section diagnosis may be specific (90 to 97 percent), it is not sensitive (60 percent). In addition, deferred diagnoses at frozen section do nothing to alter the operative procedure or guide the surgeon. Hamburger and Hamburger analyzed 359 patients who had fine needle aspirates and also intraoperative frozen sections of thyroid nodules[50]; the frozen section results influenced the surgical approach in only three cases (>1%).

Also, in the era of cost containment, it does not seem justified to perform frozen sections for the intraoperative diagnosis of thyroid nodules; this is even more true if a preoperative fine needle aspirate has been performed with malignant or suspicious results. (For assessing lymph node status, parathyroid glands, extension into soft tissue, etc., of course, intraoperative frozen section is valuable and may influence surgical management.)

Table 17–3. Facts and Statistics about FNA Thyroid*

	(Percent)
Accuracy	94
Inadequate sample	5
(reasons: nodule too small,	
nodule too deep,	
nodule too fibrous)	
Benign diagnoses	67
Malignant/Suspicious	10–20
Indeterminate diagnosis	15–18
Sensitivity	47–95
Specificity	66–93
False positive diagnosis**	7–12
False negative diagnosis**	1–9
Accuracy for individual tumors (when surgically confirmed)	
Papillary cancer	67–97
Follicular variant, papillary cancer	60–80
Medullary cancer (higher if immunostains done)	50–80
Anaplastic cancer	75–100
Malignant lymphoma	variable
Follicular cancer	up to 75
(Some authors do not differentiate among follicular neoplasms.)	

*These figures are culled from many series in the literature and should be considered estimates only. Different authors use different criteria for inclusion of suspicious samples in malignant or benign categories. Some authors exclude follicular tumors from their statistics and diagnose only "follicular neoplasm"; there is great variability about the inclusion of occult cancers as falsely negative diagnoses or excluding these entirely. In some series, surgical and histologic confirmation are the endpoint of all diagnostic comparisons; in many reports, however, "benign" fine needle aspiration diagnoses are not further confirmed. Extensive variability in lengths of follow-up is also noted among different series.

**The time frame is also important; the higher false negative rates are found in series published before 1984.

Table 17–4. Guidelines for FNA of the Thyroid: Fact and Opinion (Author's)

1. FNA is cost-effective and patient acceptable.
2. Complications of FNA are rare to nonexistent.
3. FNA is becoming and should become the primary procedure to evaluate a thyroid nodule. (Some endocrinologists feel assessing the functional state of a nodule prior to FNA is important since "hot" nodules are rarely if ever malignant—hence FNA can be avoided. Also if a nodule is "hot," hyperplastic features and nuclear atypia may lead to a false positive FNA diagnosis.)
4. Accuracy increases with increasing experience; this is true with respect to the aspiration procedure and the pathologic interpretation.
5. Inadequate samples must not be diagnosed as negative or benign. Adequacy of sample has been better defined with increasing experience.
6. Cystic lesions can produce suboptimal yields and hence false negative diagnoses.
7. Indeterminate samples decrease with increasing experience. Repeat FNA for indeterminate cases may yield diagnostic material.
8. The *diagnostic* accuracy for FNA in many thyroid lesions—benign goiter, thyroiditis, papillary cancer, medullary and anaplastic tumors—is excellent (over 90 percent).
9. For follicular lesions, FNA is a very good *screening* technique to select patients for surgery. (This applies to well-differentiated follicular lesions.)
10. Communication between pathologist and clinician should be bi-directional and frequent. (Whether this is practical or not remains an issue, however.)

SUMMARY

This chapter presents a brief overview of diagnostic approaches to thyroid disease in which the pathologist plays an important role. Fine needle aspiration, large needle biopsies, and the use of frozen section are discussed. Table 17–3 lists some facts about fine needle biopsies of the thyroid. As can be noted in this table, comparison of various series in the literature is often difficult and even impossible because of varying criteria[91] for inclusion of follicular neoplasms and occult tumors, and different criteria for defining specificity and sensitivity—e.g., are "suspicious" results included as positive or negative? However, since this is an overview, the present author felt it was appropriate to attempt some tabulation of the facts. In addition, Table 17–4 lists some known facts about fine needle aspiration cytology itself; this table includes the experience recorded in the literature and the opinions of the present author.

REFERENCES

1. Akerman, M., Tennvall, J., et al.: Sensitivity and specificity of fine needle aspiration cytology in the diagnosis of tumors of the thyroid gland. Acta Cytol. *29:*850–855, 1985.
2. Altmannsberger, M., Dralle, H., et al.: Intermediate filaments in cytological specimens of thyroid tumors. Diagn. Cytopathol. *3:*210–214, 1987.
3. Ashcraft, M. W., and van Herle, A. J.: Management of the thyroid nodule: Scanning techniques, thyroid suppressive therapy and fine needle aspiration. Head Neck Surg. *3:*297–322, 1981.
4. Asp, A. A., Georgitis, W., et al.: Fine needle aspiration of the thyroid. Use in an average health care facility. Am. J. Med. *83:*489–493, 1987.
5. Atkinson, B. F., Ernst, C. S., and LiVolsi, V. A.: Cytologic diagnosis of follicular tumors of the thyroid. Diagn. Cytopathol. *2:*1–3, 1986.
6. Baker, B. S., Gharib, H., and Markowitz, H.: Correlation of thyroid antibodies and cytologic features in suspected autoimmune thyroid disease. Am. J. Med. *74:*941–944, 1983.
7. Belanger, R., Guillet, F., et al.: The thyroid nodule: Evaluation of fine needle biopsy. J. Otolaryngol. *12:*109–11, 1983.
8. Block, M. A., Dailey, G. E., and Robb, J. A.: Thyroid nodules indeterminate by needle biopsy. Am. J. Surg. *146:*72–78, 1983.
9. Blum, M.: The diagnosis of the thyroid nodule using aspiration biopsy and cytology. Arch. Intern. Med. *144:*1140–1142, 1984.
10. Boey, J., Hsu, C., et al.: A prospective controlled study of fine needle aspiration and Tru-cut needle biopsy of dominant thyroid nodules. World J. Surg. *8:*458–465, 1984.
11. Boey, J., Hsu, C., et al.: Fine needle aspiration versus drill needle biopsy of thyroid nodules: A controlled clinical trial. Surgery *91:*611–615, 1982.
12. Bondeson, L., Bondeson, A. G., et al.: Morphometric studies on nuclei in smears of fine needle aspirates from oxyphilic tumors of the thyroid. Acta Cytol. *27:*437–440, 1983.
13. Boon, M. E., Lowhagen, T., et al.: Computation of preoperative diagnosis probability for follicular adenoma and carcinoma of the thyroid on aspiration smears. Analyt. Quant. Cytol. *4:*1–5, 1982.
14. Boon, M. E., Lowhagen, T., and Willems, J. S.: Planimetric studies on fine needle aspirates from follicular adenoma and follicular carcinoma of the thyroid. Acta Cytol. *24:*145–148, 1980.
15. Bottles, K., Miller, T. R., et al.: Fine needle aspiration biopsy. Has its time come? Am. J. Med. *81:*525–531, 1986.
16. Brauer, R. J., and Silver, C. E.: Needle aspiration biopsy of thyroid nodules. Laryngoscope *94:*38–42, 1984.
17. Broughan, T. A., and Esselstyn, C. B.: Large needle thyroid biopsy: Still necessary. Surgery *100:*1138–1141, 1986.
18. Brown, J. A., Queen, T. A., and Taub, M.: The solitary thyroid nodule: selection of patients for surgery. Am. Surg. *48:*575–576, 1982.
19. Bugis, S. P., Young, J. E. M., et al.: Diagnostic accuracy of fine needle aspiration biopsy versus frozen section in solitary thyroid nodules. Am. J. Surg. *152:*411–416, 1986.
20. Caplan, R. H., Wester, S., and Kisken, W. A.: Fine needle aspiration biopsy of solitary thyroid nodules. Minn. Med. *69:*189–192, 1986.
21. Chacho, M. S., Greenbaum, E., et al.: Value of aspiration cytology of the thyroid in metastatic disease. Acta Cytol. *31:*705–712, 1987.
22. Christ, M. L., and Haja, J.: Intranuclear cytoplasmic inclusions (invaginations) in thyroid aspirations. Frequency and specificity. Acta Cytol. *23:*327–330, 1979.

23. Chu, E. W., Thomas, T. A., et al.: Study of cells in fine needle aspirations of the thyroid gland. Acta Cytol. 23:309–314, 1979.
24. Cohen, M. B., Miller, T. R., et al.: Fine needle aspiration biopsy. Perceptions of physicians at an academic medical center. Arch. Pathol. Lab. Med. 110:813–817, 1986.
25. Crile, G., and Hawks, W. A.: Aspiration biopsy of thyroid nodules. Surg. Gynecol. Obstet. 136:241–245, 1973.
26. DeGroot, L. J.: Management of thyroid nodules: How far have we come? Hospital Pract. 21:9–10, 1986.
27. Deligeorgi-Politi, H.: Nuclear crease as a cytodiagnostic feature of papillary thyroid carcinoma in fine needle aspiration biopsies. Diagn. Cytopathol. 3:307–310, 1987.
28. Dugan, J. M., Atkinson, B. F., et al.: Psammoma bodies in fine needle aspirate of the thyroid in lymphocytic thyroiditis. Acta Cytol. 31:330–334, 1987.
29. Esselstyn, C. B., and Crile, G.: Needle aspiration and needle biopsy of the thyroid. World J. Surg. 2:321–329, 1978.
30. Esselstyn, C. B., and Crile, G.: Evaluation of various types of needle biopsies of the thyroid. World J. Surg. 8:452–457, 1984.
31. Frable, W. J.: The treatment of thyroid cancer. The role of fine needle aspiration cytology. Arch. Otolaryngol. Head Neck Surg. 112:1200–1203, 1986.
32. Frable, M. A., and Frable, W. J.: Thin needle aspiration biopsy of the thyroid gland. Laryngoscope 90:1619–1625, 1980.
33. Franklyn, J. A., Fitzgerald, M. G., et al.: Fine needle aspiration cytology in the management of euthyroid goitre. Quart. J. Med. 65:997–1003, 1987.
34. Friedman, M., Shimaoka, K., and Getaz, P.: Needle aspiration of 310 thyroid lesions. Acta Cytol. 23:194–203, 1979.
35. Friedman, M., Shimaoka, K., et al.: Parathyroid adenoma diagnosed as papillary carcinoma of thyroid on needle aspiration smears. Acta Cytol. 27:337–340, 1983.
36. Friedman, M., Shimaoka, K., et al.: Diagnosis of chronic lymphocytic thyroiditis (nodular presentation) by needle aspiration. Acta Cytol. 25:513–522, 1981.
37. Gal, R., Aronof, A., et al.: The potential value of the demonstration of thyroglobulin by immunoperoxidase techniques in fine needle aspiration cytology. Acta Cytol. 31:713–716, 1987.
38. Geddie, W. R., Bedard, Y. C., and Strawbridge, H. T. G.: Medullary carcinoma in fine needle aspiration biopsies. Am. J. Clin. Pathol. 82:552–558, 1984.
39. Gershengorn, M. C., McClung, M. R., et al.: Fine needle aspiration cytology in the preoperative diagnosis of thyroid nodules. Ann. Intern. Med. 87:265–269, 1977.
40. Gharib, H., Goellner, J. R., et al.: Fine needle aspiration biopsy of the thyroid: The problem of suspicious cytologic findings. Ann. Intern. Med. 101:25–28, 1984.
41. Goellner, J. R., Gharib, H., et al.: Fine needle aspiration cytology of the thyroid, 1980 to 1986. Acta Cytol. 31:587–590, 1987.
42. Goellner, J. R., and Johnson, D. A.: Cytology of cystic papillary carcinoma of the thyroid. Acta Cytol. 26:787–799, 1982.
43. Griffies, W. S., Donegan, E., and Abel, M. E.: The role of fine needle aspiration in the management of the thyroid nodule. Laryngoscope 95:1103–1106, 1985.
44. Guarda, L. A., and Baskin, H. J.: Inflammatory and lymphoid lesions of the thyroid gland: Cytopathology by fine needle aspiration. Am. J. Clin. Pathol. 87:14–22, 1987.
45. Haas, S. N.: Acute thyroid swelling after needle biopsy of the thyroid. N. Engl. J. Med. 307:1349, 1982 (letter).
46. Hamaker, R. C., Singer, M. I., et al.: Role of needle biopsy in thyroid nodules. Arch. Otolaryngol. 109:225–228, 1983.
47. Hamberger, B., et al.: Fine needle aspiration biopsy of thyroid nodules: Impact on thyroid practice and cost of care. Am. J. Med. 73:381–384, 1982.
48. Hamburger, J. I.: Semiquantitative criteria for fine needle biopsy diagnosis reduces false negative diagnoses. Presented at American Thyroid Association Meeting, Washington, D.C., September, 1987.
49. Hamburger, J. I.: Consistency of sequential needle biopsy findings for thyroid nodules. Arch. Intern. Med. 147:97–99, 1987.
50. Hamburger, J. I., and Hamburger, S. W.: Declining role of frozen section in surgical planning for thyroid nodules. Surgery 98:307–312, 1985.
51. Hamburger, J. I., Miller, J. M., and Kini, S. R.: Clinical-Pathological Evaluation of Thyroid Nodules: Handbook and Atlas. Privately published by author, 1979.
52. Hamlin, E., and Vickery, A. L.: Needle biopsy of the thyroid gland. N. Engl. J. Med. 254:742–746, 1956.
53. Harsoulis, P., Leontsini, M., et al.: Fine needle aspiration biopsy cytology in the diagnosis of thyroid cancer. Br. J. Surg. 73:461–464, 1986.
54. Hawkins, F., Bellido, D., et al.: Fine needle aspiration biopsy in the diagnosis of thyroid cancer and thyroid diseases. Cancer 59:1206–1209, 1987.
55. Hnilica, P., and Nyulassy, S.: Plasma cells in aspirates of goitre and overt permanent hypothyroidism following subacute thyroiditis. Endocrinol. Exp. 19:221–226, 1985.
56. Hsu, C., and Boey, J.: Diagnostic pitfalls in the fine needle aspiration of thyroid nodules: A study of 555 cases in Chinese patients. Acta Cytol. 31:699–704, 1987.

57. Jayaram, G.: Fine needle aspiration cytologic study of the solitary thyroid nodule. Acta Cytol. *29:*967–973, 1985.
58. Jayaram, G., Marwaha, R., et al.: Cytomorphologic aspects of thyroiditis: A study of 51 cases with functional, immunologic and ultrasonic data. Acta Cytol. *31:*687–693, 1987.
59. Jennings, A. S., and Atkinson, B. F.: Thyroid needle aspiration: Collecting and handling the specimen, N. Engl. J. Med. *308:*1602–1603, 1983.
60. Jones, J. D., Pittman, D. L., and Sanders, L. R.: Necrosis of thyroid nodules after fine needle aspiration. Acta Cytol. *29:*29–32, 1985.
61. Keller, M. P., Crabbe, M. M., and Norwood, S. H.: Accuracy and significance of fine needle aspiration and frozen section in determining the extent of thyroid resection. Surgery *101:*632–635, 1987.
62. Khafagi, F., Wright, G., et al.: Screening for thyroid malignancy: The role of fine needle biopsy. Med. J. Austral. *149:*302–307, 1988.
63. Kini, S. R.: Guides to Clinical Aspiration Biopsy: Thyroid. New York: Igaku-Shoin, 1987.
64. Kini, S. R., Miller, J. M., and Hamburger, J. I.: Problems in the cytodiagnosis of the "cold" thyroid nodule in patients with lymphocytic thyroiditis. Acta Cytol. *25:*506–512, 1981.
65. Kini, S. R., Miller, J. M., and Hamburger, J. I.: Cytopathology of Hürthle cells lesions of the thyroid gland by fine needle aspiration. Acta Cytol. *25:*647–652, 1981.
66. Kini, S. R., Miller, J. M., et al.: Cytopathology of follicular lesions of the thyroid gland. Diagn. Cytopathol. *1:*123–132, 1985.
67. Kini, S. R., Miller, J. M., et al.: Cytopathology of papillary carcinoma of the thyroid by fine needle aspiration. Acta Cytol. *24:*511–521, 1980.
68. Kini, S. R., Miller, J. M., et al.: Cytopathologic features of medullary carcinoma of the thyroid. Arch. Pathol. Lab. Med. *108:*156–159, 1984.
69. Koss, L. G.: Thin needle aspiration biopsy. Acta Cytol. *24:*1–3, 1980.
70. Kraemer, B. B.: Frozen section and the thyroid. Sem. Diagn. Pathol. *4:*169–189, 1987.
71. Kriete, A., Schaffer, R., et al.: Computer based cytophotometric classification of thyroid tumors in imprints. J. Cancer Res. Clin. Oncol. *109:*252–256, 1985.
72. Lawson, W., and Biller, H. F.: The solitary thyroid nodule: Diagnosis and management of malignant disease. Am. J. Otolaryngol. *4:*43–73, 1983.
73. Ljungberg, O.: Cytologic diagnosis of medullary carcinoma of the thyroid gland. Acta Cytol. *16:*253–255, 1972.
74. LoGerfo, P., Colacchio, T., et al.: Comparison of fine needle and coarse needle biopsies in evaluating thyroid nodules. Surgery *92:*835–838, 1982.
75. LoGerfo, P. L., Feind, C., et al.: The incidence of carcinoma in encapsulated follicular thyroid lesions diagnosed by large needle biopsy. Surgery *94:*1008–1010, 1983.
76. Lowhagen, T., Granberg, P. O., et al.: Aspiration biopsy cytology (ABC) in nodules of the thyroid gland suspected to be malignant. Surg. Clin. North. Amer. *59:*3–18, 1979.
77. Lowhagen, T., and Sprenger, E.: Cytologic presentation of thyroid tumors in aspiration biopsy smears. Acta Cytol. *18:*192–197, 1974.
78. Luck, J. B., Mumaw, V. R., and Frable, W. J.: Fine needle aspiration biopsy of the thyroid: Differential diagnosis by videoplan image analysis. Acta Cytol. *26:*793–796, 1982.
79. Matsuda, M., Sone, H., et al.: Fine needle aspiration cytology of malignant lymphoma of the thyroid. Diagn. Cytopathol. *3:*244–249, 1987.
80. Miller, D. A., Carrasco. C. H., et al.: Fine needle aspiration biopsy: The role of immediate cytologic assessment. Am. J. Radiol. *147:*156–158, 1986.
81. Miller, J. M.: Evaluation of thyroid nodules: Accent on needle biopsy. Med. Clin. North. Am. *69:*1063–1077, 1985.
82. Miller, J. M., Hamburger, J. I., and Kini, S. R.: Diagnosis of thyroid nodules: Use of fine needle aspiration and needle biopsy. J. A. M. A. *241:*481–484, 1979.
83. Miller, J. M., Hamburger, J. I., and Kini, S. R.: The impact of needle biopsy on the preoperative diagnosis of thyroid nodules. Henry Ford Hosp. Med. J. *28:*145–148, 1980.
84. Miller, J. M., Hamburger, J. I., and Kini, S. R.: The needle biopsy diagnosis of papillary thyroid carcinoma. Cancer *48:*989–993, 1981.
85. Miller, J. M., Hamburger, J. I., and Kini, S. R.: Thyroid nodules and needle biopsy. Ann. Intern. Med. *101:*718, 1984 (letter).
86. Miller, J. M., Kini, S. R., and Hamburger, J. I.: Needle Biopsy of the Thyroid. New York, Praeger Publishers, 1983.
87. Miller, J. M., Kini, S. R., and Hamburger, J. I.: The diagnosis of malignant follicular neoplasms of the thyroid by needle biopsy. Cancer *55:*2812–2817, 1985.
88. Miller, T. R., Abele, J. S., and Greenspan, F. S.: Fine needle aspiration biopsy in the management of thyroid nodules. West. J. Med. *134:*198–205, 1981.
89. Mishriiki, Y. Y., Lane, B. P., et al.: Hürthle cell tumor arising in mediastinal ectopic thyroid and diagnosed by fine needle aspiration: Light microscopic and ultrastructural features. Acta Cytol. *27:*188–192, 1983.
90. Muller, N., Cooperberg, P. L., et al.: Needle aspiration biopsy in cystic papillary carcinoma of the thyroid. Am. J. Radiol. *144:*251–253, 1985.
91. Nishiyama, R. H., Bigos, S. T., et al.: The efficacy of simultaneous fine needle aspiration and large needle biopsy of the thyroid gland. Surgery *100:*1133–1137, 1986.

92. Norton, L. W., Wangensteen, S. L., et al.: Utility of thyroid aspiration biopsy. Surgery 92:700–705, 1982.
93. Persson, P. S.: Cytodiagnosis of thyroiditis. Acta Med. Scand. Suppl. 483:7–100, 1967.
94. Petersen, B. W., and Griesen, O.: Fine needle aspiration biopsy of the thyroid gland. Otolaryngol. Head Neck Surg. 92:295–297, 1984.
95. Prinz, R. A., O'Morchoe, P. J., et al.: Fine needle aspiration biopsy of thyroid nodules. Ann. Surg. 198:70–73, 1983.
96. Ramacciotti, C. E., Pretorius, H. T., et al.: Diagnostic accuracy and use of aspiration biopsy in the management of thyroid nodules. Arch. Intern. Med. 144:1169–1173, 1984.
97. Reeve, T. S., Delbridge, L., et al.: The impact of fine needle aspiration biopsy on surgery for thyroid nodules. Med. J. Austral. 145:308–311, 1986.
98. Rojeski, M. T., and Gharib, H.: Nodular thyroid disease. N. Engl. J. Med.: 313:428–436, 1985.
99. Rosen, I. B., Palmer, J. A., et al.: Efficacy of needle biopsy in postradiation thyroid disease. Surgery 94:1002–1007, 1983.
100. Rosen, I. B., Provias, J. P., and Walfish, P. G.: Pathologic nature of cystic thyroid nodules selected for surgery by needle aspiration biopsy. Surgery 100:606–612, 1986.
101. Rosen, I. B., Wallace, C., et al.: Reevaluation of needle aspiration cytology in detection of thyroid cancer. Surgery 90:747–756, 1981.
102. Rothenberg, R. E., Laraja, R. D., et al.: Cold nodules of the thyroid: Current treatment. Head Neck Surg. 9:42–45, 1986.
103. Sarda, A. K., Bal, S., et al.: Diagnosis and treatment of cystic disease of the thyroid by aspiration. Surgery 103:593–596, 1988.
104. Schmid, K. W., Hofstadter, F., et al.: A fourteen year practice with fine needle aspiration biopsy of the thyroid in an endemic area. Pathol. Res. Pract. 181:308–310, 1986.
105. Schneider, V., and Frable, W. J.: Spindle and giant cell carcinoma of the thyroid: Cytologic diagnosis by fine needle aspiration. Acta Cytol. 24:184–189, 1980.
106. Schnurer, L. B., and Winstrom, A.: Fine needle biopsy of the thyroid gland: A cytohistological comparison in cases of goiter. Ann. Otol. Rhinol. Laryngol. 87:224–227, 1978.
107. Schwartz, A. E., Nieburgs, H. E., et al.: The place of fine needle biopsy in the diagnosis of nodules of the thyroid. Surg. Gynecol. Obstet. 155:54–58, 1982.
108. Silverman, J. F., West, R. L., et al.: Fine needle aspiration versus large needle biopsy or cutting biopsy in evaluation of thyroid nodules. Diagn. Cytopathol. 2:25–30, 1986.
109. Silverman, J. F., West, L. R., et al.: The role of fine needle aspiration biopsy in the rapid diagnosis and management of thyroid neoplasm. Cancer 57:1164–1170, 1986.
110. Smed, S., and Lennquist, S.: The role of aspiration cytology in the management of thyroid nodules. Eur. J. Cancer Clin. Oncol. 24:293–297, 1988.
111. Smejkal, V., Smejkalova, E., et al.: Cytologic changes simulating malignancy in thyrotoxic goiters treated with carbimazole. Acta Cytol. 29:173–178, 1985.
112. Smith, S. A., Gharib, H., and Goellner, J. R.: Fine needle aspiration; usefulness for diagnosis and management of metastatic carcinoma to the thyroid. Arch. Intern. Med. 147:311–312, 1987.
113. Suen, K. C.: How does one separate cellular follicular lesions of the thyroid by fine needle aspiration biopsy? Diagn. Cytopathol. 4:78–81, 1988.
114. Suen, K. C., and Quenville, N. F.: Fine needle aspiration biopsy of the thyroid gland: A study of 304 cases. J. Clin. Pathol. 36:1036–1045, 1983.
115. Szporn, A. H., Tepper, S., and Watson, C. W.: Disseminated cryptococcosis presenting as thyroiditis; fine needle aspiration and autopsy findings. Acta Cytol. 29:449–453, 1985.
116. VanHerle, A. J., Rich, P., et al.: The thyroid nodule. Ann. Intern. Med. 96:221–232, 1982.
117. Vickery, A. L.: Needle biopsy pathology. Clin. Endocrinol. Metab. 10:275–292, 1981.
118. Volpe, R.: The thyroid nodule—an approach to management. J. Otolaryngol. 12:107–108, 1983.
119. Walfish, P. G., Hazani, E., et al.: A prospective study of combined ultrasonography and needle aspiration biopsy in the assessment of the hypofunctioning thyroid nodule. Surgery 82:474–482, 1977.
120. Walfish, P. G., Hazani, E., et al.: Combined ultrasound and needle aspiration cytology in the assessment and management of the hypofunctioning thyroid nodule. Ann. Intern. Med. 87:270–274, 1977.
121. Wang, C., Guyton, S. P., and Vickery, A., L.: A further note on the large needle biopsy of the thyroid gland. Surg. Gynecol. Obstet. 156:509–510, 1983.
122. Wang, C., Vickery, A. L., and Maloof, F.: Needle biopsy of the thyroid. Surg. Gynecol. Obstet. 143:365–368, 1976.
123. Watts, N. B.: Carcinoma metastatic to the thyroid: Prevalence and diagnosis by fine needle aspiration cytology. Am. J. Med. Sci. 293:13–17, 1987.
124. Weymuller, E. A., Kiviat, N. B., and Duckert, L. G.: Aspiration cytology. An efficient and cost effective modality. Laryngoscope 93:561–564, 1983.
125. Willems, J. S., and Lowhagen, T.: Fine needle aspiration cytology in thyroid disease. Clin. Endocrinol. Metab. 10:247–266, 1981.
126. Willems, J. S., and Lowhagen, T.: The role of fine needle aspiration cytology in the management of thyroid disease. Clin. Endocrinol. Metab. 10:267–273, 1981.

127. Willems, J. S., Lowhagen, T., and Palombini, L.: The cytology of a giant-cell, osteoclastoma-like malignant thyroid neoplasm. Acta Cytol. *23:*214–216, 1979.
128. Wright, R. G., and Castles, H.: Variability of thyroid cell nuclear size with Romanowsky stains. Acta Cytol. *31:*526–527, 1987.
129. Wright, R. G., Castles, H., and Mortimer, R. H.: Morphometric analysis of thyroid cell aspirates. J. Clin. Pathol. *40:*443–445, 1987.
130. Zirkin, H. J., Hertzanu, Y., and Gal, R.: Fine needle aspiration cytology and immunocytochemistry in a case of intrathoracic thyroid goiter. Acta Cytol. *31:*694–698, 1987.

18

SPECIAL TECHNIQUES IN THE EVALUATION OF THYROID DISEASE

ELECTRON MICROSCOPY

The ultrastructural features of the normal thyroid gland have been described in Chapter 1. The thyroid follicle is organized so that the synthesis, storage, and subsequent secretion of thyroid hormone can occur.

Follicular neoplasms recapitulate the ultrastructure of the normal gland, since the cells show polarity to the lumen and apical terminal bars.[82, 151, 152] Johannessen et al. indicate that cytoplasmic organelles decrease as one progresses from normal thyroid through adenomas to follicular carcinomas;[81, 83] these authors postulated that this change most likely correlated with decreasing endocrine function of tumors when compared with the normal gland.

In those follicular derived tumors with Hürthle cell cytology, the voluminous mitochondria are noted;[81, 82] similarly, as noted in Chapter 15, some follicular clear cell tumors show features that may help distinguish them from metastatic renal cancers: absence of fat, and little glycogen.[167]

Most *papillary cancers* are diagnosed readily by histology alone. In keeping with their light microscopic appearance, papillary cancers of the thyroid show nuclear clearing or pores at the electron microscopic (EM) level.[13, 81, 83, 150] Of note, especially in view of the immunostaining results discussed below, Gould et al. described areas suggestive of squamous differentiation in some of the papillary tumors they examined.[61]

Small cell lesions of the thyroid have been studied extensively by EM; most reports indicate that the majority of these lesions are nonepithelial and probably lymphomas. Immunohistochemical results support the ultrastructural findings.[28, 159]

Many electron microscopic studies of *medullary carcinoma* have appeared. These tumors display the ultrastructural features of peptide hormone–producing cells and tumors.[41, 74, 125] Well-developed rough endoplasmic reticulum and Golgi complexes are found; characteristic neurosecretory granules are seen.[74, 125] In the extracellular space, amyloid fibrils are present in most but not all examples of medullary cancer.[74, 89] (See also Chapter 10.) The cells of medullary carcinoma share electron microscopic features with normal C cells; the latter are noted rarely in the normal human gland, but have been studied in patients with C cell hyperplasia.[41] In poorly differentiated medullary tumors, the features so characteristic of the classic type are less well developed.[89]

Ultrastructural studies of spindle and giant cell *anaplastic carcinomas* have confirmed the epithelial nature of most of these lesions.[57, 77, 124] (See also Chapter 11.) Their ultrastructural characteristics confirm the pleomorphic light microscopic picture; large pleomorphic nuclei, often multiple, are seen in a cytoplasm that is relatively poor in organelles. Cell to cell junctions are usually noted although they are not abundant.[77]

Reports of so-called *mixed thyroid tumors* have indicated that by electron microscopy features of both medullary and follicular differentiation are noted;[65, 71, 130] this issue is not resolved. (See Chapters 10 and 15.)

DNA ANALYSIS

Techniques to determine ploidy in thyroid lesions include both static and flow cytometry. A large literature exists of the various techniques, theories of operation, and interpretation of results.[8, 22, 39, 40, 51, 73, 109, 146, 148, 156] In this chapter, I shall review those major studies which reported the value of cytometric analysis in the diagnosis and prognosis of thyroid tumors.

Several early reports indicated that evaluation of aneuploidy in certain thyroid nodules could predict their biologic behavior, i.e., cytometric analysis could render a diagnosis.[14, 63] Further studies involving large numbers of cases proved unequivocally that this was incorrect. For example, the distinction between benign and malignant follicular thyroid nodules continues to be problematical for the pathologist. If assessment of ploidy on cells retrieved from a fine needle aspiration biopsy could distinguish between benign and cancerous follicular tumors, it would provide a major diagnostic tool. However, the work of Johannessen et al.,[84, 86] Joensuu et al.,[79] and others[6, 111] indicated that this is unfortunately not the case. By evaluating solitary follicular nodules (adenomas), nodular goiter, and even normal thyroid, Joensuu et al. found aneuploid DNA patterns in 27 percent of adenomas, 14 percent of nodular goiter and even in some normal glands.[79] The followup in this series averaged 7.2 years and was benign in each patient. Similarly, several reports[23, 48, 112] indicate that the distinction between benign and malignant Hürthle cell tumors cannot be made by flow cytometric analysis (Figs. 18–1 and 18–2; Chapter 12).

The obvious question to be asked then is: Is cytometric measurement of any use in thyroid disease? The answer is an unequivocal YES! As in other neoplasms of diverse origin, such as breast cancer, analysis of ploidy in thyroid lesions can be useful. *After a histologic diagnosis of cancer has been made,* determination of ploidy status and growth rate may have prognostic value.

Papillary Carcinoma. Although the great majority of papillary thyroid cancers are diploid, the literature suggests up to 20 percent may show aneuploid or at least nondiploid subpopulations.[7, 85, 86, 96] (However, if up to 20 percent of papillary cancers have abnormal ploidy patterns, there must be other factors at work, since surely 20 percent of papillary carcinomas do not behave in aggressive fashion.)

Occasional reports of aggressive or "anomalous" behavior in papillary carcinomas[85] have attributed the unusual biology to aneuploidy in the tumor (all other parameters suggesting usual papillary cancer).

Backdahl analyzed 40 papillary carcinomas and noted that survivors had diploid tumors[7]; hence only two of 34 patients with diploid DNA patterns developed distant metastases. In contrast, all six patients with aneuploid papillary cancers

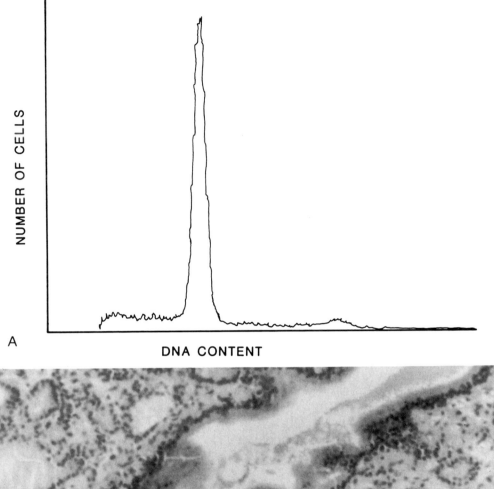

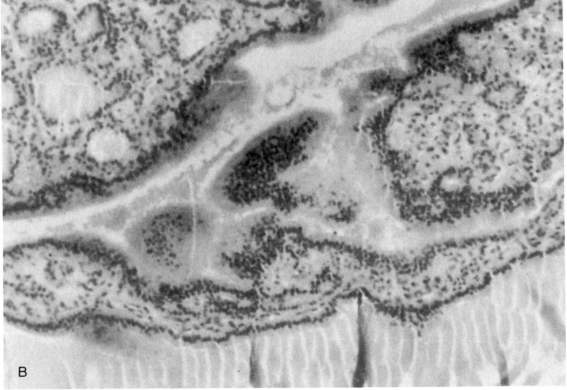

Figure 18–1. *A,* Flow cytometric analysis of multinodular goiter shows discrete diploid peak. *B,* Histologic photo of goiter. × 100, H & E.

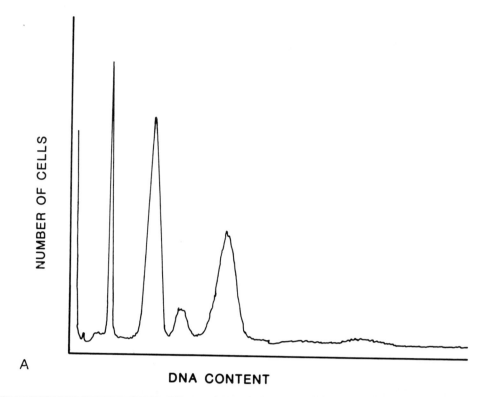

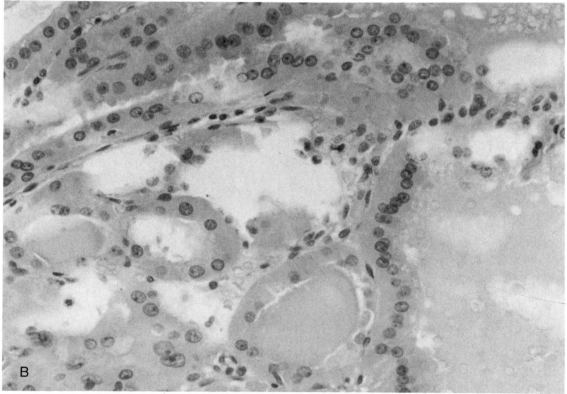

Figure 18–2. *A,* Flow cytometry of this Hürthle cell adenomatous nodule disclosed multiple peaks indicating aneuploid cell population. *B,* Histologic photo of specimen. × 150, H & E.

had distant metastases and all died of their tumors. Cohn et al. reported similar results in their series of 90 cases[38]: patients who died of tumor had lesions with abnormal (aneuploid) DNA patterns.

Follicular Carcinoma. A summary of the published studies shows that about 60 percent of follicular carcinomas will show aneuploid cell populations. Backdahl analyzed 65 follicular thyroid tumors (26 benign and 39 carcinomas).[7] He noted that, of the 20 patients with cancer who survived, 19 had diploid tumors, whereas 17 of 19 patients who died of carcinoma had tumors with aneuploid DNA patterns.

Christov reported 52 cases, in one of the few studies using fresh, not paraffin-embedded, material, and found that normal thyroid and follicular adenomas had diploid DNA patterns, whereas 65 percent (13 of 20) of follicular cancers showed aneuploid cell lines.[31] This author also identified higher growth rates in cancers than in benign nodules, and this was especially evident in less well differentiated carcinomas.

Hürthle Cell Tumors. Biologically and histologically, benign oxyphilic tumors of the thyroid can show aneuploid DNA patterns. Such a finding does not indicate malignant behavior, however.[20, 21, 23, 48, 112]

About 20 to 50 percent of Hürthle cell carcinomas are aneuploid. The studies so far reported, however, do indicate that Hürthle cell tumors which are histologically malignant and aneuploid are more aggressive biologically and clinically than diploid Hürthle cell cancers. Studies using static or flow cytometry indicate this.[20, 21, 23, 48, 112, 132] For example, Rainwater et al. evaluated 37 oncocytic thyroid tumors;[132] lesions that were diploid were never associated with a fatal outcome, whereas 58 percent of aneuploid tumors proved fatal.

Medullary Carcinoma. Schroder et al. studied a number of variables in a series of medullary thyroid carcinomas and found that aneuploid tumors were more aggressive in their biologic behavior.[142] About 50 percent of medullary cancers studied by flow cytometry contained aneuploid cell populations[142] (Fig. 18–3).

Anaplastic Carcinoma. Klemi and Joensuu analyzed 19 anaplastic thyroid tumors and found all were aneuploid[93]; these authors noted that the higher the DNA index the shorter the survival. Galera-Davidson et al. identified aneuploid cell lines in each of the 15 anaplastic carcinomas they studied.[58] An interesting finding in this report, however, was that aneuploidy was noted in the "differentiated" zones abutting the anaplastic tumors. These authors postulated that perhaps aneuploid differentiated thyroid cancers are more likely to undergo transformation to anaplastic lesions and thus have a worse prognosis.[58]

Metastatic Thyroid Carcinoma. Joensuu and Klemi reported similar DNA ploidy patterns in primary and metastatic foci of most differentiated thyroid cancers they studied.[78] However, in a few cases, variations were noted; some metastases were aneuploid from diploid primaries, and conversely, although more rarely, diploid metastases were found from aneuploid primary tumors. The reasons for this are not clear, but suggest heterogeneity of tumor populations, even in well-differentiated thyroid cancers.[78]

Malignant Lymphomas of the Thyroid. These were analyzed by Zirkin et al.,[175] and their report indicated that, in these lesions as well, diploid tumors were associated with prolonged survival, while patients with aneuploid tumors fared poorly.

In summary, aneuploidy in papillary, follicular, and medullary carcinomas is more likely in older patients, in less differentiated tumors, and in tumors infiltrating beyond the thyroid capsule. Patients with aneuploid tumors have a significantly worse survival rate than their diploid counterparts in each tumor category. The greater the DNA index, the worse the ultimate prognosis.[80]

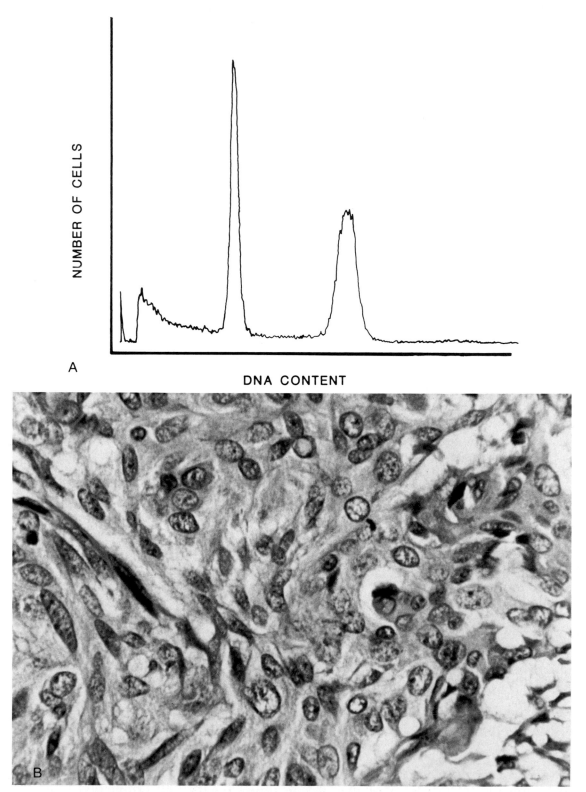

Figure 18–3. *A,* Aneuploid pattern in a medullary thyroid carcinoma. *B,* Histologic photo of specimen. × 250, H & E.

However, age, tumor type and extrathyroidal extension appear to be more important prognostic variables.

It must be remembered that all studies reported may not be exactly comparable since some utilize fresh tissue[38, 79] and others formalin-fixed paraffin-embedded archival material.[7, 23, 79, 80, 112, 132] Obviously the latter allows for prolonged follow-up periods and thus better assessment of biologic behavior. In the study of Joensuu et al. comparison of results on fresh versus fixed material showed only minor differences.[79] (Only one case showed different DNA patterns in fresh versus fixed tissue.)

As instrumentation and software become more sophisticated, further studies may reveal important prognostic information in individual cases. Evaluation of nucleolar proliferation antigens, oncogene product expression, and cell surface markers and their alterations in disease may be of diagnostic and prognostic use in the future.[9, 22, 146]

MORPHOMETRY (IMAGE ANALYSIS)

Several reports have appeared on the use of image analysis in evaluating thyroid neoplasms and in distinguishing between benign and malignant lesions. Techniques to measure shape of nuclei, area occupied by nuclei in relation to total cell size, and regularity of nuclear contour have been suggested as methods to differentiate among thyroid lesions.[22] However, certain hyperfunctioning foci,[17] Hürthle cell tumors,[21] and degenerative areas in adenomatous nodules can show great variability in nuclear shape and contour. Hence, the technique cannot indicate which nodules are benign or malignant.[20, 21, 83, 110, 111] Problems also arise because of unevenness of tissue sections, stains used, and instrumentation; it is possible that future studies using more sophisticated computers and more detailed software will be useful.

HISTOCHEMISTRY

Histochemical techniques have not proved useful in diagnostic thyroid pathology.[165] However, Cohen et al., using plastic embedded material, have reported that they can universally distinguish between benign and cancerous follicular tumors;[37] these authors found that benign nodules and normal thyroid never contained adenosine triphosphatase, whereas papillary and follicular carcinomas uniformly did. Further studies are needed to confirm these interesting results.

Lectins staining in thyroid lesions has been studied by Sobrinho-Simoes and Damjanov.[149] Although a number of lectins can be identified in benign and malignant thyroid proliferations, the staining patterns and types of lectins present are very variable. These studies tested 20 different lectins and noted inconsistent staining; the authors conclude that lectin histochemistry is of no diagnostic use in distinguishing among various well-differentiated thyroid neoplasms.[149]

Biochemical analyses by several authors have disclosed provocative results which may suggest that histochemical testing may eventually be useful.[45, 117, 100, 172] Osham et al. studied rat medullary carcinomas for different enolase isozymes and found less well differentiated tumors contained decreased levels of gamma enolase than better differentiated lesions[128]; although the significance of this work in human medullary cancer is as yet unknown, it may prove of some use in identifying poorly differentiated tumors in the thyroid. Verhagen et al. studied normal thyroid and benign and cancerous nodules for kinases (hexokinase and pyruvate kinase).[169, 170] These authors noted that papillary carcinomas contained lower concentrations of hexokinase than follicular and anaplastic tumors. Another study by this group showed that pyruvate kinase is more abundant in undifferentiated thyroid cancer than in papillary and follicular tumors.[169] Differences have been found between thyrotropin binding and adenylate cyclase activity, depending on degree of tumor differentiation.[33, 34] Whether these types of studies will be adaptable to histochemical testing and whether they will be diagnostically useful awaits further study.

IMMUNOHISTOCHEMISTRY

This discussion reviews the numerous reports that have appeared on the utility of various markers for the evaluation and diagnosis of thyroid lesions (Tables 18–1 and 18–2).

Thyroglobulin. A variety of immunologic techniques have demonstrated the presence of thyroglobulin in normal and diseased thyroid.[2, 18, 19, 24, 42, 55] Variable results in different series regarding the percentage of positive cases in specific tumor categories and the degree of positivity are probably due to differences in use of fresh versus fixed tissue, type and length of fixation, and type of antibody used (monoclonal versus polyclonal).[2, 42, 55, 95, 99, 104]

Numerous histochemical studies have appeared which show conclusively that thyroglobulin produced by nodules and neoplasms of the thyroid differs from that synthesized in the normal gland.[1, 16, 18, 19, 30, 32, 36, 44, 46, 50, 52, 64, 92, 95, 98, 129, 133, 136, 139, 141, 154, 158, 164, 166, 168] Thus, differences in protein structure, sialidase residues, and iodine content have been documented.[46, 95, 133, 136, 141, 158, 166] In addition, thyrotropin receptor[1, 45] sites may vary between normal follicles and neoplasms derived from follicular cells.[30, 32, 33, 35, 36, 50, 52]

Considering these variables, however, it is interesting to note the high degree of agreement with regard to immunostaining for thyroglobulin in thyroid lesions.[2, 42]

In the normal thyroid, staining is found within follicular cells and in the colloid. In adenomatous nodules similar results are seen, although the staining may appear less homogeneous than in the normal gland.

Thyroid carcinomas stain for thyroglobulin frequently, but the staining depends on degree of differentiation of the tumor; it has been generally reported that the more highly differentiated the tumor, the stronger the staining intensity.[2, 42] However, Harach and Franssila, who evaluated 47 primary and seven metastatic follicular carcinomas, found no absolute correlation between differentiation of the tumor and staining intensity.[66] They did note, however, weak thyroglobulin staining in poorly differentiated follicular tumors.[66] In addition, papillary carcinomas tend to stain less intensely than follicular lesions.[18, 19] In metastatic sites, thyroid carcinomas stain for thyroglobulin, confirming the origin of the lesion.[66]

Hürthle cell tumors, although positive, stain variably from area to area and usually stain weakly.[66, 87] Clear cell tumors in the thyroid often but not always stain for thyroglobulin, and this can be useful in distinguishing primary clear cell lesions from metastases. (See also Chapter 15.)

Rarely, anaplastic thyroid cancer can stain for thyroglobulin even in metastatic sites, and occasional examples of anaplastic tumors producing thyroglobulin in tissue culture are reported;[1, 121] however, most anaplastic cancers do not stain.[75, 102]

Medullary carcinomas are uniformly negative for thyroglobulin. Kameda et al.

Table 18–1. Staining of Thyroid Tissue and Its Lesions

	Thyroglobulin	Calcitonin	CEA	Low Molecular Weight Cytokeratin	High Molecular Weight Cytokeratin	LCA	Vimentin	Neurofilament	Synaptophysin	Other Hormones
Normal thyroid	+			+	–	–	+	–	–	
Hashimoto's	+			+	–	–	+	–	–	
Graves'	+			+	–	–	+	–	–	
NTNG	+			+	–	–	+	–	–	
"Adenoma"	+			+	–	–	+	–	–	
Papillary Ca.	+			+	+*	–	+	–	–	
Follicular Ca.	+			+	–	–	+	–	–	
MTC	–	+	+	+	–	–	+/–	+ (some)	+	+
Anaplastic Ca.	+			+	–	–	+/–	–	–	
Lymphoma	–			–	–	+	+/–	–	–	

*Variable.

Table 18–2. Thyroid Tissue and Lesions: Staining Patterns

	Normal Thyroid		Hashimoto's	Graves'	NTNG	Adenoma	Papillary Ca	Follicular Ca	MTC	Anaplastic Ca
	Follicles	C Cells								
Thyroglobulin	+		+	+	+	+	+	+	–	+/–
Calcitonin		+							+	
CEA		+							+	
Cytokeratin:										
Low molecular wgt.	+	+	+	+	+	+	+	+	+	+/some
"Epidermal"							+/–*			
Vimentin	+	+	+	+	+	+	+	+	+/–	+/–
Neurofilament									+/some	
Synaptophysin									+	
Other hormones									+	

*Variable in different studies.[43]

noted staining of C-cells, with medullary cancers with a substance they referred to as C-thyroglobulin.[90] The nature of this material is unclear, but it may represent an antigenically altered thyroglobulin.

The effect of diffusion of thyroglobulin into tumor cells of medullary, anaplastic, or even metastatic tumors to the thyroid can produce falsely positive results and great diagnostic problems. The issue of the existence of so-called mixed follicular and parafollicular tumors needs to be mentioned here as well,[65, 103, 130] since some of the lesions reported as mixed tumors in the thyroid may represent this diffusion phenomenon and not true dual differentiation.[71, 101]

Keratin. The intermediate filament, cytokeratin, is contained in many epithelial cells.[11, 12, 54, 119, 120, 126] Follicular and parafollicular cells of the thyroid are no exception.[69, 143] Discrepancies have appeared in the published literature, however. Permanetter et al. indicated that follicular adenomas and carcinomas did not stain for keratin.[129] Other studies indicate that low molecular weight keratins can be found in normal follicular and C cells and in almost all thyroid nodules and cancers.[69]

High molecular weight or epidermal keratins are found in papillary carcinomas but not true follicular and medullary lesions. The epidermal keratins are found in follicular and solid areas of papillary tumors, and it has been suggested that immunostaining for this type of keratin may be helpful in distinguishing follicular carcinoma from the follicular variant of papillary cancer. Why should papillary cancers contain epidermal keratin? The presence of squamous metaplasia in such lesions and the finding of squamous features by EM in some of these tumors may explain the immunostaining results.[61]

Miettenen et al.[115] and Bennett et al.[15] have suggested from their studies that keratin immunostaining may be helpful in differentiating between papillary carcinomas and papillary hyperplastic changes in follicular nodules. Thus, it appears from these reports that all papillary cancers stain intensely for monoclonal keratin, whereas hyperplastic nodules stain weakly. These results, if confirmed in large series of cases, may prove diagnostically very useful in practice.

Recent studies, however, indicate that the keratin staining in the thyroid may not be so straightforward[43, 68]; by careful biochemical and immunologic assessment of antibodies used, Dockhorn-Dworniczak et al. noted variable staining results in thyroid tumors.[43] This study found that all thyroid nodules, benign inflammatory and hyperplastic lesions as well as carcinomas, contain low molecular weight keratin; however, epidermal keratin was not identified. (See Table 18–1.) These authors do point out, however, that they did not study lesions with squamous metaplasia.

Anaplastic thyroid tumors stain for keratin in anywhere from 1 to 100 percent of cases. (In our own study it averaged about 50 percent.[102]) Such positive results for keratin may be helpful in the differential diagnosis of such anaplastic tumors from lymphoma or sarcoma.[123]

Vimentin. This intermediate filament can be found in a wide range of cells including sarcomas and carcinomas.[43, 126] Vimentin has been identified in a wide range of thyroid lesions. Coexpression of keratin and vimentin has been reported in some papillary, follicular, and even medullary carcinomas. This coexpression is seen most frequently in anaplastic thyroid tumors, although it can also be noted in differentiated thyroid carcinomas.[3, 43, 102]

Calcitonin. This hormone is found in C cells and medullary carcinomas. Staining intensity varies but is usually very strong in normal and hyperplastic C cells. Variable staining patterns are found in medullary carcinomas,[53, 70, 113, 114, 138] and some series now have shown conclusively that percentage of tumor cell stained and staining intensity can be used to prognosticate about an individual tumor. Thus tumors with 75 percent or more cells staining tend to have a biologically less aggressive course than those with small numbers of cells stained.[100, 114, 138, 142] Saad et al. divided their medullary cancers into three groups based on immuno-staining results: calcitonin-rich (>75% cells stained), calcitonin-poor (<25% cells stained) and intermediate.[138] These authors found that five-year survival rates were 100 percent, 53 percent, and 93 percent, respectively, for the groups. In addition, staining results in metastases sometimes show fewer positive cells, and with tumor progression, calcitonin staining may be minimal or even absent.[135, 138] Patients with Sipple's syndrome (multiple endocrine neoplasia type 2A) tend to have calcitonin-rich tumors and enjoy a prolonged survival.[138]

Calcitonin Gene Related Peptide (CGRP). This has also been found immuno-histologically in medullary carcinomas.[4, 72, 76, 122, 174] It is occasionally found in medullary carcinomas in which calcitonin is immunohistochemically absent.[97]

Carcinoembryonic Antigen (CEA). This substance, an oncofetal antigen, is present in normal and hyperplastic C cells and medullary carcinomas. Correlations between CEA and calcitonin staining and serum levels have been shown to be of prognostic importance in medullary cancers.[25, 26, 47, 53, 94, 97, 108, 114, 137, 142, 144, 147, 155, 163]

Although some reports indicate that nonmedullary cancers contain CEA,[171] this may represent spurious results related to antibodies used; Schroder and Kloppel addressed this question[144] and identified CEA only in C-cell hyperplasia and medullary cancers when using monoclonal antibody, but noted staining in other thyroid lesions when using a polyclonal antibody to CEA. They attributed their results to nonspecific cross reactions and affirmed that CEA is specific for C-cell lesions of the thyroid.

Other Hormone Markers. Chromogranin and neuron-specific enolase can be localized in medullary carcinoma, but these are nonspecific markers for neuroen-docrine tissues and tumors.[5, 106, 108, 140] In addition, certain examples of medullary carcinoma have been shown to contain (and secrete) adrenocorticotropin (ACTH), bombesin, synaptophysin, and other peptides, resembling the staining results of neuroendocrine tumors in general.[27, 29, 59, 62, 72, 97, 100, 125, 127, 134, 153] Some of these medullary cancers have been associated with clinical evidence of hypersecretion of these hormones, e.g., Cushing's syndrome due to secretion of ACTH. (See Chapter 10.)

Other Substances. Immunostaining for Ulex europeus lectin, a marker for endothelial cells, has been used successfully by some authors to identify vascular invasion in thyroid tumors.[60] This has been especially useful diagnostically in follicular nodules and neoplasms. However, Harach et al. found staining for factor VIII related antigen was not useful in identifying vascular invasion, since vessels completely occluded by tumor did not stain in some of their cases of follicular carcinoma.[67] Kendall et al. also found staining for laminin and basement membrane (type IV) collagen useful in this distinction.[91]

Laminin is preserved in well-differentiated tumors but not in poorly differen-tiated ones.[116]

Lactoferrin and ceruloplasmin, both substances not normally found in the thyroid, have been studied by Tuccari and Barresi.[10, 161, 162] These authors found that immunostaining for these substances could invariably distinguish between follicular adenomas and follicular carcinomas. Hence, 15 adenomas were negative for lactoferrin and ceruloplasmin, but 21 follicular carcinomas as well as six papillary carcinomas and two Hürthle cell tumors stained. Other workers have been unable to confirm these results (Bedrosian, C.—personal communication).

Markers for lymphoid cells, such as leukocyte common antigen, may prove helpful for large and small cell diffuse lymphomas of the thyroid that can be mistaken for anaplastic cancers.[123] The availability of monoclonal antibodies to distinguish B and T cell subsets in paraffin-embedded, fixed tissue allows for assessment of clonal neoplasms in lymphoid proliferations affecting the thyroid.[131] Leu-M1 antigen, a monocyte/granulocyte marker, can also be found in carcinomas. A recent study by Schroder et al. suggests that strong Leu-M1 staining in papillary carcinoma may portend a more aggressive clinical behavior.[145]

Some studies also have shown that medullary cancers can contain neurofilament proteins.[62]

ONCOGENES

A few reports have appeared that discuss the expression of oncogenes in thyroid lesions.[49, 157, 173] The study by Johnson et al. indicates that ras oncogene product p21 can be identified immunohistochemically in proliferative and benign and malignant paraffin-embedded thyroid tissue.[88] Although these authors found differences in staining intensity between normal thyroid tissue and some cancers, the immunoperoxidase results were not helpful in distinguishing between benign nodules and cancer; hence, it did not appear to represent a diagnostically useful marker. However, a study from Japan indicated that p21 staining in papillary cancers is strong and apically located, implying that this marker may be helpful in some cases.[118]

Fusco et al. described finding a novel oncogene in coculture of human papillary cancer and a transformed cell line, NIH3T3.[56] This exciting finding awaits further study to see if an oncogene unique for papillary carcinoma has indeed been identified.

Other reports indicate expression of myc and ras oncogenes in neoplastic thyroid tissue.[157, 173]

The possibility of evaluating thyroid tumors with specific oncogene products by the techniques of in situ hybridization offers promise for the future.[105, 174]

HISTOCOMPATIBILITY ANTIGENS

Immunostaining for histocompatibility antigens in thyroid lesions has been reported by Lloyd et al.[107] These authors and others[170a] found HLA-DR antigens in Hashimoto's thyroiditis, Graves' disease, and papillary cancer, including the follicular variant. Negative results were obtained in nodular goiter and follicular and anaplastic carcinomas. These studies provide further evidence for antigenic changes in thyroid epithelial cells in autoimmune disease and in some specific tumors. It is possible that immunostaining for HLA-DR may prove useful in distinguishing the follicular variant of papillary cancer from true follicular carcinoma; however, studies of larger numbers of cases appear needed to further evaluate this technique.

SUMMARY

Many markers are helpful in diagnosis of thyroid tumors. One must always remember the caution that diffusion of one or another hormone or filament or marker into a tumor in the thyroid can cause diagnostic problems. Diagnoses based solely on immunostaining results should not be tolerated if the histologic pattern, EM, or clinical picture is incompatible.

REFERENCES

1. Abe, Y., Ichikawa, Y., et al.: Thyrotropin (TSH) receptor and adenylate cyclase activity in human thyroid tumors: Absence of high affinity receptor and loss of TSH responsiveness in undifferentiated thyroid carcinoma. J. Clin. Endocrinol. Metab. 52:23–28, 1981.
2. Albores-Saavedra, J., Nadji, M., et al.: Thyroglobulin in carcinoma of the thyroid. An immunohistochemical study. Hum. Pathol. 14:62–66, 1983.
3. Altmannsberger, M., Dralle, H., et al.: Intermediate filaments in cytological specimens of thyroid tumors. Diagn. Cytopathol. 3:210–214, 1987.
4. Amara, S. G., Jonas, V., et al.: Alternative RNA processing in calcitonin gene expression generates mRNAs encoding different polypeptide products. Nature 298:240–244, 1982.
5. Angeletti, R. H.: Chromogranins and neuroendocrine secretion. Lab. Invest. 55:387–390, 1986.
6. Arps, H., Sablotny, B., et al.: DNA cytophotometry in malignant thyroid tumors—use of different evaluation schemes for prognostic statements. Virch. Arch. Pathol. Anat. 413:319–323, 1988.
7. Backdahl, M.: Nuclear DNA content and prognosis in papillary, follicular and medullary carcinomas of the thyroid. Doctoral thesis, Karolinska Medical Institute, Stockholm, Sweden, 1985.
8. Bahr, G. F.: Frontiers in quantitative cytochemistry: A review of recent developments and potentials. Anal. Quant. Cytol. 1:1–19, 1979.
9. Bakke, A. C., Sahin, A., and Braziel, R. M.: Applications of flow cytometry in surgical pathology. Lab. Med. 18:590–596, 1987.
10. Barresi, G., and Tuccari, G.: Iron binding proteins in thyroid tumours. Pathol. Res. Pract. 182: 344–351, 1987.
11. Battifora, H.: The biology of the keratins and their diagnostic applications. In: DeLellis, R. A. (ed.) Advances in Immunohistochemistry. New York, Raven Press, Inc., 1988, pp. 191–221.
12. Battifora, H.: Diagnostic uses of antibodies to keratins: A review and immunohistochemical comparison of seven monoclonal and three polyclonal antibodies. Prog. Surg. Pathol. 8:1–15, 1988.
13. Beaumont, A., Othman, S. B., and Fragu, P.: The fine structure of papillary carcinoma of the thyroid. Histopathology 5:377–388, 1981.
14. Bengtsson, A., Malmaeus, J., et al.: Measurement of nuclear DNA content in thyroid diagnosis. World J. Surg. 8:481–486, 1984.
15. Bennett, W. P., Bhan, A. K., and Vickery, A. L.: Keratin expression as a diagnostic adjunct in thyroid tumors with papillary architecture. Lab. Invest. 58:9A, 1988 (abstract).
16. Berge-LeFranc, J. L., Cartouzou, G., et al.: Quantification of thyroglobulin messenger RNA by in-situ hybridization in differentiated thyroid cancers. Cancer 56:345–350, 1985.
17. Bjelkenkrantz, K., Risberg, B. et al.: Cytophotometric determination of nuclear size and DNA distribution in different hyperfunctioning thyroid lesions. Virch. Arch. Pathol. Anat. 398:129–137, 1982.
18. Bocker, W., Dralle, H., et al.: Immunohistochemical analysis of thyroglobulin synthesis in thyroid carcinomas. Virch. Arch. Pathol. Anat. 385:187–200, 1980.
19. Bocker, W., Dralle, H., et al.: Immunohistochemical and electron microscopic analysis of adenomas of the thyroid gland. Virch. Arch. Pathol. Anat. 380:205–220, 1978.
20. Bondeson, L., Azavedo, E., et al.: Nuclear DNA content and behavior of oxyphil thyroid tumors. Cancer 58:672–675, 1986.
21. Bondeson, L., Bondeson, A. G., et al.: Morphometric studies on nuclei in smears of fine needle aspirates from oxyphilic tumors of the thyroid. Acta Cytol. 27:437–440, 1983.
22. Boon, M. E., Lowhagen, T., and Williams, J. S.: Planimetric studies on fine needle aspirates from follicular adenoma and follicular carcinoma of the thyroid. Acta Cytol. 24:145–148, 1980.
23. Bronner, M. P., Clevenger, C. V., et al.: Flow cytometric analysis of DNA content in Hürthle cell adenomas and carcinomas of the thyroid. Am. J. Clin. Pathol. 89:764–769, 1988.
24. Burt, A., and Goudie, R. B.: Diagnosis of primary thyroid carcinoma by immunohistological demonstration of thyroglobulin. Histopathology 3:279–286, 1979.
25. Burtin, P., Calmettes, C., and Fondaneche, M. C.: CEA and nonspecific cross-reacting antigen (NCA) in medullary carcinomas of the thyroid. Int. J. Cancer 23:741–745, 1979.
26. Busnardo, B., Girelli, E., et al.: Nonparallel patterns of calcitonin and carcinoembryonic antigen levels in the followup of medullary thyroid carcinoma. Cancer 53:278–285, 1984.
27. Bussolati, G., Van Noorden, S., and Bordi, C.: Calcitonin and ACTH producing in a case of medullary carcinoma of the thyroid. Virch. Arch. Pathol. Anat. 360:123–127, 1973.
28. Cameron, R. G., Seemayer, T. A., et al.: Small cell malignant tumors of the thyroid: A light and electronic microscopic study. Hum. Pathol. 6:731–740, 1975.

29. Capella, C., Bordi, C., et al.: Multiple endocrine cell types in thyroid medullary carcinoma. Virch. Arch. Pathol. Anat. *377*:111–128, 1978.

30. Carayon, P., Thomas-Morvan, C., et al.: Human thyroid cancer: Membrane thyrotropin binding and adenylate cyclase activity. J. Clin. Endocrinol. Metab. *51*:915–920, 1980.

31. Christov, K.: Flow cytometric DNA measurements in human thyroid tumors. Virch. Arch. Cell Pathol. *51*:255–263, 1986.

32. Clark, O., and Gerend, P. L.: Thyrotropin regulation of adenylate cyclase activity in human thyroid neoplasms. Surgery *97*:539–546, 1985.

33. Clark, O. H., Gerend, P. L., and Nissenson, R. A.: Mechanisms for increased adenylate cyclase responsiveness to TSH in neoplastic human thyroid tissue. World J. Surg. *8*:466–473, 1984.

34. Clark, O., Gerend, P. L., et al.: Thyrotropin binding and adenylate cyclase stimulation in thyroid neoplasms. Surgery *90*:252–261, 1981.

35. Clark, O., Gerend, P. L., et al.: Estrogen and thyroid-stimulating hormone (TSH) receptors in neoplastic and nonneoplastic human thyroid tissue. J. Surg. Res. *38*:89–96, 1985.

36. Clark, O., Gerend, P. L., et al.: Characterization of the thyrotropin receptor-adenylate cyclase system in neoplastic human thyroid tissue. J. Clin. Endocrinol. Metab. *57*:140–147, 1983.

37. Cohen, M. B., Miller, T. R., and Beckstead, J. H.: Enzyme histochemistry and thyroid neoplasia. Am. J. Clin. Pathol. *85*:668–673, 1986.

38. Cohn, K., Backdahl, M., et al.: Prognostic value of nuclear DNA content in papillary thyroid carcinoma. World J. Surg. *8*:474–480, 1984.

39. Collan, Y.: Stereology and morphometry in histopathology; Principles of application. Anal. Quant. Cytol. *7*:237–241, 1985.

40. Collan, Y., Torkkeli, T., et al.: Application of morphometry in tumor pathology. Anal. Quant. Cytol. *9*:79–86, 1987.

41. DeLellis, R. A., Nunnemacher, G., and Wolfe, H. J.: Cell hyperplasia. An ultrastructural analysis. Lab. Invest. *36*:237–249, 1977.

42. DeMicco, C., Ruf, J., et al.: Immunohistochemical study of thyroglobulin in thyroid carcinomas with monoclonal antibodies. Cancer *59*:471–476, 1987.

43. Dockhorn-Dworniczak, B., Franke, W. W., et al.: Patterns of cytoskeletal proteins in human thyroid gland and thyroid carcinomas. Differentiation *35*:53–71, 1987.

44. Dralle, H., Bocker, W., et al.: Morphometric lightmicroscopic and immunohistochemical analyses of differentiated thyroid carcinomas. Virch. Arch. Pathol. Anat. *398*:87–99, 1982.

45. Duh, Q. Y., Gum, E. T., et al.: Epidermal growth factor receptors in normal and neoplastic thyroid tissue. Surgery *98*:1000–1006, 1985.

46. Dunn, J. T., and Ray, S. C.: Changes in iodine metabolism and thyroglobulin structure in metastatic follicular carcinoma of the thyroid with hyperthyroidism. J. Clin. Endocrinol. Metab. *36*:1088–1096, 1973.

47. Ekblom, M., Valimaki, M., et al.: Familial and sporadic medullary thyroid carcinoma: clinical and immunohistological findings. Quart. J. Med. *247*:899–910, 1987.

48. El Naggar, A. K., Batsakis, J. G., et al.: Hürthle cell tumors of the thyroid: a flow cytometric DNA analysis. Arch. Otolaryngol. Head Neck Surg. *114*:520–521, 1988.

49. Fagin, J. A., Namba, H., et al.: Protooncogene mutations in human thyroid neoplasms: H-ras amplification and gene rearrangements. Clin. Res. *37*:107A, 1989 (abstract).

50. Field, J. B., Bloom, G., et al.: Effects of thyroid stimulating hormone on human thyroid carcinoma and adjacent normal tissue. J. Clin. Endocrinol. Metab. *47*:1052–1058, 1978.

51. Flint, A., Lovett, E. J., et al.: Flow cytometric analysis of DNA in diagnostic cytology. Am. J. Clin. Pathol. *84*:278–282, 1985.

52. Fragu, P., and Nataf, B. M.: Human thyroid peroxidase activity in benign and malignant thyroid disorders. J. Clin. Endocrinol. Metab. *45*:1089–1096, 1977.

53. Franc, B., and Caillou, B.: Le cancer medullaire de la thyroide: definitions morphologiques et immunohistochemiques. Le role du pathologiste en 1987. Ann. d'Endocrinol. *49*:22–33, 1988.

54. Franke, W. W., Schiller, E. L., et al.: Diversity of cytokeratins. J. Mol. Biol. *153*:933–959, 1981.

55. Franklin, W. A., Mariotti, S., et al.: Immunofluorescence localization of thyroglobulin in metastatic thyroid cancer. Cancer *50*:939–945, 1982.

56. Fusco, A., Grieco, M., et al.: A new oncogene in human thyroid papillary carcinomas and their lymph nodal metastases. Nature *328*:170–172, 1987.

57. Gaal, J. M., Horvath, E., and Kovacs, K.: Ultrastructure of two cases of anaplastic giant cell tumor of the human thyroid gland. Cancer *35*:1273–1279, 1975.

58. Galera-Davidson, H., Bibbo, M., et al.: Nuclear DNA in anaplastic thyroid carcinoma with a differentiated component. Histopathology *11*:715–722, 1987.

59. Goltzman, D., Huang, S. N., et al.: Adrenocorticotropin and calcitonin in medullary thyroid carcinoma: Frequency of occurrence and localization in the same cell type by immunocyto-chemistry. J. Clin. Endocrinol. Metab. *49*:364–369, 1979.

60. Gonzalez-Campora, R., Montero, C., et al.: Demonstration of vascular endothelium in thyroid carcinomas using Ulex europaeus I agglutinin. Histopathology, *10*:261–266, 1986.

61. Gould, V. E., Gould, N. S., and Benditt, E. P.: Ultrastructural aspects of papillary and sclerosing carcinomas of the thyroid. Cancer *29*:1613–1625, 1972.

62. Gould, V. E., Wiedenmann, B., et al.: Synaptophysin expression in neuroendocrine neoplasms as determined by immunocytochemistry. Am. J. Pathol. *126*:243–257, 1987.

63. Greenbaum, E., Koss, L. G., et al.: The diagnostic value of flow cytometric DNA measurement in follicular tumors of the thyroid gland. Cancer 56:2011–2018, 1985.
64. Gwinup, G., and Elias, A. N.: Evidence for TSH autoregulation of thyroid carcinoma. Am. J. Med. Sci. 287:42–43, 1984.
65. Hales, M., Rosenau, W., et al.: Carcinoma of the thyroid with a mixed medullary and follicular pattern. Morphological, immunohistochemical and clinical laboratory studies. Cancer 50:1352–1359, 1982.
66. Harach, H. R., and Franssila, K. O.: Thyroglobulin immunostaining in follicular thyroid carcinoma. Histopathology 13:43–54, 1988.
67. Harach, H. R., Jasani, B., and Williams, E. D.: Factor VIII as a marker for endothelial cells in follicular carcinoma of the thyroid. J. Clin. Pathol. 36:1050–1054, 1983.
68. Henzen-Logmans, S. C., Mullink, H., et al.: Expression of cytokeratins and vimentin in epithelial cells of normal and pathologic thyroid tissue. Virch. Arch. Pathol. Anat. 410:347–354, 1987.
69. Hoefler, H., Denk, H., et al.: Immunocytochemical demonstration of intermediate filament cytoskeleton proteins in human endocrine tissues and (neuro-) endocrine tumours. Virch. Arch. Pathol. Anat. 409:609–626, 1986.
70. Holm, R., Sobrinho-Simoes, M., et al.: Medullary carcinoma of the thyroid gland: an immuno-cytochemical study. Ultrastruct. Pathol. 8:25–41, 1985.
71. Holm, R., Sobrinho-Simoes, M., et al.: Concurrent production of calcitonin and thyroglobulin by the same neoplastic cells. Ultrastruct. Pathol. 10:241–248, 1986.
72. Hoppener, J. W. M., Steenbergh, P. H., et al.: Detection of mRNA encoding calcitonin, calcitonin gene related peptide and proopiomelanocortin in human tumors. Molecul. Cell. Endocrinol. 47:125–130, 1986.
73. Hostetter, A. L., Hrafnkelsson, J., et al.: A comparative study of DNA cytometry methods for benign and malignant thyroid tissue. Am. J. Clin. Pathol. 89:760–763, 1988.
74. Huang, S. N., and Goltzman, D.: Electron and immunoelectron microscopic study of thyroidal medullary carcinoma. Cancer 41:2226–2233, 1978.
75. Hurliman, J., Gardiol, D., and Scazziga, B.: Immunohistology of anaplastic carcinoma. A study of 43 cases. Histopathology 11:567–580, 1987.
76. Jacobs, J. W., Simpson, E., et al.: Characterization and localization of calcitonin messenger ribonucleic acid in rat thyroid. Endocrinology 113:1616–1622, 1983.
77. Jao, W., and Gould, V. E.: Ultrastructure of anaplastic (spindle and giant cell) carcinoma of the thyroid. Cancer 35:1280–1292, 1975.
78. Joensuu, H., and Klemi, P.: Comparison of nuclear DNA content in primary and metastatic differentiated thyroid carcinoma. Am. J. Clin. Pathol. 89:35–40, 1988.
79. Joensuu, H., Klemi, P., and Eerola, E.: DNA aneuploidy in follicular adenomas of the thyroid gland. Am. J. Pathol. 124:373–376, 1986.
80. Joensuu, H., Klemi, P., et al.: Influence of cellular DNA content on survival in differentiated thyroid cancer. Cancer 58:2462–2467, 1986.
81. Johannessen, J. V., Gould, V. E., and Jao, W.: The fine structure of human thyroid cancer. Hum. Pathol. 9:385–400, 1978.
82. Johannessen, J. V., and Sobrinho-Simoes, M.: Follicular carcinoma of the human thyroid gland: An ultrastructural study with emphasis on scanning electron microscopy. Diagn. Histopathol. 5:113–127, 1982.
83. Johannessen, J. V., Sobrinho-Simoes, M., et al.: Ultrastructural morphometry of thyroid neoplasms. Am. J. Clin. Pathol. 79:162–167, 1983.
84. Johannessen, J. V., Sobrinho-Simoes, M., et al.: The diagnostic value of flow cytometric DNA measurements in selected disorders of the human thyroid. Am. J. Clin. Pathol. 77:20–25, 1982.
85. Johannessen, J. V., Sobrinho-Simoes, M., et al.: Anomalous papillary carcinoma of the thyroid. Cancer 51:1462–1467, 1983.
86. Johannessen, J. V., Sobrinho-Simoes, M., et al.: A flow cytometric deoxyribonucleic acid analysis of papillary thyroid carcinoma. Lab. Invest. 45:336–341, 1981.
87. Johnson, T. L., Lloyd, R. V., et al.: Hürthle cell tumors: An immunohistochemical study. Cancer 59:107–112, 1987.
88. Johnson, T. L., Lloyd, R. V., and Thor, A.: Expression of ras oncogene p21 antigen in normal and proliferative thyroid tissues. Am. J. Pathol. 127:60–65, 1987.
89. Kakudo, K., Miyauchi, A., et al.: Ultrastructural study of poorly differentiated medullary carcinoma of the thyroid. Virch. Arch. Pathol. Anat. 410:455–460, 1987.
90. Kameda, Y., Harada, T., et al.: Immunohistochemical study of the medullary thyroid carcinoma with reference to C-thyroglobulin reaction of tumor cells. Cancer 44:2071–2082, 1979.
91. Kendall, C. H., Sanderson, P. R., et al.: Follicular thyroid tumours: a study of laminin and type IV collagen in basement membrane and endothelium. J. Clin. Pathol. 38:1100–1105, 1985.
92. Kim, P. S., Dunn, A. D., and Dunn, J. T.: Altered immunoreactivity of thyroglobulin in thyroid disease. J. Clin. Endocrinol. Metab. 67:161–168, 1988.
93. Klemi, P. J., Joensuu, H., and Eerola, E.: DNA aneuploidy in anaplastic carcinoma of the thyroid gland. Am. J. Clin. Pathol. 89:154–159, 1988.
94. Kodama, T., Fujino, M., et al.: Identification of carcinoembryonic antigen in the C-cell of the normal thyroid. Cancer 45:98–101, 1980.
95. Kohno, Y., Tarutani, O., et al.: Monoclonal antibodies to thyroglobulin elucidate differences in

protein structure of thyroglobulin in healthy individuals and those with papillary adenocarcinoma. J. Clin. Endocrinol. Metab. *61:*343–350, 1985.

96. Kraemer, B., Srigley, J. R., et al.: DNA flow cytometry of thyroid neoplasms. Arch. Otolaryngol. *111:*34–38, 1985.
97. Krisch, K., Krisch, I., et al.: The value of immunohistochemistry in medullary thyroid carcinoma: A systemic study of 30 cases. Histopathology *9:*1077–1089, 1985.
98. Krawiec, L., Kleiman de Pisarev, D. L., et al.: Studies on the regulation of RNA labeling and on the biochemical constituents of normal and abnormal human thyroid. Acta Physiol. Pharmacol. Lat. *34:*375–393, 1984.
99. Kurata, A., Ohta, K., et al.: Monoclonal antihuman thyroglobulin antibodies. J. Clin. Endocrinol. Metab. *59:*573–579, 1984.
100. Lippman, S. M., Mendelsohn, G., et al.: The prognostic and biological significance of cellular heterogeneity in medullary thyroid carcinoma: A study of calcitonin, L-Dopa decarboxylase and histaminase. J. Clin. Endocrinol. Metab. *54:*233–240, 1982.
101. LiVolsi, V. A.: Mixed thyroid tumors: A real entity? Lab. Invest. *57:*237–239, 1987.
102. LiVolsi, V. A., Brooks, J. J., and Arendash-Durand, B.: Anaplastic thyroid tumors: immunohistology. Am. J. Clin. Pathol. *87:*434–442, 1987.
103. Ljungberg, O., Bondeson, L., and Bondeson, A. G.: Differentiated thyroid carcinoma intermediate type: a new tumor entity with features of follicular and parafollicular cell carcinoma. Hum. Pathol. *15:*218–228, 1984.
104. Logmans, S. C., and Jobsis, A. C.: Thyroid-associated antigens in routinely embedded carcinomas. Cancer *54:*274–279, 1984.
105. Lloyd, R. V.: Use of molecular probes in the study of endocrine diseases. Hum. Pathol. *18:*119–121, 1987.
106. Lloyd, R. V., and Wilson, B. S.: Specific endocrine tissue marker defined by a monoclonal antibody. Science *222:*628–630, 1983.
107. Lloyd, R. V., Johnson. T. L., et al.: Detection of HLA-DR antigens in paraffin-embedded thyroid epithelial cells with a monoclonal antibody. Am. J. Pathol. *120:*106–111, 1985.
108. Lloyd, R. V., Sissons, J. C., and Marangos, P. J.: Calcitonin, Carcinoembryonic antigen and neuron specific enolase in medullary thyroid carcinoma. Cancer *51:*2234–2239, 1983.
109. Lovett, E. J., Schnitzer, B., et al.: Application of flow cytometry to diagnostic pathology. Lab. Invest. *50:*115–140, 1984.
110. Lukacs, G. L., Miko, T. L., et al.: The validity of some morphologic methods in the diagnosis of thyroid malignancy. Acta Chir. Scand. *149:*759–766, 1983.
111. Mattfeldt, T., Schurmann, G., and Feichter, G.: Stereology and flow cytometry of well-differentiated follicular neoplasms of the thyroid gland. Virch. Arch. Pathol. Anat. *410:*433–441, 1987.
112. McLeod, M. K., Thompson, N. W., et al.: Flow cytometric measurements of nuclear DNA and ploidy analysis in Hürthle cell neoplasms of the thyroid. Arch. Surg. *123:*849–854, 1988.
113. Mendelsohn, G., Bigner, S. H., et al.: Anaplastic variants of medullary thyroid carcinoma. Am. J. Surg. Pathol. *4:*333–341, 1980.
114. Mendelsohn, G., Wells, S. A., and Baylin, S. B.: Relationship of tissue carcinoembryonic antigen and calcitonin to tumor virulence in medullary thyroid carcinoma. An immunohistochemical study in early, localized and virulent disseminated stages of disease. Cancer *54:*657–662, 1984.
115. Miettenen, M., Franssila, K., et al.: Expression of intermediate filament proteins in thyroid gland and thyroid tumors. Lab. Invest. *50:*262–270, 1984.
116. Miettinen, M., and Virtanen, I.: Expression of laminin in thyroid gland and thyroid tumors. An immunohistologic study. Int. J. Cancer *34:*27–30, 1984.
117. Mizukami, Y., and Matsubara, F.: Correlation between thyroid peroxidase activity and histopathological and ultrastructural changes in various thyroid diseases. Endocrinol. Jpn. *28:*381–389, 1981.
118. Mizukami, Y., Nonomura, A., et al.: Immunohistochemical demonstration of ras p21 oncogene product in normal, benign and malignant human thyroid tissues. Cancer *61:*873–880, 1988.
119. Moll, R.: Diversity of cytokeratins in carcinomas. Acta Histochem. Suppl. *34:*37–44, 1987.
120. Moll, R., Franke, W. W., et al.: The catalog of human cytokeratins: Patterns of expression in normal epithelia, tumors and cultured cells. Cell *31:*11–24, 1982.
121. Monaco, F., Carducci, C., et al.: Human undifferentiated thyroid carcinoma synthesizes and secretes 19S thyroglobulin. Cancer *54:*79–83, 1984.
122. Morris, H. R., Panico, M., et al.: Isolation and characterization of human calcitonin gene related peptide. Nature *308:*746–748, 1984.
123. Myskow, M. W., Krajewski, A. S., et al.: The role of immunoperoxidase techniques on paraffin embedded tissue in determining of undifferentiated thyroid neoplasms. Clin. Endocrinol. *24:*335–341, 1986.
124. Newland, J. R., Mackay, B., et al.: Anaplastic thyroid carcinoma: An ultrastructural study of 10 cases. Ultrastruct. Pathol. *2:*121–129, 1981.
125. Normann, T., and Johannessen, J. V.: Cell types in medullary thyroid carcinoma. Acta Pathol. Microbiol. Scand. *85:*561–571, 1977.
126. Osborn, M., and Weber, K.: Tumor diagnosis by intermediate filament typing: A novel tool for surgical pathology. Lab. Invest. *48:*372–394, 1983.
127. Ohashi, M., Yanase, T., et al.: Alpha-neoendorphin like immunoreactivity in medullary carcinoma of the thyroid. Cancer *59:*277–280, 1987.

128. Oskam, R., Rijksen, G., et al.: Enolase isozymes in differentiated and undifferentiated medullary thyroid carcinomas. Cancer 55:394–399, 1985.
129. Permanetter, W., Nathrath, W. B. J., and Lohrs, U.: Immunohistochemical analysis of thyroglobulin and keratin in benign and malignant thyroid tumours. Virch. Arch. Pathol. Anat. 398:221–228, 1982.
130. Pfaltz, M., Hedinger, C., and Muhlethaler, J. P.: Mixed medullary and follicular carcinoma of the thyroid. Virch. Arch. Pathol. Anat. 400:53–61, 1983.
131. Poppema, S., Hollema, H., et al.: Monoclonal antibodies (MT1, MT2, MB1, Mb2, Mn3) reactive with leukocyte subsets in paraffin embedded tissue sections. Am. J. Pathol. 127:418–429, 1987.
132. Rainwater, L. M., Farrow, G. M., et al.: Oncocytic tumours of the salivary gland, kidney and thyroid: Nuclear DNA patterns studied by flow cytometry. Br. J. Cancer 53:799–804, 1986.
133. Ramanna, L., Waxman, A. D. F., et al.: Correlation of thyroglobulin measurements and radioiodine scans in the follow-up of patients with differentiated thyroid cancer. Cancer 55:1525–1529, 1985.
134. Roth, K. A., Bensch, K. G., and Hoffman, A. R.: Characterization of opioid peptides in human thyroid medullary carcinoma. Cancer 59:1594–1598, 1987.
135. Ruppert, J. M., Eggleston, J. C., et al.: Disseminated calcitonin-poor medullary thyroid carcinoma in a patient with calcitonin rich primary tumor. Am. J. Surg. Pathol. 10:513–518, 1986.
136. Ryff de-Leche, A., Staub, J. J., et al.: Thyroglobulin production by malignant thyroid tumors. Cancer 57:1145–1153, 1986.
137. Saad, M. F., Fritsche, H. A., and Samaan, N. A.: Diagnostic and prognostic values of carcinoembryonic antigen in the treatment of nonfamilial medullary thyroid carcinoma. J. Clin. Endocrinol. Metab. 58:889–894, 1984.
138. Saad, M. F., Ordoncz, N. G., et al.: The prognostic value of calcitonin immunostaining in medullary carcinoma of the thyroid. J. Clin. Endocrinol. Metab. 59:850–856, 1984.
139. Schlumberger, M., Charbord, P., et al.: Circulating thyroglobulin and thyroid hormones in patients with metastases of differentiated thyroid carcinoma: relationship to serum thyrotropin levels. J. Clin. Endocrinol. Metab. 51:513–519, 1980.
140. Schmid, K. W., Fischer-Colbrie, R., et al.: Chromogranin A and B and secretogranin II in medullary carcinoma of the thyroid. Am. J. Surg. Pathol. 11:551–556, 1987.
141. Schneider, A. B., Ikekubo, K., and Kuma, K.: Iodine content of serum thyroglobulin in normal individuals and patients with thyroid tumors. J. Clin. Endocrinol. Metab. 57:1251–1256, 1983.
142. Schroder, S., Bocker, W., et al.: Prognostic factors in medullary thyroid carcinoma. Cancer 61:806–816, 1988.
143. Schroder, S., Dockhorn-Dworniczak, B., et al.: Intermediate filament expression in thyroid gland carcinomas. Virch. Arch. Pathol. Anat. 409:751–766, 1986.
144. Schroder, S., and Kloppel, G.. Carcinoembryonic antigen and nonspecific cross-reacting antigen in thyroid cancer. Am. J. Surg. Pathol. 11:100–108, 1987.
145. Schroder, S., Schwarz, W., et al.: Prognostic significance of Leu-M1 immunostaining in papillary carcinomas of the thyroid gland. Virch. Arch. Pathol. Anat. 411:435–439, 1987.
146. Shapiro, H. M.: Practical Flow Cytometry. New York, Alan R. Liss, Inc., 1985.
147. Sikri, K. L., Varndell, I. M., et al.: Medullary carcinoma of the thyroid: An immunocytochemical and histochemical study of 25 cases using eight separate markers. Cancer 56:2481–2491, 1985.
148. Smeulders, A. W. M., and Dorst, L.: Measurement issues in morphometry. Anal. Quant. Cytol. 7:242–249, 1985.
149. Sobrinho-Simoes, M., and Damjanov, I.: Lectin histochemistry of papillary and follicular carcinoma of the thyroid gland. Arch. Pathol. Lab. Med. 110:722–729, 1986.
150. Sobrinho-Simoes, M., and Goncalves, V.: Nuclear bodies in papillary carcinomas of the human thyroid gland. Arch. Pathol. 98:94–98, 1974.
151. Sobrinho-Simoes, M., and Johannessen, J. V.: Surface features in human thyroid disorders, J. Microscopic Cytol. 14:187–202, 1982.
152. Sobrinho-Simoes, M., Nesland, J. M., et al.: Transmission electron microscopy and immunocytochemistry in the diagnosis of thyroid tumors. Ultrastruct. Pathol. 9:255–275, 1985.
153. Steenbergh, P. H., Hoppener, J. W. M., et al.: Expression of the proopiomelanocortin gene in human medullary thyroid carcinoma. J. Clin. Endocrinol. Metab. 58:904–908, 1984.
154. Takahashi, H., Jiang, N. S., et al.: Thyrotropin receptors in normal and pathological human thyroid tissues. J. Clin. Endocrinol. Metab. 47:870–876, 1978.
155. Talerman, A., Lindeman, J., et al.: Demonstration of calcitonin and carcinoembryonic antigen (CEA) in medullary carcinoma of the thyroid (MCT) by immunoperoxidase technique. Histopathology 3:503–510, 1979.
156. Tangen, K. O., Lindmo, T., et al.: Cellular DNA content in normal human thyroid: a flow cytometric study based on frozen biopsy material. Diagn. Histopathol. 4:343–348, 1981.
157. Terries, P., Sheng, Z. M., et al.: Structure and expression of c-myc and c-fas protooncogenes in thyroid carcinomas. Br. J. Cancer 57:43–47, 1988.
158. Thomas-Morvan, C., Nataf, B., and Tubiana, M.: Thyroid proteins and hormone synthesis in human thyroid cancer. Acta Endocrinol. 76:651–669, 1974.
159. Tobler, A., Maurer, R., and Hedinger, C. E.: Undifferentiated thyroid tumors of diffuse small cell type. Histological and immunohistochemical evidence for their lymphomatous nature. Virch. Arch. Pathol. Anat. 389:127–141, 1980.

160. Topilko, A., and Caillou, B.: Acetylcholinesterase and butylcholinesterase activities in human thyroid cancer cells. Cancer *61:*491–499, 1988.
161. Tuccari, G., and Barresi, G.: Immunohistochemical demonstration of ceruloplasmin in follicular adenomas and thyroid carcinomas. Histopathology *11:*723–731, 1987.
162. Tuccari, G., and Barresi, G.: Immunohistochemical demonstration of lactoferrin in follicular adenomas and thyroid carcinomas. Virch. Arch. Pathol. Anat. *406:*67–74, 1985.
163. Uribe, M., Grimes, M., et al.: Medullary carcinoma of the thyroid gland: clinical, pathological and immunohistochemical features with review of the literature. Am. J. Surg. Pathol. *9:*577–594, 1985.
164. Valenta, L., Kyncl, F., et al.: Soluble proteins in thyroid neoplasia. J. Clin. Endocrinol. Metab. *28:*442–450, 1968.
165. Valenta, L., and Jirasek, J. E.: Histochemistry of thyroid tumors. Arch. Pathol. *84:*215–223, 1967.
166. Valenta, L., Lissitzky, S., and Aquaron, R.: Thyroglobulin iodine in thyroid tumors. J. Clin. Endocrinol. Metab. *28:*437–441, 1968.
167. Valenta, L. J., and Michel-Bechet, M.: Electron microscopy of clear cell thyroid carcinoma. Arch. Pathol. Lab. Med. *101:*140–144, 1977.
168. Van Herle, A. J., and Uller, R. P.: Elevated serum thyroglobulin: A marker of metastases in differentiated thyroid carcinomas. J. Clin. Invest. *56:*272–277, 1975.
169. Verhagen, J. N., van der Heijden, M. C. M., et al.: Pyruvate kinase in normal human thyroid tissue and thyroid neoplasms. Cancer *55:*142–148, 1985.
170. Verhagen, J. N., van der Heijden, M. C. M., et al.: Determination and characterization of hexokinase in thyroid cancer and benign neoplasms. Cancer *55:*1519–1524, 1985.
170a. Wick, M. R., and Sawyer, M. D.: Antigenic alterations in autoimmune thyroid diseases. Arch. Pathol. Lab. Med. *113:*77–81, 1989.
171. Wilson, N. W., Pambakian, H., et al.: Epithelial markers in thyroid carcinoma: an immunoperoxidase study. Histopathology *10:*815–829, 1986.
172. Yamamoto, K., Tsuji, T., et al.: Structural changes of carbohydrate chains of human thyroglobulin accompanying malignant transformation of thyroid glands. Eur. J. Biochem. *143:*133–144, 1984.
173. Yamashita, S., Ong, J., et al.: Expression of the myc cellular proto-oncogene in human thyroid tissue. J. Clin. Endocrinol. Metab. *63:*1170–1173, 1986.
174. Zajac, J. D., Penschow, J., et al.: Identification of calcitonin and calcitonin gene related peptide messenger ribonucleic acid in medullary thyroid carcinomas by hybridization histochemistry. J. Clin. Endocrinol. Metab. *62:*1037–1043, 1986.
175. Zirkin, T. A., Baybick, J. H., et al.: Flow cytometric analysis of DNA ploidy in lymphomas of the thyroid. Head Neck Surg. *10:*324–329, 1988.

19

WHAT YOU ALWAYS WANTED TO KNOW ABOUT THYROID PATHOLOGY BUT WERE AFRAID TO ASK

The title of this final chapter may appear facetious to some readers and presumptuous to others. I include this chapter since, in my experience discussing thyroid pathology with colleagues, trainees and students, and at presentations and courses in which I have participated, these questions, or variations on these themes, keep recurring. Hence, I believe these topics in thyroid pathology must (a) be encountered often, and (b) present difficult diagnostic problems.

I have placed them together and I will attempt to discuss answers (or what I think are the answers) or offer an approach to the problems in this final chapter.

I have included this chapter for two reasons:

(a) So that the reader faced with a specific problem can conclude that the problem is not uncommon and that he or she is probably not alone; and

(b) So that the approach to an answer or the solution is outlined briefly, and reference is made to a more in-depth discussion and pertinent bibliography in specific chapters in this monograph.

In the following paragraphs, I will list and briefly discuss the ten most frequently encountered problems in thyroid pathology.

Nonneoplastic Lesions

1. What is the difference between Hashimoto's thyroiditis and nonspecific lymphocytic thyroiditis?

In my view, all lymphocytic infiltration in the thyroid is abnormal and usually reflects an immunologic reaction. In the absence of obvious inflammatory (i.e., hemorrhage) or neoplastic lesions, the reaction most likely indicates some degree of autoimmune disease. In classic Hashimoto's thyroiditis, clinical disease is often evident. Hence there is often a goiter, as well as chemical evidence, and sometimes clinical symptoms of hypothyroidism. Histologically, in addition to lymphocytic infiltration of the stroma, one finds follicular atrophy, epithelial metaplasia, and varying degrees of fibrosis. In nonspecific lymphocytic thyroiditis, there is no clinical or gross disease attributable to the thyroiditis; laboratory testing may indicate mild degrees of subclinical hypothyroidism, however. In my opinion, the autoimmune thyroid diseases represent a spectrum from nonspecific lymphocytic thyroiditis through varying grades of severity to histologically classic Hashimoto's disease. The exact interrelationships, however, need to be elucidated as knowledge of autoimmunity in general and immunologic mechanisms of endocrine disease in particular are studied with modern techniques. From the standpoint of diagnostic practice, the diagnosis of chronic lymphocytic thyroiditis with oxyphilia (i.e., Hashimoto's thyroiditis) should be rendered in cases where the histology shows all the classic features and usually there is a clinical goiter; nonspecific lymphocytic thyroiditis is diagnosed as a secondary finding in a gland surgically removed for another reason, or at autopsy. (For further discussion, see Chapter 5.)

2. What is Riedel's struma and what is its relationship to Hashimoto's thyroiditis?

Riedel's disease is not a thyroiditis per se but a collagenous proliferation with associated vasculitis similar to retroperitoneal fibrosis and inflammatory fibrosing lesions of other parts of the body. Historically, the disorder was considered among the thyroiditides, since by involving the neck and hence the thyroid (the largest organ in the neck) attention was naturally focused on the gland. However, Riedel's disease extends beyond the thyroid capsule and may involve part or all of the gland; the uninvolved thyroid is histologically normal. Depending upon the amount of thyroid tissue involved, thyroid function may be normal or not. In contrast, in the fibrosing variant of Hashimoto's thyroiditis, that disorder most commonly confused with Riedel's disease, all of the gland is involved, the disease stops at the thyroid capsule, and hypothyroidism is almost universal. (Recent studies detailing immunopathologic differences between these two disorders are discussed in Chapter 7.)

Neoplastic Disorders

3. Are all papillary lesions of the thyroid malignant? (Variation: Does papillary adenoma of the thyroid exist?)

The answer to the question is an unequivocal no! Many lesions of the thyroid manifest papillary proliferations—these include congenital goiters with hypothyroidism, diffuse toxic goiter associated with Graves' disease, and areas of papillary hyperplasia associated with nodular goiter (with or without clinical evidence of toxicity). However, from the viewpoint of the histopathologist, the differences between hyperplastic papillary lesions and papillary cancer are cytologic characteristics of the nuclei and the usually diffuse nature of the process in hyperplastic lesions. In benign follicular nodules showing papillary hyperplasia or degenerative areas taking on a papillary appearance, the lesion is encapsulated, the nuclei do not have a ground glass appearance, and the papillae show broad fibrous cores rather than the usually more delicate papillary formations seen in cancer. Whether these follicular lesions with degenerative papillary areas should be called papillary adenoma appears to be a moot point. Since papillary adenoma has been used interchangeably for small papillary cancers (not recognized as malignant) and for areas of hyperplasia, and since these two lesions are prognostically distinct, I suggest the term papillary adenoma not be used. (For further discussion and illustrations, please refer to Chapter 8.)

4. Is the follicular variant of papillary carcinoma a real entity and does that diagnosis impact on prognosis?

The answer to both questions is a definite yes! Follicular pattern is common focally in most papillary cancers of the thyroid. When that pattern predominates or is the sole pattern seen, the diagnosis of follicular variant of papillary cancer should be made if the nuclei show ground glass appearance, if psammoma bodies are present, and if the lesion shows a desmoplastic infiltrative edge. These tumors behave in a fashion much more similar to that of papillary cancer than to true follicular carcinoma; lymphatic rather than vascular spread is seen and the long-term outlook is much more favorable. Basic biologic and clinical features make it imperative that the follicular variant be diagnosed as a subset of papillary cancer rather than as a follicular cancer regardless of the degree of "follicularity" present. (For further discussion, please see Chapters 8 and 9.)

5. In considering encapsulated follicular thyroid lesions (and excluding those showing features of follicular variant of papillary cancer), how is the distinction of benign from malignant follicular neoplasm made?

This question is one of the most difficult to answer of all in the area of diagnosing thyroid neoplasms. The standard answer is: the tumor is malignant if capsular or vascular invasion is seen. However, although that answer is correct, defining capsular and vascular invasion is not easy.

Certain features need to be remembered.

(a) In a follicular carcinoma, there is usually a thick capsule (thickness is often 2 to 4 millimeters).

(b) Capsular invasion must be unequivocal and often is transcapsular and/or associated with vascular invasion.

(c) Vascular invasion involves veins in or beyond the capsule of the neoplasm; invasion of blood vessels within the substance of the tumor is not associated with malignant biologic behavior and hence should not be used as a criterion for a cancer diagnosis.

(d) Stains for elastic tissue rarely if ever help in defining vascular invasion; immunostaining for laminin or Factor VIII related antigen may on occasion be useful.

(e) Adequate numbers of sections must be examined—at least ten is recommended. The sections should be selected so as to demonstrate the tumor-capsule-thyroid interface. Looking at the middle of a follicular thyroid tumor will not give an answer as to its diagnosis.

(f) Most true follicular carcinomas look hypercellular or solid. Often mitoses are seen. However, these features should raise flags that one may be dealing with a follicular carcinoma. In and of themselves, these features are not diagnostic. Invasion of the veins and/or capsule must be identified.

(g) Similarly, cytologic atypia, usually of a few isolated groups of cells, does not mean cancer in a follicular thyroid lesion. In fact, it is probably more common to find cytologic atypia in benign nodules; it probably represents a degenerative change not unlike that seen in parathyroid adenomas. (For further discussion and illustrations, please refer to Chapter 9.)

6. Are all Hürthle cell tumors malignant?

This question is one that can cause explosive debate among members of various schools of thought. In my opinion and from our own material and that of others reported in the literature, there is no question that benign Hürthle cell tumors of the thyroid exist. In fact, the majority of single thyroid nodules composed of Hürthle cells are adenomas. The criteria for diagnosing a Hürthle cell nodule as cancer are similar to those used for follicular nodules in general, i.e., capsular or vascular invasion. However, Hürthle cell tumors do differ from ordinary follicular nodules, since a larger percentage of the former fulfill the criteria for malignancy. In addition, Hürthle cell carcinomas differ from true non-Hürthle follicular cancers in that the former may spread to lymph nodes as well as through the bloodstream. (Papillary carcinomas can occasionally be composed of Hürthle cells; these are usually not diagnostic problems). (For further discussion and reference data, see Chapter 12.)

7. What is small cell thyroid carcinoma?

Examples of small cell carcinoma include those that have an epithelial pattern; these are either medullary carcinomas without amyloid and poorly differentiated follicular carcinomas (often recognizable, better differentiated zones are seen), including the insular variant carcinoma that is follicular-derived and has a prognosis between the excellent one associated with papillary cancer and the dismal one of anaplastic carcinoma. Other so-called small cell carcinomas are those that have a diffuse pattern; virtually all of these are malignant lymphomas. The prognosis of small cell carcinoma is therefore impossible to define since it probably does not exist as an entity unto itself, and those lesions that have been diagnosed as small cell cancer have a wide range of biologic behavior. (One must always remember that small cell carcinoma of extrathyroid origin may metastasize to the gland and mimic a primary.) (For further discussion of small cell thyroid tumors, please see Chapters 10, 14, and 15.)

8. How useful is fine needle aspiration (FNA) cytology of the thyroid?

FNA is an extremely useful technique in the evaluation of thyroid nodules. It is simple, very safe, and direct; no longer do patients with solitary nodules need to undergo scans and therapeutic trials with medications; now an answer is readily obtainable. For some types of thyroid lesions, such as papillary carcinoma, including the follicular variant, medullary carcinoma, anaplastic cancer, and possibly lymphoma, FNA can be the diagnostic modality. No longer does a surgeon have to wait to plan a definitive operative procedure based upon intraoperative frozen section diagnosis; the surgeon and patient can know what procedure is needed because the diagnosis was made preoperatively by FNA. For anaplastic cancer and lymphoma, open surgical biopsy may be avoided.

However, most nodular lesions of the thyroid are follicular in pattern. Since the distinction between benign and malignant follicular lesions is based upon examination of the nodule's periphery and since FNA samples the center, a definitive diagnosis is not possible on such nodules. Hence, for the majority of nodules FNA serves as a screening procedure. It is also quite effective. Macrofollicular lesions and colloid nodules can be screened out from microfollicular or trabecular ones and those composed of Hürthle cells. The latter types require excision since, although most of these will also be benign, it is in these groups that follicular carcinomas will be found. (For further discussion of FNA and other biopsy techniques and data on specificity and sensitivity, please see Chapter 17.)

9. How helpful are mitoses in deciding benignancy from malignancy in well-differentiated thyroid tumors?

Mitoses alone are inconclusive in defining benign or malignant thyroid tumors. It is true that high grade cancers show numerous mitoses, but in these the diagnosis of malignancy is not in question.

In well-differentiated, especially follicular, nodules, the presence of mitoses even if normal is unusual. (If the nodule has recently been aspirated, however, the processes of repair and regeneration include mitoses—so the history of aspiration should be sought.) Mitotic figures are more often seen in well-differentiated follicular cancers than in benign nodules; however, they cannot be relied upon in deciding the diagnosis in an individual case. A similar situation is found in the application of flow cytometry to histologic and/or cytologic samples of thyroid nodules; lesions which are malignant in clinical behavior can show diploidy and slow growth rates, whereas lesions which behave in a clinically benign way can be aneuploid. (See also Chapter 18.)

10. Does lateral aberrant thyroid exist?

Here the answer must be equivocal. If by lateral aberrant thyroid is meant histologically benign-appearing thyroid follicles in lymph nodes which are located in the lateral neck, then the answer is *no*—lateral aberrant thyroid in these cases really indicates metastatic papillary cancer to nodes. Benign thyroid tissue can occur in the lateral neck unassociated with nodes. In some of these cases, a history of prior neck surgery or trauma can be found; in others, the patient has a significant nodular goiter and some of the most lateral nodules may be found unattached to the main gland. In these types of cases, implantation of normal thyroid tissue or acquisition of blood supply by goitrous nodules can explain the location of the tissue in aberrant sites. It is critical to recall, however, that the tissue must look normal; no psammoma bodies, papillary areas, or ground glass nuclei should be present. (See also Chapters 1 and 16.)

Other questions usually asked regard therapeutic approaches to thyroid neoplasm and the pathologic bases for these approaches. However, answers to these questions are extremely controversial and strong opinions have been expressed on all sides of virtually every issue. Rather than set forth my opinions on many of these therapeutic decisions, as a pathologist I would rather present the known pathologic data on the entities considered and let the therapist act upon these data.

Index

Note: Page numbers in *italics* refer to illustrations; page numbers followed by (t) refer to tables.

MAJOR PROBLEMS IN PATHOLOGY

The **Major Problems in Pathology (MPP) Series** provides current, accurate, and detailed information on specific areas of Diagnostic Pathology.

The volumes reflect the distilled wisdom of their authors, providing a scholarly review of the topic and practical guidance for the reader. Excellence of text, illustration, and referencing are hallmarks of the series.

Now—you can order the **MPP** volumes of your choice FREE for 30 days! Simply indicate your selections on the postage-paid order card, or call toll-free **1-800-545-2522** (8:30–7:00 Eastern time; in Fla. call 1-800-433-0001). Be sure to mention **DM#8974.**

Become an MPP series subscriber! You'll receive each new volume in the **MPP** series as soon as it's published—one to three titles per year—and save postage and handling costs!

If not completely satisfied with any volume you order through the mail, just return it with the invoice within 30 days at no further obligation. You only keep the volumes you want. *Your satisfaction is guaranteed!* ■

Valuable additions to your working library!
Available from your bookstore or the publisher

Complete and Mail Today for a FREE 30-Day Preview!

☑ **YES!** Please send me the **Major Problems in Pathology** titles I've indicated below. If not completely satisfied with any volume, I may return it with the invoice within 30 days at no further obligation.

☐ W2503-7 **Disorders of the Spleen** *(Wolf & Neiman)*

☐ W8770-9 **Immunomicroscopy: A Diagnostic Tool for the Surgical Pathologist** *(Taylor)*

☐ W1359-4 **Mucosal Biopsy of the Gastrointestinal Tract, 3rd Edition** *(Whitehead)*

☐ W1337-3 **Pathology of Neoplasia in Children & Adolescents** *(Finegold)*

☐ W7493-3 **Pathology of the Uterine Cervix, Vagina, and Vulva** *(Fu & Reagan)*

☐ W1463-9 **Problems in Breast Pathology** *(Azzopardi)*

☐ W1434-5 **Surgical Pathology of Bone Marrow: Core Biopsy Diagnosis** *(Wittels)*

☐ W1027-7 **Surgical Pathology of the Lymph Nodes and Related Organs** *(Jaffe)*

☐ W1852-9 **Surgical Pathology of Non-Neoplastic Lung Disease, 2nd Edition** *(Katzenstein & Askin)*

☐ W5782-6 **Surgical Pathology of the Thyroid** *(LiVolsi)*

☐ W1224-5 **Surgical Pathology of the Uterine Corpus, 2nd Edition** *(Hendrickson & Kempson)*

☐ W3040-5 **The Renal Biopsy, 2nd Edition** *(Striker & Olson)*

☐ W3855-X **Thin-Needle Aspiration Biopsy** *(Frable)*

☐ Enroll me in the **MPP** Subscriber Plan so that I may receive future titles immediately upon publication, and save postage & handling costs! I may preview each new volume FREE for 30 days—and keep only the volumes I want.

Name_____

Address_____

City_____ State_____ Zip_____

Staple this to your purchase order to expedite delivery. © W.B. SAUNDERS 1989. Printed in USA. Postage & Handling additional outside the USA.

C02414

DM#8974

◆ MAJOR PROBLEMS ◆ IN PATHOLOGY

- **Disorders of the Spleen** *(Wolf & Neiman)* Order #W2503-7

- **Immunomicroscopy: A Diagnostic Tool for the Surgical Pathologist** *(Taylor)* Order #W8770-9

- **Mucosal Biopsy of the Gastrointestinal Tract, 3rd Edition** *(Whitehead)* Order #W1359-4

- **Pathology of Neoplasia in Children & Adolescents** *(Finegold)* Order #W1337-3

- **Pathology of the Uterine Cervix, Vagina, and Vulva** *(Fu & Reagan)* Order #W7493-3

- **Problems in Breast Pathology** *(Azzopardi)* Order #W1463-9

- **Surgical Pathology of Bone Marrow: Core Biopsy Diagnosis** *(Wittels)* Order #W1434-5

- **Surgical Pathology of the Lymph Nodes and Related Organs** *(Jaffe)* Order #W1027-7

- **Surgical Pathology of Non-Neoplastic Lung Disease, 2nd Edition** *(Katzenstein & Askin)* Order #W1852-9

- **Surgical Pathology of the Thyroid** *(LiVolsi)* Order #W5782-6

- **Surgical Pathology of the Uterine Corpus, 2nd Edition** *(Hendrickson & Kempson)* Order #W1224-5

- **The Renal Biopsy, 2nd Edition** *(Striker & Olson)* Order #W3040-5

- **Thin-Needle Aspiration Biopsy** *(Frable)* Order #W3835-X

Enroll today!
See reverse side for details.